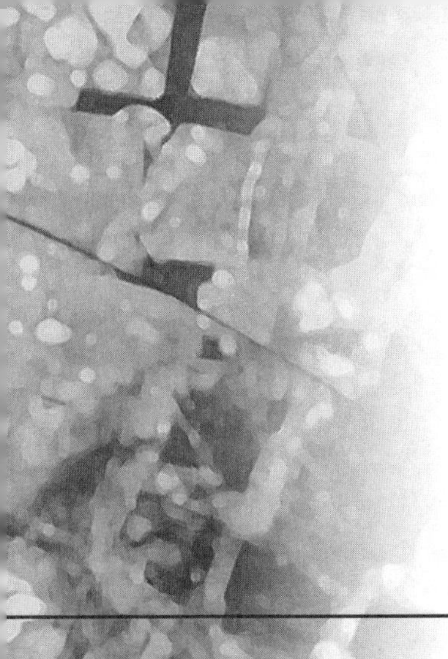

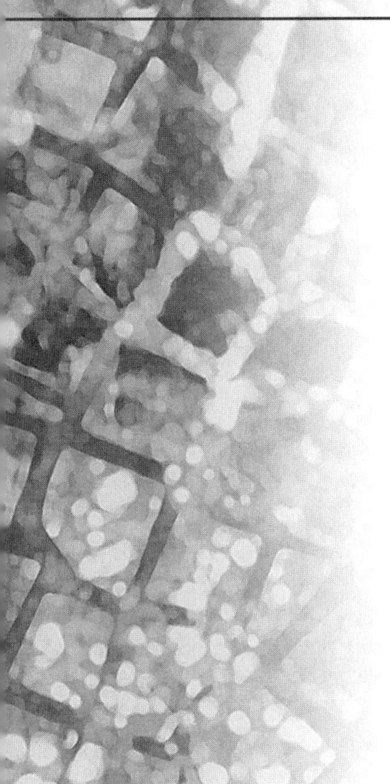

HEALTH ECONOMICS

Theories, Insights, and Industry Studies

FOURTH EDITION

REXFORD E. SANTERRE

Professor of Finance and Healthcare Management
Center for Healthcare and Insurance Studies
School of Business
University of Connecticut

•

STEPHEN P. NEUN

Professor of Economics
Assistant Vice President for Academic Affairs
Utica College

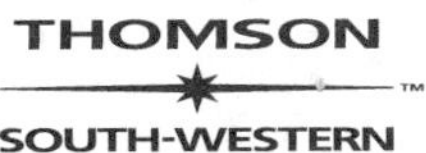

Australia · Brazil · Canada · Mexico · Singapore · Spain · United Kingdom · United States

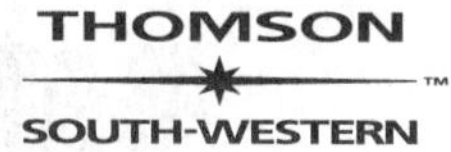

Health Economics: Theories, Insights, and Industry Studies, Fourth Edition
Rexford E. Santerre and Stephen P. Neun

VP/Editorial Director:
Jack W. Calhoun

Editor-in-Chief:
Alex von Rosenberg

Publisher:
Steve Momper

Developmental Editor:
Leslie Kauffman
LEAP Publishing Services, Inc.

Executive Marketing Manager:
Brian Joyner

Production Project Manager:
Margaret M. Bril

Manager of Technology, Editorial:
Vicky True

Technology Project Editor:
Dana Cowden

Web Coordinator:
Karen Schaffer

Senior Manufacturing Coordinator:
Sandee Milewski

Production House:
Interactive Composition Corporation (ICC)

Printer:
R. R. Donnelley
Crawfordsville, Indiana

Art Director:
Michelle Kunkler

Internal Designer:
Pagliaro Design

Cover Designer:
Pagliaro Design

Cover Images:
© Getty Images, Inc.

Printed in the United States of America
1 2 3 4 5 09 08 07 06

Student Edition: ISBN
0-324-32071-X (book only)

Student Edition: ISBN
0-324-32068-X (pkg)

Library of Congress Control Number:
2006920352

For more information about our products, contact us at:

Thomson Learning Academic Resource Center

1-800-423-0563

Thomson Higher Education
5191 Natorp Boulevard
Mason, OH 45040
USA

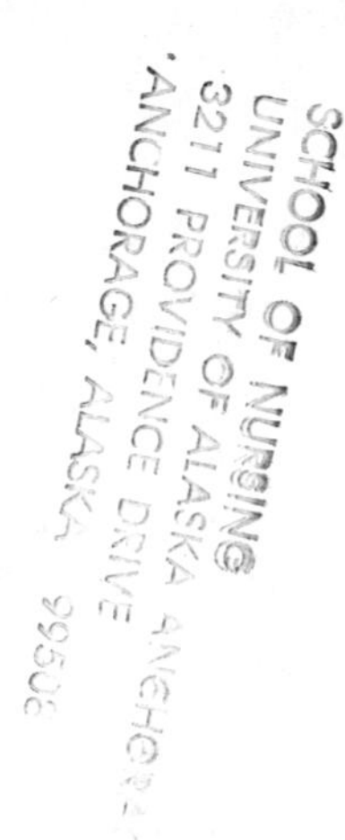

To Our Wives:

Laurie

&

Joan

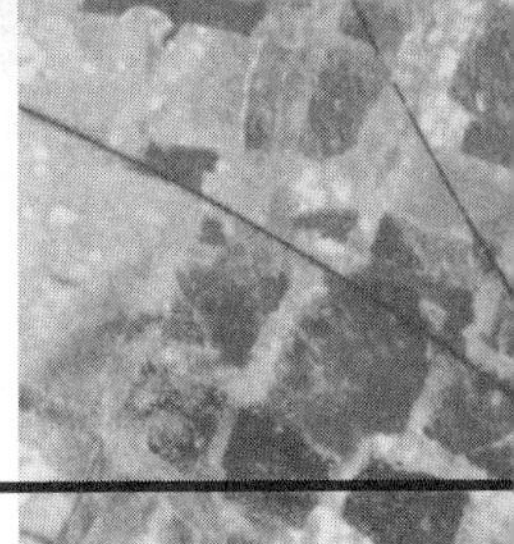

PREFACE

The health care sector, now representing more than one-seventh of the U.S. economy in terms of economic activity, continues to change in unimaginable ways. Sweeping transformations in the organizational arrangements of health care providers, newly developed medical technologies, the creation of new health insurance products, and the development and evaluation of various public policy initiatives all make the health care sector a dynamic and exciting area for applying the lens and tools of economic analysis. Indeed, not a day goes by without the unfolding of a medical event that requires the insights of economics to unravel the depths of its implications.

Our textbook, now in its fourth edition, is written expressly to capture the excitement generated by the health care field. As in the earlier editions, we take a fresh, contemporary approach to the study of health economics. We present the material in a lively and inviting manner by providing numerous and timely real-world examples throughout the text. At the same time, we resist the temptation of becoming overly encyclopedic and avoid purely technical issues that interest only academics and not students.

As a result of the approach taken, our book has wide appeal. Many business schools; liberal arts colleges; medical schools; and schools of public health, pharmacy, and health administration, at both the undergraduate and graduate levels, have chosen to use our textbook. In addition, the national Certified Employee Benefits Specialist (CEBS) program, cosponsored by the International Foundation of Employee Benefit Plans and The Wharton School of the University of Pennsylvania, has selected our text. The mix of adopters attests to the relevance and practicality of the material and the consistent and inviting manner in which various principles and concepts of health economics are presented throughout the text.

WHAT'S NEW IN THE FOURTH EDITION?

Several changes have been made in this fourth edition in response to the suggestions of various individuals.

- We have incorporated the boxed insights into the text or eliminated them because many have pointed out that they tended to disrupt the flow of material. In their place, John Schneider of the University of Iowa has graciously developed several case studies at the end of each chapter. These case studies, along with their questions, help reinforce and extend some of the concepts and principles developed in the chapter and give students the opportunity to apply some independent thought to health economics situations within a real-world context.
- Chapter 2 now includes a discussion concerning how technological changes in medicine alter the health production function. Many observers have begun to dismiss the notion of flat-of-the-curve medicine because of noticeable health improvements over time. However, that observation does not necessarily invalidate flat-of-the curve medicine, which happens at a point in time, as discussed in Chapter 2 and elsewhere in the text. Also, Chapter 2 now provides a discussion of the different approaches (such as observational studies, controlled experiments, and natural experiments) economists have used to test various hypotheses and the statistical problem of distinguishing between association and causation.

- The discussion on cost effectiveness analysis in Chapter 3 has been considerably broadened to include more coverage of quality-of-life indices. In addition, other aspects of cost effectiveness analysis are now given greater scrutiny in the revised chapter.
- Chapter 6 has been modified to include several new topics. For one, we now show in Chapter 6 how people generally gain through a pooling-of-losses arrangement. We also discuss why insurance companies are typically necessary to facilitate the pooling arrangement. Moreover, John Nyman's new theory of the demand for health insurance is given considerable coverage in Chapter 6. The difference between the conventional and Nyman theories of demand should lead to some lively and interesting classroom discussions.
- Material on the relevant product and geographical markets and measuring concentration have been added to Chapter 8. Providing this material early on better prepares the students for the industry chapters that appear later in the book.
- Exclusive dealing and tying contracts are given more attention in the antitrust section of Chapter 9. A discussion on the welfare loss of taxation has also been added to Chapter 9.
- Chapter 10 now includes material on Medicare Part D, which provides pharmaceutical insurance coverage to those who are eligible.
- Chapter 11 offers a discussion about how guaranteed renewability may solve the problems created by risk variations in individual insurance markets.
- Chapter 13 now elaborates on the economics of advertising and includes coverage of the Dorfman-Steiner condition and some empirical findings based on that model. Also, a discussion of cost shifting and hospital margins has been added to Chapter 13.
- Chapter 14 now includes a discussion of empirical studies examining the magnitude of the benefits from new pharmaceutical products.

Organization of the Textbook

The textbook contains four parts: Part I, Chapters 1 through 8, deals with basic health economic concepts, such as trade-offs, the production of health, health care systems and institutions, the demands for medical care and health insurance, the health insurance product, production and cost theories, cost and benefit analysis, and market analysis. More specifically, Chapter 2 examines theoretically and empirically the different factors that help produce health. Not surprisingly, the role of medical care in producing health is given particular attention in this chapter.

Chapter 3 covers cost-benefit and cost effectiveness analysis, among other topics. Knowledge of these two methods helps policy makers determine efficient and effective ways to keep people healthy at minimum cost. An overview of health care system elements and an introduction to the U.S. health care system is provided in Chapter 4. A general model of a health care system and the role of financing, reimbursement, and delivery are some of the issues discussed in this chapter.

Chapters 5 and 6 provide theoretical and empirical material on the demands for medical care and medical insurance. This information becomes important, for example, when asking questions concerning the utilization of medical care and why some people lack health insurance. Chapter 7 provides basic instruction on production and cost theories. These theories are crucial for understanding the behavior of any type of medical firm, regardless of its ownership type and how much competition it faces in the marketplace. Lastly, tools of market analysis are provided in Chapter 8. In this chapter, different market structures, such as perfect competition and monopoly, are discussed and compared in the context of medical care industries.

Part II, Chapters 9 and 10, focuses on the important role of government in health matters and medical care markets. In particular, Chapter 9 provides an overview of government functions, such as regulation, antitrust, and redistribution, as applied to health and medical care issues. Chapter 10 discusses government's ever-increasing role as a producer of health insurance and examines the Medicaid and Medicare programs in considerable detail.

Part III includes Chapters 11 through 15. These chapters use the concepts and theories developed in the earlier chapters to extensively analyze specific health care industries by applying the structure, conduct, and performance paradigm of industrial organization. The private health insurance, physician, hospital, pharmaceutical, and nursing home industries are covered in great depth, and the analysis is kept as current as possible. A host of different topics and issues are examined in these chapters.

Finally, Part IV, or Chapter 16, deals with health care reform. Some of the more debated plans for reforming the U.S. health care system at the federal and state levels are discussed and evaluated. The book ends with a glossary.

In most colleges and universities, a course in health economics is offered on a one-semester basis. Within one semester, it is difficult to cover all of the material in this text. The business curriculum at the University of Connecticut offers the typical health economics course in two semesters at both the undergraduate and MBA/MPH levels. (Not all students always take both courses, however.) The first-semester course is titled Health Insurance. This first course covers Chapters 4 (Health Care Systems and Institutions), 6 (The Demand for Medical Insurance), 10 (Government as Health Insurer), 11 (The Private Health Insurance Industry), and 16 (Health Care Reform). Parts of Chapter 2 (Health and Medical Care) are also covered before Chapter 6 and Chapter 8 (Structure, Conduct, Performance, and Market Analysis) is briefly reviewed before introducing Chapter 11.

The second-semester course is titled Health Care Economics, which covers Chapters 1 (Introduction), 2 (Health and Medical Care), 3 (Cost and Benefit Analysis), 5 (The Demand for Medical Services), 7 (Medical Care Production and Costs), 8 (Structure, Conduct, Performance, and Market Analysis), 9 (Government, Health, and Medical Care), and the four remaining industry chapters (12–15). Supplemental readings are assigned in both courses, and typically student presentations or point/counterpoint debates are assigned. Spreading the material over two courses means less rushing from topic to topic and provides more time to explore individual issues in greater detail. The students seem to appreciate the two-course approach.

SUPPLEMENTS

Economic Applications: Economic Applications includes South-Western's dynamic Web features: EconNews, EconDebate, and EconData Online. Organized by pertinent economic topics and searchable by topic or feature, these features are easy to integrate into the classroom. EconNews, EconDebate, and EconData all deepen students' understanding of theoretical concepts through hands-on exploration and analysis of the latest economic news stories, policy debates, and data. These features are updated on a regular basis. For more information, visit www.thomsonedu.com.

InfoTrac: With InfoTrac College Edition, students can receive anytime, anywhere online access to a database of full-text articles from thousands of popular and scholarly periodicals, such as *Newsweek, Fortune,* and *Nation's Business*. InfoTrac is a great way to expose students to online research techniques, with the security that the content is academically based and reliable. For more information, visit www.thomsonedu.com.

Web Site: The support site for *Health Economics* can be accessed at www.thomsonedu.com/economics/santerre and contains chapter-by-chapter web links, term paper tips, instructor resources, and other teaching and learning resources.

If a 1pass access card came with this book, you can start using many of these resources right away by following the directions on the card. One username and password gives you multiple resources. Get started today at www.thomsonedu.com!

Web-Based Instructor's Manual: The *Health Economics* support site (www.thomsonedu.com/economics/santerre) contains password-protected material for instructors only, including answers to end-of-chapter questions in the text, teaching notes for the case studies, a sample syllabus with web links, a list of readings for each chapter, and ideas for course projects.

PowerPoint™ Slides: PowerPoint slides, developed by Linda Ghent of Eastern Illinois University, are also located on the support site and are available for use by instructors for enhancing lectures. Each chapter's slides include a lecture outline illustrated with key tables and graphs.

Instructor's Resource CD-ROM: Get quick access to the Instructor's Manual and PowerPoint slides from your desktop via one CD-ROM.

ACKNOWLEDGMENTS

Our goal is to create the best possible learning device for students and teaching tool for professors. We are profoundly grateful to all of the reviewers for helping us bring this goal to fruition. For reviewing this fourth edition and providing numerous comments and suggestions, we thank Richard Beil of Auburn University; Diane M. Dewar of University at Albany, State University of New York; Maya Federman of Pitzer College; Stephan F. Gohmann of University of Louisville; Glenn Graham of SUNY–Oswego; Darren Grant of University of Texas–Arlington; Jessica Wolpaw Reyes of University of Texas; Windsor Westbrook Sherrill of Clemson University; Marie Truesdell of Marian College; Aaron Yelowitz of University of Kentucky; and Nicole Yurgin of University of Toledo. In addition, we would like to thank John Nyman of the University of Minnesota for reviewing the material in Chapter 6 relating to his theory of the demand for health insurance.

We also appreciate the reviewers of past editions and others who have provided us with comments for improving the text over the years, including Steven Andes, Jay Bae, Mary Ann Bailey, Laurie Bates, Sylvester Berki, Bruce Carpenter, Sewin Chan, Partha Deb, Diane Dewar, Randall Ellis, Alfredo Esposto, Andrew Foster, A. Mark Freeman, Dennis Heffley, Vivian Ho, Robert Jantzen, Donald Kenkel, Frank Musgrave, Albert Oriol, Irene Powell, Jeffrey Rubin, James Thornton, Kay Unger, Gary Wyckoff, and Donald Yett. We also thank Vivian Ho for providing the PowerPoint slides that were used with previous editions of this text. The time-consuming and exhaustive review and appraisal of the original manuscript by Steven Andes, Mary Ann Bailey, and Gary Wyckoff continues to receive our deepest appreciation.

At Thomson South-Western we thank Leslie Kauffman, our developmental editor. Leslie expertly guided the revision from beginning to end. Our thanks are also extended to all of the production staff and marketing personnel who face the important and overwhelming task of packaging and selling the final product. We are very appreciative for their professional support. Lastly, we thank our families for their understanding and love.

As mentioned in the previous editions, if you have any comments or suggestions for improving the text, please bring them to our attention. We are only an email message away. We thank you in advance.

Rex Santerre
rsanterre@business.uconn.edu
Stephen Neun
sneun@utica.edu

The Certified Employee Benefit Specialist® (CEBS) Program

The International Foundation of Employee Benefit Plans (IFEBP), located in Brookfield, Wisconsin, and The Wharton School of the University of Pennsylvania cosponsor the CEBS Program. The IFEBP is the largest educational association serving the employee benefits and compensation industry. For over 50 years, the International Foundation has served as the premier source of education and information to the industry. The Wharton School, the world's first collegiate school of management, was founded in 1881 and is today widely regarded as a leader in preparing students to succeed in a globally competitive business environment.

For more than 25 years, CEBS has been recognized as the most respected credential in the employee benefits industry. CEBS also offers candidates the opportunity to earn specialty designations. The Compensation Management Specialist (CMS), the Group Benefits Associate (GBA), and the Retirement Plans Associate (RPA) are the three specialty designations that form the core of the CEBS curriculum. Each designation stands on its own, delivering specialized knowledge in group benefits, group retirement, and compensation. However, when combined, the three designations form a comprehensive, integrated curriculum that leads to the only professional certification in total compensation.

To qualify for the CEBS designation, students must successfully complete an exam for the following six required courses and any of the two electives:

Six Required Courses

Course 1—Employee Benefits: Concepts and Health Care Benefits
Course 2—Employee Benefits: Design, Administration and Other Welfare Benefits
Course 3—Retirement Plans: Basic Features and Defined Contribution Approaches
Course 4—Retirement Plans: Defined Benefit Approaches and Plan Administration
Comp 1—Compensation Concepts and Principles
Course 8—Human Resources and Compensation Management

Two Electives

(any of the following CEBS courses)

Course 7—Asset Management
Course 9—Health Economics
Comp 2—Executive Compensation and Compensation Issues
PFP 1—Personal Financial Planning 1: Concepts and Principles
PFP 2—Personal Financial Planning 2: Tax and Estate Planning Techniques

CEBS candidates are a diverse group holding positions such as: human resource managers, benefits consultants, compensation specialists, insurance agents, trust plan administrators, and health care providers. CEBS graduates combine academic education with professional experience to fulfill employer and client needs at the highest level. Upon completing the CEBS Program, graduates continue their professional development by joining the International Society of Certified Employee Benefit Specialists and participating in educational activities sponsored by the Society. As members of the Society, graduates can build on their employee benefits and compensation knowledge through continuing education courses and examinations on emerging issues and statutory changes. Membership in the Society also is open to those individuals who hold the CMS, GBA, and/or RPA designations.

A CEBS Catalog of Information can be obtained from:

CEBS Program
IFEBP
18700 W. Bluemound Road
P.O. Box 1270
Brookfield, WI 53008–1270
(262) 786–6710, Ext. 8579
http://www.cebs.org

CEBS Program
The Wharton School
Lauder-Fischer Hall, Suite 304
256 South 37th Street
Philadelphia, PA 19104–6330

The **Review Questions and Problems** sections of selected chapters in the textbook include sample Questions on Subject Matter from the CEBS Study Manual for Course 9 and sample CEBS Exam Questions.

BRIEF CONTENTS

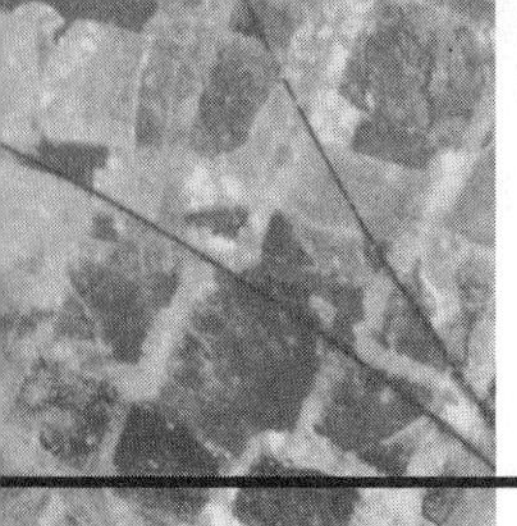

CONTENTS

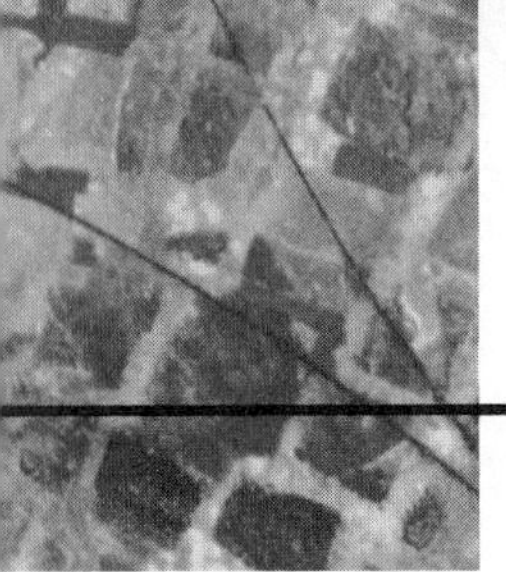

CASE STUDIES ACKNOWLEDGMENT

Case studies written by:

John E. Schneider, Ph.D.
Department of Health Management and Policy
University of Iowa College of Public Health

Acknowledgments:

Very helpful research assistance was provided by Lauren Tucker Huber, Janet Benton, and Andrew Barth.

PART 1

BASIC HEALTH CARE ECONOMIC TOOLS AND INSTITUTIONS

CHAPTER 1

INTRODUCTION

Like millions of Americans at some point in their lives, Joe awoke one night feeling a crushing weight on his chest. As the pain spread down his arm, he realized he was experiencing his worst dread: a heart attack. His wife, Angela, called the paramedics. While the ambulance was rushing Joe to the hospital, she anguished over the kind of care he would receive. Angela's anxiety starkly illustrates the basic questions any health care system faces:

1. Who should receive the medical goods and services? Would a person like Joe receive care merely because he is a citizen, or would he receive care only if he worked for a large company that provides health insurance for its employees?
2. What types of medical goods and services should be produced? Should the most expensive tests (such as angiograms) be performed without regard to cost? What treatments (such as balloon angioplasties) should be provided?
3. What inputs should be used to produce the medical goods and services? Should the hospital use high-tech medical equipment, a large nursing staff, or both?[1]

This chapter examines these fundamental questions. In addition, the chapter:

- introduces the discipline of health economics
- discusses the design and purpose of models and analysis in health economics
- explains how economic decisions are typically driven by a cost-benefit calculation

1. We are indebted to Gary Wyckoff of Hamilton College for providing us with this example.

What Is Health Economics?

For many of you, this textbook provides your first exposure to the study of health economics. Perhaps the ongoing controversy regarding health care reform or the prospect of a career in the health care field motivated you to learn more about health economics. Or perhaps you need only three more credits to graduate. Whatever the reason, we are sure you will find health economics to be challenging, highly interesting, and personally rewarding.

The study of health economics involves the application of various microeconomics tools, such as demand or cost theory, to health issues and problems. The goal is to promote a better understanding of the economic aspects of health care problems so that corrective health policies can be designed and proposed. A thorough understanding of microeconomic analysis is essential for conducting sound health economics analyses. If you lack a background in microeconomics, don't worry. This textbook is intended to help you learn and apply basic microeconomic theory to health economics issues. Before long, you will be thinking like a health economist!

The tools of health economics can be applied to a wide range of issues and problems pertaining to health and health care. For example, health economics analysis might be used to investigate why 29 of every 1,000 babies born in Turkey never reach their first birthday, whereas all but 3 of every 1,000 babies born in Japan live to enjoy their first birthday cake. The tools of health economics analysis might also be used to examine the economic desirability of a hotly contested merger between two large hospitals in a major metropolitan area. The burning question is, Will the merger of the two hospitals result in lower hospital prices due to overall cost savings or higher prices due to monopoly power?

Health economics is difficult to define in a few words because it encompasses such a broad range of concepts, theories, and topics. The *Mosby Medical Encyclopedia* (1992, p. 361) defines *health economics* as follows:

> ***Health economics*** *. . . studies the supply and demand of health care resources and the impact of health care resources on a population.*

Notice that health economics is defined in terms of the determination and allocation of *health care resources*. This is logical, because medical goods and services cannot exist without them.[2] Health care resources consist of *medical supplies*, such as pharmaceutical goods, latex rubber gloves, and bed linens; *personnel*, such as physicians and lab assistants; and *capital inputs*, including nursing home and hospital facilities, diagnostic and therapeutic equipment, and other items that provide medical care services. Unfortunately, health care resources, like resources in general, are limited or scarce at a given time, and wants are limitless. Thus, tradeoffs are inevitable and a society, whether it possesses a market-driven or a government-run health care system, must make a number of fundamental but crucial choices. These choices are normally couched in terms of four basic questions, discussed next.

The Four Basic Questions

As just noted, resources are scarce. Scarcity means that each society must make important decisions regarding the consumption, production, and distribution of goods and services as a way of providing answers to the four basic questions:

2. Even health care services produced in the home, such as first aid (therapeutic services) or home pregnancy tests (diagnostic services), require resources.

1. What combination of nonmedical and medical goods and services should be produced in the macroeconomy?
2. What particular medical goods and services should be produced in the health economy?
3. What specific health care resources should be used to produce the chosen medical goods and services?
4. Who should receive the medical goods and services that are produced?

How a particular society chooses to answer these four questions has a profound impact on the operation and performance of its health economy.

The first two questions deal with **allocative efficiency:** What is the best way to allocate resources to different consumption uses? The first decision concerns what combination of goods and services to produce in the overall economy. Individuals in a society have unlimited wants regarding nonmedical and medical goods and services, yet resources are scarce. As a result, decisions must be made concerning the best mix of medical and nonmedical goods and services to provide, and this decision-making process involves making trade-offs. If more people are trained as doctors or nurses, fewer people are available to produce nonmedical goods such as food, clothing, and shelter. Thus, more medical goods and services imply fewer nonmedical goods and services, and vice versa, given a fixed amount of resources.

The second consumption decision involves the proper mix of medical goods and services to produce in the health economy. This decision also involves trade-offs. For example, if more health care resources, such as nurses and medical equipment, are allocated to the production of maternity care services, fewer resources are available for the production of nursing home care for elderly people. Allocative efficiency in the overall economy and the health economy is achieved when the best mix of goods is chosen given society's underlying preferences.

The third question—what specific health care resources should be used?—deals with **production efficiency.** Usually resources or inputs can be combined to produce a particular good or service in many different ways. For example, hospital services can be produced in a capital- or labor-intensive manner. A large amount of sophisticated medical equipment relative to the number of patients served reflects a capital-intensive way of producing hospital services, whereas a high nurse-to-patient ratio indicates a labor-intensive process. Production efficiency implies that society is getting the maximum output from its limited resources because the best mix of inputs has been chosen to produce each good.

Production and Allocative Efficiency and the Production Possibilities Curve

The most straightforward way to illustrate production and allocative efficiency is to use the **production possibilities curve (PPC).** A PPC is an economic model that depicts the various combinations of any two goods or services that can be produced efficiently given the stock of resources, technology, and various institutional arrangements. Figure 1–1 displays a PPC. The quantities of maternity services, *M*, and nursing home services, *N*, are shown on the vertical and horizontal axes, respectively.[3] Points on the bowed-out PPC depict the various combinations of maternity and nursing home care services that can be efficiently produced within a health economy assuming that the amounts of health care resources and technology are fixed at a given point in time.

Every point on the PPC implies production efficiency, since all health care resources are being fully utilized. For example, notice points *A*, *B*, *C*, *D*, and *E* on the PPC. At each of these points,

3. We assume society has already made its choice between medical and nonmedical goods.

FIGURE 1–1
Production Possibilities Curve for Maternity and Nursing Home Services

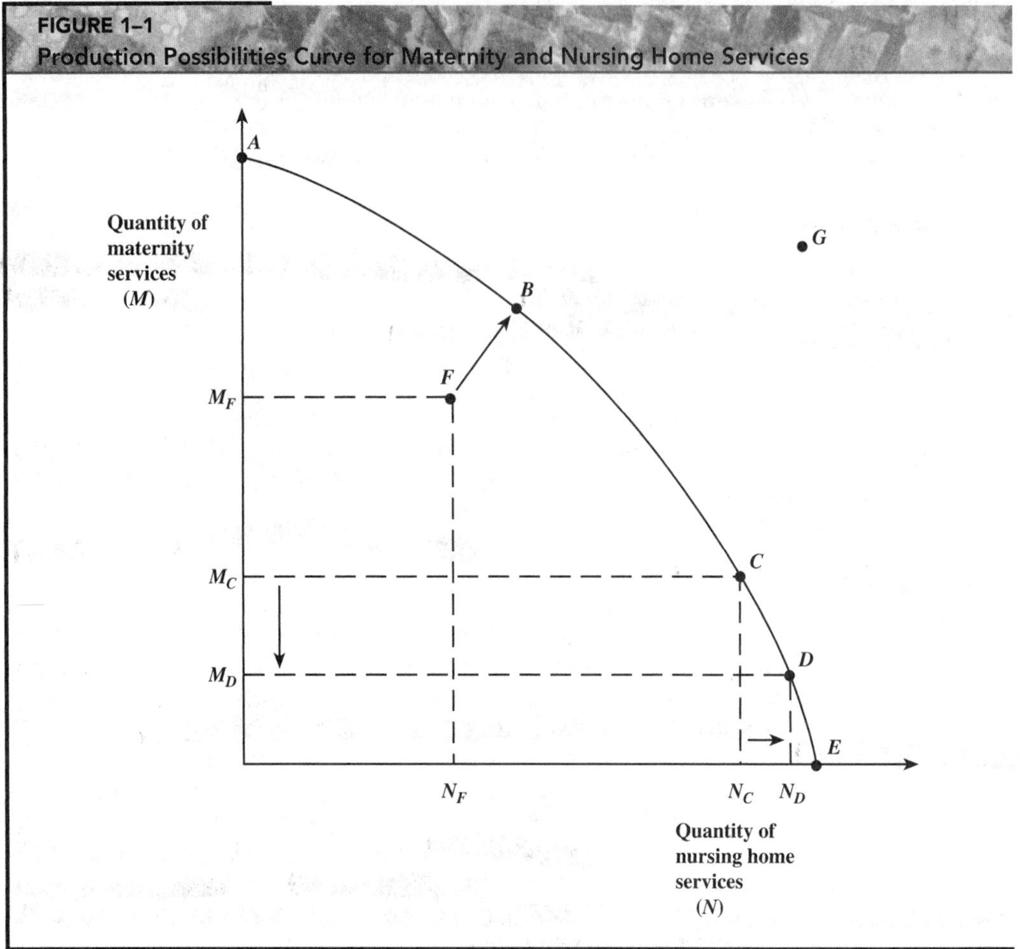

The PPC shows the trade-off between any two goods given a fixed stock of resources and technology. Any point on the PPC, such as points *A* through *E*, reflects efficiency because units of one good must be given up to receive more of the other. A point in the interior, such as *F*, reflects inefficiency because more of one good can be attained without necessarily reducing the other. A point outside the PPC, such as *G*, is not yet attainable but can be reached with an increase in resources or through institutional or technological changes that improve productivity.

medical inputs are neither unemployed nor underemployed (for example, a nurse involuntarily working part time rather than full time) and are being used in the most productive manner so that society is getting their maximum use. If a movement along the curve from one point to another occurs, units of one medical service must be forgone to receive more units of the other medical service.

Specifically, assume the health economy is initially operating at point *C* with M_C units of maternity care services and N_C units of nursing home services. Now suppose health care decision makers decide that society is better off at point *D* with one more unit of nursing home services, $N_D - N_C$. The movement from point *C* to point *D* implies that $M_C - M_D$ units of maternity care services are given up to receive the additional unit of nursing home services. Because medical resources are fully utilized at point *C*, a movement to point *D* means that medical inputs must be drawn or reallocated from the maternity care services market to the nursing home services market. As a result, the quantity of maternity care services must decline if an additional unit of nursing home services is produced. The forgone units of maternity care services, $M_C - M_D$, represent the **opportunity cost** of producing an additional unit of nursing home services.[4] Generally, opportunity cost is the value of the next best alternative that is given up.

The bowed-out shape of the PPC implies that opportunity cost is not constant but increases with a movement along the curve. Imperfect substitutability of resources is one reason for this so-called **law of increasing opportunity cost**. For example, suppose the nursing home services market expands downward along the PPC. To produce more nursing home services, employers must bid resources away from the maternity care services market. Initially, the least productive inputs in the maternity care services market are likely to be bid away, because they are available at a lower cost to nursing home employers. Consequently, very few maternity care services are given up at first. As the nursing home services market continues to expand, however, increasingly productive inputs in the maternity care services market must be drawn away. The implication is that society gives up ever-increasing units of maternity care services. Thus, the law of increasing opportunity cost suggests that ever-increasing amounts of one good must be given up to receive successively more equal increments of another good.

If medical inputs are not fully utilized because some inputs are idle or used unproductively, more units of one medical service can be produced without decreasing the amount of the other medical service. An example of an underutilization of resources is indicated by point *F* in the interior of the PPC. At point *F*, the health care system is producing only M_F units of maternity services and N_F units of nursing home services. Notice that by moving to point *B* on the PPC, both maternity care services and nursing home services can be increased without decreasing the other. The quantities of both goods increase only because some resources are initially idle or underutilized at point *F*. Health care resources are inefficiently employed at point *F*.

A point outside the current PPC, such as *G*, is attainable in the future if the stock of health care resources increases, a new, productivity-enhancing technology is discovered, or various economic, political, or legal arrangements change and improve productive relationships in the health economy. If so, the PPC shifts out and passes through a point like *G*. For example, technological change may enable an increased production of both maternity and nursing home services from the same original stock of health care resources. Alternatively, a greater quantity of maternity and nursing home services can be produced and the PPC shifts outward if more people enter medical professions (possibly at the expense of all other goods and services).

Production efficiency is attained when the health economy operates at any point on the PPC, since medical inputs are producing the maximum amount of medical services and no unproductive behavior or involuntary unemployment exists. Allocative efficiency is attained when society chooses the best or most preferred point on the PPC. All points on the PPC are possible candidates for allocative efficiency. The ideal, or optimal, point for allocative efficiency depends on society's underlying preferences for the two medical services.

The Distribution Question

The answer to the fourth question—who should receive the medical goods and services?—deals with **distributive justice** or **equity**. It asks whether the distribution of services is equitable, or fair, to everyone involved. In practice, countries around the world have chosen to address this distribution question involving medical care in many different ways.

4. As economists are fond of reminding noneconomists, "There is no such thing as a free lunch!"

When thinking about the distribution question, it is sometimes useful to consider two theoretically opposite ways of distributing output: the **pure market system** and a **perfect egalitarian system.** Goods and services are distributed in a pure market system based solely on each person's willingness and ability to pay because decisions concerning the four basic questions are answered on a decentralized basis within a system of markets. That is, goods and services are distributed, or rationed, to only those people who are both willing and able to purchase them in the marketplace. Because people face an incentive to earn income to better afford goods and services in a pure market system, they tend to work hard and save appropriately for present and future consumption. Consequently, productive resources tend to be allocated efficiently in a pure market system. In other words, the incentives associated with a pure market system typically mean that the economy operates on the PPC.

In many cases, differences in ability to pay among individuals reflect that some have consciously chosen to work harder and save more than others. Unfortunately, differences in ability to pay may also indicate that some people have less income because of unfortunate life circumstances such as a mental, physical, or social limitation. Regardless of the specific reason, it follows that people without sufficient incomes face a financial barrier to obtaining goods and services in a pure market system in which price serves as a rationing mechanism. Given income disparities some people may be denied access to needed goods and services. Consequently the pure market system is typically viewed as inherently unfair by many when it comes to the distribution of important goods and services such as health care.

In direct contrast, a central committee, such as a federal or subnational unit of government, may answer the distribution question by ensuring that everyone receives an equal share of goods and services. In an egalitarian system of this kind, everyone has access to the same goods and services without regard to income status or willingness to pay. Therefore, no one is denied access to needed goods and services. But an incentive may exist for people to choose to work and save less because the consumption decision is divorced from the distribution of earned income. Because of this inefficient allocation of resources, fewer goods and services may be available for distribution in an egalitarian system. In this case, the economy may operate inside the PPC.

In practice, most countries have adopted a mixed distribution system, with the reliance on central versus market distribution varying by degree across countries. For example, in the United States, many goods and services are distributed by both the market and the government. The food stamp, temporary assistance for needy families, and Medicaid programs represent some of the many policies adopted by the government to redistribute goods and services in the United States. Some people applaud these programs, whereas others argue that they worsen both efficiency and equity. They argue that efficiency and equity are compromised when those who choose to commit fewer resources to production are rewarded through redistributive programs and productive individuals are penalized via taxation. The efficiency and equity implications of various redistributive policies are constantly debated in the United States and elsewhere. In the context of health care, the consequence of this debate regarding distribution might determine who lives and who dies. For this reason, among others, more discussion on the redistributive function of government is taken up in Chapters 9 and 10.

Implications of the Four Basic Questions

Given a scarcity of economic resources, a society generally wishes to produce the best combination of goods and services by employing least-cost methods of production. Trade-offs are inevitable. As the PPC illustrates, some amount of one good or service must be given up if the production and consumption of another good or service increases. As a result, each society must make hard choices concerning consumption and production activities because scarcity exists. Choices may involve sensitive trade-offs, for example, between the young and the old, between prevention and treatment, or between men (prostate cancer) and women (breast cancer).

In addition, some individuals lack financial access to necessary goods and services such as food, housing, and medical care. Because achieving equity is a desirable goal, a society usually seeks some redistribution of income. Normally, the redistribution involves taxation. However, a tax on labor or capital income tends to create a disincentive for employing resources in their most efficient manner.[5] Inefficient production suggests that fewer goods and services are available in the society (production inside the PPC). Thus, a trade-off often exists between equity and efficiency goals, and, consequently, hard choices must be made between the two objectives. The design of a nation's health care system normally reflects the way the society has chosen to balance efficiency and equity concerns.

Economic Models and Analysis

Economic Models

As mentioned earlier, the production possibilities curve is an example of an **economic model.** Models are abstractions of reality and are used in economics to simplify a very complex world. Economic models can be stated in descriptive (verbal), graphical, or mathematical form. Usually an economic model like the PPC describes a hypothesized relation between two or more variables. For example, suppose the hypothesis is that health care expenditures, E, are *directly* (as opposed to *inversely*) related to consumer income, Y. That hypothesis simply means that expenditures on health care services tend to rise when consumer income increases. Mathematically, a health care expenditure function can be stated in general form as

$$E = f(Y). \quad (1\text{–}1)$$

Equation 1–1 implies that health care spending is a *f*unction of consumer income. In particular, health care expenditures are expected to rise with income.

An assumption underlying economic models is that all factors, other than the variables of interest, remain unchanged. For example, our hypothesis that health care expenditures are directly related to income assumes that all other likely determinants of health care spending, such as prices, tastes, and preferences, stay constant. As another example, notice in the previous analysis that the stocks of resources and technology are held constant when constructing the PPC. Indeed, economists normally qualify their hypotheses with the Latin phrase *ceteris paribus,* meaning "all other things held constant." By holding other things constant, we can isolate and describe the pure relation between any two variables.

The expenditure function in Equation 1–1 is expressed in general mathematical form, but a hypothesis or model is often stated in a specific form. For example, the following equation represents a linear expenditure function for health care services:

$$E = a + bY, \quad (1\text{–}2)$$

where a and b are the fixed parameters of the model. This equation simply states that health care expenditures are directly related to consumer income in a linear (rather than nonlinear) fashion. Mathematically, the parameter a reflects the amount of health care expenditures when income is

5. This point is discussed in more detail in Chapter 9.

zero, whereas b is the slope of the expenditure function. The slope measures the change in health care expenditures that results from a one-unit change in income, or $\Delta E/\Delta Y$.

For example, let us assume the parameter a equals \$1,000 per year and b equals one-tenth, or .1. The resulting health care expenditure function is thus

$$E = 1{,}000 + 0.1Y. \tag{1–3}$$

Equation 1–3 implies that health care expenditures rise with income. In fact, the slope parameter of 0.1 suggests that each \$1,000 increase in consumer income raises health care spending by \$100.

The health care expenditure function in Equation 1–3 is represented graphically in Figure 1–2. Yearly consumer income per household is shown on the horizontal axis, and annual health care spending per household is shown on the vertical axis. According to the function, health care spending equals \$3,000 when household income is \$20,000 per year. Consumers earning \$50,000 per year spend \$6,000 per year on health care services. Note that the expenditure function clearly represents our hypothesis concerning the direct relation between income and health care spending.

Now suppose some other determinants of health care expenditures change. Although this assumption violates our implicit *ceteris paribus* condition, we can incorporate changes in other

FIGURE 1–2
Health Care Expenditure Function

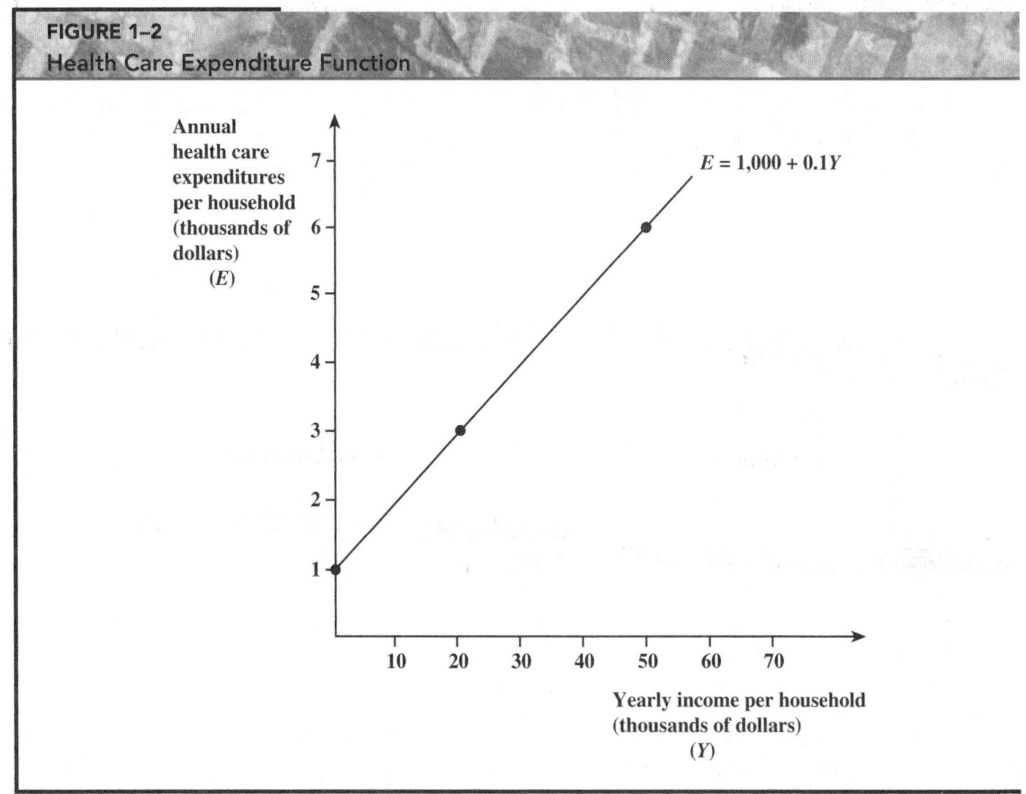

According to the expenditure function, health care spending increases with income. For example, health care spending equals \$3,000 when household income equals \$20,000 per year and \$6,000 when household income equals \$50,000 per year.

FIGURE 1–3
A Shift in the Health Care Expenditure Function

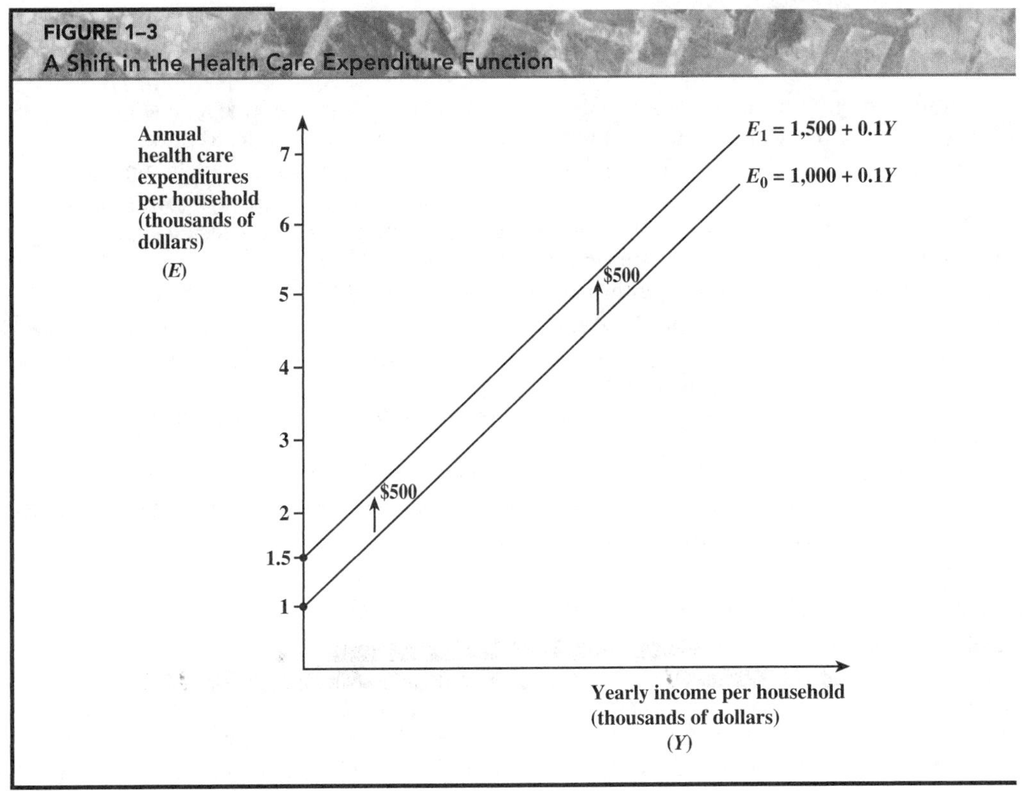

Yearly health care spending is assumed to increase by $500 for a reason other than a change in income. Thus, the expenditure function shifts upward at each level of income by $500 to E_1.

factors into the health care expenditure model fairly simply. For example, suppose people generally become sicker than before, perhaps because households have become older on average. Obviously, this change tends to increase health care spending. Assuming that the "aging" effect influences only the intercept term and not the value of the slope parameter, the expenditure function shifts upward by the yearly increase in health care spending due to the aging population. Figure 1–3 shows an example of this effect.

Yearly medical costs are assumed to increase by $500 for the typical household. Thus, the health care expenditure function shifts upward at each level of income by $500 to E_1. If the aging effect also influences the percentage of additional income that people spend on health care services, the slope of the function changes as well. An increase (decrease) in the marginal propensity to spend out of income raises (lowers) the slope and rotates the expenditure function to the left (right).[6]

As you can see, a model, such as this expenditure function or the PPC, is useful because it helps simplify an otherwise complex world so we can better and more easily understand the relation among key variables. Models are also useful because they often offer valuable insights

6. Problem 3 at the end of the chapter asks you to complete an exercise of this type.

into the necessity or relative effectiveness of various public policies. For example, we saw from the PPC that policy changes typically involve trade-offs that public policy makers should heed.

In the case of our health care expenditure function, suppose that some government agency, such as the General Accounting Office or Congressional Budget Office, determines that $4,000 of annual household spending on health care is necessary to maintain the health of family members in the typical household. Further suppose that a study by this same government agency finds that our health care expenditure model, as reflected in Equation 1–3, represents the true relation between household income and health care spending. If so, our model suggests that households with incomes less than $30,000 tend to spend less than the necessary amount on health care. The government might use this information to determine the subsidy needed at each level of family income to reach the targeted amount of $4,000. For example, a household with $10,000 of income would require a $2,000 subsidy to reach the targeted amount of health care spending whereas a household with $28,000 would need only $200.

Consequently, economic models are useful because they help simplify complex situations so we can more easily understand how things fit together. Models are also useful, however, because they often can be used for policy purposes.

Empirical Testing of Health Economic Theories

Health economists often use statistical methods to test their theories. Statistical tests are conducted either to verify the theories or to quantify the magnitude of the relation among economic variables. For example, empirical methods might be used to estimate values for the parameters *a* and *b* in Equation 1–2. A statistical study of this type could support our hypothesis that income and health care expenditures are directly related by finding empirically that the slope parameter, *b*, has a positive value. In addition, an empirical study could provide some useful information concerning how strongly income affects health care spending. Is *b* equal to 0.1 or 1.2? As we just learned, this information might be useful for determining the amount of a health care subsidy, for example.

Throughout this book, we refer to a host of empirical studies using multiple regression analysis. In the simplest terms, **multiple regression analysis** is a statistical technique used to estimate lines or curves such as Equation 1–2. The only difference is that a number of independent variables are specified on the right-hand side of the equation—hence *multiple* regression. Reviewing multiple regression studies should give you a better understanding of the underlying theories and also help you learn how to interpret multiple regression findings. Most of you have probably studied multiple regression analysis in your statistics classes; an elementary discussion of regression analysis is provided in an appendix at the end of this chapter. For those desiring a more advanced treatment of regression analysis, an additional appendix is provided at www.thomsonedu.com/economics/santerre. The material provides a general overview of the technique and some pitfalls commonly encountered in multiple regression studies.

Positive and Normative Analysis

Health economists perform two types of analysis. **Positive analysis** uses economic theory and empirical analysis to make statements or predictions concerning economic behavior. It seeks to answer the question "What is?" or "What happened?" For example, we might investigate the exact relation between income and health care spending. Because positive analysis provides explanations or predictions, it tends to be free of personal values.

Normative analysis, on the other hand, deals with the appropriateness or desirability of an economic outcome or policy. It seeks to answer the question "What ought to be?" or "Which is better?" For example, an analyst might conclude that households with incomes less than $30,000 per year should be subsidized by the government because they are unable to maintain a proper level of health care spending. Naturally, this implies that the analyst is making a value judgment. Because opinions vary widely concerning the desirability of any given economic outcome and the role government should play in achieving outcomes, it is easy to see why normative statements generally spark more controversy than positive ones. For instance, when 518 health economists were asked whether the Canadian health care system is superior to the U.S. system, there was much disagreement. Fifty-two percent of the economists agreed and 38 percent disagreed with the statement. The remaining 10 percent had no opinion or lacked the information needed to respond to the question (Feldman and Morrisey, 1990).

The following sets of positive and normative economic statements should give you a better understanding of the difference between the two. Notice that the positive statements deal with what is or what will be, whereas the normative statements concern what is better or what ought to be.

> ***Positive:*** According to Becker and Murphy (1988), a 10 percent increase in the price of cigarettes leads to a 6 percent reduction in the number of cigarettes consumed.
> ***Normative:*** The government should increase the tax on cigarettes to prevent people from smoking.

> ***Positive:*** A study by Hellinger (1991) estimates that the average yearly cost of treating someone with AIDS is $38,300, while the lifetime costs equal $102,000.
> ***Normative:*** It is in our country's best interests that the federal government take a more active role in the prevention of AIDS.

> ***Positive:*** National health care expenditures per capita are higher in the United States than Canada.
> ***Normative:*** To control health care expenditures, the United States should adopt a national health insurance program similar to Canada's.

THE NET BENEFIT CALCULUS

As we saw from the PPC analysis, resource scarcity forces society to make choices. For example, an entire economy must collectively decide how much medical care to produce and who is to receive it, while each health care provider must determine the most appropriate method to produce health care services. Even the consumer who has complete medical insurance coverage faces scarcity and choices because time is a finite commodity. In this situation, the consumer must consider the opportunity cost of time. The consumer must decide whether the time needed to make a doctor's appointment, travel to the physician's office, and receive medical services is worth the value of forgone activities. Thus, scarcity necessitates choice, and economics is the social science that analyzes the process by which society makes these choices.

Economists treat people as *rational* decision makers. **Rationality** means people know how to rank their preferences from high to low or best to worst. It also means people never purposely choose to make themselves worse off. Consequently, it stands to reason that people will make choices based on their self-interests and choose those activities they expect will provide them with the most net satisfaction. Pursuing self-interests does not mean people are always selfish, however. For example, giving money to charity or volunteering one's time at a local hospital gives even the most devout Good Samaritan a considerable amount of pleasure.

The decision rule people follow when choosing activities is straightforward and involves an assessment of the expected benefits and costs associated with each choice. If expected benefits exceed expected costs for a given choice, it is in the economic agent's best interest to make that choice. In formal terms, the optimizing rule looks like this:

$$\text{NB}^e(X) = \text{B}^e(X) - \text{C}^e(X) \tag{1–4}$$

where X represents a particular choice or activity under consideration, B^e stands for the expected benefits associated with the choice, C^e equals the expected costs resulting from the choice, and NB^e represents the expected net benefits.

Expected values take both the probability of occurrence and the magnitude of the loss or gain into consideration. For example, the expected benefit of activity X can be expressed in the following manner:

$$\text{B}^e(X) = \pi(X) \times \text{B}(X), \quad \text{where } 0 \leq \pi(X) \leq 1. \tag{1–5}$$

$\pi(X)$ measures the probability or degree of certainty that activity X will provide actual benefits, and $\text{B}(X)$ reflects the dollar magnitude of the actual benefits. If $\pi(X)$ equals 1, the actual benefits of activity X are known with perfect certainty. Oppositely, if $\pi(X)$ equals zero, the true benefits of X are completely unknown. Intermediate values for $\pi(X)$ mean the benefits of X are uncertain to some degree. For example, in deciding whether to purchase an over-the-counter cold remedy, a person implicitly considers both the probability that the cold remedy will be effective and the benefit of being relieved of cold symptoms.

Expected costs are calculated in an analogous manner. In the decision to purchase a cold remedy, the monetary costs are known, a priori, so the probability of occurrence is 100 percent, or 1. In that case, the expected cost equals the actual cost of the cold remedy. In some instances, however, the true costs may be unknown when the activity initially takes place, so expected costs are either implicitly or explicitly estimated. For example, actual physician charges are never known until after the episode of care is completed. One office visit may result in numerous tests and many follow-up visits.

If NB^e is larger than zero, the economic agent's well-being is enhanced by choosing the activity. Your reading of this textbook indicates that the book's expected benefits outweigh its expected costs (unless, of course, your professor forced you to buy and read it). That is, you expect this book to provide benefits in excess of the money you spent on it, plus the forgone use of your time. Nonreaders of this book obviously believe the costs outweigh the benefits.

Health care providers, government agencies, and individual consumers employ cost-benefit analysis on either an informal or a formal basis to guide them in the decision-making process. The formal approach is to estimate the monetary value of the expected costs and benefits associated with a policy proposal. If the benefits exceed the costs, the policy may warrant adoption. More likely, however, several proposals are under consideration, so the best proposal is associated with the highest net benefit or payoff. Chapter 3 discusses formal cost-benefit analysis in detail.

Equation 1–4 can also be used to illustrate how government policies sometimes attempt to alter behavior by manipulating the expected costs or benefits associated with a health care decision. For example, the primary purpose of "sin taxes" on cigarettes and alcohol is to discourage the consumption of both products by increasing their actual costs. Government warnings on cigarette packages and alcoholic beverages aim to lower the expected benefits associated with these consumption practices and thereby reduce the amount of medical care services directed toward alcohol- and tobacco-induced illnesses.

SUMMARY

Health economics is concerned with the determination and allocation of health resources and distribution of medical services in a society. Because resources are scarce, society must determine what amounts of medical services to produce, what kinds of medical services to produce, what mix of health care resources should be used, and who should receive the output of health care services. Answering these four basic questions involves tough trade-offs.

Essential to the study of health economics is the use of microeconomic models. Economic models are necessary to simplify a very complex world. Models or hypotheses can be expressed in descriptive, mathematical, or graphical form and can be used to conduct positive analysis or draw normative conclusions.

A major assumption in economics is that people are rational; that is, people are able to rank their preferences from high to low and never purposely make themselves worse off. People choose activities that offer the greatest benefits at the lowest possible cost.

CASE STUDIES

1-1 Information[7]

According to a 2005 Harris Interactive poll, an increasing number of Americans are using the Internet to search for health or other medical information. The U.S. Census Bureau reported that nearly 117 million adults have been online to look for health care information, showing an increase of about 111 million from previous years. Those who used the Internet to gain health care information were successful in finding what they needed and 90 percent believed that the information they found was reliable. Around 57 percent of the people responding to the poll also said they discussed the health care information they received online with their physician at least once. Overall, 58 percent of Americans with Internet access reported that they looked for health or medical information online "sometimes" or "often," which was up 50 percent from the previous year.

Questions for Discussion

1. *This report suggests that more people are turning to the Internet to retrieve health-related information. Discuss the future role of the Internet in providing such information. What are its main strengths and limitations?*
2. *Some people argue that medical information should be handled mainly by physicians, who have the expertise required to interpret scientific findings. Do you agree or disagree? Justify your position.*
3. *Can the Internet improve health care? Why or why not?*

1-2 Is Health Care Different?

Health policy experts have often argued that the health industry is different from other industries. The "differentness" argument says that that health care is too important to be treated as a commodity and that the health industry does not function like a market in any meaningful way (see, for example, Rice, 1998). One of the most often cited reasons for the latter—that health care markets are not anything like normally functioning markets—is the prevalence of high levels of

7. Source: "More Americans Go Online for Health-Care Information," *The Wall Street Journal,* July 15, 2005.

information asymmetry in most health care transactions (Arrow, 1963). Patients know more about their health than the employers who pay for their health insurance, the insurance companies that pay their bills, and the doctors that they visit; doctors know more about diagnosis and treatment than patients. In the era of selective contracting, one could extend the information asymmetry argument to other kinds of transactions, such as those between health plans and hospitals and between health plans and physician organizations. According to the differentness argument, moral hazard, adverse selection, supplier-induced demand, opportunism, and fraud are in large part the result of asymmetrically distributed information.

Critics of this viewpoint, on the other hand, submit that health care is really not all that different from other industries, and that information asymmetry alone explains very few of the unique features of the U.S. health care system (Robinson, 2001). Although health care is essential to health, Robinson notes that so too are food and shelter, yet those industries are not normally considered "different" and, perhaps more important, do not exhibit the high levels of organizational heterogeneity, laws, and entry barriers common to the health care industry. In other words, they are essential to health but allowed to function more or less as free markets.

Questions for Discussion

1. *List three to five points in favor of and against the differentness conjecture.*
2. *What are the advantages and disadvantages to thinking of health care as an industry like many other industries? Are there research findings from other industries that might be applied fruitfully to the health sector?*

REVIEW QUESTIONS AND PROBLEMS

1. Draw a bowed-out production possibilities curve (PPC) with an *aggregate* measure of medical services, Q, on the horizontal axis and an *aggregate* measure of all other goods (and services), Z, on the vertical axis. Discuss the implications of the following changes on the quantities of medical services and all other goods.
   A. A movement down along the curve.
   B. A movement from the interior of the curve to a northeasterly point on the curve.
   C. An increase in the quantity of labor in the economy.
   D. A technological discovery that increases the production of Z.

   If it were your choice, where would you choose to produce on the PPC? Why?
2. Determine whether the following statements are based on positive or normative analysis. Be sure to substantiate your answers.
   A. Prices of physician services should be controlled by the government because many citizens cannot afford to pay for a visit to a physician.
   B. According to Tosteson et al. (1990), a 25 percent drop in the number of people who smoked in 1990 would reduce the incidence of coronary heart diseases by 0.7 percent by the year 2015.
   C. Rising health care costs have forced numerous rural hospitals to close their doors in recent years.
   D. According to government statistics, in 1989 7.2 deaths per 100,000 residents were alcohol induced. To decrease this number, the government should impose higher taxes on alcohol.
3. Suppose a health expenditure function is specified in the following manner:

$$E = 500 + 0.2Y,$$

where E represents annual health care expenditures per capita and Y stands for income per capita.

A. Using the slope of the health expenditure function, predict the change in per capita health care expenditures that would result from a $1,000 increase in per capita income.
B. Compute the level of per capita health care spending when per capita income takes on the following dollar values: 0; 1,000; 2,000; 4,000; and 6,000.
C. Using the resulting values for per capita health care spending in part B, graph the associated health care expenditure function.
D. Assume that the fixed amount of health care spending decreases to $250. Graph the new and original health care functions on the same graph. What is the relation between the original and new health care expenditure functions?
E. Now assume that the fixed amount of health care spending remains at $500 but the slope parameter on income decreases to .1. Graph both the original and new health care expenditure functions. Explain the relation between the two lines.

4. Assume the following facts at a particular point in time:
   A. There is a 20 percent, or .20, probability that the appropriate dosage of a painkiller will relieve your headache.
   B. Headache relief provides you with $30 worth of actual benefits.
   C. The monetary cost of the appropriate dosage is $7.50. Would you purchase the painkiller? Why or why not?
   D. Would you purchase the painkiller if headache relief provides you with $50 of actual benefits because of an important job interview? Why or why not?
5. Victor Fuchs (1996) lists the following questions in an article in *The Wall Street Journal.* Identify whether the following questions involve positive or normative analysis. All the questions deal with a Republican plan to reform Medicare, the public health insurance program for the elderly.
   A. How many Medicare beneficiaries will switch to managed care?
   B. How much should the younger generation be taxed to pay for the elderly?
   C. Should seniors who use less care benefit financially, or should they subsidize those who use more care?
   D. How many Medicare beneficiaries will switch to medical savings accounts (see Chapter 16)?
   E. What effect will these changes have on utilization?
   F. How much should society devote to medical interventions that would add one year of life expectancy for men and women who have already passed the biblical "three score and ten"?
   G. Will senior citizens' choices about types of coverage depend on their health status?
   H. If the rate of spending growth is reduced to 6 percent from 10 percent a year, what will happen to the growth of medical services? To physician incomes?
6. Congratulations! Upon graduating you accept a well-deserved job with XER Consulting. Your first job involves a consulting gig with a state subcommittee on health care issues. The senate health care subcommittee is considering the expansion of two existing public health programs. One program concerns additional funding for nursing homes around the state. The other program involves additional funding for community health centers around the state. In both cases the funding is supposed to be used to attract more nurses for expansion purposes. Your job involves the following four tasks:
   A. Draw and use a production possibilities curve to graphically show and verbally explain to the subcommittee members the opportunity cost at a point in time of expanding any one of the programs, assuming that both of them are initially operating efficiently. Be sure to correctly label the axes and all points. Refer to the points on the graph in your explanation.

B. Use the production possibilities curve to graphically show and verbally explain how one or both programs could be expanded at a lower opportunity cost if some inefficiency or slack initially exists in the overall public health system. Refer to various points on the graph in your explanation.
C. Use the production possibilities curve to graphically show and verbally explain how both programs could be expanded at a lower opportunity cost if growth is expected for the public health care system. Refer to points on the graph in your explanation.
D. Verbally explain to the subcommittee members what factors might cause the public health care system to grow.

CEBS QUESTIONS*

■ *CEBS Sample Question on Subject Matter from CEBS Course 9 Study Manual*

1. Using the mathematical terminology in the text and the model, $E = a + bY$, how much will health care expenditures change when income increases from \$30,000 to \$50,000 if when income is zero, health care expenditures equal \$2,000, and the slope is 0.05? (pages 9–11)

■ *CEBS Sample Exam Questions*

1. Which of the following statements characterizes the concept of distributive justice or equity in a health economy?
   A. The concept is based on rewarding individuals who have chosen to work harder and save more with more health care goods and services.
   B. In theory, equitable distribution of health care services and goods is accomplished through a central committee such as a federal or subnational unit of government.
   C. Most countries have chosen to solve health care distribution issues using the pure market system.
   D. Most health care experts agree that U.S. Medicaid programs are both efficient and equitable.
   E. The concept draws attention to the health care needs of individuals with mental, physical, or social limitations.
2. Which of the following statements regarding a production possibilities curve is (are) correct?
   I. Points on the curve show the combinations of production that can be efficiently produced.
   II. Points under the curve illustrate combinations with the highest opportunity cost.
   III. Points above the curve can be achieved in the future with better technology.
   A. I only
   B. II only
   C. I and II only
   D. I and III only
   E. I, II, and III
3. All the following statements regarding regression analysis are correct EXCEPT:
   A. The purpose of regression analysis is to isolate the cause and effect among variables.
   B. The "ordinary least squares" is a popular method of fitting a line to data in a scatter diagram.
   C. t-statistics identify the fraction of the variation in the dependent variable that is explained by the independent variable.
   D. Multiple linear regression has more than one independent variable.
   E. A rule of thumb is that when the t-statistic is 2 or more we can place about 95 percent confidence in the estimated average value of the estimated parameter.

*The CEBS designation stands for the Certified Employee Benefit Specialist program.

■ *Answer to Sample Question from Study Manual*

At an income level of $30,000 expenditures will be ($2,000 + 0.05 ($30,000)) or $3,500. At an income level of $50,000, expenditures will be ($2,000 + 0.05 ($50,000)) or $4,500. The difference, or increase, is $1,000, i.e., $4,500 − $3,500.

■ *Answers to Sample Exam Questions*

1. E. is the correct answer. See pages 7–8 of the text.
2. D. See pages 5–7 of the text.
3. C. The coefficient of determination, R^2, shows the percentage of the variation in the dependent variable that is explained by the independent variable. See pages 19–22 of the text.

ONLINE RESOURCES

To access Internet links related to the topics in this chapter, please visit our web site at **www.thomsonedu.com/economics/santerre**.

REFERENCES

Arrow, K. J. "Uncertainty and the Welfare Economics of Medical Care." *American Economic Review* 53, no. 5 (1963), pp. 941–73.

Becker, Gary S., and Kevin M. Murphy. "A Theory of Rational Addiction." Journal of Political Economy 96 (August 1988), pp. 675–700.

Feldman, Roger, and Michael A. Morrisey. "Health Economics: A Report on the Field." *Journal of Health Politics, Policy and Law* 15 (fall 1990), pp. 627–46.

Fuchs, Victor R. "The Tofu Triangle." *The Wall Street Journal,* January 26, 1996, p. A16.

Hellinger, Fred J. "Forecasting the Medical Care Costs of the HIV Epidemic: 1991–1994." *Inquiry* 28 (fall 1991), pp. 213–25.

Rice, T. *The Economics of Health Reconsidered.* Chicago, Ill.: Health Administration Press, 1998.

Robinson, J. C. "The End of Asymmetric Information." *Journal of Health Politics, Policy and Law* 26, no. 5 (2001), 1045–53.

The Mosby Medical Encyclopedia. New York: C. V. Mosby, 1992.

Tosteson, Anna, et al. "Long-Term Impact of Smoking Cessation on the Incidence of Coronary Health Disease." *American Journal of Public Health* 80 (December 1990), pp. 1481–86.

APPENDIX TO CHAPTER 1

Regression Analysis

As mentioned in Chapter 1, empirical testing of economic theories is important for two reasons. First, economic hypotheses require empirical validation, especially when a number of competing theories exist for the same real-world occurrence. For example, some people believe medical illnesses occur randomly whereas others believe medical illness is largely a function of lifestyle. The "random" and "lifestyle" explanations represent two competing theories for medical illnesses. Empirical studies can potentially ascertain which theory does a better job of explaining illnesses.

Second, even well-accepted theories are unable to establish the magnitude of the relation between any two variables. For example, suppose we accept the theory that lifestyle is a very important determinant of health status. A question remains about the magnitude or strength of the impact lifestyle has on health status. Does a young adult who adopts a sedentary lifestyle face a 10, 20, or 50 percent chance of dying prematurely compared to an otherwise comparable individual? Empirical studies can help provide the answer to that question.

There are many different ways for researchers to conduct an empirical analysis. The method we emphasize in this book, which most economists also use, is **regression analysis.** Regression analysis is a statistical method used to isolate the cause-and-effect relation among variables. Our goal in this appendix is to provide the reader with an elementary but sufficient understanding of regression analysis so the regression results discussed in this book can be properly interpreted. Regression analysis is explained through an example.

The example used concerns the relation between health care expenditures, E, and consumer income, Y, which was briefly introduced in Chapter 1. Suppose we hypothesize that health care expenditures rise with household income and want to test our theory. Health care expenditures represent the dependent variable, and income is the independent variable. Furthermore, suppose we expect a linear (or straight-line) relationship between income and health care expenditures, or

(A1–1) $$E = a + bY,$$

where a is the constant or intercept term and b is the slope parameter. If you recall, the slope parameter in this case identifies the change in health care expenditures that results from a one-unit change in income.

Because we are interested in the actual or real-world magnitudes of the parameters a and b, we now collect a random sample of observations relating information on both medical expenditures and income. The data might be series observations on income and expenditures for a particular household over time or cross-sectional observations on income and expenditures across different households at a particular point in time. In this case we collect cross-sectional data on income and medical expenditures from a random survey of 30 households.

Exhibit A1–1 shows a scatter diagram illustrating our random sample of observations (only 5 of the 30 observations are illustrated for easier manageability). Notice that the scatter diagram of observations does not automatically show a linear relation between income and health care expenditures because of omitted factors that also influence spending on health care, some

EXHIBIT A1–1
Scatter Diagram of Income and Health Care Expenditures

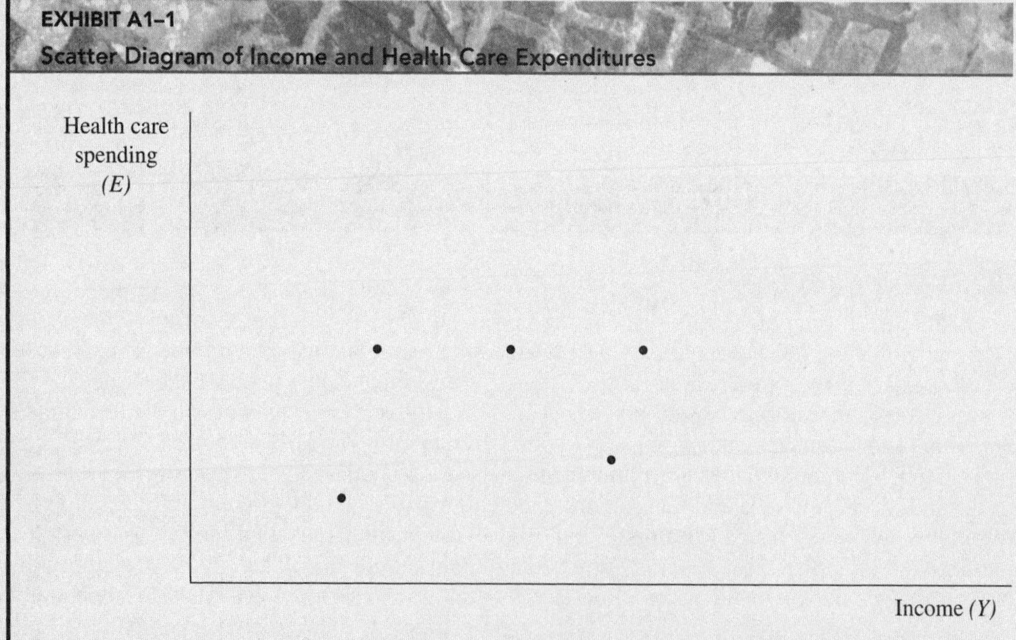

EXHIBIT A1–2
Fitted Line

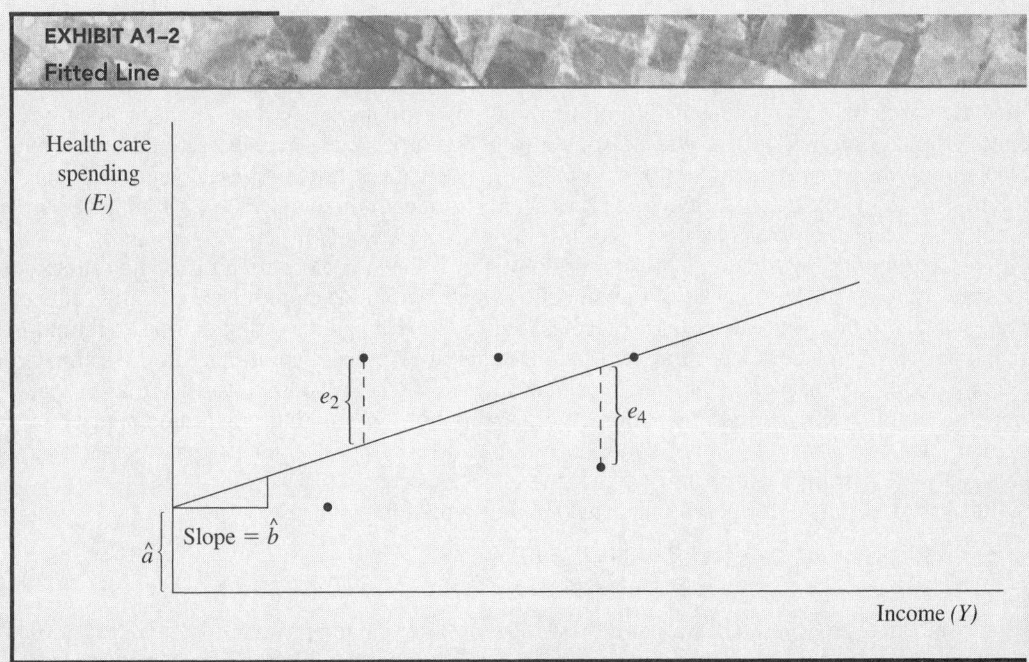

randomness to economic behavior, and measurement error. Our objective is to find the line that passes through those observations and provides the best explanation of the relation between Y and E. One can imagine numerous lines passing through the set of observations. What we want is the line that provides the best fit to the data.

A criterion is necessary to determine which line constitutes the best fit. One popular criterion is ordinary least squares, or OLS. OLS finds the best line by minimizing the sum of the squared deviations, e_i, from the actual observations and a fitted line passing through the set of observations, or

(A1–2) $$\text{Minimize } \Sigma\, e_i^2 = \Sigma\, (E_a - E_f)^2 = \Sigma\, (E_a - \hat{a} - \hat{b}Y)^2,$$

where E_a is the actual observation on medical expenditures and E_f is fitted (or predicted) expenditures from the estimated regression line, $\hat{a} + \hat{b}Y$. In Exhibit A1–2, we show an example of a fitted line and the resulting deviations between actual and fitted expenditures. Based upon the sample of observations, a computer program (such as SAS, SPSS, or TSP) searches for the best line using the OLS procedure. In the process of finding the best line, the intercept and slope are determined, and thus we estimate the best magnitudes for a and b that minimize the sum of the squared deviations from the actual observations.

Let's suppose the following results are obtained from the regression analysis:

(A1–3) $$E = 2{,}000 + 0.2Y.$$

The results would tell us that the best fitted line to the data has an intercept of $2,000 and a slope of 0.2. Although the fitted or estimated regression line provides the "best" fit compared to all other lines, we do not know yet whether it represents a "good" fit to the actual data. Fortunately, the computer estimation procedure also provides us with some goodness-of-fit information that we can use to determine if the best fit is also a reasonably good one.

The two most common and elementary goodness-of-fit measures are the coefficient of determination, R^2, and the t-statistic, t. The coefficient of determination identifies the fraction of the variation in the dependent variable that is explained by the independent variable. Thus, the R^2

ranges between 0 and 1. Researchers tend to place more faith in a regression line that explains a greater proportion of the variation in the dependent variable.

The values for the parameters $\hat{a}$ and $\hat{b}$ are average estimates rather than true values because they are based on a sample instead of all possible observations; thus, they are associated with some error. Accordingly, there will be some deviations around the average estimate for a and also around the average estimate for b. In fact, if the deviations are very large, we cannot place much faith in the estimated value for the parameters. Indeed, the true value for b may be zero. If so, no relationship exists between income and health care expenditures.

The computed t-statistic helps us identify how much deviation occurs around the estimated average value for the parameters of the model. A t-statistic of 2 or more means that the value of the estimated parameter was at least twice as large as its average deviation. A rule of thumb is that when the t-statistic is 2 or more, we can place about 95 percent confidence in the estimated average value for the parameter, meaning that only a 5 percent likelihood exists that the relationship could have occurred by chance. Another rule of thumb is that when the t-statistic is 3 or more, we can place 99 percent confidence in our estimated value for the parameter. In this case, only a 1 percent likelihood exists that the relation occurred by chance.

Regression results are generally reported similar to the following:

(A1–4)
$$\underset{(2.52)}{E = 2{,}000} + \underset{(3.40)}{0.2Y} \qquad R^2 = 0.47 \quad N = 30$$

The t-statistics are reported in parentheses below the parameter estimates. Because the t-statistic associated with income is greater than 3, we can place a high degree of confidence in the parameter estimate of 0.2. Also, according to the regression results, income explains about 47 percent of the variation in health care expenditures. The number of observations, N, is 30.

Before we move on we need to interpret the parameter estimates for Equation A1–4. The intercept term of 2,000 tells us the level of health care expenditures when income is zero. The parameter estimate of 0.2 on the income variable is much more telling and suggests that expenditures on health care will increase by 20 cents if income increases by one-dollar. If the estimated parameter was instead –0.2, it would mean that a one-dollar increase in income causes health care expenditures to decrease by 20 cents. Thus, both the sign and value of the parameter estimate convey important information to the researcher.

The regression analysis we have been discussing thus far is an example of a simple regression because there is only one independent variable. Multiple regression refers to an analysis in which more than one independent variable is specified. For example, theory might tell us that price or tastes and preferences should also be included in an expenditure equation. The OLS procedure behind multiple regression is the same as that for simple regression and finds the best line that minimizes the squared deviations between the actual and fitted values. The computed R^2 identifies the variation in the dependent variable, say, health care expenditures, explained by the set of independent variables, which in our example would be price, income, and tastes and preferences. Each independent variable would be associated with an estimated parameter and t-statistic. For example:

(A1–5)
$$\underset{(2.32)}{E = 1{,}000} - \underset{(0.42)}{0.2P} + \underset{(3.23)}{0.13Y} + \underset{(4.00)}{0.8A} \qquad R^2 = 0.75 \quad N = 30$$

where P represents the price of medical services and A represents the average age in the household as a proxy for tastes and preferences. According to the regression results, the independent variables collectively explain 75 percent of the variation in health care expenditures. Also, the regression results suggest that income and age both have a statistically significant direct impact on health care expenditures. Price, on the other hand, has no impact on health care expenditures according to the regression findings.

CHAPTER 2

HEALTH AND MEDICAL CARE: AN ECONOMIC PERSPECTIVE

The disintegration of the Soviet Union, which many Americans viewed on their televisions with the collapse of the Berlin Wall on November 6, 1989, emerged as a major turning point in the twentieth century and radically changed the lives of millions of people. As a case in point, in just five short years, from 1989 to 1994, the life expectancy of men in Russia fell by 6.6 years. For women over the same time period, life expectancy fell by 3.3 years. Brainerd and Cutler (2005) investigate the impact of five major trends on the increase in mortality rates in Russia: the deterioration of the health care system, the increase in traditional risk factors for cardiovascular disease such as smoking, the increase in alcohol consumption, changes in diet, and material deprivation. Overall, they find that about half of the increase in mortality in Russia was brought about by increased alcohol consumption and the stress that accompanied the transition to a market economy. The other three major trends did not appear to statistically impact the increase in mortality rates.

The study by Brainerd and Cutler illustrates the important roles that medical care, lifestyle, socioeconomic conditions, and the environment play in the overall health of the people in a country. This chapter explores these relationships by establishing the theoretical and empirical connection between health and various factors such as medical care. In particular, this chapter:

- discusses the concepts of health and medical care
- introduces utility analysis to explain why people desire health
- utilizes production theory to explain the making of health
- reviews the empirical results concerning the factors that influence health

What Is Health?

The *Mosby Medical Encyclopedia* (1992, p. 360) defines **health** as "a state of physical mental and social well-being and the absence of disease or other abnormal condition." Economists take a radically different approach. They view health as a durable good, or type of capital, that provides services. The flow of services produced from the stock of health "capital" is consumed continuously over an individual's lifetime (see Grossman, 1972a, 1972b). Each person is assumed to be endowed with a given stock of health at the beginning of a period, such as a year. Over the period, the stock of health depreciates with age and may be augmented by investments in medical services. Death occurs when an individual's stock of health falls below a critical minimum level.

Naturally, the initial stock of health, along with the rate of depreciation, varies from individual to individual and depends on many factors, some of which are uncontrollable. For example, a person has no control over the initial stock of health allocated at birth, and a child with a congenital heart problem begins life with a below-average stock of health. However, we learn later that medical services may compensate for many deficiencies, at least to some degree. The rate at which health depreciates also depends on many factors, such as the individual's age, physical makeup, lifestyle, environmental factors, and the amount of medical care consumed. For example, the rate at which health depreciates in a person diagnosed with high blood pressure is likely to depend on the amount of medical care consumed (is this person under a doctor's care?), environmental factors (does he have a stressful occupation?), and lifestyle (does the person smoke or have a weight problem?). All these factors interact to determine the person's stock of health at any point in time, along with the pace at which it depreciates.

Regardless of how you define it, health is a nebulous concept that defies precise measurement. In terms of measurement, health depends as much on the quantity of life (that is, number of life-years remaining) as it does on the quality of life. Quality of life has become an increasingly important issue in recent years due to the life-sustaining capabilities of today's medical technology. The issue gained national prominence in 1976 when, in a landmark court decision, the parents of Karen Ann Quinlan were given the right to remove their daughter, who was in a persistent vegetative state, from a ventilator. Because the quality of life is a relative concept that is open to wide interpretation, researchers have wrestled with developing an instrument that accurately measures health. As we will see, health economists often use the inverse of mortality or morbidity rates as a measure of health.

Why Good Health? Utility Analysis

As mentioned earlier, health, like any other durable goods, generates a flow of services. These services yield satisfaction, or what economists call **utility.** Your television set is another example of a durable good that generates a flow of services. It is the many hours of programming, or viewing services, that your television provides that yield utility, not the set itself.

As a good, health is desired for consumption and investment purposes. From a consumption perspective, an individual desires to remain healthy because she receives utility from an overall improvement in the quality of life. In simple terms, a healthy person feels great and thus is in a better position to enjoy life. The investment element concerns the relation between health and time. If you are in a positive state of health, you allocate less time to sickness and therefore have more healthy days available in the future to work and enhance your income or to pursue other activities, such as leisure. Economists look at education from the same perspective. Much as a person invests in education to enhance the potential to command a higher wage, a person invests in health to increase the likelihood of having more healthy days to work and generate income.

The investment element of health can be used to explain some of the lifestyle choices people make. A person who puts a high value on future events is more inclined to pursue a healthy lifestyle to increase the likelihood of enjoying more healthy days than a person who puts a low value on future events. A preference for the future explains why a middle-aged adult with high cholesterol orders a salad with dressing on the side instead of a steak served with a baked potato smothered in sour cream. In this situation, the utility generated by increasing the likelihood of having more healthy days in the future outweighs the utility received from consuming the steak dinner. In contrast, a person who puts a much lower value on future events and prefers immediate gratification may elect to order the steak dinner and ignore the potential ill effects of high cholesterol and fatty foods.

Naturally, each individual chooses to consume that combination of goods and services, including the services produced from the stock of health, that provides the most utility. The isolated relation between an individual's stock of health and utility is captured in Figure 2–1, where the quantity of health, *H*, is measured on the horizontal axis and the level of utility, *U*, is

FIGURE 2–1
The Total Utility Curve for Health

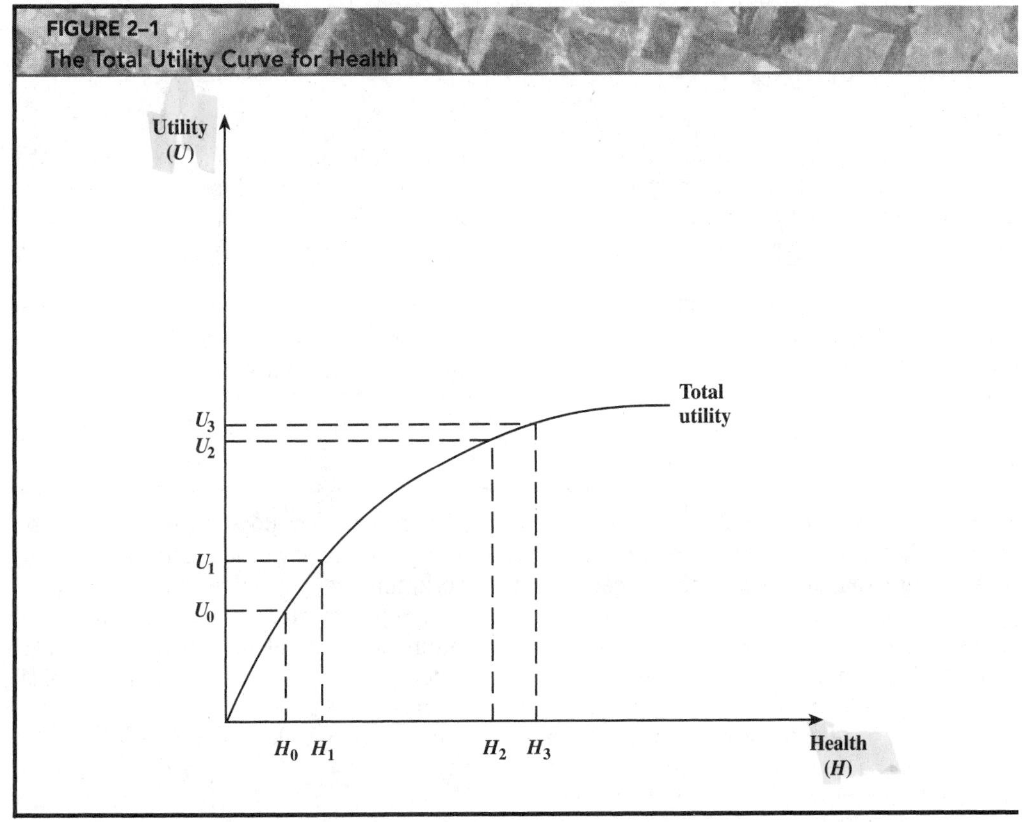

The total utility curve is upward sloping and depicts the relation between an individual's stock of health and utility. The positive slope indicates that total utility increases as an individual's stock of health improves; the bowed shape of the curve captures the impact of the law of diminishing marginal utility. This law is a fundamental principle of economics that states that each additional improvement in health generates an ever smaller increase in utility. Notice that the increase in health from H_0 to H_1 causes utility to increase from U_0 to U_1, while an equal increase in health for H_2 to H_3 results in a smaller increase in utility from U_2 to U_3.

represented on the vertical axis.[1] The positive slope of the curve indicates that an increase in a person's stock of health directly enhances total utility. The shape of the curve is particularly important because it illustrates the fundamental economic principle of the **law of diminishing marginal utility.** This law states that each successive incremental improvement in health generates smaller and smaller additions to total utility; in other words, utility increases at a decreasing rate with respect to health.

For example, in Figure 2–1 an increase in health from H_0 to H_1 causes utility to increase from U_0 to U_1, while an equal increase in health from H_2 to H_3 generates a much smaller increase in utility, from U_2 to U_3. In the second case, the increase in utility is less when the stock of health is greater because of the law of diminishing marginal utility. The implication is that a person values a marginal improvement in health more when sick (that is, when having a lower level of health) than when healthy. This does not mean that every individual derives the same level of utility from a given stock of health. It is possible for two or more people to receive a different amount of utility from the same stock of health. The law of diminishing marginal utility requires only that the addition to total utility decreases with successive increases in health for a given individual.

Another way to illustrate the law of diminishing marginal utility is to focus on the marginal utility associated with each unit of health. Marginal utility equals the addition to total utility generated by each successive unit of health. In mathematical terms,

$$MU_H = \Delta U / \Delta H, \qquad (2\text{–}1)$$

where MU_H equals the marginal utility of the last unit of health consumed and Δ represents the change in utility or health. In Figure 2–1, Equation 2–1 represents the slope of a tangent line at each point on the total utility curve. The bowed shape of the total utility curve implies that the slope of the tangent line falls as we move along the curve, or that MU_H falls as health increases.

Figure 2–2 captures the relation between marginal utility and the stock of health. The downward slope of the curve indicates that the law of diminishing marginal utility holds because each new unit of health generates less additional utility than the previous one.

WHAT IS MEDICAL CARE?

Medical care is composed of myriad goods and services that maintain, improve, or restore a person's physical or mental well-being. For example, a young adult might have shoulder surgery to repair a torn rotator cuff so that he can return to work, an elderly woman may have hip replacement surgery so that she can walk without pain, or a parent may bring a child to the hygienist for an annual cleaning of his teeth to prevent future dental problems. Prescription drugs, wheelchairs, and dentures are examples of medical goods, while surgeries, annual physical exams, and visits to physical therapists are examples of medical services.

Because of the heterogeneous nature of medical care, units of medical care are difficult to measure precisely. Units of medical care are also hard to quantify because most represent services rather than tangible products. As a service, medical care exhibits the four *Is* that

1. To simplify matters, we ignore the intermediate step between the health stock, the services it provides, and the utility received from these services and assume that the stock of health directly yields utility.

FIGURE 2–2
The Marginal Utility Curve for Health

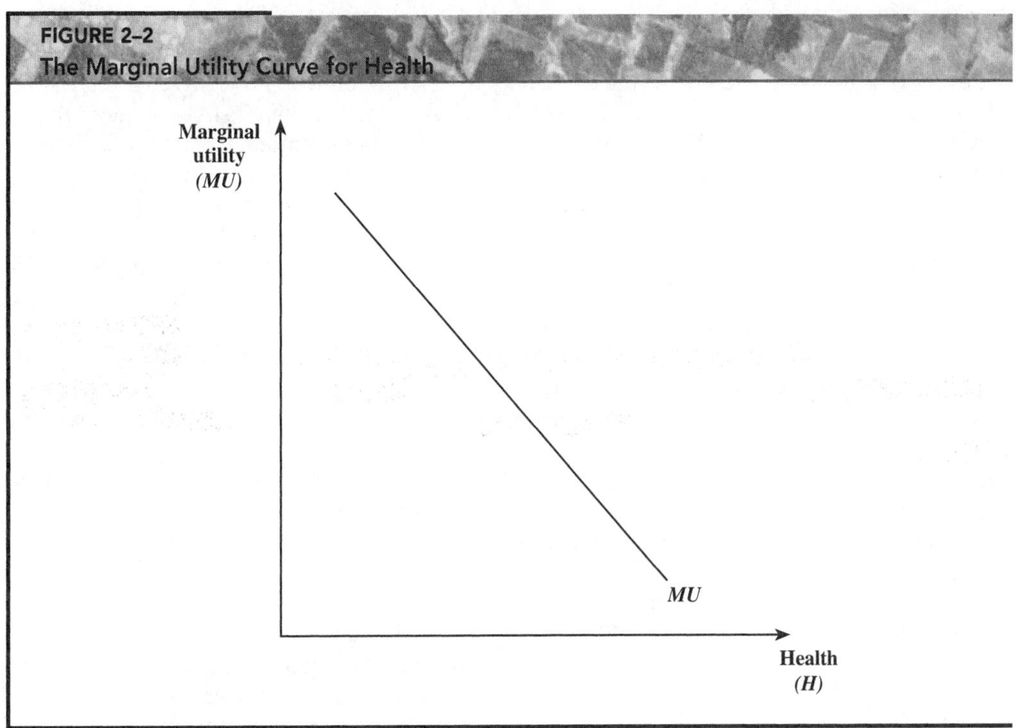

The *MU* curve illustrates the relation between marginal utility and the stock of health, and it is downward sloping because of the law of diminishing marginal utility. The shape of curve reflects the notion that each additional improvement in health results in a smaller increase in utility than the previous one.

distinguish it from a good: intangibility, inseparability, inventory, and inconsistency (Berkowitz et al., 1989).

The first characteristic, **intangibility,** means that a medical service is incapable of being assessed by the five senses. Unlike a new car, a steak dinner, or a new CD, the consumer cannot see, smell, taste, feel, or hear a medical service.

Inseparability means that the production and consumption of a medical service take place simultaneously. For example, when you visit your dentist for a checkup, you are consuming dental services at the exact time the dentist is producing them. In addition, a patient often acts as both producer and consumer. Without the patient's active participation, the medical product is likely to be poorly produced.[2]

Inventory is directly related to inseparability. Because the production and consumption of a medical service occur simultaneously, health care providers are unable to stockpile or maintain an inventory of medical services. For example, a dentist cannot maintain an inventory of dental checkups to meet demand during peak periods.

2. Educational services, like medical services, require the consumer's active participation; that is, education is likely to be poorly provided when the student plays a passive role in the process.

Finally, **inconsistency** means that the composition and quality of medical services consumed vary widely across medical events. Although everyone visits a physician at some time or another, not every visit to a physician is for the same reason. One person may go for a routine physical, while another may go because he needs heart bypass surgery. The composition of medical care provided or the intensity at which it is consumed can differ greatly among individuals and at different points in time.

The quality of medical care is also difficult to measure. Quality differences are reflected in the structure, process, and/or outcome of a medical care provider (Donabedian, 1980, 1988). **Structural quality** is reflected in the physical and human resources of the medical care provider, such as the facilities (level of amenities), medical equipment (type and age), personnel (training and experience), and administration (organization structure). **Process quality** reflects the specific actions health care providers take on behalf of patients in delivering and following through with care. Process quality might include access (waiting time), data collection (background history and testing), communication with the patient, and diagnosis and treatment (type and appropriateness). **Outcome quality** refers to the impact of care on the patient's health and welfare as measured by patient satisfaction, work time lost to disability, or postcare mortality rate. Because it is extremely difficult to keep all three aspects of quality constant for every medical event, the quality of medical services, unlike that of physical goods, is likely to be inconsistent.

As you can see, medical care services are extremely difficult to quantify. In most instances, researchers measure medical care in terms of either availability or use. If medical care is measured on an availability basis, such measures as the number of physicians or hospital beds available per 1,000 people are used. If medical care is measured in terms of use, the analyst employs data indicating how often a medical service is actually delivered. For example, the quantity of office visits or surgeries per capita is often used to represent the amount of physician services rendered, whereas the number of inpatient days is frequently used to measure the amount of hospital or nursing home services consumed.

The Production of Good Health

Health economists take the view that the creation and maintenance of health involves a production process. Much as a firm uses various inputs, such as capital and labor, to manufacture a product, an individual uses medical inputs and other factors, such as a healthy lifestyle, to produce health. The relation between medical inputs and output can be captured in what economists call a production function. A **health production function** indicates the maximum amount of health that an individual can generate from a specific set of inputs in a given period of time. In mathematical terms it shows how the level of output (in this case, health) depends on the quantities of various inputs, such as medical care. A generalized short-run health production function for an individual takes the following form:

$$\text{Health} = H(\text{medical care, technology, profile, lifestyle, socioeconomic status, environment}) \quad \textbf{(2–2)}$$

where *health* reflects the level of health at a point in time; *medical care* equals the quantity of medical care consumed; *technology* refers to the state of medical technology at a given point in time; *profile* captures the individual's mental and physical profile as of a point in time; *lifestyle* represents a set of lifestyle variables, such as diet and exercise; *socioecononomic status* reflects the joint effect of social and economic factors, such as education, income and

FIGURE 2–3
The Total Product Curve for Medical Care

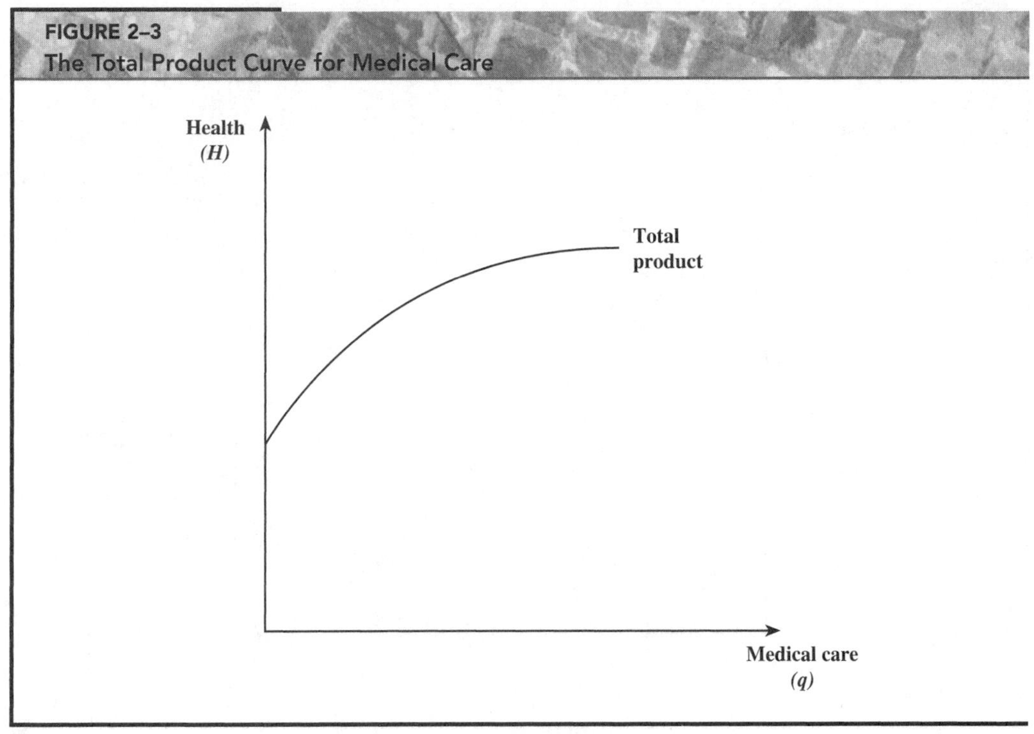

The total product curve is upward sloping and indicates that as an individual consumes more medical care, overall health improves. The positive intercept term represents the individual's level of health when no medical care is consumed and is a function of other factors such as lifestyle and the environment. The law of diminishing marginal productivity accounts for the bowed shape of the curve. This law is a fundamental principle of production theory and it implies that health increases at a decreasing rate when additional units of health care are consumed, holding all other inputs in the health production process constant.

poverty; and *environment* stands for a variety of environmental factors, including air and water quality.

To focus on the relation between health and medical care, we assume initially that all other factors in the health production function remain constant. Figure 2–3 depicts this relation, where q is a hypothetical measure of health care, holding technology constant, and H represents the level of health. The intercept term represents the individual's level of health when zero medical care is consumed. As drawn, the **total product curve** implies that an individual's level of health is positively related to the amount of medical care consumed.[3] The shape of the curve is very similar to that in Figure 2–1 and reflects the **law of diminishing marginal productivity.** This law implies that health increases at a decreasing rate with respect to additional amounts of

3. However, we should not rule out the possibility that poor health status or an illness might be created by additional medical services. An illness created by a medical care encounter is referred to as an *iatrogenic disorder,* "a condition caused by medical personnel or procedures or through exposure to the environment of a health-care facility" (*Mosby Medical Encyclopedia,* p. 401). For example, a physician may accidentally harm a patient by prescribing the wrong medicine for a given medical condition.

FIGURE 2–4
The Marginal Product Curve for Medical Care

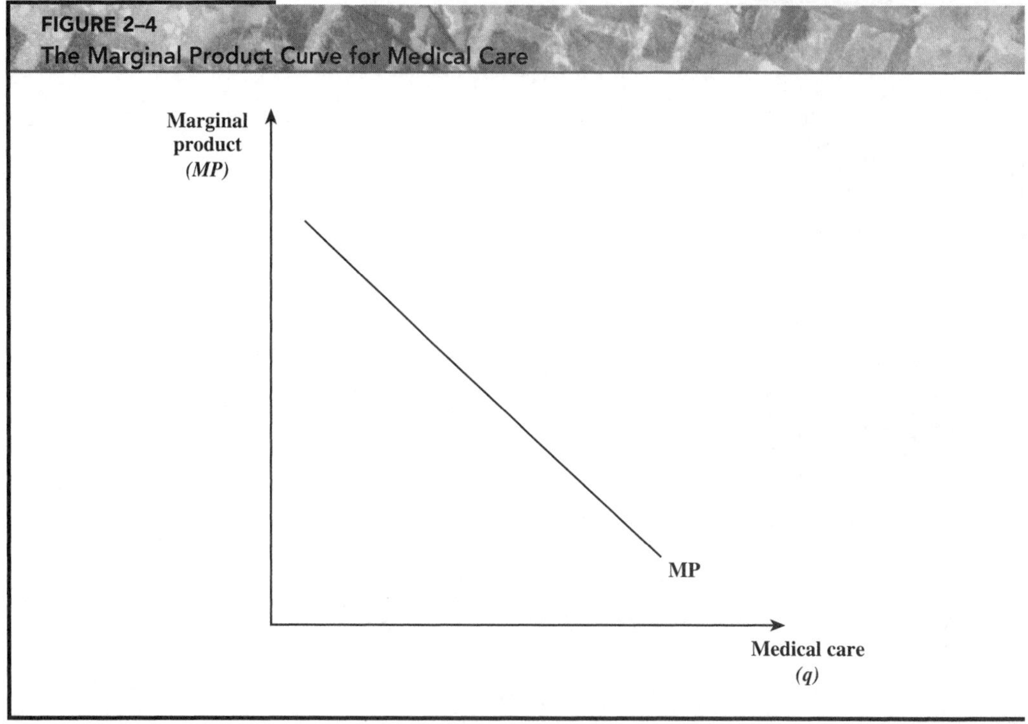

The MP curve establishes the relation between the marginal product of medical care and the amount of medical care consumed. The curve is downward sloping because the marginal product of the last unit of medical care consumed decreases as the individual consumes more medical care, reflecting the law of diminishing marginal productivity.

medical care, holding other inputs constant. For example, suppose an individual makes an initial visit and several follow-up visits to a physician's office for a specific illness or treatment over a given period of time. It is very likely that the first few visits have a more beneficial impact on the individual's stock of health than the later visits. Thus, each successive visit generates a smaller improvement in health than the previous one.

The relation between health and medical care can also be viewed from a marginal perspective, where the marginal product of medical care represents the incremental improvement in health brought about by each successive unit of medical care consumed, or

$$\text{MP}_q = \Delta H/\Delta q, \quad (2\text{–}3)$$

where MP_q equals the marginal product of the last unit of medical care services consumed. The law of diminishing marginal productivity holds that the marginal product of medical care diminishes as the individual acquires more medical care. A graph of this relationship appears as a negatively sloped curve in Figure 2–4.[4]

4. As in utility analysis, the marginal product of medical care equals the slope of a tangent line drawn to every point on Figure 2–3.

The other variables in the health production function can also be incorporated into the analysis. In general terms, a change in any one of the other variables in the production function alters the position of the total product curve. The total product curve may shift in some instances and/or rotate in others. In the latter case, the curve rotates because the marginal productivity of medical care has changed in response to the change in the other factors.

New medical technologies have profoundly affected all aspects of the production of medical care. In the broadest of terms, examples of new technologies include the development of sophisticated medical devices, the introduction of new drugs, the application of innovative medical and surgical procedures, and most recently, the use of computer-supported information systems, just to name a few. According to Cutler and Huckman (2003) and Cutler and McClellan (2001), technological change can result in *treatment expansion, treatment substitution,* or some elements of both. Treatment expansion occurs when more patients are treated by a new medical intervention, perhaps because of a higher success rate or lower risks to health. Treatment substitution occurs when the new technology substitutes for or replaces an older one.

In the context of our health production model, the development and application of a new medical technology causes the total product curve to pivot and rotate upward because the marginal productivity of each unit of medical care consumed increases, as illustrated in Figure 2–5.

FIGURE 2–5
The Effect of Technological Change on the Total Product Curve for Medical Care

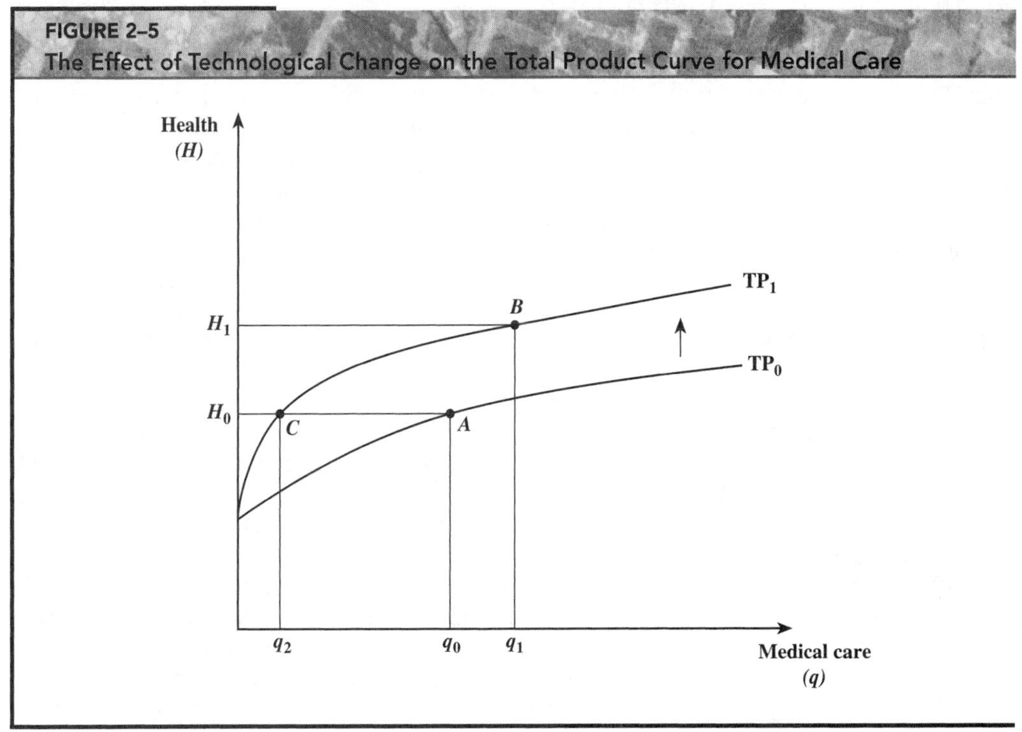

The total product curve shifts upward with the development and application of new medical technology because of an increase in the marginal product of medical care. A movement from point *A* to point *B* illustrates the case in which a new technology results in a simultaneous increase in the amount of medical care consumed and improvement in health. A movement from point *A* to point *C* depicts the case in which the new medical technology has no impact on health but results in less consumption of medical care.

Notice that the total product curve rotates upward from TP_0 to TP_1 and each unit of medical care consumed now generates a greater amount of health. The movement from point *A* to point *B* in Figure 2–5 illustrates the case in which the improvement in medical technology brings about an increase in the amount of medical care consumed from q_0 to q_1 along with an improvement in health from H_0 to H_1. This movement represents the treatment expansion resulting from the new medical technology. Movement from point *A* to point *C* illustrates the situation in which the new technology has no impact on health but results in less consumption of medical care from q_0 to q_2. In this case, the new technology is cost saving, everything else held constant. It should be noted that the increase in the marginal product of medical care brought about by the medical technology also causes the marginal product curve to shift to the right.

The profile variable in Equation 2–2 depends on a host of variables and controls for such items as the person's genetic makeup, mental state, age, gender, and race/ethnicity as of a given point in time (such as the beginning of the year). Any change in the profile variable affects both the intercept term and the slope of the health production function. For example, an individual's genetic makeup may make him or her a candidate for prostate or breast cancer. If this individual gets cancer for that reason, then his or her total product curve shifts downward. That is because overall health has decreased regardless of the amount of medical care consumed. The total product curve is also likely to rotate downward at the same time because the marginal product of medical care should decrease as the profile worsens. The total product curve rotates downward because an otherwise healthy person is likely to respond more favorably to medical treatments *for a given medical complication* than one who is less healthy. Both of these changes are represented in Figure 2–6, where the total product curve shifts and rotates downward at the same time from TP_0 to TP_1. The marginal product curve for medical services also shifts to the left, because each incremental unit of medical care now brings about a smaller improvement in health.

The effect of age on the production of health is relatively straightforward. Age affects health through the profile variable. As an individual ages and deteriorates physically, both health and the marginal product of medical care are likely to fall. In addition, the rate at which health depreciates over the period is also likely to increase with age. This causes the total product curve to shift downward and flatten out. The decrease in the marginal product of medical care also causes the marginal product curve to shift to the left.[5]

Lifestyle variables consider the impact of personal health habits on the production of health. Personal habits include such things as whether the person smokes, drinks excessively, leads a sedentary lifestyle, is overweight, or has an improper diet. For example, consider a newly health-conscious individual who decides that a change in lifestyle is in order. After a regimen of diet and exercise, this person loses some weight and improves his physical conditioning. As a result of this change in lifestyle, the individual's level of health and the marginal product of medical care should increase. This causes the total product curve to shift and rotate upward.

As is the case with improvements in personal habits, improved socioeconomic conditions cause the intercept term and the marginal product of medical care to increase. For example, since education is likely to make the individual a more efficient producer of health independently of the amount of medical care consumed, the total product curve shifts upward. An individual with more education is likely to better understand the positive impact of a healthy diet on health. The total product curve also steepens, or the marginal product of medical care increases, because education allows the person to utilize each unit of medical care consumed more effectively. For example, an educated individual may be more inclined to understand and

5. The impact of gender on the total and marginal product curves is left to the reader and is the focus of a review question at the end of this chapter.

FIGURE 2–6
A Shift in the Total Product Curve for Medical Care

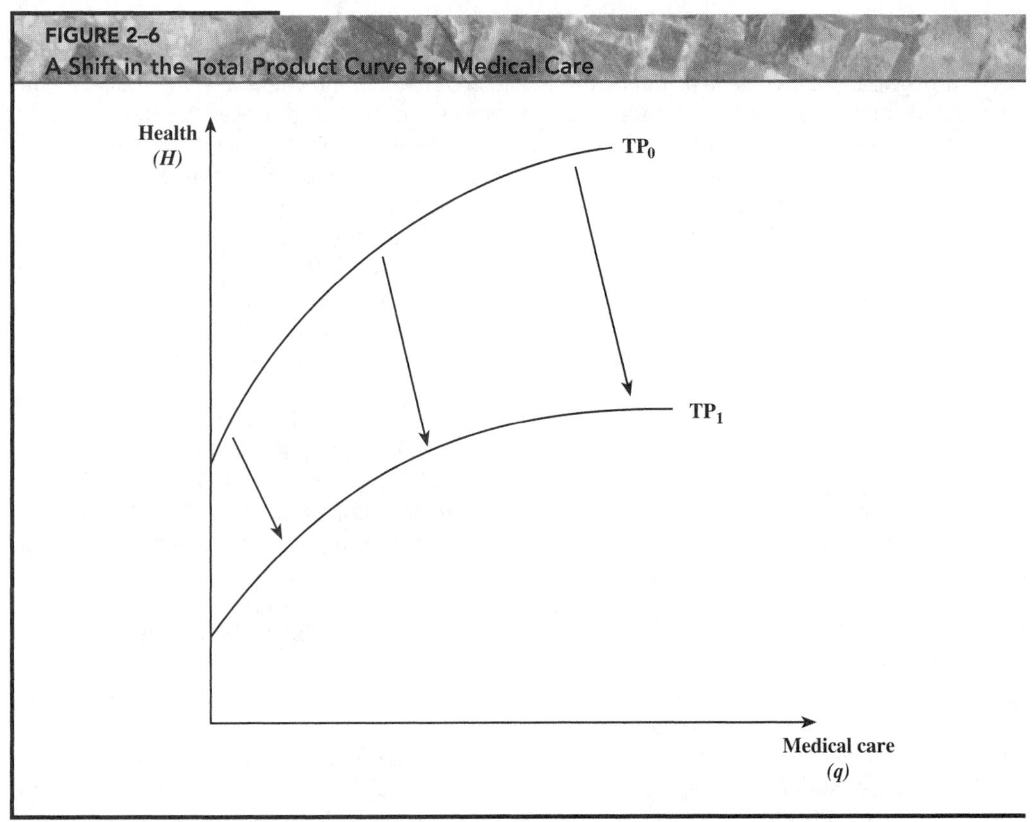

The graph illustrates what happens to the total product curve when an individual gets an illness such as cancer for a reason other than improper medical care. The curve shifts downward because at each level of medical care consumed the individual is less healthy than previously was the case. The curve also rotates downward and becomes flatter, reflecting the likelihood that the now ill individual is going to respond less favorably to a given amount of medical care consumed, such as an office visit, than previously was the case when she was healthy.

follow a physician's advice concerning diet and exercise after undergoing a heart bypass operation. In addition, she may be able to recognize a medical problem early and seek medical care quickly when the effectiveness of medical treatment is generally at its maximum.

Some analysts have hypothesized that the relation between education and health is far more complex. For example, Fuchs (1979) argues that the acquisition of education and health depends on the value people place on future events, or the rate at which they discount future events. Individuals who place a high value on future benefits and are willing to postpone gratification are inclined to acquire more education and pursue a healthier lifestyle when they are young. This is because they want to reap the rewards of a higher income and a longer life that more education and a healthier lifestyle can bring. On the other hand, individuals who place a low value on future events and desire immediate gratification are not likely to acquire significant amounts of education or to follow a healthy lifestyle because they have adopted a "live for today" attitude. Thus, according to Fuchs, higher levels of education may be associated with better health not because there is a direct link between the two variables but because both variables are directly correlated with a third factor, the degree to which future events are valued.

The impact of income on health is also complex and is referred to as the "income gradient" in the literature "to emphasize the gradual relationship between the two: health improves with income throughout the income distribution" (Deaton, 2002, p. 14). Income is likely to indirectly impact health through a number of pathways. An increase in income provides the individual the means to consume more medical care. In addition, a more affluent individual is likely to be more educated, pursue a healthier lifestyle, and live in a safer environment, all of which contribute to improved health. For example, a more affluent individual may live in a suburban community where the crime rate is low, access to drugs and alcohol is limited, and quality medical care is available just around the corner. Income may also have a direct impact on health, although the net effect is far from clear. On the one hand, a wealthier individual may be employed in a safer work environment where the risk of a work-related accident or illness is slim. On the other hand, a wealthier individual may be employed in a more stressful occupation, which can adversely impact health.

In recent years an extensive body of literature has developed that examines whether the distribution of income impacts health, and the income-health hypothesis has taken on a variety of forms. According to the literature (Lynch et al., 2004; Wagstaff and van Doorslaer, 2000), the various hypotheses that have been offered over time can be classified into four broad categories: the absolute income hypothesis, the relative income or deprivation hypothesis, the relative position hypothesis, and the income inequality hypotheses.

The absolute income hypothesis simply states that an individual's absolute income is positively related to health for the reasons discussed previously. The relative income or deprivation hypothesis posits that an individual's income relative to some social group average impacts overall health. Put in more definable terms, it is a person's income relative to some critical level such as the poverty line in the United States that matters. The presumption is that anyone with an income below the poverty line lacks the ability to acquire the basic necessities, such as health care.

The relative position hypothesis emphasizes that one's social position in the income distribution also impacts health. For example, those at the bottom of the income scale in the United States may become frustrated and feel left behind by the "American dream" despite the fact that they have enough income to live in reasonable housing and receive adequate health care. Out of a sense of discouragement, these people may tend to give up and pursue a lifestyle detrimental to their health that could involve increased alcohol consumption, smoking, and obesity.

Finally, the income inequality hypothesis states that the distribution of income itself directly impacts health. For example, greater income inequality may create an incentive for government to limit spending on social programs that have a direct bearing on health in an attempt to lower taxes. Greater income inequality may also lead to an erosion of social capital, defined as "those features of social organizations—such as the extent of interpersonal trust between citizens, norms of reciprocity, and vibrancy of civic organizations—that facilitate cooperation for mutual benefit" (Kawachi and Kennedy, 1999, p. 221). As a result, the poor may find their public health needs largely ignored by society at large.

An adjustment in a person's physical environment is also likely to affect the total product curve. For example, an individual with an asthmatic condition might move from Los Angeles, where smog is intense, to a community on the far outskirts of the city. Or the person's spouse may give up smoking to decrease the level of secondhand smoke in the home. As a result, the probability that this person will succumb to a respiratory ailment diminishes. Both of these changes cause the total product curve to shift and rotate upward.

In short, health production theory suggests that a variety of factors, such as the individual's profile, medical care, state of medical technology, lifestyle, socioeconomic status, and environment, interact to determine health. The theory also suggests that health increases at a diminishing rate with respect to greater amounts of medical care consumed, provided all other inputs remain constant. If any other inputs in the production process change, the impact of medical care on health is also likely to change. The effect of any one nonmedical input on health is also likely to exhibit diminishing returns, all other inputs held constant. For example, running two miles a day may reduce someone's weight by 15 pounds over a six-month period. It is doubtful, however, that an additional two miles per day of running could produce additional 15 pounds of weight loss during the next six-month period.

Before we conclude this section, you should be aware that recently Jacobson (2000), Bolin et al. (2002), and others have extended the Grossman model and developed a number of sophisticated mathematical models that focus on the family rather than the individual as the main producer of health. While these models are beyond the scope of this book, they represent a valuable addition to the literature. The common theme is that individual decisions to invest in health are made within the context of a family and that any decision on the part of one family member regarding investments in health impacts the health investment decisions of others in the family. For example, a learning-disabled child may provide an incentive to a mother to invest more in her own health to ensure that she will have the time to aid her child. These theoretical developments provide a number of challenges to researchers as they strive to understand the complex relationships between family members and individual health-related decisions.

Empirical Evidence on the Production of Health in the United States

The production of health has been the focus of numerous empirical studies. In most instances, a specification similar to Equation 2–2 is estimated using multiple regression analysis. Health is usually represented by the inverse of an age-, gender-, and race-adjusted mortality rate. Using the literature as our guide, we will review the empirical evidence concerning the characteristics associated with the production of health for adults and infants.

The Determinants of Health among Nonelderly Adults

To no one's surprise, the literature has found that the consumption of medical care has a positive impact on the production of adult health. However, the results also indicate that quantitatively, the impact is relatively small. For example, Hadley (1982) finds that a 10 percent increase in per capita medical care expenditures results in only a 1.5 percent decrease in the adult mortality rate. His result confirms those of an earlier study conducted by Auster et al. (1969), who estimate that a 10 percent increase in medical services leads to a 1 percent drop in the age-adjusted mortality rate. Finally, Sickles and Yazbeck (1998) find that a 10 percent increase in health-related consumption leads to about a 0.3 percent improvement in health as measured by a comprehensive health index that considers a number of quality-of-life variables. Enthoven (1980) has referred to the small marginal impact of medical care services on the health status of adults as "flat-of-the-curve" medicine. In the context of Figure 2–3, this means that the typical adult consumes medical services at the point where the slope of the total product curve or marginal product of medicine is near zero.

If, as the empirical evidence indicates, the overall contribution of medical care to health is rather modest at the margin, what determines marginal improvements in health? The answer lies in the other factors associated with the production of health, with education, income, lifestyle, and the environment being the major contributing factors.[6]

6. A discussion of the impact of technology on health is postponed until Chapter 3.

The positive relation between education and health is well documented in the literature. For example, Guralnik et al. (1993) find that education positively impacts life expectancy among older adults. Adults 65 years old with at least 12 years of education had a life expectancy approximately three years longer than those of similar age with less than 12 years of education. Elo and Preston (1996) find that education had a significant impact on mortality for both men and women in the United States during the early 1980s, with the impact of education greater for men and those of working age than for women and the elderly. Finally, Lleras-Muney (2001) finds a significant relation between education levels and health. In particular, she finds that one more year of schooling decreases the probability of dying within 10 years by 3.6 percent.

Empirical studies have also documented a positive connection between income and health. Ettner (1996) finds that increases in income enhance both mental and physical health, while Lantz et al. (2001) find that income and education are both associated with improved health. More specifically, they find that people with less than a high school education and incomes below $10,000 are between two and three times more likely to have functional limitations and poorer self-rated health than their more advantaged counterparts.

While the positive relation between income and health is well established in the literature, a question remains concerning how temporary changes in the macroeconomy impact health. In other terms, what is the relationship between cyclical changes in the macroeconomy and overall health? Your first inclination is to assume that a procyclical relationship holds between the state of the economy and health. In other words, as an economy emerges from a recession and the unemployment rate begins to fall, overall health should improve. You might argue that higher per capita incomes should translate into improved health as people have more discretionary income to spend on medical care. In addition, as more people acquire jobs with employer-financed health insurance, the out-of-pocket price of medical care should drop, causing people to consume more health care. An improved economy may also be associated with healthier lifestyles because as unemployed workers find employment, stress levels are likely to fall along with alcohol consumption and smoking.

Ruhm (2000, 2003) argues that just the opposite may occur: an improved economy may be linked to poorer health. He cites three reasons why health may decline during a cyclical economic expansion. First, the opportunity cost of time is likely to increase with an improved economy. As workers find employment, the amount of leisure time they have to perform what Ruhm refers to as health-producing activities (such as exercise and eating right) diminishes. Second, the act of work may adversely impact the production of health. As the economy improves and more workers find employment, the number of work-related accidents and work-related stress increase. Third, an economic expansion may cause an increase in other types of unintentional injuries such as traffic fatalities, homicide, and suicides.

To test the relationship between cyclical conditions and health, Ruhm estimates the impact that various economic indicators such as unemployment and personal income have on a number of health indicators. The author utilizes a state-based data set for the years 1972 through 1991 and estimates a number of equations utilizing a variety of health measures. Among the measures of health included in the analysis were overall mortality rates, age-based mortality rates, and deaths due to specific causes such as cardiovascular diseases, chronic liver disease and cirrhosis of the liver, motor vehicle accidents, and suicide.

The results are illuminating and suggest an inverse relationship between the strength of the economy and health in the short run. Overall, Ruhm finds that a 1 percent drop in the unemployment rate, relative to the state historical average, results in an increase in the total mortality rate of between 0.5 and 0.6 percent. In addition, Ruhm finds that the impact of changes in the unemployment rate on mortality rates appears to concentrate among the relatively young, between ages 20 and 44. This makes intuitive sense given that they are the ones likely to be hit hardest by temporary changes in economic conditions. The author also finds fluctuations in state unemployment rates to be inversely related to a number of specific causes of death. For example, Ruhm finds decreases in state unemployment rates to be associated with increased fatalities from auto accidents, others types of accidents, homicides, cardiovascular disease, and influenza. Ruhm (2003) also finds that a one-percentage-point decrease in the unemployment rate is associated with acute morbidity and ischemic heart disease increases of 1.5 and 4.3 percent, respectively. Ruhm's empirical results are compelling because they suggest that cyclical, or temporary, changes in economic activity inversely impact health.

Lynch et al. (2004) and Wagstaff and van Doorslaer (2000) provide two excellent reviews of literature regarding the relation between income inequality and health. Both papers agree that there is significant support in the literature for the absolute income hypothesis. The same cannot be said for the other alternative hypotheses, however. According to Wagstaff and van Doorslaer, there is "no support for the relative-income hypotheses and little or no support for the income–inequality hypothesis" (p. 543). They conclude that there is no empirical support for the relative position hypothesis. Lynch et al. (2004) come up with the substantially the same conclusions. However, they state that there is some support among studies that concentrate on the United States that greater income inequality worsens health outcomes. The most consistent support comes from studies that measure income inequality at the state level.

The literature abounds with studies that illustrate the important role lifestyle plays in determining health. Among the risky lifestyle behaviors found to negatively impact health are smoking, excessive alcohol consumption, lack of physical activity, and poor diet. For example, Leigh and Fries (1992) estimate that the typical one-pack-a-day smoker experiences 10.9 more sick days every six months than comparable nonsmokers, while a person who consumes two or more drinks a day has 4.6 more sick days than a comparable light drinker (one or fewer drinks a day). Strum (2002) analyzes the impact of obesity, being overweight, smoking, and problem drinking on health and the consumption of health care for a sample of adults between ages 18 and 65 in 1997–1998. He finds that all four risk behaviors impact health to some degree, with obesity having the greatest impact. In fact, Strum estimates that obesity has the same impact on health as 20 years of aging when health status is measured by the number of seventeen common chronic conditions present. The impact increases to 30 years when health is measured by a quality-of-life index. Strum also finds a correlation between the four risky behaviors and the level of medical care consumed. For example, obesity is related to an average increase in expenditures on inpatient and ambulatory care of $395 a year. In the context of Figure 2–6, these results suggest that obesity causes the total product curve for medical care to shift downward and possibly flatten out. To partially compensate for the loss in health, an obese person slides up the total product curve by consuming more medical care.

Taken together these studies illustrate the fundamental role that lifestyle plays in the production of health for adults. Such information is important if we are to develop appropriate public policies to improve health.

The relation between environmental factors and health is mixed and, as a result, it is difficult to draw overall conclusions from the literature. Auster et al. (1969) included two variables in the regression equation to capture the impact of environmental factors on health: an index of industrialization and a variable that measured the extent of urbanization. Both measures were hypothesized to be positively associated with such factors as air and water pollution, and therefore negatively related to health. The index of industrialization was found to cause higher mortality, but the level of urbanization had no influence.

Hadley (1982) undertook one of the more comprehensive assessments of the impact of environmental factors on health. Included in the regression analysis were variables representing water quality, air quality, climate, and occupational hazards. The results are inconclusive, which Hadley attributes mainly to "the lack of good quality data" (p. 73).

Other variables found to contribute to health are age and marital status. The impact of marital status on health is interesting and merits a brief discussion. Married adults appear to experience better health than their single counterparts, everything else held constant. Most likely, this is because a spouse augments the production of health within the home. Marriage may also have a positive effect on health by altering preferences for risky behavior. Manor et al. (2000) find the mortality rate of married women to be lower than unmarried women for a sample of Israeli adult women, while more recently Kravdal (2001) finds that married people have a higher chance of survival of twelve common forms of cancer in Norway than their unmarried counterparts.

The Determinants of Health among Children and the Elderly

Numerous studies have investigated the factors that influence health among children. Employing county-level data, Corman and Grossman (1985) regress the neonatal mortality rates for blacks and whites on a host of factors including education of the mother, the prevalence of poverty (a measure of income), and the availability of public programs.[7] Some of the public programs included in the analysis are the existence of neonatal intensive care facilities, the availability of abortion services, organized family planning, and Medicaid. Overall, the results are robust and enlightening. Lack of schooling and the existence of poverty are found to raise the neonatal mortality rate for both white and black infants. Together, they account for an increase in neonatal mortality rates by 0.950 and 0.786 per 1,000 live births for whites and blacks, respectively. Access to health care also plays a role, as the presence of neonatal intensive care has caused the neonatal mortality rate to fall by 0.631 and 0.426 per 1,000 live births for white and black infants, respectively. Moreover, the results indicate that various government programs are associated with a reduced mortality rate for black as well as white infants. For example, Medicaid accounts for a decrease in the mortality rate by 0.632 per 1,000 live births for white children and 0.359 per 1,000 live births for black children.

Two recent articles point to the significance of environmental factors on infant health. Chay and Greenstone (2003) use county data from 1981–1982 to estimate the impact of total suspended particulates (TSPs) on infant mortality. TSPs are minute pieces of dust, soot, dirt, ash, smoke, liquid vapor, or other matter in the atmosphere that can cause lung and heart disease. The authors find that a 1 percent reduction in TPS causes the infant mortality rate to fall by 0.35 percent at the county level. Currie and Neidell (2005) find that reductions in carbon monoxide also impact infant mortality. In particular, they find that reductions in carbon monoxide in California throughout the 1990s saved approximately 1000 infant lives. Interestingly, Fuchs and Frank (2002) find an increased use of medical care, both inpatient and outpatient care, among Medicare recipients living in highly polluted metropolitan areas of the United States. The relationship holds even after controlling for population, education, income, racial composition, cigarette use, and obesity. These studies are part of a growing body of literature that illustrates the importance of environmental factors in determining health.

7. The infant mortality rate equals the number of deaths from the first to the 364th day of life per 1,000 live births. The neonatal mortality rate represents the number of deaths from the first to the 27th day of life per 1,000 live births.

Case et al. (2002) focus on the impact of socioeconomic status on children's health.[8] To no one's surprise, the authors find a strong positive relation between the education of the parents and the health of their children. For example, the health of children is positively related to the education of mothers for children living with a mother. Education, in this case, is measured by whether the mother did not complete high school, had a high diploma, or had more than a high school education. The education of fathers is also found to positively contribute to improved health among children, implying that parental education positively impacts the production of a child's health at all age levels.

The study also finds that household income is a strong predictor of children's health. More specifically, the authors find that when household income doubles, the probability that a child 3 years old or younger is in excellent or very good health increases by 4 percent. Comparable improvements for children between ages 4 and 8, 9 and 12, and 13 and 17 are 4.9 percent, 5.9 percent, and 7.2 percent, respectively. Just as interesting, the authors find that permanent income is a strong determiner of children's health. In particular, they find that family income before a child is born is positively related to the child's health for all ages.

Finally, the authors find that healthier parents tend to have healthier children. Why that is the case, however, remains to be determined. However, the authors do estimate a series of equations for children with adoptive and biological parents and find that the impact of income on health is not significantly different across the two populations. While this evidence is not definitive, it does suggest that genetics may explain only part of the reason why healthier parents have healthier children. Could it be that the production of health takes place at the household level and that healthier parents are simply more efficient producers of health for all members of the household? Clearly, more research needs to be done before we fully understand how parental behavior coupled with socioeconomic factors impacts children's health.

The literature concerning uninsured versus insured status and health outcomes offers additional insights into the effect of medical care on infant health as well as on other groups. However, we couch the discussion in terms of the relation between medical care and health because the only plausible pathway from insurance to health outcomes is through medical care (Levy and Meltzer, 2001). In their survey of the literature on this topic, Levy and Meltzer acknowledge that three types of empirical studies have examined whether the consumption of medical care "causes" better health outcomes. Observational studies, the first type, use a technique such as multiple regression analysis to explore the relation between medical care and health outcomes while carefully controlling for all other nonmedical inputs or factors belonging in a health production function. Levy and Meltzer explain that an observational study is hindered by its inability to distinguish between a causal relationship and an association, as illustrated in Figure 2–7.

The figure shows a simple health production function where all nonmedical inputs are collapsed and captured in the variable X. If the multiple regression analysis yields a direct and statistically significant relation between medical care and some favorable health outcome measure, we cannot be certain whether the evidence supports an association or a causal relationship. A third unobservable factor Z, that we are unable to include in X, may simultaneously affect both medical care usage and health status and thereby produce the observed association. For instance, people with better baseline health may be physically more capable of visiting physicians than those with a worse underlying initial endowment of health. Hence an observed correlation, in the presence of an important omitted unobservable variable, may not necessarily

8. Consult Case and Paxson (2002) for a nontechnical overview of the study.

FIGURE 2–7
Association Rather Than Causation

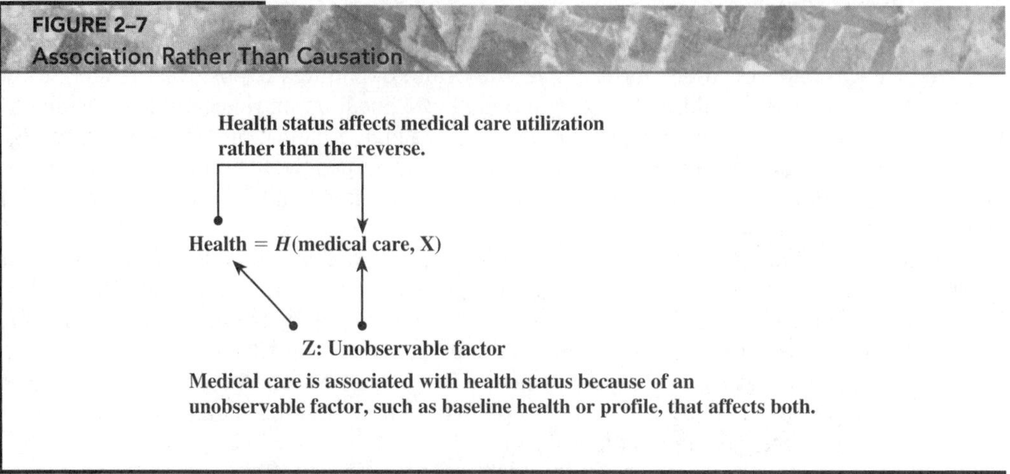

mean that more office visits cause better health. Also, reverse causality may pose a problem when attempting to draw inferences about causal relationships from the regression results. That is, poorer health status, the dependent variable in Figure 2–7, may influence the availability and utilization of medical care. For example, state governments may pursue policies to encourage more doctors per person in areas with the highest infant mortality rates. Pregnant mothers may be more likely to seek out physicians when they suspect that the health of their infants may be at greater risk. Hence, an observational study might show an inverse correlation between the number of visits and infant health in this case.

As a result, investigators sometimes use other methods to identify causal relationships. Basically, some type of identification strategy is necessary to distinguish a causal relationship from an association. One strategy randomly assigns people or households to different categories and conducts a controlled behavioral experiment. For instance, on a random basis, various households might be allowed to visit the doctor only a certain number of times per year. Some households might not be allowed to visit the doctor at all, and others may be allowed office visits ranging from one to ten times per year, regardless of their income, initial endowment of health, or other personal characteristics. The random assignment of households corrects for any self-selection bias that results when households with lower baseline health select a category that allows for more doctor visits.

Periodically, the analyst studies the relation between the number of office visits and various measures of health status, while controlling for other nonmedical inputs in the health production function. The hypothesis is that health improves with more office visits, *ceteris paribus.* As you might expect, randomized social experiments of this kind offer valuable insights but are very expensive to conduct. In addition, the health of some households might be seriously compromised if they are not permitted to visit the doctor a reasonable number of times per year. Hence large-scale social experiments are rarely conducted.[9]

A natural experiment, the third method, arises when some type of external global policy, unrelated to the nonmedical determinants of health outcomes, produces a change in the

9. In Chapter 5 we discuss the RAND Health Insurance Study of the 1970s, which represented a randomized social experiment. Interestingly, the RAND study found evidence of flat-of-the-curve medicine for average adult patients, which agrees with the results of the observational studies previously discussed.

medical care of a treatment group. Changes in the health outcomes of the treatment group are then compared to health outcomes of some control group that did not experience that same external policy but otherwise faced fairly similar circumstances. For example, Levy and Meltzer point to several natural experiments that studied the effect of medical care program terminations (such as veteran or maternal health benefits) on health outcomes in a treatment group to that of an otherwise similar control group in which the terminations did not take place.

Hanratty (1996) examines the impact of Canada's national health insurance program on health outcomes. Her identification strategy involves the fact that Canadian provinces adopted national health insurance at different times between 1962 and 1972. She observed changes in the mortality and birth weights of infants across Canadian counties at different introduction dates for the national health insurance program while controlling for other nonmedical determinants of infant health. Her results suggest a significant reduction in the infant mortality rate and a smaller reduction in the low birth weight rate after the introduction of national health insurance in the various provinces of Canada.

As another example, Lichtenberg (2002) analyzes the effect of Medicare on the health of elderly individuals by looking for sudden discontinuities in medical care utilization and health outcomes at age 65, when people typically become eligible for the federal program. Notice that chronological age is an external factor that cannot be altered by the nonmedical determinants of health or influenced by health status. He finds evidence that the utilization of ambulatory and inpatient care increases sharply at age 65. Lichtenberg also finds evidence that people spend less time in bed and face a reduced probability of dying compared to what would have occurred in the absence of Medicare. His results suggest a relatively large marginal productivity of medical care on the health of elderly individuals.

Based on their review of the literature, Levy and Meltzer conclude that observational studies typically find an association but not necessarily a causal relation between health insurance (and therefore medical care) and health outcomes. Furthermore, they note that small-scale natural experiments have produced mixed results, but large-scale natural experiments find more consistent evidence that health insurance (through medical care) produces better health outcomes. Levy and Meltzer note that the size of the improvements in health depends on whom we are talking about, however. Medical care seems to produce more meaningful improvements in health among more vulnerable populations such as the poor, infants, and elderly.

In summary, health production studies illustrate that while the total impact of medical care on health may be significant, particularly for vulnerable populations such as infants and the elderly, the marginal impact may be relatively small. At the margin, socioeconomic conditions and lifestyle factors may play a greater role in determining health than does medical care, especially among insured adults. These results have some rather interesting policy implications. They suggest that any public policy aimed at improving health should be directed toward raising education levels, reducing the amount of poverty, or improving lifestyles rather than simply providing additional medical care. Naturally, the specifics of any policy should be based on sound cost-benefit analysis.

The Ten Major Causes of Death in the United States in 2002

As mentioned earlier, individual choices, socioeconomic status, and environmental factors play a significant role in the production of health. If so, one might suspect that national disease-specific mortality rates would reflect the importance of these variables. That is, mortality rates should be high for diseases that are more sensitive to adverse lifestyles, low

TABLE 2–1
The Ten Leading Causes of Death in the United States in 2002

	Cause	Number of Deaths
1.	Diseases of the heart	696,947
2.	Malignant neoplasms	557,271
3.	Cerebrovascular diseases (stroke)	162,672
4.	Chronic lower respiratory diseases	124,816
5.	Unintentional injuries	106,742
6.	Diabetes mellitus	73,249
7.	Influenza and pneumonia	65,681
8.	Alzheimer's disease	58,866
9.	Nephritis, nephritic syndrome, and nephrosis (kidney disease)	40,974
10.	Septicemia	33,865
	TOTAL	2,443,387

SOURCE: *Health, United States, 2004* (Hyattsville, Md.: National Center for Health Statistics, 2004), Table 31.

socioeconomic status, or unhealthy environments. With this in mind, Table 2–1 lists the top ten causes of death in the United States for 2002. Over the course of the year, more than 2.4 million individuals died in the United States. Of this number, approximately 79 percent succumbed to the ten most common causes of death listed in the table. By far the number one cause of death is diseases of the heart, accounting for almost 29 percent of all deaths in the United States in 2002. Although researchers are still unclear as to what determines an individual's risk for heart disease, they are certain that the blood level of cholesterol, smoking, level of physical activity, stress, and obesity play a major role in determining the risk of heart disease. Each of these factors is influenced by lifestyle choices, socioeconomic status, and environmental settings.

The second leading cause of death is malignant neoplasms, or cancers. Lifestyle choices often have an impact on this type of illness as well. For example, Edlin and Golanty (1988) point out that approximately 80 percent of all lung cancer deaths, the most common form of cancer, can be attributed to smoking. Socioeconomic status and environmental factors also come into play in determining the likelihood of contracting lung cancer through exposure to such items as asbestos and radon. The third leading cause of death is stroke and the medical community is in agreement that lifestyle, such as whether a person follows a proper diet and exercises, impacts the chances of having a stroke.

The fourth leading cause of death is chronic lower respiratory diseases, which includes chronic obstructive pulmonary disease, emphysema, and chronic bronchitis. Air pollution plays a critical role in the progression of these diseases. The next leading cause of death is unintentional injuries, which deals with deaths directly related to individual behavior such as automobile and industrial accidents rather than natural causes.

Finally, the list is interesting for what it does not include. In 1995 the human immunodeficiency virus (HIV) was the eighth leading cause of death and accounted for 32,655 deaths. By 2003 that number had dropped to 18,017. This dramatic decrease in the number of deaths can be attributed to a series of factors including improved therapies and changes in lifestyle brought about by great public awareness of the disease.

This rather simple exercise underscores the importance that lifestyle choices, socioeconomic status, and environmental factors play in determining deaths in the United States. It is worth noting that the information in Table 2–1 can also be used to illustrate the importance that an individual's mental and physical profile play in the making of health. For example, age is a critical factor in determining the onset of Alzheimer's disease, while the environment, genetics, and age contribute to development of diabetes.

SUMMARY

Health, like any other good or service, is desired because it generates utility. Also like other goods and services, health is subject to the law of diminishing marginal utility. This law stipulates that each additional unit of health provides less marginal utility than the previous unit.

The making, or production, of health is influenced by a variety of factors, including the amount of medical care consumed. The positive relation between health and medical care, however, is nonlinear due to the law of diminishing marginal productivity. This law underlies a fundamental production relation stating that health increases at a decreasing rate with additional amounts of medical care, holding other inputs constant. Some of the other factors determining health are the state of medical technology, the individual's initial health profile, socioeconomic status, lifestyle, and environmental factors.

The empirical evidence for adults indicates that good health depends only moderately on the consumption of medical care. Socioeconomic status and lifestyle appear to play a much greater role in the production of good health of adults.

CASE STUDIES

2-1 Health Utility[10]

Evidence supporting the notion that exercise is good for the brain as well as the body continues to surface. The science behind the evidence illustrates that exercise can boost a person's ability to process data, reduce depression and anxiety, and reduce illnesses that can affect a person's mental functioning, such as Alzheimer's. A 2005 study of 884,715 fifth-, seventh-, and ninth-graders published in the *Journal of Exercise Physiology* shows that students in the best physical shape have the best test scores. The results indicate a good relationship between fitness and academic achievement, but exercise cannot replace intellectual exertion; it can only strengthen it. Evidence also points to the long-term benefits of exercise and indicates that exercise can make the brain act younger. The results of a study at the University of Illinois show that when seniors exercise, it produces patterns of brain activity usually seen in 20-year-olds.

10. Source: Kevin Helliker, "Exploring the Bicycle-Brain Connection: How Exercise Boosts Cognitive Function," *The Wall Street Journal*, August 30, 2005.

Questions for Discussion

1. *Workplace health promotion is becoming an important issue as employers seek ways to reduce the high costs of health insurance. This study suggests that employers may also benefit from sharper on-the-job thinking by employees who exercise. In addition to a lunch break, should employers allow an extra hour each day for exercise?*
2. *Health can be thought of as a personal asset. We invest in health by consuming medical care and other health-related inputs, such as exercise. Discuss how the results of these studies are likely to impact the role of exercise in the "production" of health.*
3. *We know two things for sure in public health: smoking is bad and exercise is good. But we have had trouble stopping the bad behavior and encouraging the good. Smoking is addictive, which adds to the complexities of figuring out how to stop it. Why has it been so difficult to encourage people to exercise?*

2-2 Beauty and Health[11]

Beauty supplements that can be taken orally have long been marketed for various things, such as hair strengthening and skin lightening, but published evidence to confirm the success of these products has long been lacking. Nevertheless, beauty industry experts claim that people will continue to look for a quick fix to their cosmetic needs. Doctors have encouraged patients who insist on taking the supplements to discuss the products with their physician, going over the ingredients and determining compatibility with other medications they might be taking at the time. According to a market research company, ingestible beauty supplements have more than doubled in sales since 2000. The American Society of Plastic Surgeons warned in 2005 that the supplements were not as effective as traditional cosmetic surgery, and research about their safety is basically nonexistent. Additionally, the Food and Drug Administration still had not approved the supplements. One of the supplements, a tanning pill that contained a color additive called canthaxanthin, was found to be associated with eye disorders and could cause liver damage and skin itching. Doctors warned patients to be cautious of the supplements, saying that if these products worked as effectively as advertised, doctors would prescribe them themselves.

Questions for Discussion

1. *We derive utility from obtaining health in its many forms; we invest in health by going to the doctor, exercising, and so on. Is the consumption of over-the-counter health and beauty aids considered investing in health? Is it health care? Why or why not?*
2. *Are cosmetic procedures and beauty aids a waste of increasingly scarce health care dollars? Why or why not?*
3. *Should these kinds of expenditures be counted along with doctor and hospital services in national health care spending accounts? Why or why not?*

2-3 A Healthy Marriage[12]

A study released at a national marriage conference in 2005 shows that being divorced may be linked to unhealthy conditions later in life. The 2005 study of 8,652 people aged 51 to 61 shows that a person's "marital biography," meaning a person's experience with marriage, divorce, and

---

11. Source: Loretta Chao, "Beauty: Searching for a Quick Fix" *The Wall Street Journal*, October 11, 2005.

12. Source: Sue Shellenbarger, "Another Argument for Marriage: How Divorce Can Put Your Health at Risk," *The Wall Street Journal*, July 16, 2005.

remarriage, has a growing effect on health, indicating that the longer a person is divorced or widowed, the higher the likelihood of heart or lung disease, cancer, high blood pressure, diabetes, stroke, and difficulties with mobility. Those married at the time of the study and who had never been divorced or widowed had less chronic conditions than those who had been divorced, as the stresses of divorce tend to trigger conditions associated with chronic disease. Additionally, the study suggests that when considering remarriage, people must choose carefully, because those in low-quality remarriages are no healthier than those who remain divorced. The only exception to the study was obesity, which appeared more often with married than single people. Researchers have not been able to completely control the study results for the effect of marital selection, which is the likelihood that people who are healthier will be more likely to form lasting, happy marriages in the beginning. However, it seems clear that the healthier state of those who are married comes not only from selection, but from the protective, calming effect of marriage as well.

Questions for Discussion

1. *In addition to marriage, what are some other non–health care factors (for example, income) that are likely to affect one's health? For the factors that you identify, rank-order them according to what you believe are the most important and least important. For now, defend your rankings with logic rather than data.*
2. *Why does marriage have a positive effect on health? What are some of the likely mechanisms? In your answers, avoid the temptation to stereotype the structural characteristics of marriage—there are many different kinds out there.*
3. *The article mentions possible "selection bias," that people who are healthier and more robust may be more likely to form lasting relationships. Discuss the extent to which this selection bias might influence the results of this study.*

Review Questions and Problems

1. Describe the factors that make it difficult to measure output in medical care markets.
2. As mentioned at the beginning of the chapter, the life expectancy rate in Russia fell significantly from 1989 through 1994. Use health production theory to explain what would happen to the relationship between good health and medical care in Russia if alcohol consumption diminished and the market economy strengthened. Provide a graph to illustrate your explanation.
3. Use health production theory to explain the role gender plays in the production of health during pregnancy. Provide a graph to illustrate your answer.
4. Use production theory to graphically illustrate the case in which a medical innovation improves health without any change in the consumption of medical care.
5. In your own words, use utility analysis to explain why people demand health. How does the law of diminishing marginal utility fit into the analysis?
6. Explain how an increase in income would affect the level of health in a relatively affluent country like the United States compared to a relatively poor country like Haiti.
7. You have just been appointed to the post of surgeon general of the United States. The president wants you to develop an advertising campaign called "A Healthy America by the Year 2010" that encourages Americans to lead a healthier lifestyle. What types of behavior would you try to influence? Why?
8. You have just been hired by a major metropolitan city as a health policy analyst. Your assignment is to devise a plan that city authorities could implement to lower the infant

mortality rate. Based on the results cited in this chapter, what types of policies would you recommend? Substantiate your answer.

9. Explain how a change in each of the following factors would alter the shape of the total product curve for medical care.
   A. An increase in education.
   B. An improvement in lifestyle.
   C. An improvement in the environment.
10. Some people believe that cigarette and alcohol advertisements should be banned completely in the United States. If this were the case, what would likely happen to the shapes of the total and marginal product curves for medical care?

Online Resources

To access Internet links related to the topics in this chapter, please visit our web site at **www.thomsonedu.com/economics/santerre**.

References

Auster, Richard, Irving Leveson, and Deborah Sarachek. "The Production of Health: An Exploratory Study." *Journal of Human Resources* 9 (fall 1969), pp. 411–36.

Berkowitz, Eric N., Roger A. Kerin, and William Rudelius. *Marketing*, 2nd ed. Homewood, Ill.: Richard D. Irwin, 1989.

Bolin, Kristian, Lena Jacobson, and Bjorn Lindgren. "The Family as the Health Producer—When Spouses Act Strategically." *Journal of Health Economics* 21 (May 2002), pp. 475–95.

Brainerd, Elizabeth, and David M. Cutler. "Autopsy on an Empire: Understanding Mortality in Russia and the Former Soviet Union." *Journal of Economic Perspectives* 19 (winter 2005), pp. 107–130.

Case, Anne, Darren Lubotsky, and Christina Paxson. "Economic Status and Health in Childhood: The Origins of the Gradient." Working paper, Center for Health and Well-being, Princeton University, February 2002.

Case, Anne, and Christina Paxson. "Parental Behavior and Child Health." *Health Affairs* 21 (March/April 2002), pp. 164–78.

Chay, Kenneth Y., and Michael Greenstone. "The Impact of Air Pollution on Infant Mortality: Evidence from Geographic Variation in Pollution Shocks Induced by a Recession." *Quarterly Journal of Economics* 118 (August 2003), pp. 1121–67.

Corman, Hope, and Michael Grossman. "Determinants of Neonatal Mortality Rates in the U.S." *Journal of Health Economics* 4 (September 1985), pp. 213–36.

Currie, Janet, and Matthew Neidell. "Air Pollution and Infant Health: What Can We Learn from California's Recent Experience?" *Quarterly Journal of Economics*. 120 (August 2005), pp. 1003–30.

Cutler, David M., and Robert S. Huckman. "Technological Development and Medical Productivity: The Diffusion of Angioplasty in New York State." *Journal of Health Economics* 22 (2003), pp. 187–217.

Cutler, David M., and Mark McClellan. "Is Technological Change in Medicine Worth It?" *Health Affairs* 20 (September/October 2001), pp. 11–29.

Deaton, Angus. "Policy Implications of the Gradient of Health and Wealth." *Health Affairs* 21 (March/April 2002), pp. 13–30.

Donabedian, Avedis. *The Definition of Quality and Approaches to Its Assessment*. Ann Arbor, Mich.: Health Administration Press, 1980.

———. "The Quality of Care: How Can It Be Assessed?" *Journal of the American Medical Association* 260 (September 23–30, 1988), pp. 1743–48.

Edlin, Gordon, and Eric Golanty. *Health and Wellness: A Holistic Approach*. Boston: Jones and Bartlett, 1988.

Elo, Irma T., and Samuel H. Preston. "Educational Differentials Immortality: United States, 1979–1985." *Social Science and Medicine* 42 (1996), pp. 47–57.

Enthoven, Alain C. *Health Plan*. Reading, Mass.: Addison-Wesley, 1980.

Ettner, Susan L. "New Evidence on the Relationship between Income and Health." *Journal of Health Economics* 15 (1996), pp. 67–85.

Fuchs, Victor R. "Economics, Health and Post-Industrial Society." *Millbank Memorial Fund Quarterly* 57 (1979), pp. 153–82.

Fuchs, Victor R., and Sarah Rosen Frank. "Air Pollution and Medical Care Use by Older Americans: A Cross-Areas Analysis." *Health Affairs* 21 (November/December 2002), pp. 207–14.

Grossman, Michael. *The Demand for Health: A Theoretical and Empirical Investigation*. New York: National Bureau of Economic Research, 1972a.

______. "On the Concept of Health Capital and the Demand for Health." *Journal of Political Economy* 80 (March–April 1972b), pp. 223–55.

Guralnik, Jack M., et al. "Education Status and Active Life Expectancy among Older Blacks and Whites." *New England Journal of Medicine* 329 (July 8, 1993), pp. 100–16.

Hadley, Jack. *More Medical Care, Better Health*. Washington, D.C.: Urban Institute Press, 1982.

Hanratty, Maria. "Canadian Health Insurance and Infant Health." *American Economic Review* 86 (1996): 276–84.

Health, United States, 2004. Hyattsville, Md.: National Center for Health Statistics, 2004.

Jacobson, Lena. "The Family as Producer of Health—An Extended Grossman Model." *Journal of Health Economics* 19 (September 2000), pp. 611–37.

Kawachi, Ichiro, and Bruce P. Kennedy. "Income Inequality and Health: Pathways and Mechanisms." *Health Services Research* 34 (April 1999, Part II), pp. 215–27.

Kravdal, Oystein. "The Impact of Marital Status on Cancer." *Social Science and Medicine* 52 (2001), pp. 357–68.

Lantz, Paula M., et al. "Socioeconomic Disparities in Health Change in a Longitudinal Study of US Adults: The Role of Health-Risk Behaviors." *Social Science and Medicine* 53 (2001), pp. 29–40.

Leigh, Paul J., and James F. Fries. "Health Habits, Health Care Use and Costs in a Sample of Retirees." *Inquiry* 29 (spring 1992), pp. 44–54.

Levy, Helen, and David Meltzer. "What Do We Really Know about Whether Insurance Affects Health." Mimeo, University of Chicago, 2004.

Lichtenberg, Frank. "The Effects of Medicare on Utilization and Outcomes." *Frontiers in Health Policy Research* 5 (January 2002), pp. 27–52.

Lleras-Muney, Adriana. "The Relationship between Education and Adult Mortality in U.S." Working paper, Center for Health and Wellbeing, Princeton University, May 2001.

Lynch, John, et al. "Is Income a Determinant of Population Health? Part 1. A Systematic Review." *Milbank Quarterly* 82 (2004), pp. 5–99.

Manor, Orly, Zvi Eisenbach, Avi Israeli, and Yechiel Friedlander. "Mortality Differentials among Women: The Israel Longitudinal Mortality Study." *Social Science and Medicine* 51 (2000), pp. 1175–88.

Mosby Medical Encyclopedia, 2nd ed. New York: C. V. Mosby, 1992.

Ruhm, Christopher. "Are Recessions Good for Your Health?" *Quarterly Journal of Economics* 115 (May 2000), pp. 617–50.

Ruhm, Christopher J. "Good Times Make You Sick." *Journal of Health Economics* 22 (2003), pp. 637–58.

Sickles, Robin C., and Abdo Yazbeck. "On the Dynamics of Demand for Leisure and the Production of Health." *Journal of Business and Economic Statistics* 16 (April 1998), pp. 187–97.

Strum, Roland. "The Effect of Obesity, Smoking, and Drinking on Medical Problems and Costs." *Health Affairs* 21 (March/April 2002), pp. 245–53.

Wagstaff, Adam, and Eddy van Doorslaer. "Income Inequality and Health: What Does the Literature Tell Us?" *Annual Review of Public Health* 21 (2000), pp. 543–67.

COST AND BENEFIT ANALYSIS

CHAPTER 3

Every day decisions are made in the health care sector concerning the best, or most efficient, amount of medical care to provide. At some juncture in the decision-making process, the all-important question becomes: At what point do the added costs of providing more medical care outweigh the benefits in terms of improved health? In practice, the answer to this question is complex because costs and benefits depend on such factors as the availability of medical resources, patient preferences, and the severity of illnesses.

Consider an adult who complains to her physician about chest pains during an annual physical exam. The first thing the physician must do is determine the seriousness of the problem. The pain could simply be the result of stress or could be a sign of more serious trouble, such as an impending heart attack (remember Joe at the beginning of Chapter 1?). When confronted with a patient's chest pains, a physician faces several options. For example, one clinical professor of medicine says,

> *To assess chest pain, . . . we can take a history and a physical examination for \$100; do an exercise test for \$500; perform a nuclear stress test for \$1,500; or do coronary angiography for \$5,000. Each escalation in diagnostic approach improves the accuracy of diagnosis from 50 percent to 60 to 80 to 100 percent. (Rubenstein, 1994)*

Basically, the best medical procedure is chosen by comparing the incremental costs of progressively more expensive medical tests with the benefits of additional medical information provided by greater diagnostic capabilities.

This chapter examines how costs and benefits affect medical decisions from the point of view of a health policy maker who is attempting to make informed choices concerning the production or allocation of medical care services. The information provided will make you more knowledgeable about such important concepts as costs, benefits, and efficiency. Specifically, this chapter:

- introduces cost identification analysis
- reviews the theory underlying cost-benefit analysis
- illustrates how cost-benefit analysis can be used to make health care decisions
- explains the concept of discounting to take into account those costs and benefits resulting from health care decisions that occur over time
- discusses the monetary value of a life using the human capital and willingness-to-pay approaches
- introduces cost effectiveness analysis as an alternative to cost-benefit analysis
- introduces cost-utility analysis and the concept of a quality-adjusted life-year

COST IDENTIFICATION ANALYSIS

The first type of analysis we will consider is cost identification. Generally speaking, **cost identification studies** measure the total cost of a given medical condition or type of health behavior on the overall economy. The total cost imposed on society by a medical condition or a health behavior can be broken down into three major components:

1. Direct medical care costs
2. Direct nonmedical costs
3. Indirect costs

Direct medical care costs encompass all costs incurred by medical care providers, such as hospitals, physicians, and nursing homes. They include such costs as the cost of all necessary medical tests and examinations, the cost of administering medical care, and the cost of any follow-up treatments.

Direct nonmedical costs represent all monetary costs imposed on any nonmedical care personnel, including patients. For the patient, direct nonmedical costs include the cost of transportation to and from the medical care provider, in addition to any other costs borne directly by the patient. For example, the patient may require home care or have specific dietary restrictions. Others may also be influenced by the treatment. For example, the cost of instituting a substance abuse program in the workplace includes not only the direct medical costs of drug and alcohol rehabilitation but also any nonmedical costs the firm incurs while implementing and overseeing the program. Family members may be financially affected as well.

Indirect costs consist primarily of the time costs associated with implementation of the treatment. Indirect costs include the opportunity cost of the patient's (or anyone else's) time that the program affects, especially because many health behaviors and medical conditions result in lost productivity due to injury, disability, or loss of life. Consider the substance abuse program previously discussed. Costs should reflect the opportunity costs of the time needed to educate workers about the potential dangers of substance abuse. The time cost is borne by the employer and equals the value of forgone production.

By and large, cost identification studies consider the direct medical care and indirect costs associated with medical actions or adverse health behaviors. For example, Druss et al. (2001) estimated the total economic cost of five chronic medical conditions—mood disorders, diabetes, heart disease, asthma, and hypertension—in 1996. In their estimates, the authors considered medical costs as well as work loss. Out of the five conditions, hypertension was by far the most costly medical condition with a total cost of $121.8 billion annually, of which slightly more than 90 percent was accounted for in health care costs. The next largest was mood disorders, $66.4 billion, followed by diabetes, $57.6 billion, heart disease, $42.4 billion, and asthma, $31.2 billion. In another study, Meltzer et al. (1999) estimated that an influenza pandemic in the United States would result in 89,000 to 207,000 deaths, 314,000 to 734,000 hospitalizations, 18 to 42 million outpatient visits, and 20 to 47 million other illnesses. The economic impact of such an outbreak would be between $71.3 and $165.5 billion.

The American Diabetes Association (2003) estimated the direct and indirect costs of diabetes in 2002 at $132 billion, with almost $92 billion attributed to direct medical costs and the remaining $40 billion to indirect expenses such as lost work days and permanent disability. The American Heart Association set the cost of cardiovascular disease and stroke at $394 billion in 2005. Finally, Sander and Bergemann (2003) estimated the cost of obesity in Germany between 2.7 billion and 5.7 billion euros, with direct medical costs accounting for between 1.3 billion and 2.7 billion of the total.

Cost identification studies like these are enlightening because they provide a sense of the total costs associated with various medical conditions or health behaviors. However, they provide little guidance for decision making. For example, what is the best, or most efficient, method to treat Alzheimer's disease? To answer questions like this, we must turn to other types of decision-making techniques, such as cost-benefit and cost effectiveness analysis.

COST-BENEFIT ANALYSIS

In Chapter 1, we introduced the net benefit calculus or decision rule that economic actors use when making rational decisions. In a nutshell, it is in the economic agent's best interests to make a particular choice when the decision's expected benefits exceed its expected cost. Recall that the equation looks like the following:

$$NB^e(X) = B^e(X) - C^e(X), \tag{3–1}$$

where NB^e represents the expected net benefits, X equals the individual decision or choice under consideration, B^e stands for the expected benefits from that choice, and C^e equals the expected costs resulting from that choice.

Formal cost-benefit analysis utilizes the same net benefit calculus to establish the monetary value of all the costs and benefits associated with a given health policy decision. Such information is invaluable to policy makers who are under pressure to utilize scarce resources to generate the most good for society. To illustrate this point, let's suppose that an all-knowing benevolent dictator, called the "surgeon general," is responsible for ensuring the economic happiness of the people in some hypothetical society. The surgeon general realizes that people possess unlimited wants and that numerous goods and services, such as food, clothing, housing, medical care, and automobiles, provide them with satisfaction. The surgeon general also knows that scarcity of resources involves trade-offs; that is, more of one good means less of the others.

The surgeon general's task is to maximize the social utility of the population by choosing the best aggregate mix of goods and services to produce and consume.[1] To accomplish this objective, the surgeon general has the power to allocate land, labor, and capital resources to any and all uses. Consistent with the maximization of the social utility received from all goods and services, we can think of the surgeon general as trying to maximize the **total net social benefit (TNSB)** from each and every good and service produced in the economy. The total net social benefit derived from a good or service is the difference between its total social benefit (TSB) in consumption and its total social cost (TSC) of production. The difference represents the net benefit, or gain, that the society receives from producing and consuming a particular amount of some good or service. The total social benefit can be treated as the money value of the satisfaction generated from consuming the good or service. The total social cost can be looked at as the money value of all the resources used in producing the good or service.

For example, the total net social benefit from medical services can be written as

$$TNSB(Q) = TSB(Q) - TSC(Q). \tag{3–2}$$

Equation 3–2 allows for the fact that the levels of benefits, costs, and net social benefit depend on the quantity of medical services, Q. The surgeon general maximizes TNSB by choosing the quantity

1. In the context of the production possibilities curve, the surgeon general is trying to find the specific point that maximizes the collective well-being of the population. The surgeon general is assumed to accept the current distribution of income.

FIGURE 3–1
Determination of the Efficient Level of Output

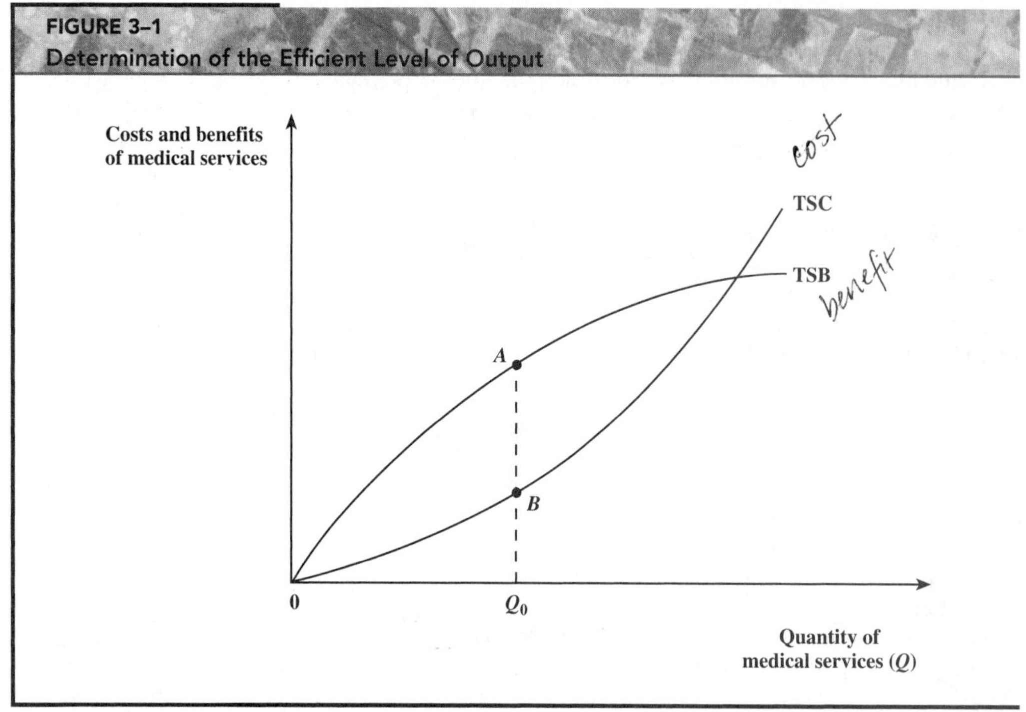

The TSB curve represents the monetary value of the total social benefit generated from consuming medical care. The curve is positively sloped to reflect the added monetary benefits that come about by consuming more medical care. The curve bows downward to capture the fact that society experiences diminishing marginal benefit with regard to medical care. The TSC curve represents the total social cost of producing medical care and is upward sloping because total costs increase as more medical care is produced. The curve bows toward the vertical axis because the marginal cost of producing medical care increases as more medical care is produced. Total net social benefit is maximized when the vertical distance between the two curves is greatest and that occurs at Q_0 level of medical services.

of medical services at which the difference between total social benefit and total social cost reaches its greatest level. Figure 3–1 presents a graphical representation of this maximization process.

Notice in the figure that total social benefits increase at a decreasing rate with respect to the quantity of medical services. This shape reflects an assumption that people in society experience diminishing marginal benefit with respect to medical services and indicates that successive incremental units generate continually lower additions to social satisfaction. Total social costs increase at an increasing rate and reflect the increasing marginal costs of producing medical services.

The slope of the TSB curve can be written as

(3–3) $$\text{MSB}(Q) = \Delta\text{TSB}/\Delta Q,$$

where MSB stands for the marginal social benefit from consuming a unit of medical services. Obviously, MSB decreases with quantity since the slope of the TSB curve declines due to diminishing marginal benefit. Similarly, the slope of the TSC curve is

(3–4) $$\text{MSC}(Q) = \Delta\text{TSC}/\Delta Q,$$

where MSC represents the marginal social cost of producing a unit of medical services. MSC increases with output as the slope of the TSC curve gets steeper due to increasing marginal cost.

Total net social benefit is maximized where the vertical distance between the two curves is the greatest at distance *AB*. A common principle in geometry is that the distance between two curves is maximized when their slopes are equal. That condition holds at output level Q_0 and implies that allocative efficiency, or the best quantity of medical services, results where

$$\text{MSB}(Q) = \text{MSC}(Q). \quad \text{(3–5)}$$

Thus, the surgeon general chooses output Q_0 because it maximizes TNSB.

To illustrate this point in a slightly different manner, Figure 3–2 graphs the MSB and MSC curves. Notice that the negatively sloped MSB and the positively sloped MSC reflect diminishing marginal benefit and increasing marginal costs, respectively. The efficient amount of medical services is at Q_0 in Figure 3–2 because MSB equals MSC. Let us consider why Q_0 is the efficient or best level of medical services by examining the figure more closely.

FIGURE 3–2
Under- and Overprovision of Medical Services

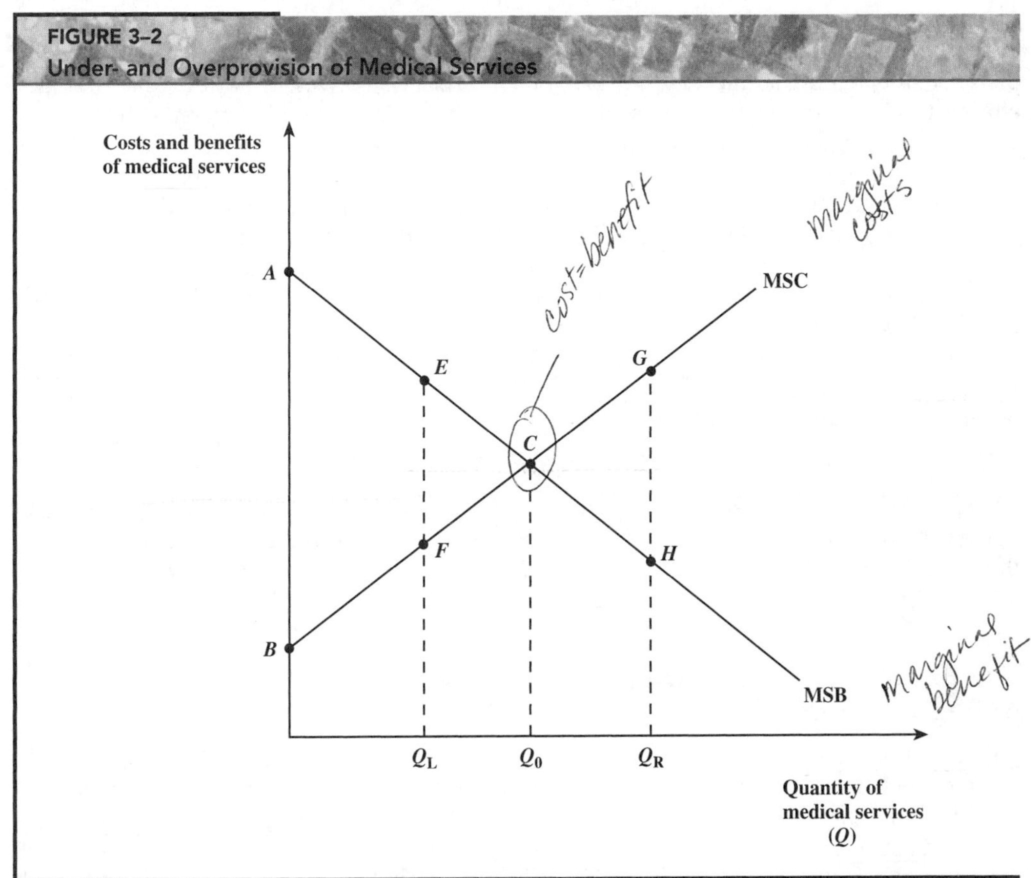

The MSB curve stands for the marginal social benefit generated from consuming medical care and is downward sloping because of the notion of diminishing marginal benefit. The MSC curve stands for the marginal social cost of producing medical care and is upward sloping because of increasing marginal costs. Total net social benefit is maximized at Q_0 level of medical care where the two curves intersect. At that point, the marginal social benefit of consuming medical care equals the marginal social cost of production. If Q_L amount of medical care is produced, then the MSB exceeds the MSC and society would be better off if more medical services were produced. If Q_R amount of medical care is produced, then the MSB is less than the MSC and too much medical care is produced.

In the figure, units of medical services to the left of Q_0, such as Q_L, imply that too few medical services are being produced because MSB (point *E*) is greater than MSC (point *F*). At Q_L, an additional unit of medical services generates positive additions to TNSB because the marginal net social benefit, the difference between MSB and MSC, is positive. Society is made better off if more medical services are produced. At Q_0, where MSB equals MSC, the marginal net social benefit is equal to zero and TNSB is maximized.

In contrast, output levels to the right of Q_0 suggest that too many medical services are being produced. For example, at Q_R, MSC (point *G*) exceeds MSB (point *H*) and marginal net social benefit is negative, subtracting from maximum total net social benefits. The cost of producing unit Q_R exceeds the benefits at the margin, and society could be made better off by not producing this unit. This same argument applies to all units of medical services to the right of Q_0.

TNSB is represented by the area below the MSB curve but above the MSC curve in Figure 3–2. This is because TNSB is equal to the sum of the marginal net social benefits, or the difference between MSB and MSC for every unit of medical services actually produced. Thus, in Figure 3–2, the area *ABC* represents the maximum TNSB that society receives if resources are allocated efficiently. (Conceptually, this area is equal to the vertical distance *AB* in Figure 3–1.)

If the surgeon general decides to produce Q_L instead of Q_0 units of medical services, society fails to receive the part of the TNSB indicated by area *ECF*. In economics, the lost amount of net social benefits is referred to as a **deadweight loss.** In this example, it measures the cost associated with an underallocation of resources to medical services. Similarly, if the surgeon general chooses to produce Q_R units of medical services, a deadweight loss of area *GCH* results. Area *GCH* indicates the net cost to society from producing too many units of medical services and therefore too few units of all other goods and services.

The preceding discussion can be easily couched in terms of the net benefit calculus in Equation 3–1. For example, if we solve Equation 3–5 for the difference between the marginal social benefit and the marginal social cost, we get

$$\text{NMSB}(Q) = \text{MSB}(Q) - \text{MSC}(Q), \quad (3\text{–}6)$$

where NMSB equals the **net marginal social benefit** the society derives from consuming a unit of the good. If NMSB is larger than zero, total net social benefit increases if an additional unit of the good is consumed. Naturally, if NMSB is negative, the society is made worse off if an additional unit of the good is produced and consumed.

The Practical Side of Using Cost-Benefit Analysis to Make Health Care Decisions

Public policy makers concerned with formulating health policies that affect the overall well-being of society, or total net social benefit, must wrestle with the problem of operationalizing Equation 3–6. That is no easy task, as it requires that they establish the monetary value of all the costs and benefits associated with a given health policy decision. The problem is complicated by the fact that some of the costs and benefits may be of an indirect nature and therefore difficult to quantify. For example, suppose you are responsible for estimating the net benefits associated with a rehabilitation program that requires one hour of exercise a day for people who recently had a heart bypass operation. One of the costs you will have to measure is the opportunity cost of the patients' time. Your first inclination may be to base your estimate on the average hourly wage of the people in the program. But what if the people conduct their daily exercise regime on their own time rather than while at work? You now face the problem of determining the opportunity cost of leisure time.[2] As you can see, indirect costs or benefits may be hard to quantify. The benefits, or diverted costs, of a medical intervention fall into four broad categories:

1. The medical costs diverted because an illness is prevented.
2. The monetary value of the loss in production diverted because death is postponed.
3. The monetary value of the potential loss in production saved because good health is restored.
4. The monetary value of the loss in satisfaction or utility averted due to a continuation of life or better health or both.

The first benefit is usually the easiest to calculate and involves estimating the medical costs that would have been incurred had the medical treatment not been implemented. The next two benefits involve projecting the value of an individual's income that would be lost due to illness or death.

The last benefit is the most subjective and therefore the most difficult to quantify, because it involves estimating the monetary value of the pleasure people receive from a longer life and good health. For example, how does one attach a dollar value to the decrease in pain and suffering an individual may experience after hip replacement surgery? Or what is the monetary value of the satisfaction a parent receives from watching a child grow up? Given the difficulty involved in measuring the pleasure of life, many studies simply calculate the other three types of benefits. The resulting figure is considered to reflect a lower-bound estimate of total benefits.[3]

Discounting

The costs and benefits of any medical decision are likely to accrue over time rather than at a single point in time. For example, the benefits of a polio vaccination are felt primarily in terms of allowing children who might otherwise have been afflicted with polio to lead normal, healthy, active lives. The benefits in this case accrue over many decades. Therefore, an adjustment must be made to account for the fact that a benefit (or a cost) received today has more value than one received at a future date. That is, the net benefit of an activity yielding a stream of future returns must be expressed in **present value** terms before proper comparisons can be made.

In simplest terms, present value means that an individual prefers \$100 today rather than a year from now. Even if the individual wants to spend the money a year from now, he or she is still made better off by accepting the money today. For example, \$100 deposited in a savings account offering a 4 percent annual return yields \$104 a year later. We say that the present value of \$104 to be received a year from now at a 4 percent rate of interest equals \$100. In more formal terms, we can state present value, PV, using the following equation:

(3–7)
$$PV = \frac{F}{(1 + r)}$$

where F equals a fixed sum of money and r represents the annual rate of interest, or the rate at which the sum is discounted. In our example, F equals \$104 and r is 4 percent, or .04, so PV equals

2. Although no hard-and-fast rule exists, the opportunity cost of leisure time is most often estimated at some fraction, usually one-half, of the average hourly wage.

3. In this simple example, we considered the costs and benefits associated with a new medical treatment where one never existed before. As a result, we considered the total costs and benefits experienced by society. In some instances, however, that approach is not appropriate. Consider a new medical treatment that potentially displaces, or complements, an existing one. In this situation, the appropriate practice is to focus on the incremental, or marginal, costs and benefits associated with the new treatment rather than the total costs and benefits. As such, only the added costs and benefits of the new treatment are considered.

\$100. Notice that a higher interest rate means the present value of a fixed sum falls. For example, if the rate of interest increases to 5 percent, the present value of \$104 decreases to \$99.05. Thus, the present value of a fixed sum is inversely related to the rate at which it is discounted.

When referring to sums of money received over a number of periods, the present value formula becomes slightly more complicated. If different sums of money, or net benefits, are to be received for a number of years, n, at the close of each period, the formula looks like the following:

$$\text{(3–8)} \qquad PV = \frac{F_1}{(1 + r)^1} + \frac{F_2}{(1 + r)^2} + \frac{F_3}{(1 + r)^3} + \cdots + \frac{F_T}{(1 + r)^T}$$

where F_t ($t = 1, 2, 3, \ldots, T$) equals the payment, or net benefit, received annually for T years. For simplicity's sake, we normally assume the discount rate is fixed over time. Each annual payment is expressed in today's dollars by dividing it by the discounting factor. The discounting factor equals 1 plus the rate of interest raised to the appropriate power, which is the number of years in the future when the payment is to be received. The sum total, or PV, represents the present value of all annual payments to be received in the future.

If Equation 3–8 is rewritten in summation form and specifically in terms of benefits and costs over time, it looks like the following:

$$\text{(3–9)} \qquad NB = \sum_{t=1}^{T} \frac{(B_t - C_t)}{(1 + r)^t}$$

where NB equals the present value of net benefits.

In every cost-benefit study in which the effects of a medical treatment or project occur over time, careful consideration must be given to choosing the discount rate. That is because the rate at which future payments are deflated can profoundly affect the present value of a project, especially when the costs or benefits do not accrue until far into the future. The earlier polio vaccination example is a case in point. A cost-benefit analysis of a polio vaccination project involves taking the present value of benefits potentially received 70 years into the future (the average American can expect to live about 75 years). Selecting an interest rate that is too high results in the choice of medical interventions that offer short-term net benefits. Conversely, choosing an interest rate that is too low leads to the choice of medical projects that provide long-term net benefits.

Theoretically, the chosen interest rate should equal the rate at which society collectively discounts future consumption, or society's time preference. In an industrial economy, however, there are many interest rates to choose from, including the prime business lending rate, the residential mortgage rate, and the U.S. government bond or T-bill rate. So naturally, the "correct" interest rate is open to interpretation. Most studies choose a discount rate of between 3 and 5 percent or look to private financial markets for guidance. In the latter instance, the interest rate on government bonds is the typical choice. The T-bill interest rate is chosen because it supposedly represents a risk-free rate of return and therefore reflects the rate at which the private sector discounts future streams of income in the absence of risk. Some studies circumvent this problem by presenting a range of estimates based on alternative rates of interest. It is then left to the ultimate decision maker to choose the appropriate rate of discount.

The Value of Life

To properly estimate the total benefits of a medical intervention, we must be able to measure the value of a human life, because many medical interventions extend or improve the quality of life. The most common method used to determine the monetary worth of a life is the human capital

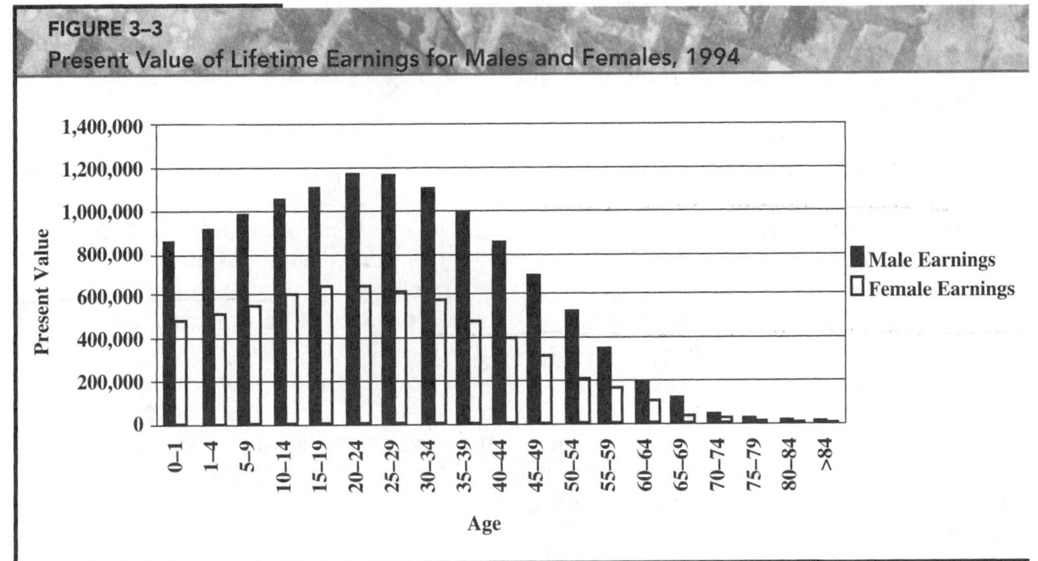

FIGURE 3–3
Present Value of Lifetime Earnings for Males and Females, 1994

SOURCE: Ted R. Miller et al. *The Consumer Product Safety Commission's Revised Injury Cost Model.* Calverton, Md.: U.S. Consumer Protection Safety Commission, 2000, Table 15.

approach.[4] The **human capital approach** essentially equates the value of a life to the market value of the output produced by an individual during his or her expected lifetime. The technique involves estimating the discounted value of future earnings resulting from an improvement in or an extension of life.

Figure 3–3 provides some average estimates of the present value of lifetime earnings (including fringe benefits) by age and gender, discounted using a 2.5 percent real discount rate. Notice that the discounted value of lifetime earnings initially increases with age and then decreases. The present value figures increase at first because as an individual ages beyond infancy, the value of lifetime earnings that accrue mainly in the middle adult years are discounted over a shorter period of time. For both males and females the discounted value of lifetime earnings peaks between the ages of 20 and 24 years, $1.16 million for males and $644,000 for females. Eventually, lifetime earnings decrease with age as productivity and the number of years devoted to work decrease.

Although the human capital approach is the most widely accepted method for determining the value of a life, the technique is not without shortcomings. One concern is that the approach is unable to control for labor market imperfections. For example, from Figure 3–3, it is apparent that the discounted value of lifetime earnings for males is substantially greater than that for females. Gender discrimination in the workplace may account for part of the difference. As a result, women may be penalized and assigned a lower value of life because of their gender. Also, racial and other forms of discrimination may result in an inappropriate estimate of the value of life when the human capital approach is used.

The human capital approach can also be criticized because it fails to consider any nonmarket returns the individual might receive from other activities, such as leisure. As such, it does not

4. Economists view expenditures on education and health as personal investments that enhance an individual's ability to command a higher salary in the marketplace; hence the term *human capital.*

take into account the value of any pain and suffering averted because of a medical treatment, nor does it consider the value an individual receives from the pleasure of life itself. For example, take an extreme view. According to the human capital approach, a chronically unemployed person has a zero or near-zero value of life.

An alternative approach used to measure the value of a life is the willingness-to-pay approach. The **willingness-to-pay approach** is based on how much money people are willing to pay for small reductions in the probability of dying. This kind of information is revealed when, for example, people install or fail to install smoke detectors in their homes, wear or do not wear automobile seat belts, or smoke or do not smoke cigarettes. For example, assume that people in society choose to spend \$100 per person per year on some device that improves environmental quality and reduces the probability of a person dying by 1 in 10,000. In this case, the imputed value of the average person's life equals \$1 million (\$100 ÷ 1/10,000).

To understand how the willingness-to-pay approach works, consider a person who is deciding whether to purchase a potentially life-saving medical service. The benefit of the life-saving medical service equals the reduced probability of dying, π, times the value of the person's life, V. Using a cost-benefit approach, the "marginal" person purchases the medical service if the benefit, $\pi \times V$, just compensates for the cost, C, or

(3–10) $$\pi \times V = C,$$

although "inframarginal" consumers might perceive greater benefits because they value their lives more highly. Dividing both sides by π results in

(3–11) $$V = C/\pi.$$

Equation 3–11 implies that a lower-bound estimate can be calculated for the value of a human life by dividing the cost of a life-saving good or service by the reduced probability of dying.

The advantage of the willingness-to-pay approach is that it measures the total value of life and not just the job market value. The imputed value of life generated by the willingness-to-pay approach includes the value of forgone earnings plus the nonmarket value received from life and good health. As a result, the willingness-to-pay approach generally estimates the value of a life to be higher than that generated by the human capital approach. For example, based on a survey conducted in 1999, Alberini et al. (2002) estimated the mean value of a statistical life to equal \$933,000 in Canada and \$1.5 million in the United States for a 5 in 1,000 reduction in risk. The mean estimates jumped to \$3.7 million in Canada and \$4.8 in the United States for a 1 in 1,000 reduction in risk. Viscusi (1993) found the willingness-to-pay estimates to range between \$3 and \$7 million in 1990 dollars, while Mrozek and Taylor (2002) reviewed more than 40 studies and found the statistical value of a life to be between \$1.5 and \$2.5 million in 1998 dollars. All indications are that the willingness-to-pay estimates are higher than the human capital estimates.

Keeler (2001) recently illustrated how the human capital approach can be reconciled with the willingness-to-pay approach by estimating the discounted value of life and considering the monetary value of all time, not just work time. As such, he estimated the value of life by assuming that all time is valued at the market wage rate and controlling for the total number of hours remaining for an individual at a given age, rather than simply the remaining number of work hours. Given that the average worker under 50 years of age is likely to spend only between one-tenth and one-fifth of future hours working, you can imagine how this increased the discounted value of a remaining life. For a 30-year-old male, Keeler estimated the value of all future hours to equal slightly more than \$2.6 million in 1990 dollars, which is more than five times the discounted value of future earnings, and in line with willingness-to-pay estimates. While his figures are crude, they illustrate that people place a significant monetary value on the amount of time spent outside work, and that researchers need to consider that when estimating the value of a life.

An Application of Cost-Benefit Analysis—Should College Students Be Vaccinated?

An increase in the number of reported cases of meningococcal disease in the United States has prompted a discussion as to whether college students should be vaccinated for the disease. Jackson et al. (1995) utilize cost-benefit analysis to determine if such a policy would be an appropriate use of scarce health care resources. That is done by comparing the benefits that would result from a decrease in the number of cases of meningococcal disease to the cost of implementing a vaccination program for all college students.

The cost of this medical intervention equals the cost of the vaccine multiplied by the number of doses needed plus the estimated cost of any side effects occurring because of the vaccine. The total cost of the vaccine was assumed to equal $30 per dose, which accounted for the actual cost of the vaccine plus the cost of administering the vaccine. The authors also assumed that 2.3 million freshmen would enter college every year and that 80 percent of those would receive the vaccine. Regarding side effects, the authors assumed that there would be one severe reaction to the vaccine per 100,000 students vaccinated, which would cost $1,830 per case. Based on these factors, the authors calculate that it would cost $56.2 million a year to administer a vaccination program among college students.

The benefits include the medical costs diverted plus the estimated value of the lives saved because of the vaccine. Treatment costs per case were assumed to equal $8,145, which included seven days of hospitalization and one physician visit per day, and costs for cases occurring in the second, third, and fourth years of college were discounted at a rate of 4 percent. Because there is no way of knowing the rate at which college students contract meningococcal disease, the authors used varying multiples of the baseline rate (the national average for that age group) to calculate the benefits. A total of 58 cases would be prevented at 2 times the baseline rate for a savings of $500,000 in direct medical costs. The cost savings equal $3.1 million at 15 times the baseline rate.

The human capital approach was used to determine the value of lost earnings, and it was assumed that each life saved was worth $1 million. The total benefit from lives saved was $8.8 million for 2 times the baseline rate and $60.7 million for 15 times the baseline rate.

Table 3–1 summarizes the findings for the scenarios where students contract meningococcal disease at 2 times and 15 times the national average. According to the estimates, the net

TABLE 3–1
Estimated Benefits and Costs for the Vaccination of College Students against Meningococcal Disease (in millions of dollars)

	Baseline times 2	Baseline times 15
Cost of the Vaccination Program	$ 56.2	$56.2
Total Benefits	9.3	63.8
Direct Medical Benefits	0.5	3.1
Indirect Benefits—Value of Lives Saved	8.8	60.7
Net Benefits—(Benefits – Cost)	−46.9	7.6

SOURCE: Lisa Jackson et al. "Should College Students Be Vaccinated against Meningococcal Disease? A Cost-Benefit Analysis." *American Journal of Public Health* 85 (June 1995), Table 1.

benefit for vaccinating college students is −\$46.9 million, assuming a baseline rate of 2 times the national average for that age group. In other words, the estimated costs of this program outweigh the benefits by more than \$46 million. Under the assumption that students contract the disease at 15 times the national average, the net benefits equal \$7.6 million. In fact, a student rate of 13 times the national average must be employed before the estimated benefits generated by a vaccination program equal the costs. Using a rate of 2.6 times the national average for that age group, which the authors feel is the maximum possible rate for students, Jackson et al. conclude that the costs of any vaccination program are likely to far outweigh the benefits. Thus, while one cannot ignore the fact that lives would be saved through a vaccination policy, the estimates indicate that such a policy may not be the most efficient way to spend scarce medical care dollars.

The Costs and Benefits of Medical Technology

Most analysts would agree that advances in medical technology have been the driving force behind rising medical costs in the United States over the last few decades. A cursory look at health statistics also appears to confirm that these new technologies have had a profound effect on the health and well-being of millions of people. For example, overall mortality and disability rates in the United States have fallen consistently since World War II. New surgical and diagnostic techniques, medical devices, pharmaceutical products, and the like are introduced each year and recent advances in such areas as biomedical research and information technology almost ensure that the pace of technological development will not abate anytime soon.

The impact of medical technology on health can best be illustrated by the total product curve for medical care discussed in the previous chapter. Recall that the total product curve as depicted in Figure 2–5 shows the relationship between health and amount of medical care consumed. Also recall that any new medical technology that improves health causes the total product curve for medical care to rotate upward. The curve rotates upward because each unit of medical care consumed now has a greater impact on overall health. For example, take the person who is suffering from emphysema and depression. Now assume that this individual begins taking a new antidepressant drug that is far more effective at combating depression and has fewer side effects than her previous medication. In this case the total product curve rotates upward, capturing the enhanced ability of the new drug to counteract depression and the fact that the medical care she is consuming as a result of her emphysema now becomes that much more effective.

Some have argued that new expensive technologies are developed and adopted with little regard to whether the benefits justify the costs. While that is clearly a debatable premise, Cutler and McClellan (2001) analyzed the costs and benefits associated with technological change in five specific health conditions: heart attack, low-birthweight infants, depression, cataracts, and breast cancer. In all cases they found that the benefits of technological change are not less than the costs.

For example, from 1984 through 1998 technological advances in treatment of heart attacks increased the life expectancy for the average heart attack victim by one year. Assuming each added year of life is worth \$100,000 and subtracting out the yearly cost of consumption at \$25,000, because most heart attack victims cease to work, the added benefit to society of an additional year of life is \$75,000, or \$70,000 in present value terms. Given that the costs of treating heart attacks increased by approximately \$10,000 from 1984 to 1998 in present value terms, the net benefit of enhanced technology in the treatment of heart attacks is roughly \$60,000 per patient. In other words, there is a 7 to 1 payoff in terms of benefits to costs. This finding supports a convincing argument that the increase in spending brought about by technology is more than justified in terms of health benefits.

As another example, Cutler and McClellan also found that in the case of low-birthweight infants, the net benefits equal $200,000 per infant with a payoff of approximately 6 to 1. To further bolster their claim concerning the value of medical technology, the authors state that "if one takes just the medical component of reduced mortality for low-birthweight infants and ischemic heart disease, medical care explains about one-quarter of overall mortality reduction" (p. 24).

While one should be careful not to overgeneralize from their results, it is fair to say that Cutler and McClellan developed a compelling case for the positive net benefits associated with new medical technologies. In most cases, the benefits of technological change in recent years appear to justify the costs. The authors concluded their article with a word of caution concerning cost containment policies. While everyone benefits when resources are used efficiently in the production of health, any policy change that halts or slows the rate of technological innovation should be examined with a skeptical eye. That is, serious attempts at cost containment may come at the expense of new medical technologies and thereby compromise the quality and longevity of future lives.

COST EFFECTIVENESS ANALYSIS

The difficulty of measuring benefits is one major drawback of cost-benefit analysis. The problem is even more pronounced in the health care field because the benefits associated with the adoption of a new technology or medical intervention are often in terms of intangible long-term benefits such as the dollar value of prolonging life or an enhancement in the quality of life. As we learned earlier, considerable debate surrounds the most appropriate way to determine the value of a human life. When the benefits that accrue from a particular policy are clearly defined and deemed desirable, cost effectiveness analysis (CEA) is often employed.

McGuigan and Moyer (1986, pp. 562–563) suggest that the primary difference between cost-benefit and cost effectiveness analysis lies in the basic question being asked: "Cost-benefit analysis asks the question: What is the dollar value of program costs and benefits, and do the benefits exceed the costs by a sufficient amount, given the timing of these outcomes to justify undertaking the program?" In contrast, the question asked in cost effectiveness analysis is, "Given that some prespecified object is be attained, what are the cost associated with the various alternatives means for reaching that objective?"

With CEA, the analyst estimates the costs associated with two or more medical treatment options or clinical strategies for a given health care objective, such as life-years saved, to determine the relative value of one medical treatment or technology over another.[5] In most cases, the comparison is done through the calculation of an **incremental cost effectiveness ratio** or **ICER.** For example, assume that a new medical treatment, *new,* is being compared to an existing treatment, *old,* and the cost and medical effectiveness of each treatment are C_{new}, C_{old} and E_{new}, E_{old}, respectively. In this case:

$$\text{ICER} = \frac{C_{new} - C_{old}}{E_{new} - E_{old}} \qquad (3\text{–}12)$$

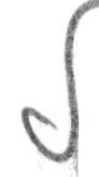

5. Other objectives, such as reducing cholesterol levels of blood pressure, may also be specified.

FIGURE 3–4
The Cost Effectiveness Plane

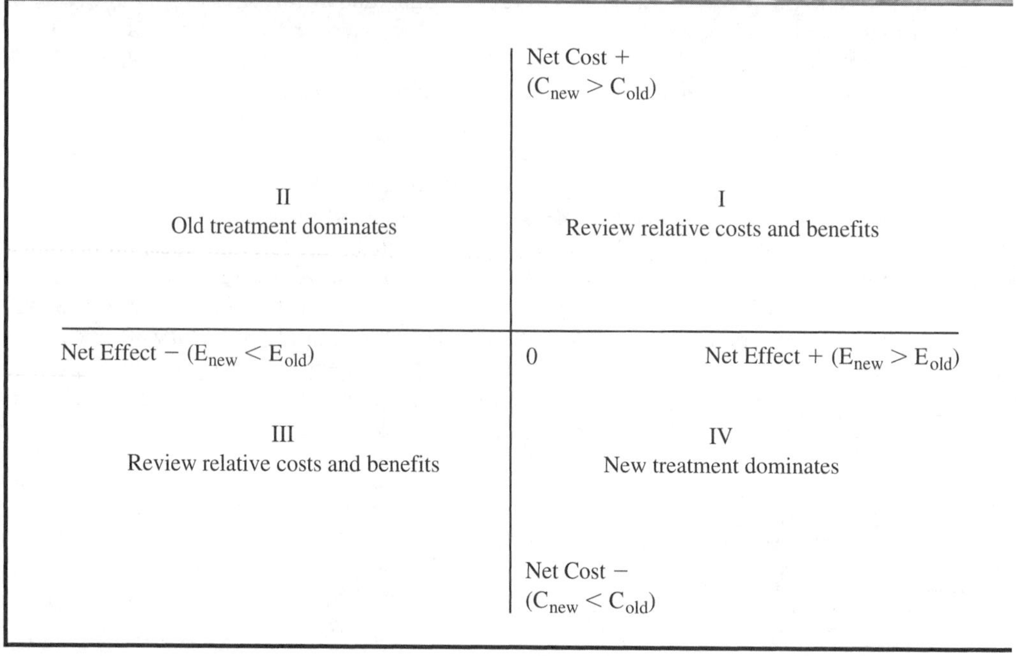

The cost-effectiveness plane shows how CEA can be used to determine whether a new medical technology or treatment should be adopted. The horizontal axis measures the net impact of a new medical treatment or technology on health outcomes. To the right of the origin, the new treatment enhances health or life expectancy, and to the left of the origin it diminishes health when compared to the current treatment. Net costs are measured on the vertical axis with positive net costs scored above the origin and negative net costs scored below the origin. Quadrant I depicts the situation in which a new medical option is more effective and more costly than the current procedure. In quadrant II the new option is less effective and more costly than the current one. In this case, the current medical option should be retained. Moving counterclockwise, quadrant III shows the case in which the new medical option is less costly and less effective than the current one. The relevant question is whether the reduction in cost is worth the loss in health associated with the new medical option. In quadrant IV the new medical option dominates the old one because it is more effective and less costly.

SOURCE: Adapted from Michael F. Drummond et al. *Methods for the Economic Evaluation of Health Care Programmes,* 2nd ed. Oxford: Oxford University Press, 1997; and MedPAC. *Issues in a Modernized Medicare Program.* Washington, D.C., June 2005.

If the new treatment is less costly than the old ($C_{new} < C_{old}$) and more effective ($E_{new} > E_{old}$), then the new treatment is said to dominate the old and should be adopted. This situation is depicted in quadrant IV of Figure 3–4, where the net effect ($E_{new} - E_{old}$) is measured on the horizontal axis and the net cost ($C_{new} - C_{old}$) is measured on the vertical axis. On the other hand, if the new treatment is both more costly and less effective than the old, then the old is dominant (quadrant II in Figure 3–4). In this situation, the new treatment should not be adopted.

The most interesting case is when the new treatment is more effective than the old and at the same time more costly. This situation is captured in quadrant I of Figure 3–4. Cost effectiveness analysis becomes an important tool of analysis under this circumstance because a decision has to be made regarding whether the new treatment is worth adopting. The basic question becomes, is the gain in improved health brought about by the new treatment worth the additional cost in dollars? For example, assume that the new treatment costs $5,000 per additional life-year saved. This seems like a rather small price to pay for a life-year and most would conclude that the new treatment should be adopted. But what happens if the cost is $150,000 per additional life-year saved? Is the cost of the new treatment worth the benefits in terms of life-years saved? Or, put in other terms, what is the threshold point at which a particular medical treatment or technology is simply too costly to adopt? Clearly, there is no straightforward answer. However, many agree that if the cost of a new medical treatment is less than $50,000 per additional year of life saved it is generally viewed favorably.

Finally, we have the case where the new technology is less costly and less effective than the old. This situation is depicted in quadrant III of Figure 3–4 and the relevant question becomes whether the decrease in health is worth the cost savings. Cost effectiveness analysis is needed to provide the relative cost savings per life-year. Given that the major emphasis in medical care is on improving or extending life, very little attention is paid in literature regarding this possibility.

If a new medical treatment or technology is being examined where none previously existed, then Equation 3–12 becomes

$$\text{ICER} = \frac{C_{\text{new}}}{E_{\text{new}}} \tag{3–12}$$

and Figure 3–4 is still relevant. The only difference is that the net change in terms of cost and effectiveness now becomes the total change and quadrants I and III still remain the focus of attention.

As an example, Lindfors and Rosenquist (1995) examined the cost-effectiveness of breast cancer screening using mammography. According to their estimates, the cost of breast cancer screening per year of life saved varies between $16,000 and $31,900, with the most cost-effective strategy being a biennial mammogram for women between ages 50 and 59. The most costly strategy ($31,900) is an annual screening for high-risk women between ages 40 and 49, a biennial screening for low-risk women in the same age bracket, and an annual screening for all women between ages 50 and 79. These results are similar to other findings in the literature and are part of an ongoing debate as to whether women in their forties should receive a regular mammogram. Over the years a number of studies like this one have been published in medical and economics journals. Tengs et al. (1995) reviewed the findings of five hundred cost effectiveness life-saving interventions and found the median intervention to cost $42,000 per life-year saved with the median medical intervention costing $19,000 per life-year saved.

Even cost effectiveness analysis is not without its critics. Some argue that life-years are not homogenous. Sometimes a medical intervention is associated with a significant number of life-years saved but a reduced quality of life. Conversely, a medical intervention may result in few life-years saved but an enhanced quality of life. For example, some analysts claim that coronary bypass operations do more to enhance the quality of life than they do to extend life.

As a result, another technique, called **cost-utility analysis,** has been used frequently in recent years. Cost-utility analysis considers the number of life-years saved from a particular medical intervention along with the quality of life. As result, it adjusts the number of life-years gained by some type of index that reflects health status, or quality of life. While a few different rating scales are in use, the most common is **quality-adjusted life-years (QALYs)**.[6]

6. For example, the World Health Organization uses DALYs, or disability-adjusted life-years, which measures potential life lost due to premature death and the years of productive life lost due to disability.

In mathematical terms, a QALY equals the product of life expectancy times a measure of the quality of remaining life-years. The latter is referred to a **health-utility index** and it is normally measured on a scale from 1 to 0, where 1 equals one year of full health and 0 represents death.[7] For example, consider an individual who will die within one year without a given medical procedure. Assume that this individual could expect to live an additional eight years with a quality of life equal to 0.75 if he were to receive a particular medical procedure. In this case, the medical procedure generates 6.0 QALYs, or 8 times 0.75. Notice that the number of QALYs depends on both the number of life-years generated by the medical procedure and the ensuing quality of life.

Three survey techniques are generally used by researchers to develop a health-utility index (Drummond et al., 1997). The first is a **rating scale** where individuals are asked to rate various health outcomes. The researcher then converts the responses to a scale from 0 to 1. The second is a **standard gamble** whereby an individual is given two hypothetical health alternatives. The first alternative is a health outcome that is less than perfect, such as being unable to walk or hear. The second alternative is that the individual undergoes a medical procedure that has a probability of success equal to π. If the procedure is successful, the individual will be in perfect health. However, if the procedure is unsuccessful with probability $(1 - \pi)$, the individual dies. The individual is then asked to choose the probability of success π that generates an indifferent response between the two alternatives; living with the disability or undergoing the procedure with π probability of success. In most cases, the probability provided in the standard gamble equals the value of the health-utility index for the health outcome under discussion.

The third method is referred as the **time trade-off.** In its simplest terms, an individual is given a hypothetical choice: she can live for x years in perfect health followed by death, or she can live y years with a particular chronic condition such as the inability to walk, where $y > x$. The number of healthy years x is then varied until the person is indifferent between the two outcomes. The health utility index in this simple example equals x/y. For example, suppose that an individual feels that fifteen years of perfect health is worth twenty years of life with the inability to walk. Using the time trade-off approach, this individual is giving the inability to walk a health utility index of 0.75 (Dranove, 2003).

Equation 3–13 can be used to calculate the cost-utility ratio from a new medical treatment or technology:

$$\text{(3–13)} \qquad \frac{\text{Cost}_{\text{new}} - \text{Cost}_{\text{old}}}{\text{No. of QALYs}_{\text{new}} - \text{No. of QALYs}_{\text{old}}}$$

Notice that Equation 3–13 is very similar to Equation 3–11. The only major difference is that the denominator now has the number of quality-adjusted life-years for each intervention rather than the number of life-years. Figure 3–4 is also relevant. The only change is that the net effectiveness of the new treatment on the horizontal axis is now measured in terms of quality-adjusted life-years. As before, cost-utility analysis becomes an important part of the decision-making process in quadrants I and III.

The cost-utility approach is not without its critics. Some question whether the survey techniques used to develop the health utility indexes accurately reflect any changes in the quality of life. Others are concerned that certain segments of society may be discriminated against because they have a shorter life expectancy (the elderly) or a lower quality of life (the disabled) (Dranove, 2003). Finally, like cost-effectiveness analysis, cost-utility analysis does not tell us whether the

7. It is conceivable that a score of less than one could be generated. For example, some may prefer death to living one year as a quadriplegic.

overall well-being of society is increased, as with cost-benefit analysis. It can only tell us whether one medical treatment or technology is more cost effective than another.

Cost-utility analysis has emerged as an accepted and common form of analysis in recent years. As an example, Neumann et al. (2000) examined the results of almost 230 studies that used cost-utility analysis to see if prescription drugs are a cost-effective means of improving overall health. According to their analysis, pharmaceutical studies generated a mean ratio of $11,000 per quality-adjusted life-year. As a category, immunization had the lowest mean ratio of $2,000 per QALY, while medical procedures had the highest ratio of $140,000 per QALY. Other categories included surgery at $10,000 per QALY and screening at $12,000 per QALY. In another study, Stone et al. (2000) reviewed the findings of fifty studies that used cost-utility analysis to examine the effectiveness of clinical preventive services. They found the median cost utility ratio to equal $14,000 per QALY.

By the Numbers: Cost-Effectiveness and Cost-Utility Analysis

Table 3–2 provides a simple example of cost effectiveness and cost-utility analysis. The current medical option costs $20,000 and generates 2 life-years and 1.4 QALYs (2 × 0.7), while the new medical option under consideration results in 8 life-years gained and 3.2 QALYS (8 × 0.4). The incremental cost-effectiveness ratio for the new medical procedure equals $15,000 per life-year gained, or ($110,000 − $20,000) divided by (8 years − 2 years). Given the relatively low ICER, it would appear that the new medical option should be adopted. When the quality of life is factored into the analysis, the cost-utility ratio equals $50,000 per quality-adjusted life-year gained, or ($110,000 − $20,000) divided by (3.2 QALYs − 1.4 QALYs). In this case, the cost per quality-adjusted life-year is much higher than the cost per life-year because the new procedure results in a decrease in the quality of life. For example, the new procedure may leave the patient with moderate pain or discomfort or decreased mobility. Now the decision to adopt the new treatment deserves further reflection because the cost per quality-adjusted life is considerably higher.

The opposite would occur if the quality of life is significantly enhanced by the new technology. Assume for argument's sake that the new medical procedure improves health and the health utility index equals 0.95. In this case, there are 7.6 QALYs (8 × 0.95) generated by the new medical option and the cost-utility ratio equals $11,842, which is marginally lower than the ICER.

Before we move on, two points are worth stressing. First, notice that the cost of any medical procedure or technology is the same regardless of whether it is judged on a cost effectiveness or cost-utility basis. Second, the quality of life associated with any medical option plays a critical role in determining its relative worth.

TABLE 3–2
An Example of Cost Effectiveness and Cost-Utility Analysis

Treatment option	Cost	Life-years gained	Health-utility index	QALY
Current procedure	$20,000	2 years	0.7	1.4
New procedure	$110,000	8 years	0.4	3.2

An Application of Cost Effectiveness Analysis: Autologous Blood Donations—Are They Cost Effective?

Since the rise in the number of cases of acquired immunodeficiency syndrome (AIDS), there has been a growing concern about the safety of the U.S. blood supply. Many are worried that they may receive tainted blood through a transfusion and contract an infectious disease, such as HIV or hepatitis C. This has led to an increase in the number of autologous blood donations.[8] Although more costly than traditional community blood donations, autologous donations are safer because the risk of receiving any contaminated blood is zero. Unfortunately, autologous blood donations are also more costly because they involve more administrative and collection expenses and have higher discarding costs than allogeneic donations. The question now becomes whether the increase in safety brought about by using autologous blood donations is worth the additional costs.

Using cost effectiveness analysis, Etchason et al. (1995) estimate the cost per quality-adjusted life-year saved through autologous blood donations for four different surgical procedures: total hip replacement, coronary-artery bypass grafting, abdominal hysterectomy, and transurethral prostatectomy. The added, or marginal, costs of using autologous blood donations are provided in the first row of Table 3–3. As you can see, the marginal cost of autologous blood donations varies from $68 to $4,783 per unit. The difference results mostly from the disposal cost of discarded units of blood. The second row of Table 3–3 provides the quality-adjusted life-years gained from using autologous donated blood for each of the four procedures. The authors arrived at these figures by first estimating the probabilities of acquiring a number of infections, such as hepatitis C and HIV, through transfusions of allogeneic blood and then estimating the number of disease outcomes that would result from those infections. These figures were used to determine changes in life expectancy for each of the four surgical procedures. Finally, the authors consulted the medical literature and adjusted their life expectancy figures to arrive at estimates for quality-adjusted life-years (QALY). For example, using autologous blood donations for a hip replacement would result in .00029 quality-adjusted life-years saved, or approximately 2.5 hours of perfect health.

8. An autologous blood donation is one in which the donor and the recipient of the blood are the same person. An allogeneic donation is one in which the donor and the recipient are different people.

TABLE 3–3
Estimated Cost Effectiveness of Autologous Blood Donations

	Total Hip Replacement	Coronary-Artery Bypass Grafting	Abdominal Hysterectomy	Transurethral Prostatectomy
Additional cost per unit of autologous blood transfused	$68	$107	$594	$4,783
QALY per unit transfused	0.00029	0.00022	0.00044	0.00020
Cost effectiveness (row one/row two)	$235,000	$494,000	$1,358,000	$23,643,000

SOURCE: Jeff Etchason et al. "The Cost Effectiveness of Preoperative Autologous Blood Donations." *New England Journal of Medicine* 332 (March 16, 1995), Table 4.

The cost effectiveness per unit of autologous blood for each procedure can be arrived at by dividing the marginal cost of using autologous blood by the QALY saved per unit. For example, according to Table 3–3, the cost effectiveness for using autologous blood for a hip replacement equals $235,000 per quality-adjusted life-year, or $68/.00029.

As you can see, the cost effectiveness per unit of autologous blood runs from $235,000 per quality-adjusted life-year saved for a total hip replacement to more than $23 million for a transurethral prostatectomy. Although there is no rule concerning what constitutes a cost-effective expenditure for a medical intervention, the estimates generated by Etchason et al. (1995) seem to be high and suggest that the use of autologous blood donations represents a costly way of saving a life.

SUMMARY

Because resources are limited, allocation decisions must be made based on cost-benefit analysis. If the benefits resulting from a health care decision exceed the costs, it is in the economic agent's best interests to pursue that decision. One problem that frequently arises when utilizing formal cost-benefit analysis is that of determining the monetary worth of a human life. The human capital approach is the most common method used to translate the value of a life into dollars. It involves estimating the discounted value of earnings gained through an extension of life. The willingness-to-pay approach is an alternative method that has been gaining wider acceptance in recent years. With the willingness-to-pay approach, the monetary value of a life is based on the amount people are willing to pay for small reductions in the probability of dying. The advantage of this approach is that it captures the total value of a life rather than simply the market value, as is the case with the human capital approach. Unfortunately, data limitations preclude the widespread use of the willingness-to-pay approach.

Cost effectiveness analysis is another method commonly used to determine the merits of health care policy options. Because the benefits of improved health are difficult to quantify, many analysts elect to use cost effectiveness analysis. The analysis involves estimating the cost of achieving a given health care objective, usually a life-year saved. Another more sophisticated method analysis called cost-utility analysis takes into consideration both the quality and quantity of life-years saved. The most common rating scale is quality-adjusted life-years (QALYs), which equals the product of life expectancy and an index of the quality of remaining life-years.

The various techniques discussed in this chapter represent a sampling of the tools health care economists have at their disposal for analyzing the economic aspects of resource allocation. These tools provide policy makers with the information they need to make informed decisions concerning the allocation of scarce health care resources across competing ends.

CASE STUDIES

3-1 Digital Mammograms[9]

A recent study in *The New England Journal of Medicine* considers the comparative ability of digital versus traditional film X-ray technology in detecting breast cancer. The study involved more than 40,000 women and finds digital mammograms more precise than traditional film X-rays in

9. Source: Kathryn Kranhold, "Digital Mammograms Excel in Study," *The Wall Street Journal*, September 17, 2005.

detecting breast cancer in women under age 50, women with denser breasts, and women who are near menopause. Both digital and film-based mammograms take pictures in the same way, but the digital technology records the images faster and uses less radiation. The new technology appears more sensitive to breast cancer in specific groups, but the study does not resolve whether it is cost-effective to use digital mammography. Additionally, the study does not determine whether digital mammograms can reduce the number of deaths from breast cancer. The digital mammogram machines cost nearly five times as much as traditional X-ray machines, and insurers may not pay more for the more expensive digital exams.

Questions for Discussion

1. *This technology appears to have advantages over the prevailing (nondigital) approaches. But as the article suggests, it is not clear whether the new technology is "cost effective." What does it mean for something to be considered "cost effective?" Does it mean that the benefits exceed the costs? What additional information might we need to determine whether this new technology is cost effective?*
2. *As we assess the value of digital mammograms, how important is it that digital mammograms have the long-term effect of reducing death rates from breast cancer? Why?*
3. *In the health care sector of the economy, one policy concern has been that new technologies do not typically substitute for older technologies as they normally do in other industries. An example is that MRI scans have not replaced CT scans, as providers have determined that each type of scan yields different (and in some cases complementary) kinds of information. Are digital mammograms likely to be substitutes for nondigital mammograms? Why or why not? What are the implications for cost effectiveness findings?*

3-2 Are Stents Overrated?[10]

A study released by the *New England Journal of Medicine* finds that stent-and-angioplasty procedures are not as helpful as bypass surgery for heart patients with two or three blocked arteries. The study involved nearly 60,000 patients with serious heart disease and calls into question the effectiveness of angioplasty, saying it carries a higher risk of death in the long run and that those who underwent angioplasty were more likely to need another procedure within three years as opposed to those who had bypass surgery. The companies that make the stents used in angioplasties say the research does not include newer drug-coated stents that may produce better outcomes. Experts anticipate that the study will result in more bypass surgeries and fewer angioplasties being conducted, which in turn will increase the cost of care since bypass surgery costs significantly more than angioplasty. This study is not the first to find an advantage to bypass surgery, which has been seen as more effective over the long run because it creates a new pathway in the heart, as opposed to simply opening up a diseased artery that may be prone to future blockages as is done in angioplasty.

Questions for Discussion

1. *How might these results be interpreted by the medical community? Will more patients undergo bypass? In answering this question, consider (a) how treatment decisions are typically made and (b) the desire to seek less invasive forms of treatment.*
2. *This article describes a classic cost effectiveness problem: one procedure is more expensive and appears to have better outcomes in the long run, whereas the alternative treatment is less*

10. Source: John Hechinger, "The Growing Case for Heart Surgery," *The Wall Street Journal*, May 26, 2005.

expensive but appears to have worse outcomes in the long run. Describe how you would determine which procedure is optimal from (a) the patient's perspective, (b) the hospital's perspective, and (c) society's perspective.

3. *Which "variables" might tip the scale in favor of one procedure versus the other? (For example, is the quality of life the same after each procedure? Do older patients respond better to one or the other?)*

Review Questions and Problems

1. We have learned that production efficiency is achieved when society is receiving the maximum amount of output from its limited resources. Explain how cost-benefit analysis can be used to achieve that outcome.
2. You have just been hired by your city's department of health. Your first task is to use cost-benefit analysis to evaluate a smoking awareness program that the department has been promoting for two years. Under the smoking awareness program, the department of health sends a team of health care professionals to various private firms free of charge to lecture to employees about the risks of smoking. The lecture takes one hour and is given during the workday. Describe the costs and benefits you should consider in your analysis.
3. In your own words, describe the difference between cost-benefit and cost effectiveness analysis.
4. According to a study by Boyle et al. (1983), it costs $2,900 per life-year gained and $3,200 per quality-adjusted life-year gained to use neonatal intensive care to increase the survival rates of low-birthweight infants weighing from 1,000 to 1,499 grams. For newborns weighing between 500 and 999 grams, the figures are $9,300 and $22,400, respectively. Based on these figures, for which group of low-birthweight infants does neonatal intensive care have the most cost effectiveness results? Why?
5. Think of a situation in which cost effectiveness analysis and cost-utility analysis would give you contrary results. Substantiate your answer.
6. As of March 1, 1994, children riding bicycles in New York must wear safety helmets. Assuming that the decision to enact this law was based on cost-benefit analysis, what types of costs and benefits do you think were included in the study?
7. The commissioner of health is concerned about the increasing number of reported cases of preventable childhood diseases, such as polio and rubella. It appears that a growing number of young children are not being vaccinated against childhood diseases as they should be. Two proposals to address the problem are sitting on the commissioner's desk. The programs have equal costs, but the commissioner has funding for only one. The first proposal involves providing free vaccinations at clinics around the country. The benefits from a free vaccination program are likely to be experienced immediately in terms of a drop in the number of reported cases of illness. The second program calls for educating young married couples about the benefits of vaccination. The benefits in this instance will not be felt for some years. The commissioner wants to use cost-benefit analysis to determine which proposal should be implemented. Explain to the commissioner the critical role the discount rate plays in determining which program is chosen. In particular, which program is more likely to be chosen if a relatively low discount rate is selected? Why?
8. Distinguish between the human capital and willingness-to-pay approaches for determining the value of a life. Why does the willingness-to-pay approach generally estimate the value of a life to be higher than the human capital approach does?
9. According to Chase (1993), TPA, a heart drug produced by Genentech, Inc., costs ten times more at $2,200 a dose than streptokinase, an alternative heart drug sold by Astra AB and

Kabi Farmacia AB of Sweden and by Hoechst AG of Germany. A trial of 41,000 heart attack patients found that the TPA treatment saves 1 more life out of 100 than streptokinase does. Assume that a person pays full cost for either drug and chooses TPA over streptokinase. Another otherwise identical person makes the opposite choice. Use the willingness-to-pay approach to calculate the difference in the value of their lives (assume that dosage requirements are the same).

10. Read the following passage from an article in *The Wall Street Journal* (October 3, 1995, p. B1) and answer the following questions.

    Diabetic Toby Warbet quit her secretarial job last year because of physical problems, including blurred vision and a general loss of sensation. Such was her desperation that when she heard about an unproven treatment that might help her, she decided to borrow $20,000 from relatives to pay for it. . . . "Even if the chances are one in a million, I was hoping I would be the one," says the Livingston, NJ resident.

    A. Use the human capital approach to provide a monetary estimate of the value of Toby Warbet's life as of October 3, 1995. Explain.
    B. Use the willingness-to-pay approach to estimate the value of Toby Warbet's life. Explain.
    C. Provide a reason for the discrepancy between the two approaches.
    D. How might you measure the value of Toby Warbet's life using the human capital approach and attain a figure close to the willingness-to-pay approach?

11. According to Russell (1992), $1 million spent on two medical interventions yields the following life-years for elderly persons:

Pneumococcal pneumonia vaccine	100 life-years
Influenza vaccine	11,000 life-years

    Given this information, what is the opportunity cost of $1 million spent on the pneumococcal pneumonia vaccine? What is the opportunity cost of $1 million worth of influenza vaccine? If $1 million were available to spend on medical care for elderly people, how would it be spent based on the data provided if the goal is to save the greatest number of life-years?

12. Given this information, answer the following questions.

	Cost	Effectiveness
Current treatment	$100,000	4 life-years gained
New treatment	$250,000	10 life-years gained

    A. Calculate the ICER for the new treatment, assuming that the new treatment would replace the old one.
    B. In what quadrant is the ICER located in Figure 3–4? Is cost effectiveness analysis relevant?
    C. How does your answer change if the cost of the new treatment equals $75,000?

13. Given the information for question 11, calculate the number of QALYs for the current and new treatment, assuming that the health-utility index is 0.5 for the current treatment and 0.8 for the new treatment. Also, calculate the cost-utility index for new treatment. Should the new treatment be adopted? Why?

Online Resources

To access Internet links related to the topics in this chapter, please visit our web site at **www.thomsonedu.com/economics/santerre**.

REFERENCES

Alberini, Anna, Maureen Cropper, Alan Krupnick, and Nathalia B. Simon. *Does the Value of a Statistical Life Vary with Age and Health Status? Evidence from the United States and Canada.* Washington, D.C.: Resources of the Future, April 2002.

American Diabetes Association. "Economic Costs of Diabetes in the U.S. in 2002." *Diabetes Cares* 26 (March 2003), pp. 917–32.

American Heart Association, http://www.americanheart.org.

Boyle, H. Michael, George W. Torrance, John C. Sinclair, and Sargent P. Horwoord. "Economic Evaluation of Neonatal Intensive Care of Very-Low-Birth-Weight Infants." *New England Journal of Medicine* 308 (June 2, 1983), pp. 1330–37.

Chase, Marilyn. "Genentech Drug Raises Question of a Life's Value." *The Wall Street Journal,* May 3, 1993, p. B1.

Cutler, David M., and Mark McClellan. "Is Technological Change in Medicine Worth It?" *Health Affairs* 20 (September/October 2001), pp. 11–29.

Dranove, David. *What's Your Life Worth?* Upper Saddle River, N.J.: Prentice Hall, 2003.

Drummond, Michael F., Bernie J. O'Brien, Greg L. Stoddart, and George W. Torrance. *Methods for the Economic Evaluation of Health Care Programmes,* 2nd ed. Oxford: Oxford University Press, 1997.

Druss, Benjamin, et al. "Comparing the National Economic Burden of Five Chronic Conditions." *Health Affairs* 20 (November/December 2001), pp. 233–41.

Etchason, Jeff, et al. "The Cost Effectiveness of Preoperative Autologous Blood Donations." *New England Journal of Medicine* 332 (March 16, 1995), pp. 719–24.

Jackson, Lisa A., et al. "Should College Students Be Vaccinated against Meningococcal Disease? A Cost-Benefit Analysis." *American Journal of Public Health* 85 (June 1995), pp. 843–46.

Keeler, Emmett B. "The Value of Remaining Lifetime Is Close to Estimated Values of Life." *Journal of Health Economics* (January 2001), pp. 141–43.

Lindfors, Karen K., and John Rosenquist. "The Cost-Effectiveness of Mammographic Screening Strategies." *Journal of the American Medical Association* 24 (September 20, 1995), pp. 881–84.

McGuigan, James R., and R. Charles Moyer. *Managerial Economics,* 4th ed. St. Paul, Minn.: West, 1986.

Medicare Payment Advisory Commission (MedPAC). *Issues in a Modernized Medicare Program.* Washington D.C., June 2005.

Meltzer, Martin J., Nancy J. Cox, and Keiji Fukuda. "The Economic Impact of Pandemic Influenza in the United States: Priorities for Intervention." *Emerging Infectious Diseases* 5 (September/October 1999), pp. 659–71.

Miller, Ted R., et al. *The Consumer Product Safety Commission's Revised Injury Cost Model.* Calverton, Md.: U.S. Consumer Protection Safety Commission, 2000.

Mishan, E. J. *Cost-Benefit Analysis: An Informal Introduction,* 3rd ed. London: Allen and Unwin, 1982.

Mrozek, Janusz R., and Laura O. Taylor. "What Determines the Value of Life? A Meta-Analysis." *Journal of Policy Analysis and Management* 21 (2002), pp. 253–70.

Neumann, Peter J., Eileen A. Sandberg, Chaim M. Bell, Patricia W. Stone, and Richard H. Chapman. "Are Pharmaceuticals Cost-Effective: A Review of the Evidence." *Health Affairs* 19 (March/April 2000), pp. 92–109.

Rubenstein, Joel L. "The High Cost of Marginal Benefits." *Boston Globe,* May 12, 1994, p. 70.

Russell, Louise B. "Opportunity Costs in Modern Medicine." *Health Affairs* 11 (summer 1992), pp. 162–69.

Sander, Beate, and Rito Bergemann. "Economic Burden of Obesity and Its Complications in Germany." *European Journal of Health Economics* 4 (2003), pp. 248–53.

Stone, Patricia W., Steven Teutsch, Richard H. Chapman, Chaim Bell, Sue J. Goldie, and Peter J. Neumann. "Cost-Utility Analysis of Clinical Preventive Services." *American Journal of Preventive Medicine* 19 (2000), pp. 15–23.

Tengs, Tammy O., Miriam E. Adams, Joseph S. Pliskin, Dana Gelb Safran, Joanna E. Siegel, Milton C. Weinstein, and John D. Graham. "Five-Hundred Life-Saving Interventions and Their Cost-Effectiveness." *Risk Analysis* 15 (1995), pp. 369–90.

Viscusi, W. Kip. "The Value of Risks to Life and Health." *Journal of Economic Literature* 31 (December 1993), pp. 1912–46.

HEALTH CARE SYSTEMS AND INSTITUTIONS

CHAPTER 4

PPOs, HMOs, and DRGs are just a few of the many health care acronyms bandied around in the popular press. To the uninformed, they are simply the ingredients in an alphabet soup. Those familiar with them know that they stand for preferred provider organizations, health maintenance organizations, and diagnosis-related groups. They, like many other health care institutions, have evolved over the last several decades and have greatly contributed to the ongoing and wide-sweeping transformation of the U.S. health care system.

This chapter introduces and explains the structure and purpose behind various institutions and payment systems that typically compose a health care system. The knowledge you gain will help you better understand how the different parts of a health care system are interrelated. In addition, the material will provide you with a greater appreciation for the remaining chapters of the book and help make you a more informed consumer or producer of health care services. Specifically, this chapter:

- constructs a general model of a health care system
- discusses the reasoning for and responsibilities of third-party payers
- introduces and explains some of the different reimbursement methods used by third-party payers
- identifies some structural features associated with the production of medical services and the role of health care provider choice
- uses the general model to describe the health care systems in Canada, Germany, and the United Kingdom
- provides an overview of the U.S. health care system

ELEMENTS OF A HEALTH CARE SYSTEM

A **health care system** consists of the organizational arrangements and processes through which a society makes choices concerning the production, consumption, and distribution of health care services. How a health care system is structured is important because it determines who actually makes the choices concerning the basic questions, such as what medical goods to produce and who should receive the medical care. At one extreme, the health care system might be structured such that choices are decided by a centralized government, or authority, through a single individual or an appointed or elected committee. At the other extreme, the health care system might be decentralized. For example, individual consumers and health care providers, through their interaction in the marketplace, may decide the answers to the basic questions.

From a societal point of view, it is difficult to determine whether a centralized or decentralized health care system is superior. A normative statement of that kind entails value judgments, and trade-offs are inevitably involved. On the one hand, a centralized authority with complete and coordinated control over the entire health care system may be more capable of distributing output more uniformly and have a greater ability to exploit any economies associated with large size. At the same time, a single centralized authority may lack the competitive incentive to innovate or respond to varied consumer-voter demands. A central authority may also face high costs of collecting information about consumer needs.

On the other hand, a health care system with a decentralized decision-making process, such as the marketplace (or a system of local governments), may provide more alternatives and innovation but may result in high costs in the presence of economies of size, nonuniformity, or lack of coordination. Determining the best structure for a health care system involves quantifying the value society places on a number of alternative and sometimes competing outcomes, such as choice, innovation, uniformity, and production efficiency, among other things. A study of that kind is difficult at best because it involves so many normative decisions. Indeed, alternative health care systems exist throughout the world because people place different values on each of the various outcomes (Reinhardt, 1996). Reflecting the trade-offs involved, most health care systems today are neither purely centralized nor decentralized but rather take on elements of both systems of decision making. In any case, as we discuss the elements of various health care systems, it is important to keep in mind that understanding how and at what level decisions are made is critical to grasping how any health care system works.

Health care systems are huge, complex, and constantly changing as they respond to economic, technological, social, and historical forces. For example, the structure of the U.S. health care system involves a seemingly endless list of participants, some of which were foreign to us only a decade ago, such as preferred provider organizations. The list includes more than 800,000 physicians and dentists, about two million nurses, nearly 7,000 hospitals, and more than 80,000 nursing homes and mental retardation facilities, not to mention the millions of people who purchase medical care, the thousands of health insurers, and the multitude of government agencies involved in health care issues.

Because of the vastness and complexity of health care systems, many people have trouble understanding how they function. With that problem in mind, Figure 4–1 presents a general model of a health care system. Notice that the diagram possesses a triangular shape reflecting the three major players in any health care system: patients or consumers, health care providers or producers, and insurers or third-party payers. Sponsors, such as employers or the government, are also included in the general model because they act as intermediaries or brokers. As brokers, sponsors

FIGURE 4–1
A Model of a Health Care System

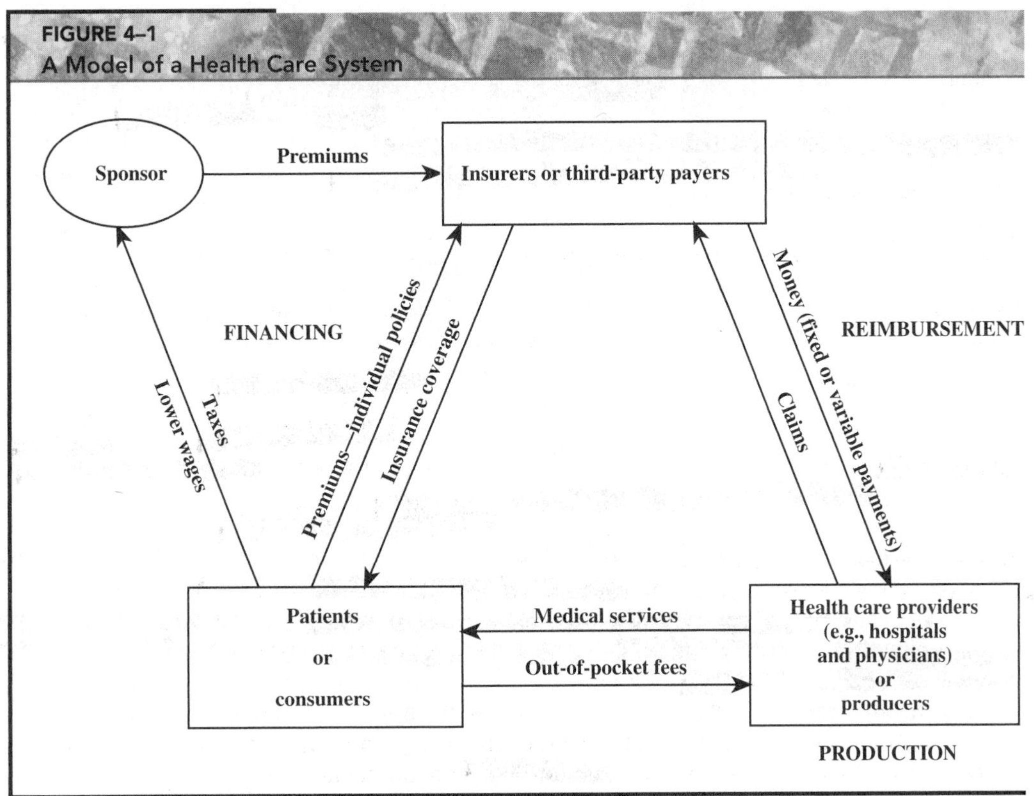

structure coverage, manage enrollment, contract and negotiate risk-sharing arrangements, and collect and submit the contributions of insured (Van de Ven and Ellis, 2000). Contributions show up as forgone wage income resulting from either taxes or premium payments. The figure also illustrates the three elements common to all health care systems: financing, reimbursement, and production or delivery.

For a typical market transaction, the individual consumer and producer are the only ones involved in the exchange as shown in the bottom flow of the diagram. In that instance, the consumer's out-of-pocket price equals the full cost of the service provided. Buyer and seller are equally well informed, and the buyer pays the seller directly for the good or service. For example, the purchase of a loaf of bread at a local convenience store involves a normal market transaction. Both consumer and seller have the same information regarding the price and quality of the bread, and the transaction is anticipated and planned by the consumer. An unexpected outcome is not likely to occur, and, if it did, it could be easily rectified (for example, stale bread can be easily returned).

In a medical market, the corresponding situation is a prespecified patient fee paid directly to a doctor or a hospital for some predetermined and expected quantity and quality of medical services. In the case of medical services, however, the transaction is often not anticipated, and the price, quantity, and quality of medical services are unknown until after the medical event occurs. The transaction is unanticipated because medical illnesses occur irregularly and unexpectedly

(Arrow, 1963). The price, quality, and quantity of medical services are not known initially because much uncertainty surrounds the diagnosis and proper treatment of a medical problem. In addition, health care providers possess a greater amount of information relative to patients regarding the provision of medical services, giving rise to an asymmetry of information. Because no simple relation exists between diagnosis and treatment, and much is left to the discretion of health care providers, possibilities for opportunistic behavior arise. That is, health care providers may produce more treatments or a higher-quality treatment than economic considerations warrant.[1]

The Role and Financing Methods of Third-Party Payers

Because the timing and amount of medical treatment costs are uncertain from an individual consumer's perspective, third-party payers, such as private health insurance companies or the government, play a major role in medical care markets. Third-party payers often serve as intermediaries between the consumer and the health care producer and monitor the behavior of health care providers as a means of controlling medical costs.

Also, third-party payers are responsible for managing the financial risk associated with the purchase of medical services. A third-party payer faces a much lower level of risk than does an individual consumer because it can pool its risk among various subscribers by operating on a large scale. The law of large numbers implies that whereas single events may be random and largely unpredictable, the average outcome of many similar events across a large population can be predicted fairly accurately. For example, it is difficult for one individual to predict whether he or she will experience a heart attack. An insurance company, on the other hand, can be reasonably sure about the heart attack rate by judging from past experiences involving a large number of individuals. Third-party payers can use indicators such as occupational and demographic averages to forecast expected medical claims for a large group of individuals. A risk-averse consumer is made better off by making a certain preset payment to an insurer for coverage against an unforeseen medical event rather than facing the possibility of paying some unknown medical costs. Essentially, consumers receive a net benefit from the financial security that third-party payers supply.[2]

Third parties make the health care system much more complex because the source of third-party financing and the method of reimbursement must be worked into the model. If the third-party payer is a private health insurance company, the consumer pays a premium in exchange for some amount of medical insurance coverage. As part of the health insurance plan, the consumer may be responsible for paying a deductible portion as well as a copayment or coinsurance. The deductible provision requires the consumer to pay the first $\$X$ of medical costs, after which the health insurance company is responsible for reimbursement. With a coinsurance provision, the consumer pays a fixed percentage of the cost each time he or she receives a medical service. A copayment refers to a fixed amount per service.

When a government agency (or a public health insurance company) acts as a third-party payer, the financing of medical care insurance usually comes from taxes. Premiums and taxes differ in the way risk is treated and the voluntary nature of the payment.[3] Premiums are paid

1. This so-called **supplier-induced demand theory** is explained in great detail in Chapter 12.
2. Health insurance principles are developed more fully in Chapters 5 and 6.
3. See Bodenheimer and Grumbach (1992) for an in-depth comparison of taxes and premiums for financing universal health insurance.

voluntarily and often depend on the risk category of the buyer of health insurance. Tax payments are mandatory and represent a single fee without reference to risk category.

Some alternative ways to finance health care can be gleaned by examining the different methods used in Canada, Germany, and the United Kingdom.[4] We chose these particular countries because their health care systems possess unique features. In addition, most proposals for health care reform in the United States are based to some extent on the health care systems of these three countries.

Canada has a compulsory **national health insurance (NHI)** program administered (somewhat differently) by each of its 10 provinces. The NHI program provides first-dollar coverage, and no limit is imposed on the level of medical benefits an individual can receive during his or her lifetime. **First-dollar coverage** means complete health insurance coverage in that the health insurer reimburses for the first and every dollar spent on medical services (that is, there is no deductible or copayment amount). For all practical purposes, taxes finance the NHI program in each province.[5] In addition, the Canadian government provides up to 40 percent in direct cost sharing and makes hospital construction grants available to provinces. Private insurance is available for some forms of health care in Canada, although private coverage is prohibited for services covered by the NHI plan. Because the public sector rather than the private sector insures against medical costs, there are no marketing expenses, no administrative costs of estimating risk status or determining whom to cover, and no allocation for profits.

The **socialized health insurance (SI)** program in Germany is based on government-mandated financing by employers and employees. The premiums of unemployed individuals and their dependents are paid by former employers or come from various public sources (the Federal Labor Administration and public pension funds). Private not-for-profit insurance companies, called **Sickness Funds**, are responsible for collecting funds from employers and employees and reimbursing physicians and hospitals. The statutory medical benefits are comprehensive, with a small copayment share for some services. Affluent and self-employed individuals are allowed to go outside the system and purchase private health insurance coverage.

Mechanic (1995) and others refer to the health care system in the United Kingdom (U.K.) as a **public contracting** model because the government contracts with various providers of health care services on behalf of the people. The U.K. health care system, under the auspices of the National Health Service (NHS), offers universal health insurance coverage financed through taxation. The NHS provides global budgets to district health authorities (DHAs). Each DHA is responsible for assessing and prioritizing the health care needs of about 300,000 people and then purchasing the necessary health care services from public and private health care providers. Hospital services are provided by nongovernmental trusts, which compete among themselves and with private hospitals for DHA contracts. Community-based primary care givers also contract with the DHAs. In addition, general practitioner (GP) fundholders apply for budgets from the DHAs, and, with the budgets, service a minimum group of 5,000 patients by providing primary care and purchasing elective surgery, outpatient therapy, and specialty nursing services. There is some limited competition among GP fundholders for patients.

4. See Raffel (1997) for discussion on the health care systems in various industrialized countries. For manageability, we confine the discussion to the insurance, physician, and hospital services industries. No mention is made of the existing systems in the pharmaceutical and long-term care markets, for example.

5. Three provinces charge insurance premiums that are related to family size rather than risk. These premiums are not compulsory for coverage and will be paid by the province if individuals are unable to pay. Because these premiums are not adjusted for risk, they are essentially taxes.

Risk Management, Reimbursement, and Consumer Cost Sharing

Another important element of a health care system concerns the manner in which health care providers are reimbursed and the share of medical costs paid by consumers. Reimbursement is important because some payment methods shift much more financial risk onto health care providers than others. As Figure 4–1 indicates, insurers may reimburse health care providers with either a fixed or variable payment, although in practice the payment methods are sometimes combined. A fixed payment is set independent of the amount of medical services actually provided to patients for a given and defined treatment episode. If the actual costs of delivering services to patients are less than the level of the fixed payment, health care providers are normally allowed to keep the surplus. However, health care providers also face the possibility that actual costs are greater than the fixed payment. Thus, some financial risk is shifted to health care providers when reimbursement takes place on a fixed-payment basis. A prospectively set fixed annual budget to a hospital or nursing home or a fixed annual salary for an employee are examples of fixed-payment systems. Regardless of how many resources a hospital or nursing home employs, or the number of hours an employee works during a given period, the payment remains the same.

Under a variable-payment system, the reimbursement amount varies with the quantity of services actually delivered to patients. Retrospective reimbursement, in which the health care provider bills for actual costs incurred, and fee-for-service, in which a price is paid for each unit of a medical service, are two common examples of a variable-payment system. A few state governments still reimburse nursing homes on a retrospective basis for caring for Medicaid patients. The price paid for each physician office visit is an example of a fee-for-service payment. When reimbursement takes on a variable-payment basis, health care providers face much less risk from cost overruns.

Similarly, the share of medical costs paid by consumers is important because a greater amount of cost sharing puts more financial risk on them. For example, take the extreme cases. The typical consumer faces very little financial incentive, if any, to care about the costs associated with his or her medical treatment if fully insured with no out-of-pocket expenses. Even if the medical costs equal $100, $1,000, or $10,000, the consumer pays a zero out-of-pocket price if fully insured. Conversely, that same consumer faces much more financial incentive to be concerned with the cost if required to pay the entire bill (that is, 100 percent out-of-pocket price) associated with the medical treatment. No one disagrees that the opportunity cost of paying $200 for an office visit is much greater than paying $100.

The matrix in Figure 4–2 helps illustrate the importance of risk sharing. The matrix shows how the two reimbursement schemes just discussed and the consumer's out-of-pocket price interact and affect the likelihood that a large volume of medical services will be supplied and demanded. The probability of a high volume of medical services is given inside each cell of the matrix for each combination of reimbursement method and consumer out-of-pocket price.

We can identify the opportunity for a large volume of medical services per patient by considering how the different provider reimbursement schemes and consumer payment plans affect the incentives of health care providers and consumers. For example, a health care provider that is reimbursed on a fixed-payment basis is very unlikely to supply a large volume of medical services to a patient unnecessarily. The cost of additional medical services immediately subtracts from the fixed payment and puts the health care provider at risk for cost overruns. In contrast, for the variable-payment schemes, health care providers do not absorb the financial risk of the higher costs associated with additional services.

FIGURE 4–2
The Likelihood of a Large Volume of Medical Services for Different Reimbursement and Consumer Copayment Schemes

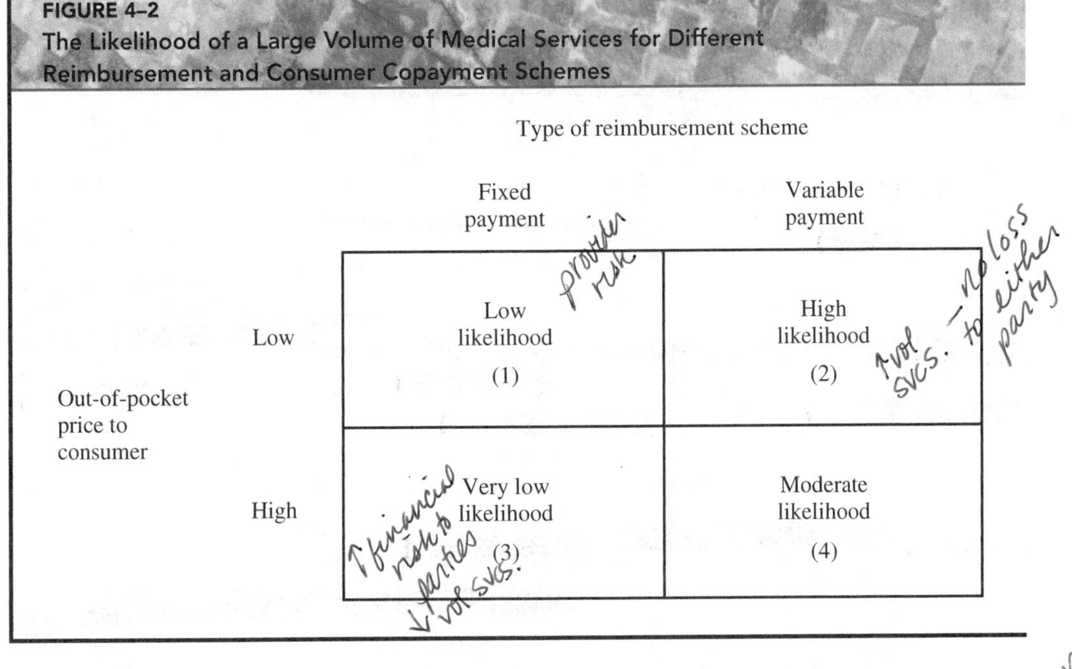

We can conduct a similar analysis for the consumer. Consumers who face a low out-of-pocket price of obtaining medical services are more likely to seek out additional medical services (this is referred to as the moral hazard problem in Chapter 5). On the other hand, consumers who face a high out-of-pocket price are less inclined to seek out medical services given the greater opportunity cost of their money.

Combining the reimbursement and out-of-pocket payment schemes, the likelihood of a large volume of medical services per patient is the greatest in cell 2, where a variable-payment scheme interacts with a low consumer out-of-pocket plan. Neither party loses much financially in the exchange of dollars for medical services. Conversely, a large volume of medical services is least likely in cell 3, where a fixed-payment plan coexists with a large consumer out-of-pocket scheme. Both parties in the exchange lose financially. Cell 4 offers a moderate likelihood of a large volume of medical services, because the provider is not made financially worse off by providing additional services. For this to happen, however, either the consumer's out-of-pocket price must not be too high or the consumer must be relatively insensitive to price (that is, highly inelastic demand). Finally, in cell 1, the health care provider is made worse off while the consumer is relatively unaffected by additional medical services, so the probability of a large volume of medical services is low.

A major current concern of health care policy makers is that a variable reimbursement system, when combined with a modest consumer out-of-pocket plan, results in excessive medical services that provide low marginal benefits to patients but come at a high marginal cost to society. For example, medical care providers may offer expensive diagnostic tests to low-risk patients. The tests come at a high marginal cost to society but yield only small marginal benefits to patients given their low-risk classification. Small marginal medical benefits coincide with the "flat-of-the-curve" medicine observed in several empirical studies, as discussed in Chapter 2.

As a result, many health policy analysts believe that fee-for-service or retrospective payments and small consumer out-of-pocket payments are responsible for high-cost, low-benefit medicine. Policy makers typically argue that some cost sharing is needed on the supply and/or demand side of the market to reduce the potential for excess medical services (Ellis and McGuire, 1993). That is, they believe that fixed-payment reimbursement plans and nontrivial consumer payments are required to control unnecessary medical services.

Canada

We can appreciate the importance of the reimbursement method by examining and contrasting the countrywide reimbursement schemes practiced in Canada, Germany, and the United Kingdom. In Canada, everyone is eligible for the same medical benefits, and there are no copayments for most medical services. Patients essentially drop out of the reimbursement picture, and reimbursement exclusively takes place between the public insurer (the government) and the health care provider. In terms of Figure 4–1, this means that the monetary exchange is virtually nonexistent between patient and health care provider. The ministry of health in each province is responsible for controlling medical costs. Cost control is attempted primarily through fixed global budgets for hospitals and predetermined fees for physicians. Specifically, the operating budgets of hospitals are approved and funded entirely by the ministry in each province, and an annual global budget is negotiated between the ministry and each individual hospital. Capital expenditures must also be approved by the ministry, which funds the bulk of the spending.

Physician fees are determined by periodic negotiations between the ministry and provincial medical associations (the Canadian version of the American Medical Association). With the passage of the Canada Health Act of 1984, the right to **extra billing** was removed in all provinces. Extra billing or balance billing refers to a situation in which the physician bills the patient some dollar amount above the predetermined fee set by the third-party payer. For the profession as a whole, negotiated fee increases are implemented in steps, conditional on the rate of increase in the volume of services. If volume per physician rises faster than a predetermined percentage, subsequent fee increases are scaled down or eliminated to cap gross billings—the product of the fee and the volume of each service—at some predetermined target. The possible scaling down of fee increases is supposed to create an incentive for a more judicious use of resources. Physicians enjoy nearly complete autonomy in treating patients (for example, there is no mandatory second opinion for surgery) because policy makers believe there is no need for intrusive types of controls given that the hospital global budgets and physician expenditure targets tend to curb unnecessary services.

The Sickness Funds in Germany, which collect employer and employee insurance premiums, pay negotiated lump-sum funds equal to the product of a capitation (per-patient) payment and the number of insured individuals to regional associations of ambulatory care physicians. These regional associations, in turn, reimburse individual physicians for services on the basis of a fee schedule. The fee schedule is determined through negotiation between the regional associations of Sickness Funds and physicians. To determine the fee schedule, each physician service is assigned a number of points based on relative worth. The price per point is established by dividing the lump-sum total budget by the actual number of points billed within a quarter by all physicians. The income to an individual physician equals the number of points billed times the price per point.

The Sickness Funds that operate in a given state also negotiate fixed prices for various procedures (based on the diagnosis-related group, or DRG) with local hospitals. Because hospitals can make profits or incur losses because of the fixed prices, there is an incentive for hospitals to save resources and specialize in certain procedures. For some procedures, hospital accommodations are reimbursed on a per diem basis but funds are limited by an overall budget. Hospital-based physicians are paid on a salary basis. Most of the hospital funds for capital acquisitions come from state and local governments and are reviewed and approved through a state planning process.

In the United Kingdom, the district health authorities are allocated funds by the NHS on a weighted capitation basis, which considers age, sex, and health-risk factors as well as geographical cost differences. Independent community-based family practitioners contract with the NHS and are uniformly paid throughout the United Kingdom, primarily on a capitation basis. The DHAs prospectively reimburse individual hospital trusts based on the actual cost of providing the services. All hospital-based physicians and consultants are paid on a fixed salary basis by the trusts. Trusts are required to earn a 6 percent return on assets and the residual is returned to the DHA. Capital funding for the trusts is determined by the DHA and is based on its regional allocation.

Any funds allocated to GP fundholders are deducted from the DHA's allocation. GP fundholders annually negotiate funds to purchase elective and nonemergency services for their subscribers. About 41 percent of the population in England is served by GP fundholders. Any savings made by a fundholder may be reinvested in the practice or new services but cannot directly increase the GP's personal income. GP fundholders are not at personal financial risk as they are protected against any legitimate cost overruns by the DHAs.

In sum, these three countries have shied away from relying on an uncontrolled fee-for-service reimbursement scheme because of the concern that it creates incentives for high-cost, low-benefit medicine. The payment is on either a per diem, per-person, or negotiated fee-for-service basis. In addition, the payment for medical services is determined by a single payer—the government in Canada and the United Kingdom and representatives of the Sickness Funds in Germany. Policy makers in these countries believe that a single-payer, controlled-payment system can reduce the incentive to provide high-cost, low-benefit medicine and better contain health care costs.

The Production of Medical Services

The mode of production also differs across health care systems. Several distinguishing features of production are worth mentioning. We normally think of health care services as being produced on an inpatient care basis in hospitals or nursing homes or on an outpatient (ambulatory) care basis at physician clinics or in the outpatient department of a hospital. However, health care services are also produced in the home. Preventive care (such as exercise, dieting, and flossing) and first aid are two prime examples of home-produced health care services. In addition, long-term or chronic care services are often produced in the home rather than in an institution, such as a nursing home. Although acute care services can also be produced in the home, the cost of producing these services is usually prohibitive for the individual consumer because of the high per-person labor and capital expenses.[6] As a result, it is almost always cheaper for the individual consumer to purchase acute care services at a hospital because such an organization can exploit various economies associated with large size.

Outside the home, health care providers may be organized in a number of ways. For example, a hospital may be a freestanding, independent institution or part of a multihospital chain. Similarly, a physician may operate in a solo practice or belong to a group practice. Usually the size and scope of the medical organization depend on whether any economies exist from operating on a small or large scale. In addition, some physicians, such as radiologists and anesthesiologists, may be employees of the hospital. In contrast, some physicians on the medical staff may not be employees of the hospital but instead are granted admitting privileges.

6. According to the *Mosby Medical Encyclopedia* (1992), long-term care is "the provision of medical care on a repeated or continuous basis to persons with chronic physical or mental disorders" (p. 471). Acute care is "treatment for a serious illness, for an accident, or after surgery. . . . This kind of care is usually for only a short time" (p. 11).

Health care services may be produced in the private or public sector by health care providers in the medical services industry. If produced in the private sector, the health care provider may offer medical services on a not-for-profit or a for-profit basis. A not-for-profit organization is required by law to use any profits exclusively for the charitable, educational, or scientific purpose for which it was formed. For example, a hospital may use profits to lower patient prices or finance medical equipment or hospital expansion.

Institutional Differences between For-Profit and Not-for-Profit Health Care Providers

Because not-for-profit institutions are so prevalent in the health care sector, it is important that we examine the institutional differences between for-profit and not-for-profit firms. There are five basic institutional differences between these two classes of organizations.

First, when for-profit firms are established, they acquire initial capital by exchanging funds for ownership with the private sector. Ownership gives the private sector a claim on future profits. Not-for-profit firms must rely on donations for their initial capital because they are not privately owned. In a broad sense, they are owned by the community at large. Second, for-profit providers are capable of earning accounting profits and distributing cash dividends to their owners, whereas not-for-profit firms face a **non-distribution constraint** and are prohibited from distributing profits. A non-distribution constraint means that not-for-profit firms cannot legally distribute any revenues in excess of costs to individuals without regard to the charitable purpose for which the organization was formed. Third, for-profit organizations can easily be sold or liquidated for compensation by their owners, whereas it is very difficult to sell a not-for-profit organization. Fourth, not-for-profit providers are exempt from certain types of taxes and are eligible to receive subsidies from the government. In fact, it has been argued that the tax exemption and subsidies give not-for-profit firms an unfair advantage over for-profit firms. Finally, not-for-profit providers are restricted by law in the types of goods and services they can provide.

Why Are Not-for-Profit Health Care Providers So Prevalent?

Now that we understand the differences between for-profit and not-for-profit providers, the next item to address is why not-for-profit providers are so prevalent in the health care sector. Weisbrod (1988) discusses the issue in general terms, but his analysis can easily be applied to the health care sector. Not-for-profit firms exist primarily as a result of market failure in the private sector. The market failure results from three factors.

First, the private sector works best when all market participants are perfectly informed. However, given the complexity of medical technology and the difficulty of assessing the appropriateness of medical care, consumers typically possess imperfect information about the health care sector. As a result, many consumers believe they are in a vulnerable situation and can easily be exploited by medical providers for the sake of profits. For that reason, they prefer to deal with not-for-profit providers, which presumably are driven by more altruistic motives.

The second reason for market failure concerns equity. Society as a whole believes that each citizen has a right to some minimum level of medical care that would not be provided if health care resources were allocated by the for-profit sector. The profit motive ensures that health care is allocated based on the ability to pay and not on need. As a result, some argue that not-for-profit providers are necessary to meet the needs of those who cannot pay for medical care.

The third reason for market failure involves the presence of externalities as discussed further in Chapter 9. When externalities exist, resources are not efficiently allocated because the for-profit sector does not consider all the costs and benefits associated with production. Thus, for these three reasons, the for-profit sector may fail to address the collective need for health care.

The next question that comes to mind is why the public sector does not simply take over the allocation of health care resources in the presence of market failure. The answer, Weisbrod contends, is that consumer needs are heterogeneous. When needs are widely diverse, the government has difficulty developing an appropriate overall policy that meets the desires of all consumers in a cost-effective manner. For example, "one-size-fits-all" medicine most likely would not appeal to everyone. Hence, a multitude of not-for-profit health care providers, such as hospital and nursing homes, are required to satisfy heterogeneous demands. Each institution can be tailored to fit the individual demands of its constituents. For example, the Shriners run not-for-profit hospitals aimed at orthopedic pediatric care, while some religious organizations operate nursing homes specifically for elderly members of their own religion.

One last question deserves some discussion. If these market failures are substantial, why is the for-profit sector allowed to operate at all in the health care field? Consumer knowledge and preferences provide the answer to this question. Although some consumers lack the information they need to make informed decisions, others are much more informed. Informed consumers may "have no institutional preferences" and "prefer to deal with any organization, regardless of ownership form, that provides the wanted outputs at the lowest price" (Weisbrod, 1988, p. 124). Thus, the for-profit sector exists in the health care market primarily to satisfy the demands of these types of consumers.

Production of Health Care in the Three Systems

The organizations of production in the three health care systems we have been discussing have some slight differences. In Canada, medical services are produced in the private sector. Most hospitals in the private sector are organized on a not-for-profit basis and are owned by either charitable or religious organizations. In Germany, medical services are produced primarily in the private sector, because most physicians operate in private practices. Public hospitals control about 51 percent of all hospital beds in Germany. The remaining beds are managed by not-for-profit (35 percent) and for-profit hospitals (13 percent). Office-based physicians are normally prohibited from treating patients in hospitals, and most hospital-based physicians are not allowed to provide ambulatory care services in Germany.

The structure of production in the United Kingdom now largely takes place in the private, although mostly not-for-profit, sector. The present situation in the United Kingdom is in stark contrast to the method of production that prevailed before the passage of the National Health Service and Community Act of 1990. Up to 1990, almost all hospitals were publicly owned and operated and most doctors were employees of the NHS. Even before 1990, however, family practitioners were community-based in solo or small group practices and simply contracted with the NHS.

Physician Choice and Referral Practices

Important differences in the availability and utilization of medical services can also result from the degree of physician choice the health care consumer possesses and the types of referral practices used within the health care system. More choice typically provides consumers with increased satisfaction (Schmittdiel et al., 1997). However, greater choice may come at a cost if it leads to a large number of fragmented health care providers that are unable to sufficiently coordinate care or exploit any economies that come with large size (Halm et al., 1997).

In some health care systems, patients have unlimited choice of and full access to any physician or health care provider within any type of setting (such as a clinic or hospital). For example, at one time in the United States, insured individuals could directly seek out any general practitioner or specialist without financial penalty. Moreover, at one time in the United States, it was not unusual for a general practitioner to review the care of a patient referred for hospital services. We will see later that conditions regarding physician choice and referral practices have changed a great deal in the United States.

Other countries have adopted different referral practices. Although the Canadian and German health care systems allow free choice of provider, general practitioners in the United Kingdom act as "gatekeepers" and must refer patients to a specialist or a hospital. Once the patient is referred to a hospital, the patient–general practitioner relationship is severed for any particular illness in both the United Kingdom and Germany. Unlike in Germany, however, patients are allowed to go directly to a family practitioner or a hospital for primary care in the United Kingdom, unless they are registered with a GP fundholder.

The Three National Health Care Systems Summarized

Based on our generalized model of a health care system, Table 4–1 provides a capsulized summary of the current national health care systems in the three countries we have been discussing. Each national health care system is differentiated according to the degree of health insurance coverage,

TABLE 4–1
A Comparison of Health Care Systems

	Country (Type of System)			
Feature	Canada (NHI)*	Germany (SI)†	United Kingdom (PC)‡	United States (Pluralistic)
Health insurance coverage	Universal	Near universal	Near universal	84 percent
Financing	General taxes	Payroll and general taxes	General taxes	Voluntary premiums or general taxes
	Single-payer system	Single-payer system§	Single-payer system	Multipayer system
Reimbursement	Global budgets to hospitals	Fixed payments to hospitals	Global budgets to hospitals	Mostly fixed payments to hospitals
	Negotiated fee-for-service to physicians	Negotiated point-fee-for-service to physicians	Salaries and capitation payments to physicians	Mostly fee-for-service to physicians
Consumer out-of-pocket price	Negligible	Negligible	Negligible	Positive, but generally small
Production	Private	Private	Private but public contract	Private
Physician choice	Unlimited	Unlimited	Limited	Relatively limited

*NHI = national health insurance program.
†SI = socialized insurance.
‡PC = public contracting.
§Multiple third-party payers are responsible for paying representatives of the health care providers, but the universal fees are collectively negotiated by the third-party payers.

type of financing, reimbursement scheme, consumer out-of-pocket price, mode of production, and degree of physician choice. The essential features of the Canadian health care system are national health insurance, free choice of health care provider, private production of medical services, and regulated global budgets and fees for health care providers. The dominating features of the German health care system include socialized health insurance financed through Sickness Funds, negotiated payments to health care providers, free choice of provider, and private production of health care services. In the case of Great Britain, the distinguishing characteristics include restrictions on choice of provider, public contracting of medical services, global budgets for hospitals, fixed salaries for hospital-based physicians, and capitation payments to family practitioners.

The U.S. health care system is discussed in detail in the next section, and the last column in Table 4–1 gives a quick preview. The pluralistic U.S. health care system contains some structural elements found in most of the other three systems (such as private production) but relies more heavily on a fee-for-service reimbursement scheme. In addition, health care providers are reimbursed through multiple payers, including the government and thousands of private insurance companies, in contrast to the single-payer system in Canada (government), Germany (Sickness Funds), and the United Kingdom (government).

AN OVERVIEW OF THE U.S. HEALTH CARE SYSTEM

Some analysts argue that the multifaceted nature of the health care system accounts for the relatively high expenditures devoted to medical care in the United States. Although this may be true and is a topic of discussion throughout this book, it most certainly is true that this diversity makes it very difficult to describe the U.S. health care system in sufficient detail. This section presents a brief overview of the current system in the United States based on the generalized model of a health care system. The remainder of the book discusses the operation and performance of the U.S. health care system in much greater detail, albeit on a piecemeal basis.

Financing of Health Care in the United States

The United States has no single nationwide system of health insurance. Health insurance is purchased in the private marketplace or provided by the government to certain groups. Private health insurance can be purchased from various for-profit commercial insurance companies or from nonprofit insurers, such as Blue Cross/Blue Shield. About 84 percent of the population is covered by either public (27 percent) or private (68 percent) health insurance.[7]

Approximately 60 percent of health insurance coverage is employment related, largely due to the cost savings associated with group plans that can be purchased through an employer. Employers voluntarily sponsor the health insurance plans. Nearly all privately insured individuals belong to some type of managed care plan. As discussed in Chapter 6, managed care plans are designed to practice cost-effective medicine and place varying degrees of restrictions on consumer choices.

In addition to private health insurance, some portion of the U.S. population is covered by public health insurance. The two major types of public health insurance, both of which began in 1966, are **Medicare** and **Medicaid.**[8] Medicare is a uniform, national public health insurance

7. U.S. Census Bureau, " Income, Poverty, and Health Insurance Coverage in the United States: 2004," http://www.census.gov/prod/2005pubs/p60-229.pdf (accessed September 21, 2005). The figures for private and public insurance coverage do not sum to 86 percent because of double-counting. For example, some people receiving public insurance coverage also purchase private health insurance.

8. See Chapter 10 for a more detailed discussion on the Medicare and Medicaid programs. The federal government is also responsible for providing health insurance to individuals in the military and to federal employees.

program for aged and disabled individuals (such as those with kidney failure). Administered by the federal government, Medicare is the largest health insurer in the country, covering about 14 percent of the population, and is primarily financed through taxes. The Medicare plan consists of two parts. Part A is compulsory and provides health insurance coverage for inpatient hospital care, very limited nursing home services, and some home health services. Part B, the voluntary or supplemental plan, provides benefits for physician services, outpatient hospital services, outpatient laboratory and radiology services, and home health services.

The second type of public health insurance program, Medicaid, provides coverage for certain economically disadvantaged groups. Medicaid is jointly financed by the federal and state governments and is administered by each state. The federal government provides state governments with a certain percentage of matching funds ranging from 50 to 83 percent, depending on the per capita income in the state. Individuals who are elderly, blind, disabled, or members of families with dependent children must be covered by Medicaid for states to receive federal funds. In addition, although the federal government stipulates a certain basic package of health care benefits (hospital, physician, and nursing home services), some states are more generous than others. Consequently, in some states individuals receive a more generous benefit package under Medicaid than in others. Medicaid is the only public program that finances long-term nursing home care. Approximately 13 percent of the population is covered by Medicaid.

In summary, the financing of health care falls into three broad categories: private health insurance, Medicare, and Medicaid. However, another category of individuals exists: those who are uninsured. Approximately 16 percent of the U.S. population is estimated to lack health insurance coverage at any point in time. This does not mean these individuals are without access to health care services. Many uninsured people receive health care services through public clinics and hospitals, state and local health programs, or private providers that finance the care through charity and by shifting costs to other payers. Nevertheless, the lack of health insurance can cause uninsured households to face considerable financial hardship and insecurity. Furthermore, the uninsured often find themselves in the emergency room of a hospital, sometimes after it is too late for proper medical treatment. We take up this discussion in later chapters.

Reimbursement for Health Care in the United States

Unlike in Canada and Europe, where a single-payer system is the norm, the United States possesses a multipayer system in which a variety of third-party payers, including the federal and state governments, commercial health insurance companies, and Blue Cross/Blue Shield, are responsible for reimbursing health care providers. Naturally, reimbursement takes on various forms in the United States, depending on the nature of the third-party payer. The most common form of reimbursement is fee-for-service, although most health care providers accept discounted fees from private health insurance plans.

Physician services under Medicare (and most state Medicaid plans) are also reimbursed on a fee-for-service basis, but the fee is set by the government based on the time and effort involved in providing the care. Since 1983, the federal government has reimbursed hospitals on a prospective basis for services provided to Medicare patients. This Medicare reimbursement scheme, called the **diagnosis-related group (DRG)** system, contains 500 or so different payment categories based on the characteristics of the patient (age and sex), primary and secondary diagnosis, and treatment.[9] A prospective payment is established for each DRG. The prospective payment is claimed to provide hospitals with an incentive to contain costs (cells 1 and 3 of Figure 4–2).

Beginning in the early 1980s, many states, such as California, instituted **selective contracting,** in which various health care providers competitively bid for the right to treat Medicaid patients. In fact, much of the favorable experience with selective contracting in the United States led to the adoption of the public contracting model in the United Kingdom (Mechanic, 1995). Under selective contracting, recipients of Medicaid are limited in the choice of health care provider. In addition, to better contain health care costs and coordinate care, the federal government and various state governments have attempted to shift Medicare and Medicaid beneficiaries into managed care organizations (MCOs). As of 2004, about 61 percent of all Medicaid recipients and roughly 11 percent of all Medicare beneficiaries were enrolled in MCOs.

Production of Health Services and Provider Choice in the United States

Like the financing and reimbursement schemes, the U.S. health care system is very diversified in terms of production methods. Government, not-for-profit, and for-profit institutions all play an important role in health care markets. For the most part, primary care physicians in the United States function in the private for-profit sector and operate in group practices, although some physicians work for not-for-profit clinics or in public organizations. In the hospital industry, the not-for-profit is the dominant form of ownership. Specifically, not-for-profit hospitals control about 70 percent of all hospital beds. The ownership structure is the reverse in the nursing home industry, however. More than 70 percent of all nursing homes are organized on a for-profit basis. One should also keep in mind that mental retardation facilities, dialysis facilities, and even insurance companies possess different ownership forms. The variety of ownership forms helps make health care a very difficult, but challenging and interesting, industry to analyze.

In addition, we previously mentioned that provider choice matters. Consumers typically receive greater satisfaction from facing more choices. We also discussed, however, that more choices may come at greater costs if small, differentiated providers are unable to fully exploit any economies associated with size. Hence, it is important to know how much choice consumers have over health care providers in the United States.

Up to the early 1980s most insured individuals had full choice of health care providers in the United States. Consumers could choose to visit a primary care giver or the outpatient clinic of a hospital, or see a specialist if they chose to. The introduction of restrictive health insurance plans and such new government policies as selective contracting have limited the degree to which consumers can choose their own health care provider. For example, some health care plans require that patients receive their care exclusively from a particular network; otherwise they are fully responsible for the ensuing financial burden. Furthermore, the primary care giver acts as a gatekeeper and must refer the patient for additional care. Of course, the lower premiums of a restrictive plan compensate consumers at least to some degree for the restriction of choice. There are arguments for and against free choice of provider and once again trade-offs are involved. This issue will be discussed throughout the text in more depth. For now let us just say that these trade-offs must be given serious thought when determining what degree of consumer choice is best from a societal point of view.

9. The DRGs are based on 23 major diagnostic groups centered on a different organ of the body.

SUMMARY

Every health care system must answer the four basic questions concerning the allocation of medical resources and the distribution of medical services. Some systems rely on centralized decision making whereas others answer the basic questions through a decentralized process. Health care systems are complex largely because third-party payers are involved. Third-party payers help reduce the financial risk associated with the irregularity and uncertainty of many medical transactions. Third-party payers also help monitor the behavior of health care providers.

The financing, reimbursement, and production methods and the degree of choice over the health care provider are important elements that make up a health care system. Medical care is financed by out-of-pocket payments, premiums, and/or taxes. Medical care providers are reimbursed on a fixed or variable basis. The production of medical care may take place in a for-profit, a not-for-profit, or a public setting, and medical care providers may operate in independent or large group practices. Choice of provider may be limited. All these features are important because they affect incentives and thereby often influence the operation and performance of a health care system. For example, many economists predict that fee-for-service insurance plans provide an incentive for medical care providers to produce a large volume of services.

The U.S. health care system is very pluralistic. For instance, considerable variation exists in the financing, reimbursement, and production of medical care. The remainder of this book provides a better understanding about how each of these elements affects the functioning of the U.S. health care system.

CASE STUDIES

4-1 Physician Utilization Rates and Payment Mechanisms

Physician payment method influences the quality and intensity of services supplied to patients. Fee-for-service (FFS) payment schemes reward providers financially for performing more services (higher volume, greater intensity, or both) (column 2 in Figure 4–2). In some cases, the "extra" services provided under FFS may be excessive or wasteful. In contrast, the connection between volume and payment is muted in salary-based systems. In fact, physicians could actually face the opposite incentive: to discourage office visits and reduce workloads as a way to receive on-the-job leisure time (column 1 in Figure 4–2). Studies of the effects of these payment systems are challenging, primarily because it is difficult to adjust for organizational differences in practice settings, patient severity, treatment outcomes, and patient costs.

Hickson et al. (1987) overcome some of these problems. Specifically, nine pairs of closely matched medical residents at a Vanderbilt pediatric clinic were randomly assigned to an FFS or salary-based reimbursement group over a nine-month period. The common clinic setting and random assignment of physicians controlled for the organizational form, patient payment methods, and physician characteristics, so any utilization differences could be attributed solely to the method of reimbursing physicians. At the end of the nine months, records were consulted to determine the utilization rates of the residents in the two groups. Although the average number of patient visits per physician did not differ significantly between the FFS (111.6) and salaried (104.8) physician groups, the results show that FFS patients are more likely to see their regular physicians. In the study, almost 87 percent of FFS visits were attended by the primary physician, whereas the comparable figure for the salaried group was only about 78 percent. In addition, FFS patients were less likely to visit the emergency room than those patients assigned to salaried physicians, supporting the contention that FFS physicians direct their patients away from the emergency room to their offices, where it is easier for them to personally treat the patients. Thus Hickson, et al. note that an FFS plan may provide more "continuity" of care given that patients are more likely to see their regular doctors. The results also suggest that FFS physicians schedule and attend 22 percent more visits than salaried physicians.

Questions for Discussion

1. *The conventional wisdom for many years has been that FFS results in a "fragmented" system, but managed care, which often is associated with salary and other prepayment mechanisms, results in more continuity of care. This study, however, finds essentially the opposite: under certain circumstances, continuity of care appears to be better when physicians are paid on an FFS basis. Discuss the most plausible economic rationale for this finding.*
2. *The study also shows that physicians paid on an FFS basis tend to work more hours. Is that a good thing? Why or why not?*

4-2 Medical Technology

The availability of medical technologies affects the production of medical care services and health care costs. Medical technologies, such as drugs, medical devices, and procedures, may offer cost savings or higher-quality services. Four stages are associated with the development and diffusion of medical technology: (1) basic research, (2) applied research, (3) clinical investigation and testing, and (4) diffusion and imitation. The clinical benefit of new medical technologies is typically demonstrated in the third stage, and the "business case" for new technology, if there is any, is typically demonstrated in the diffusion stage. Some health policy analysts (such as Aaron, 1991), however, have expressed concern that unconstrained health care markets encourage the diffusion of medical technologies that offer low benefits at high costs. As a result, many countries have adopted policies to either directly or indirectly control the adoption and diffusion of medical technologies. But is technological change in medicine worth it? That question is posed by Cutler and McClellan (2001), who examine the costs and benefits of new technologies used to treat heart attacks, low-birthweight infants, depression, cataracts, and breast cancer. They found that, for all conditions except breast cancer, "medical spending as a whole is worth the increased cost of care" (p. 11). For example, the authors determine that "around 70 percent of the survival improvement in heart attack mortality is a result of changes in technology" (p. 18).

Questions for Discussion

1. *Cutler and McClellan focus mainly on the costs and benefits of new technologies aimed at the five conditions. Do you think their results would hold if the list of conditions were expanded? What kinds of conditions are less likely to show positive rates of return on technology?*
2. *Even if many new medical technologies are "worth it," what kinds of unique problems do technological advances pose in health care? Does the prevalence of third-party payers complicate matters? Is everyone willing to pay equally for new medical technology?*

Review Questions and Problems

1. Answer the following questions pertaining to health care systems.
   A. Why isn't the market for health care services organized according to a typical consumer (patient) and producer (health provider) relationship?

B. What are the basic differences between insurance premiums and taxes as sources of medical care financing?
C. How might the reimbursement method differ among health care providers? Why might the reimbursement method make a difference?
D. Identify the four basic kinds of health care systems discussed in the chapter.
E. Point out some unique institutions (compared to the United States) associated with the health care systems of the various countries discussed in the chapter.

2. Suppose you had the opportunity to organize the perfect health care system. Explain how you would organize the financing method, reimbursement scheme, mode of production, and physician referral procedure.
3. Which of the following reimbursement and consumer copayment schemes would have the greatest and lowest likelihood of producing high-cost, low-benefit medicine? Explain your answers.
   A. Fee-for-service plan with 40 percent consumer copayment.
   B. Prepaid health plan with 40 percent consumer copayment.
   C. Fee-for-service plan with no consumer cost sharing.
   D. Fixed-salary plan with no consumer cost sharing.
   E. Prepaid health plan with no consumer cost sharing.
   F. Fixed-salary plan with 40 percent consumer cost sharing.
4. Answer the following questions regarding the U.S. health care system.
   A. What are the basic differences between conventional health insurance and managed care health insurance in terms of type of insurance offered and reimbursement practice?
   B. What is the difference between Medicare and Medicaid? How is Medicare financed? How is Medicaid financed?
   C. What is the DRG system? How are physicians currently reimbursed under the Medicare system?

CEBS Questions

■ *CEBS Sample Question on Subject Matter from CEBS Course 9 Study Manual*

1. Why does a third-party payer face a much lower level of risk than an individual health care consumer does? (page 76)

■ *CEBS Sample Exam Questions*

1. In the Canadian health care system, cost containment is accomplished primarily through:
   A. Copayments
   B. High deductibles
   C. Cost sharing with the government
   D. Voluntary restraint in raising prices
   E. Fixed budgets for hospitals and predetermined fees for physicians
2. Which of the following statements regarding health insurance systems in foreign countries is (are) correct?
   I. Canada has a national health insurance program that provides first-dollar coverage with no limit on lifetime benefits.
   II. Germany has socialized health insurance financed by employers and employees.

III. The primary health service in the United Kingdom is much the same as the Medicaid program in the United States.
   A. II only
   B. III only
   C. I and II only
   D. II and III only
   E. I, II, and III

3. All of the following statements describe the impact provider reimbursement and consumer co-payment methods are likely to have on the supply and demand of medical services EXCEPT:
   A. A health care provider reimbursed on a fixed-payment basis is unlikely to supply a large volume of medical services to a patient unnecessarily.
   B. A large volume of unnecessary medical services is likely to be provided when the out-of-pocket price to consumers is low regardless of the provider type of reimbursement scheme.
   C. A health care provider reimbursed on a variable-payment basis is more likely to supply a large volume of medical services to a patient unnecessarily than one reimbursed on a fixed-payment scheme.
   D. The likelihood of a large volume of medical services is the greatest when a variable-payment scheme interacts with a low consumer out-of-pocket plan.
   E. Fee-for-service payments combined with small consumer out-of-pocket payments are likely to produce high-cost, low-benefit medicine.

■ *Answer to Sample Question from Study Manual*

Third-party payers face much lower risk than individual consumers because of the law of large numbers. That is, third-party payers can pool the experience of many individuals and use indicators such as occupational and demographic averages to predict aggregate medical costs.

■ *Answers to Sample Exam Questions*

1. E is the correct answer. See page 80 of the text.
2. C is the correct answer. The primary health care system in the United Kingdom is not only for the economically disadvantaged. See page 77 of the text.
3. B is the correct answer. See pages 78–79 of the text.

Online Resources

To access Internet links related to the topics in this chapter, please visit our web site at **www.thomsonedu.com/economics/santerre**.

References

Arrow, Kenneth J. "Uncertainty and the Welfare Economics of Medical Care." *American Economic Review* 53 (December 1963), pp. 941–73.

Bodenheimer, Thomas, and Kevin Grumbach. "Financing Universal Health Insurance: Taxes, Premiums and the Lessons of Social Insurance." *Journal of Health Politics, Policy and Law* 17 (fall 1992), pp. 439–62.

Cutler, D. M., and M. McClellan. "Is Technological Change in Medicine Worth It?" *Health Affairs* 20, no. 5 (2001), pp. 11–29.

Ellis, Randall P., and Thomas G. McGuire. "Supply-Side and Demand-Side Cost Sharing in Health Care." *Journal of Economic Perspectives* 7 (fall 1993), pp. 135–51.

Halm, Ethan A., Nancyanne Causino, and David Blumenthal. "Is Gatekeeping Better Than Traditional Care?" *Journal of the American Medical Association* 278 (November 1997), pp. 1677–81.

Mechanic, David. "Americanization of the British NHS." *Health Affairs* 14 (summer 1995), pp. 51–67.

Mosby Medical Encyclopedia. New York: C. V. Mosby, 1992.

Raffel, Marshall W., ed. *Health Care and Reform in Industrial Countries.* University Park: Pennsylvania State University Press, 1997.

Reinhardt, Uwe. "Economics." *Journal of the American Medical Association* 275 (June 1996), pp. 23–25.

Schmittdiel, Julie, Joe V. Selby, Kevin Grumbach, and Charles P. Quesenberry. "Choice of Personal Physician and Patient Satisfaction in a Health Maintenance Organization." *Journal of the American Medical Association* 278 (November 1997), pp. 1596–99.

Van de Ven, Wynand, P. M. M., and Randall P. Ellis. "Risk Adjustment in Competitive Health Plan Markets." In *Handbook in Health Economics,* eds. A. J. Calger and J. P. Newhouse. Amsterdam: North-Holland, 2000, chap. 14, pp. 755–845.

Weisbrod, Burton A. *The Nonprofit Economy.* Cambridge, Mass.: Harvard University Press, 1988.

THE DEMAND FOR MEDICAL CARE

CHAPTER 5

Many people have the misconception that economic theory has little relevance to the demand for medical care because economic factors are not important when an individual needs urgent medical attention. Recall Joe in Chapter 1, who awoke one night with a pain in his chest and realized he was having a heart attack. It is highly unlikely that he and his wife considered the price of medical care as Joe was rushed to the hospital.

However, most visits to a physician's office and the majority of visits to a hospital emergency room are not of a life-threatening nature. Thus, for many medical care transactions, there is sufficient time to make conscious choices, and price often plays an important role in the determination of choices. Results of a survey of various types of health care providers and insurers substantiate the critical role price plays in determining the demand for medical care (Winslow, 1994). According to the survey, price was ranked as more important than patient satisfaction or access to doctors, among other factors, in determining the economic success of health care providers.

This chapter explores the demand side of the medical care market. The chapter highlights:

- the theoretical derivation of the demand curve for medical services
- economic and noneconomic variables that influence the demand for medical services
- the impact of health insurance on the demand for medical services
- the concept of elasticity of demand
- a review of the empirical literature concerning the factors that determine the demand for medical care
- an examination of health spending in the United States
- a review of the sources and uses of health care funds in the United States

The Demand for Medical Care and the Law of Demand

To derive the demand curve for medical care, we must first establish the relation between the quantity of medical services and utility. Recall from Chapter 2 that the stock of health can be treated as a durable good that generates utility and is subject to the law of diminishing marginal utility.[1] This means that each incremental improvement in health generates successively smaller additions to total utility. We also know that medical services are an input in the production of health because a person consumes medical care services for the express purpose of maintaining, restoring, or improving health. However, the law of diminishing marginal productivity causes the marginal improvement to health brought about by each additional unit of medical care consumed to decrease.

From this discussion, it follows that medical care indirectly provides utility. Specifically, medical care helps to produce health, which in turn generates utility. Consequently, utility can be specified as a function of the quantity of medical care. Figure 5–1 depicts the relation between the level of medical care consumed and utility. Utility is specified on the vertical axis, and the quantity of medical care (q) is measured on the horizontal axis. The shape of the total utility curve indicates that utility increases at a decreasing rate with respect to medical care, or that medical care services are subject to diminishing marginal utility. Marginal utility decreases because (1) each successive unit of medical care generates a smaller improvement in health than the previous unit (due to the law of diminishing marginal productivity) and (2) each increase in health, in turn, generates a smaller increase in utility (due to the law of diminishing marginal utility).

The Utility-Maximizing Rule

Given market prices at a point in time, consumers must decide which combination of goods and services, including medical care, to purchase with their fixed incomes. According to microeconomic theory, each consumer chooses the bundle of goods and services that maximizes utility. Without working through the mathematics underlying the process, logic dictates that consumer utility is maximized when the marginal utility gained from the last dollar spent on each product is equal across all goods and services purchased.[2] This condition is known as the **utility-maximizing rule,** and it basically states that total utility reaches its peak when the consumer receives the maximum "bang for the buck" in terms of marginal utility per dollar of income from each and every good. In mathematical terms, the rule states that utility is maximized when

(5–1) $$MU_q/P_q = MU_z/P_z,$$

where MU_q represents the marginal utility received from the last unit of medical care purchased, q, and MU_z equals the marginal utility derived from the last unit of all other goods, z. The latter good is often referred to as a *composite good* in economics. To illustrate why the utility-maximizing rule must hold, suppose that

(5–2) $$MU_q/P_q > MU_z/P_z.$$

1. As a reminder, note that we continue to ignore the intermediate step between the stock of health, the services it provides, and utility.

2. That is, assuming all prices are known, income is spent over the period in question, and all products are subject to the law of diminishing marginal utility.

FIGURE 5–1
The Relationship between Utility and Medical Care

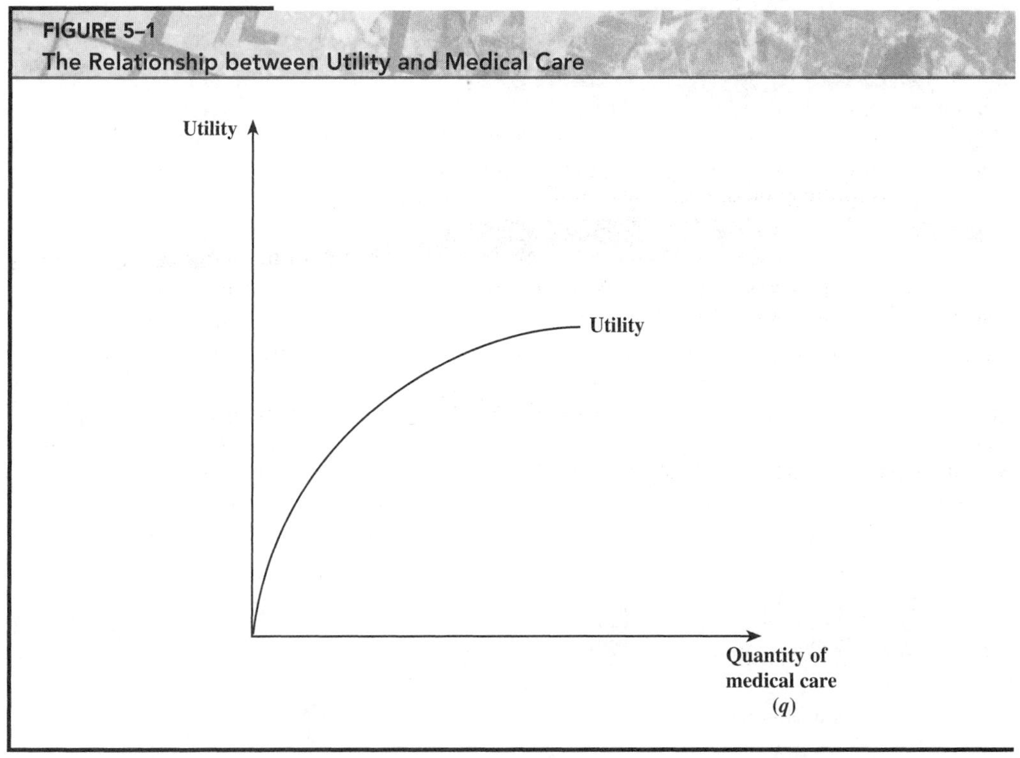

The shape of the utility curve illustrates that total utility increases at a decreasing rate with respect to the level of medical care consumed. The curve has a bow shape for two reasons. First, each additional unit of medical care consumed results in a smaller increase in health than the previous unit because of the law of diminishing marginal productivity. Second, each additional improvement in health generates a smaller increase in utility because of the law of diminishing marginal utility.

In this case, the last dollar spent on medical care generates more additional utility than the last dollar spent on all other goods. The consumer can increase total utility by reallocating expenditures and purchasing more units of medical care and fewer units of all other goods. As the consumer purchases more medical services at the expense of all other goods (remember that the consumer's income and the composite good's price are fixed), the marginal utility of medical care falls and the marginal utility of other goods increases. This, in turn, causes the value of MU_q/P_q to fall and the value of MU_z/P_z to increase. The consumer purchases additional medical services until the equality in Equation 5–1 again holds, or the last dollar spent on each product generates the same amount of additional satisfaction. At this point, total utility is maximized and any further changes in spending patterns will negatively affect total utility.

The Law of Demand

The equilibrium condition specified in Equation 5–1 can be used to trace out the demand curve for a particular medical service, such as physician services. For simplicity, assume the prices of all other goods and income remain constant and initially the consumer is purchasing the optimal mix of physician services and all other goods. Now assume the price of physician services increases. In this case, MU_q/P_q is less than MU_z/P_z (where MU_q and P_q represent the marginal utility and price of physician services, respectively). Consequently, the consumer receives more satisfaction per dollar from consuming all other goods. In reaction to the price increase, the consumer purchases fewer units of physician services and more units of all other goods. This reallocation continues until MU_q/P_q increases and MU_z/P_z decreases and the equilibrium condition of Equation 5–1 is again in force such that the last dollar spent on each good generates an equal amount of utility. Thus, an inverse relation exists between the price and the quantity demanded of physician services.

If the price of physician services continually changes, we can determine a number of points representing the relation between the price and the quantity demanded of physician services. Using this information, we can map out a demand curve like the one depicted in Figure 5–2, where the horizontal axis indicates the amount of physician services consumed (as measured by the number of visits, for example) and the vertical axis equals the price of physician services. The curve is downward sloping and reflects the inverse relation between the price and the quantity demanded of physician services, *ceteris paribus*. For example, if the price of physician services equals P_0, the consumer is willing and able to purchase q_0. Notice that if the price falls to P_1, the consumer purchases q_1 amount of physician services.

In this case, price represents the per-unit out-of-pocket expense the consumer incurs when purchasing medical services from a physician. As such, it equals the amount the consumer must

FIGURE 5–2
The Individual Demand Curve for Physician Services

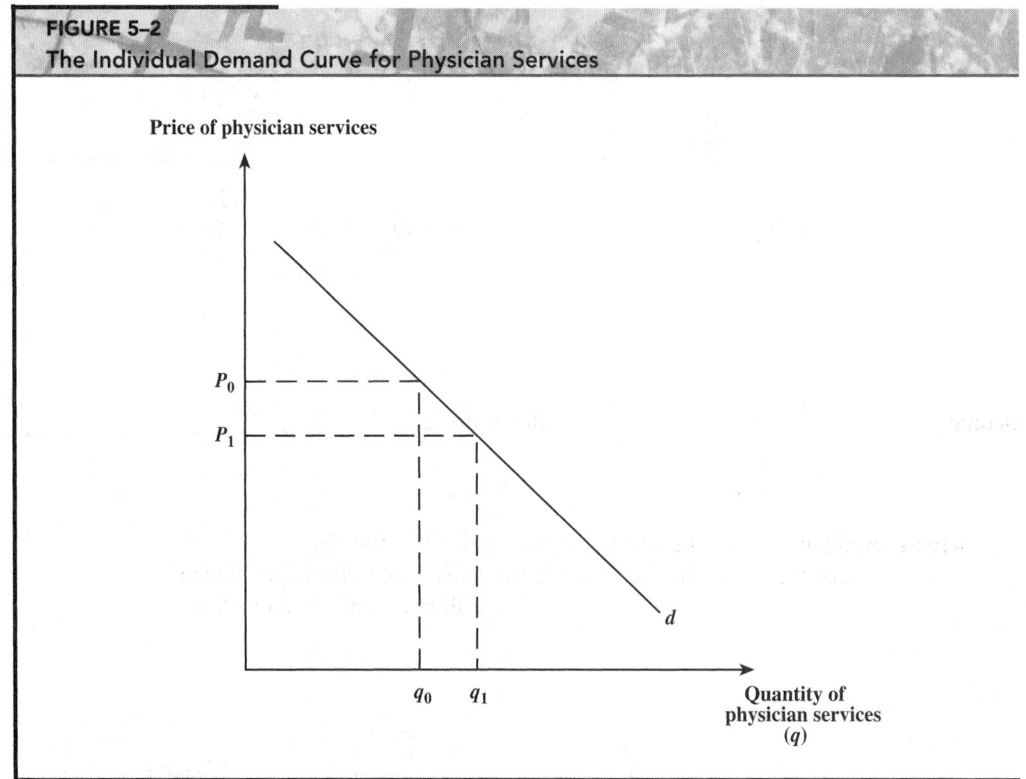

The individual demand curve for physician services is downward sloping, illustrating that quantity demanded increases as the price of physician services drops. Utility analysis, or the income and substitution effects, can be used to derive this inverse relationship, which is called the *law of demand*.

pay after the impact of third-party payments has been taken into account. Naturally, if the visit to the physician is not covered by a third party, the actual price of the visit equals the out-of-pocket expense.

The substitution and income effects associated with a price change offer another theoretical justification of the inverse relationship between price and quantity demanded. Both of these effects predict that a higher price will lead to a smaller quantity demanded and, conversely, a lower price will result in a greater quantity demanded. According to the substitution effect, a decrease in the price of physician services causes the consumer to substitute away from the relatively higher-priced medical goods, such as hospital outpatient services, and purchase more physician services. That is, lower-priced services are substituted for higher-priced ones. As a result, the quantity demanded of physician services increases as price decreases.

According to the income effect, a lower price also increases the real purchasing power of the consumer. Because medical care is assumed to be a normal good (that is, the quantity demanded of medical services increases with income), the quantity demanded of physician services increases with the rise in purchasing power. That also generates an inverse relation between price and quantity demanded because as price falls, real income increases and quantity demanded rises. Taken together, the substitution and income effects indicate that the quantity demanded of physician services decreases as price increases.

In summary, Figure 5–2 captures the inverse relationship between the price the consumer pays for medical care (in this instance, physician services) and the quantity demanded. The curve represents the amount of medical care the consumer is willing and able to purchase at every price. Utility analysis, or the income and substitution effects, can be used to generate this relationship. This inverse relationship is sometimes referred to as the **law of demand.** It is important to note that the demand for medical care is a *derived* demand, because it depends on the demand for good health. A visit to a dentist illustrates this point. An individual receives no utility directly from having a cavity filled. Rather, utility is generated from an improvement in dental health.

Of course, other economic and noneconomic variables also influence the demand for health care. Unlike price, which causes a movement along the demand curve, other factors influence quantity demanded by altering the position of the demand curve. These other economic and noneconomic determinants of demand are the topic of the next section.

Other Economic Demand-Side Factors

Income is another economic variable that affects the demand for medical services. Because medical care is generally assumed to be a normal good, any increase in income, which represents an increase in purchasing power, should cause the demand for medical services to rise. Figure 5–3 illustrates what happens to the demand for physician services when income increases. The increase in income causes the demand curve to shift to the right, from d_0 to d_1, because at each price the consumer is willing and able to purchase more physician services. Similarly, for each quantity of medical services, the consumer is willing to pay a higher price. This is attributable to the fact that at least some portion of the increase in income is spent on physician services. Conversely, a decrease in income causes the demand curve to shift to the left.[3]

3. Some goods are referred to as *inferior* goods. This is because the demand for these goods decreases as income increases. A classic nonmedical example is hamburger. As real income increases, the consumer may prefer to buy more expensive cuts of meat and purchase less hamburger. In the medical sector, hospital outpatient services may be an example of an inferior good. As income increases, the consumer may prefer to visit a private physician to receive individual care rather than outpatient services. As a result, the demand for outpatient services may decrease as income increases. Some researchers have found that tooth extractions represent an inferior dental service.

FIGURE 5–3
Shifts in the Individual Demand Curve for Physician Services

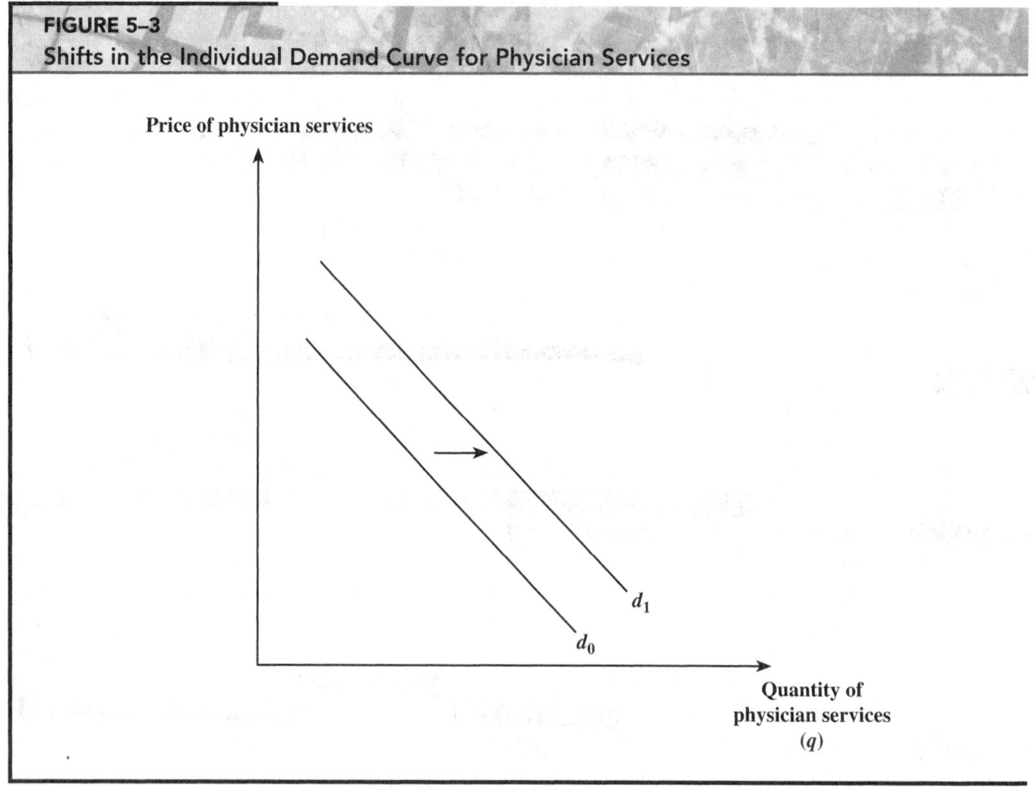

Medical care is assumed to be a normal good, which means that as income increases the consumer spends at least a portion of the increase in purchasing power on additional physician services. As a result, the individual demand curve for physician services shifts to the right, from d_0 to d_1, when income increases. At each price, the consumer is now willing and able to purchase more physician services.

The demand for a specific type of medical service is also likely to depend on the prices of other goods, particularly other types of medical services. If two or more goods are jointly used for consumption purposes, economists say that they are **complements in consumption**: Because the goods are consumed together, an increase in the price of one good inversely influences the demand for the other. For example, the demand for eyewear (that is, glasses or contact lenses) and the services of an optometrist are likely to be highly complementary. Normally, an individual has an eye examination before purchasing eyewear. If these two goods are complements in consumption, the demand for optometric services should increase in response to a drop in the price of eyewear. As a result, the demand curve for optometric services shifts to the right. Another example of a complementary relation exists between obstetric and pediatric services. An increase in the price of pediatric services should inversely influence the demand for obstetric services. If, for example, a woman postpones pregnancy because of the high cost of pediatric services, her demand for obstetric services also falls. The demand curve for obstetric services shifts to the left.

It is also possible for two or more goods to satisfy the same wants or provide the same characteristics. If that is the case, economists say that these goods are **substitutes in consumption**:

The demand for one good is directly related to a change in the price of a substitute good. For example, suppose physician services and hospital outpatient services are substitutes in consumption. As the price of outpatient services increases, the consumer is likely to alter consumption patterns and purchase more physician services because the price of a visit to the doctor is cheaper in relative terms. That causes the demand curve for physician services to shift to the right. Generic and brand-name drugs provide another example of two substitute goods. The demand for brand-name drugs should decrease with a decline in the price of generic drugs. If so, the demand curve for brand-name drugs shifts to the left. Finally, eyeglasses and contact lenses are likely to be substitutes in consumption.

Time costs also influence the quantity demanded of medical services. Time costs include the monetary cost of travel, such as bus fare or gasoline, plus the opportunity cost of time. The opportunity cost of an individual's time represents the dollar value of the activities the person forgoes when acquiring medical services. For example, if a plumber who earns $50 an hour takes two hours off from work to visit a dentist, the opportunity cost of the time equals $100. The implication is that the opportunity cost of time is directly related to a person's wage rate. Given time costs, it is not surprising that children and elderly people often fill doctors' waiting rooms. Time costs can accrue while traveling to and from a medical provider, waiting to see the provider, and experiencing delays in securing an appointment. In other words, travel costs increase the farther an individual has to travel to see a physician, the longer the wait at the doctor's office, and the longer the delay in getting an appointment. It stands to reason that the demand for medical care falls as time costs increase (that is, as the demand curve shifts to the left).

The Relationship between Health Insurance and the Demand for Medical Care

The growth of health insurance coverage is one of the most significant developments in the health care field over the past several decades. It has had a profound influence on the allocation of resources within the medical care market, primarily through its impact on the out-of-pocket prices of health care services. Out-of-pocket payments for health care dropped from almost half of total expenditures in 1960 to approximately one-seventh in 2003. Even more striking, out-of-pocket payments for hospital care fell from 20.7 percent in 1960 to a mere 3.2 percent in 2003. Given that various features are associated with health insurance policies, it is impossible to discuss the economic implications of each one. Here we will focus on three of the more common features of health insurance policies: coinsurance, copayments, and deductibles.

Coinsurance and Copayments. Many health insurance plans, particularly private plans, have a **coinsurance** component. Under a coinsurance plan, the consumer pays some fixed percentage of the cost of health care and the insurance carrier picks up the other portion. For example, under a plan with a coinsurance rate of 20 percent (a common arrangement), the consumer pays 20 cents out of every dollar spent on health care and the carrier picks up the remaining 80 cents. As you can imagine, an insurance plan like this one has a significant impact on the demand for health care because it effectively lowers the out-of-pocket price of health care by 80 percent.

Let's begin our discussion of coinsurance coverage by looking at the demand curve for medical care from an alternative perspective. We normally think of the demand curve as revealing the amount of a good that a consumer is willing and able to buy at various prices. However, a

FIGURE 5–4
The Demand Curve for Physician Visits with Coinsurance

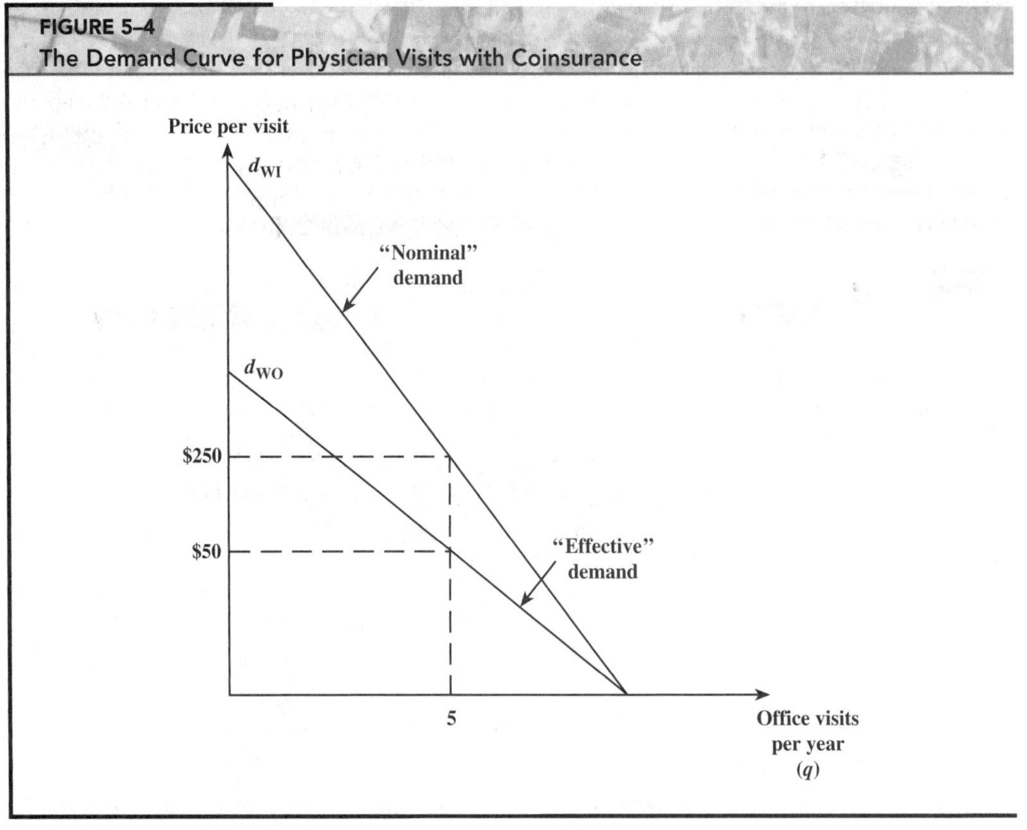

The graph illustrates how a coinsurance health plan impacts the individual demand curve for physician visits. The demand curve labeled d_{WO} is the individual's effective demand without coinsurance while the demand curve labeled d_{WI} is with coinsurance. The nominal demand curve d_{WI} traces out the total price for various physician visits and captures that portion paid by consumers as out-of-pocket payments as well as that portion paid by the insurance carrier. If you draw a vertical line from any point on the nominal demand curve to the horizontal axis, you can break down the amount paid by consumers (from the horizontal axis to the d_{WO} curve) and the amount paid by the insurance carrier (the wedge between the d_{WI} and d_{WO} curves). As the coinsurance rate falls, d_{WI} rotates upward and pivots off the point where the two curves cross the horizontal axis.

demand curve also shows the consumer's willingness to pay (or marginal benefit) for each unit of a good. The negative slope of the curve indicates that the willingness to pay falls as more of the good is consumed due to the law of diminishing marginal utility.

For example, the demand curve d_{WO} (WO = without insurance) in Figure 5–4 represents the consumer's demand or willingness to pay for office visits in the absence of health insurance coverage. This "effective" demand curve reveals that the consumer is willing to pay $50 for the fifth office visit. If $50 is the market price paid by the consumer, she visits the physician five times during the year in the process of maximizing utility because any additional office visits do not yield benefits that compensate for their higher out-of-pocket costs. Notice that the consumer's willingness to pay for the first four visits, as revealed by the effective demand curve, exceeds the market price of $50. The difference between the willingness to pay and the market price paid is referred to as a customer surplus and, in this example, reflects the net benefits received from visiting the doctor the first four times.[4]

Now suppose the consumer acquires a health insurance plan that requires her to pay a certain fraction, C_0, of the actual price, P. In this case, the insurance coverage drives a wedge between the willingness to pay, or effective demand, and the actual price, or "nominal" demand, for the office visits. Because the utility-maximizing consumer determines the optimal number of times to visit the physician by equating her willingness to pay (or marginal benefit) to the out-of-pocket price (marginal cost), the relationship between the actual and out-of-pocket price can be specified by the following equation:

$$P_W = C_0 P. \tag{5–3}$$

Here P_W stands for the consumer's willingness to pay for the last visit, and C_0 represents the coinsurance amount. If we solve Equation 5–3 for the actual price, we get

$$P = P_W / C_0. \tag{5–4}$$

Because the coinsurance, C_0, is less than 1, it follows that the actual price paid, or nominal demand, for office visits is greater than the out-of-pocket price the consumer pays. For example, if she is willing to pay \$50 for five visits to a doctor and the coinsurance is 20 percent of the full price, the actual price equals \$250 per visit, or \$50/0.2.

The nominal demand curve labeled d_{WI} (WI = with insurance) in Figure 5–4 reflects the total price paid for medical services that takes into account the coinsurance paid by the insured. The vertical distance between d_{WI} and the horizontal axis represents the total price for office visits. That can be broken down into the amount the consumer pays and the amount the insurance carrier pays. The portion of the total price the consumer pays as an out-of-pocket payment equals the distance between the horizontal axis and the d_{WO} demand curve. The remaining distance between the two curves represents the amount the insurance carrier pays. It represents the wedge that coinsurance drives between the consumer's willingness to pay, or effective demand, and the total price paid, or nominal demands.

It is easy to see from this analysis that a reduction in the coinsurance rate causes the nominal demand curve d_{WI} to rotate clockwise and pivot off the point where d_{WO} crosses the horizontal axis. At a zero willingness-to-pay price, insurance has no bearing on quantity demanded because medical care is a free good to the individual. In addition, the nominal demand curve d_{WI} becomes steeper as the coinsurance, C_0, decreases in value as indicated by Equation 5–4. That makes intuitive sense, because we expect the consumer to become less sensitive to changes in the total price as the coinsurance declines.

In the case where the consumer has full coverage ($C_0 = 0$), the nominal demand curve d_{WI} rotates out to its fullest extent and becomes completely vertical. This is shown in Figure 5–5. Because the consumer faces a zero price, she consumes medical care as though it were a free good, when in reality it has a nonzero price. Equation 5–4 can be used to illustrate that point. As C_0 approaches zero, the total price is potentially infinity even when P_W equals zero.

Coinsurance should not be confused with a copayment. A **copayment** represents a fixed amount paid by the consumer that is independent of the market price or actual costs of medical care. For example, a person may be required to pay \$10 for each office visit regardless of the actual

4. As discussed in Chapter 8, market price considers both supply and demand conditions. The demand curves in Figure 5–4 represent the effective and nominal demands of an individual. Individual demands must be horizontally summed to arrive at a market demand and then interacted with supply to determine the market price.

FIGURE 5–5
The Demand Curve for Physician Visits with 100 Percent Coverage

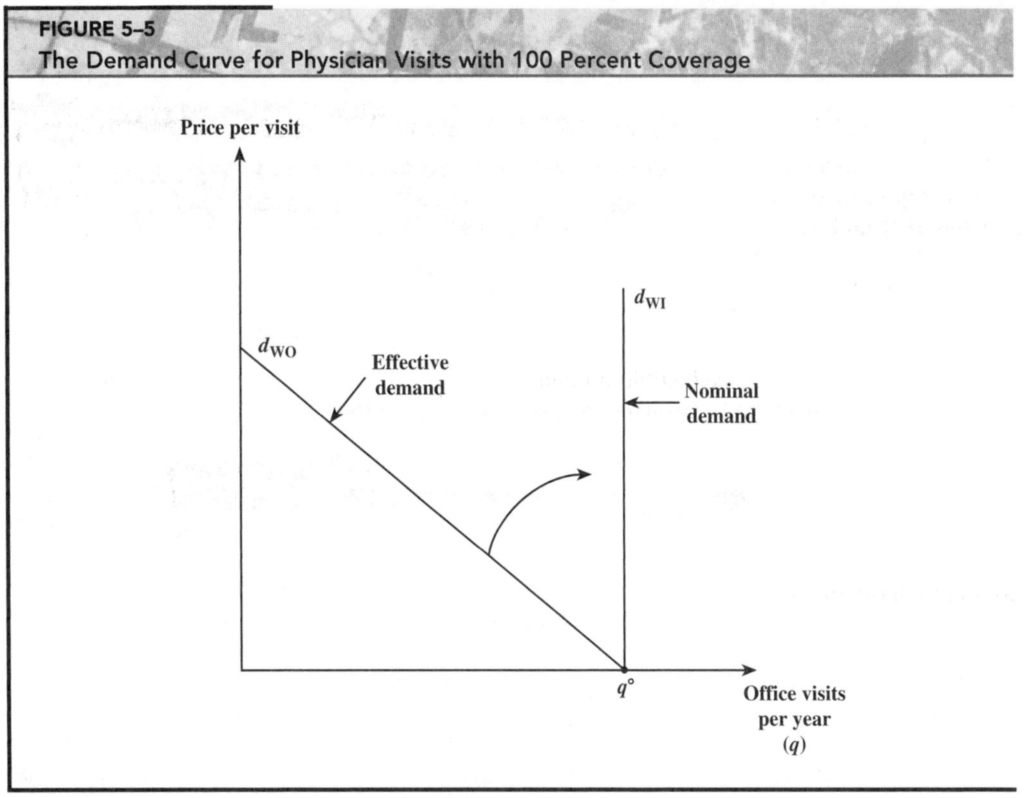

The graph illustrates the situation in which the individual has complete medical coverage and the coinsurance rate is zero. Notice that the nominal demand curve is vertical because the individual faces a zero out-of-pocket price and visits the physician without regard to the actual price.

fee negotiated by the health insurer with the physician. Like a lower coinsurance rate, a reduced copayment results in a movement down the effective demand curve and typically leads to greater quantity of care demanded. But unlike a change in the coinsurance rate, a change in the copayment does not cause a rotation of the nominal demand because the consumer's portion of the bill is independent rather than proportional to nominal demand (that is, the actual price paid).

Also unlike coinsurance, a copayment does not automatically change with an adjustment in the costs of providing medical care. For example, suppose, in response to higher production costs, a physician negotiates a higher price with the insurer for each office visit so that the market price increases from $100 to $150. An insured individual who is responsible for paying 20 percent of the cost now faces a $10 increase in his coinsurance from $20 to $30 per office visit. However, an insured individual who is required to pay a copayment of $10 per office visit is unaffected by the higher negotiated price for an office visit (at least until the insurance policy is renegotiated). Thus, compared to a copayment, coinsurance makes consumers more sensitive to the actual market price of medical care.

Deductibles. Many insurance policies have a deductible whereby the consumer must pay out of pocket a fixed amount of health care costs per calendar year before coverage begins. For example, the plan may call for the individual to pay the initial $200 of health care expenses with a limit of $500 per family per year. Once the deductible is met, the insurance carrier pays all or some portion of the remaining medical bills, depending on how the plan is specified. From the insurance carrier's perspective, the purpose of a deductible is to lower costs. This is accomplished in two ways.

First, the deductible is likely to lower administrative costs because fewer small claims will be filed over the course of a year. Second, the deductible is likely to have a negative impact on the demand for health care. The extent to which this is true, however, is difficult to determine and depends on such factors as the cost of the medical episode, the point in time when the medical care is demanded, and the probability of needing additional medical care for the remainder of the period. To illustrate, assume a new deductible is put in place at the beginning of each calendar year and once the deductible is met, the consumer has full medical coverage. It is easy to see that the extent to which a deductible influences the demand for medical services for any one medical episode is likely to be inversely related to the cost of the medical services involved. For example, if the consumer faces a potentially large medical bill for an operation, the existence of a deductible is likely to have little impact on demand. This is because in relative terms, the deductible represents very little money. On the other hand, a deductible may play a crucial role in the decision to purchase medical care if the cost of such care is relatively inexpensive. In this case, the out-of-pocket cost is substantial relative to the total cost, and the consumer may elect not to purchase the medical care or postpone the purchase to a later date.

It is slightly more difficult to understand how the health of the individual, along with the time of the year, influences the impact of a deductible on demand. The best way to explain this is with an example. Consider a normally healthy individual who contracts the flu late in November and has incurred no medical expenses up to this point. Under these circumstances, he may be less inclined to visit the doctor. This is because he will have little opportunity to take advantage of the fact that health care is a free good after he makes his initial visit to the physician and fulfills the deductible. On the other hand, this same individual is much more likely to visit the physician if he catches the flu early in February and his overall health is such that he can expect to visit the physician three or four more times over the remainder of the year. By visiting the doctor and meeting the deductible, he lowers the cost of any future visits to zero for the rest of the year. Therefore, a deductible is likely to have the greatest negative impact on the demand for medical care when the cost of the medical episode is low, the need for care is late in the calendar year, and the probability of needing future care is slight because the person is in good health.

Moral Hazard

Before we leave the subject of the impact of insurance on the demand for medical care, we need to introduce the concept of moral hazard. **Moral hazard** refers to the situation in which consumers alter their behavior when provided with health insurance. For example, health insurance may induce consumers to take fewer precautions to prevent illnesses or to shop very little for the best medical prices. In addition, insured consumers may purchase more medical care than they otherwise would have without insurance coverage. Let's illustrate this point by referring to Figure 5–4. According to the graph, a consumer without insurance purchases five units of medical services at a price of $50 per unit. If that consumer acquires full medical coverage such that the insurer's coinsurance rate, C_0, equals zero, the quantity demanded of medical care increases to the point where the demand curve crosses the horizontal axis. At this point, the consumer consumes medical care as though it were a free good because she faces a zero price. Thus, any extension of medical insurance coverage has the potential to increase the consumption of medical care because consumers no longer pay the full price. The availability and extensiveness of health insurance may have a profound effect on medical care expenditures. Chapter 6 examines the implications of moral hazard in more detail.

Noneconomic Determinants of the Demand for Medical Care

Four general noneconomic factors influence the demand for medical services: tastes and preferences, physical and mental profile, state of health, and quality of care.

Taste and preference factors include personal characteristics such as marital status, education, and lifestyle, which might affect how people value their healthy time (that is, their marginal utility of health), or might lead to a greater preference for certain types of medical services. Marital status is likely to impact the demand for health care in the marketplace primarily through its effect on the production of health care in the home. A married individual is likely to demand less medical care, particularly hospital care, because of the availability of a spouse to care for him at home, such as when recuperating from an illness.

The impact of education on the demand for medical care is difficult to predict. On the one hand, a consumer with additional education may be more willing to seek medical care to slow down the rate of health depreciation because that consumer may have a better understanding of the potential impact of medical care on health. As an example, an individual with a high level of education may be more inclined to visit a dentist for periodic examinations. Thus, we should observe a direct relation between educational attainment and demand.

On the other hand, an individual with a high level of education may make more efficient use of home-produced health care services to slow down the rate of health depreciation and, as a result, demand fewer medical care services. For example, such an individual may be more likely to understand the value of preventive medicine (such as proper diet and exercise). In addition, the individual may be more likely to recognize the early warning signs of illness and be more apt to visit a health care provider when symptoms first occur. As a result, health care problems are addressed early when treatment has a greater probability of success and is less costly. That means that we should observe an inverse relation between the level of education and the demand for medical care, particularly acute care.

Finally, lifestyle variables, such as whether the individual smokes cigarettes or drinks alcohol in excessive amounts, affect health status and consequently the amount of health care demanded. For example, a person may try to compensate for the detrimental health impact of smoking by consuming more health care services. That translates into an increased demand for medical care.

The *profile* variable considers the impact of such factors as gender, race/ethnicity, and age on the demand for medical services. For example, females generally demand more health care services than males primarily because of childbearing. In addition, certain diseases, such as cardiovascular disease, osteoporosis, immunologic diseases (such as thyroid disease and rheumatoid arthritis), mental disorders, and Alzheimer's disease, are more prevalent in women than men (Miller, 1994). Age also plays a vital role in determining the demand for medical care. As we stated in Chapter 2, as an individual ages, the overall stock of health depreciates more rapidly. To compensate for this loss in health, the demand for medical care is likely to increase with age, at least beyond the middle years (the demand curve shifts to the right). Thus, we should observe a direct relation between age and the demand for medical care.

State of health controls for the fact that sicker people demand more medical services, everything else held constant. As you might expect, health status and the demand for health care are also likely to be directly related to the severity of the illness. For example, a person who is born with a medical problem, such as hemophilia, is likely to have a much higher than average demand for medical care. In economics jargon, an individual who is endowed with less health is likely to demand more medical care in an attempt to augment the overall stock of health.

Finally, although nebulous and impossible to quantify, the *quality of care* is also likely to impact the demand for medical care. Because quality cannot be measured directly, it is usually assumed to be positively related to the amount and types of inputs used to produce medical care. Feldstein (1967, pp. 158–62) defines the quality of care as "a catch-all term to denote the general level of amenities to patients as well as additional expenditures on professional staff and equipment." For example, a consumer may feel that larger hospitals provide better-quality care than smaller ones because they have more specialists on staff along with more sophisticated equipment. Or, that same individual may think that physicians who have graduated from prestigious medical schools provide a higher quality of care than those who have not. It matters little whether the difference in the quality of medical care provided is real or illusory. What matters is that the consumer perceives that differences in quality actually exist.

With regard to the previous example, it is certainly not the case that larger hospitals provide better care for all types of hospital services. However, if the consumer generally feels that larger hospitals provide better services, the demand for medical services at larger hospitals will be higher than at smaller ones. As Feldstein's definition indicates, quality can also depend on things that have little to do with the actual production of effective medical care. For example, the consumer may prefer a physician who has a pleasant office with a comfortable waiting room along with courteous nurses. Thus, any increase in the quality of care provided is likely to increase that consumer's demand for medical care regardless of whether it affects the actual production of health care.

Before we move on, we must distinguish between a movement along the demand curve and a shift of the curve. A change in the price of medical services generates a change in the quantity demanded, and this is represented by a movement along the demand curve. If any of the other factors change, such as income or time costs, the demand curve for medical services shifts. This shift is referred to as a change in demand. Thus, a change in the quantity demanded is illustrated by a movement along the demand curve, while a change in demand is illustrated by a shift of the curve.

In summary, let's review the variables we expect to influence an individual's demand for medical care. Economic theory indicates that the demand equation should look something like the following:

(5–5) Quantity demanded = *f*(out-of-pocket price, income, time costs, prices of substitutes and complements, tastes and preferences, profile, state of health, and quality of care)

Equation 5–5 states that the quantity demanded of medical services is a function of, or depends on, the general factors listed. Note that a change in the first factor results in a movement along a given demand curve, whereas an adjustment in the other factors produce a shift of the demand curve. A rightward shift indicates a greater demand and a leftward shift reveals a lower demand.

The Market Demand for Medical Care

Up to now, we have been discussing the individual's demand for medical care services. The market demand for medical care, such as physician services, equals the total demand by all consumers in a given market. In graphical terms, we can construct the market demand curve for medical care services by horizontally summing the individual demand curves. This curve represents the amount of medical services that the entire market is willing and able to purchase at every given price. For example, if the average price of a visit to a doctor is $50 and at this price consumer A is willing to see a physician three times over the course of a year while consumer B is willing to make four visits, the total, or market, demand for physician services is seven visits per year at $50 per visit. The market demand curve is downward sloping for the same reasons the individual demand curves are downward sloping. In addition, the factors that shift the individual demand curves also shift the overall market demand curve, providing the changes take place on a marketwide basis. The market demand curve also shifts if the overall number of consumers in the market increases or decreases. For example, the demand for medical care in a particular community may increase if an influx of new residents occurs. This causes the market demand curve to shift to the right.

The development of a market demand curve allows us to distinguish between the intensive and extensive margins. The **intensive margin** refers to how much more or less of a product consumers buy when its price changes. The **extensive margin** captures how many more or fewer people buy a product when its price changes. Obviously, this is an important distinction to make for a product like medical care. Many medical purchases such as surgeries happen only once for a particular individual. As another example, an individual can have a particular tooth pulled only once. This is also a one-shot purchase that either happens or does not happen. If the price of tooth extraction falls, however, we may still observe a inverse relationship between the price and number of teeth extracted. That is because at the extensive margin, more consumers elect to purchase this onetime form of dental services as price falls. Consequently, quantity demanded may increase with a reduction in price because of changes that occur at the intensive and extensive margins.

The Fuzzy Demand Curve

Up to this point, we have assumed the market demand curve for medical care is a well-defined line, implying a precise relation between price and quantity demanded. In reality this is usually not the case, and we need to refer to the derivation of the demand curve for medical care to see why. Recall that the demand for medical care is a derived demand and depends on the demand for health and the extent to which medical care influences the production of health. The relation between medical care and health, however, is far from exact. That is because there is a considerable lack of medical knowledge concerning the efficacy of certain types of medical interventions. As a result, health care providers disagree about the treatment of some types of medical problems, and the demand for medical services becomes fuzzy. For example, there is debate among physicians concerning when surgery is necessary for elderly males with prostate cancer.

In addition, in some instances consumers may lack the information or medical knowledge they need to make informed choices. Consequently, consumers tend to rely heavily on the advice of their physicians when making such decisions as when a particular medical test or surgery is necessary. The implication is that physicians rather than consumers choose medical services, which makes the demand curve fuzzier. Further complicating matters is the inability to accurately measure medical care, an issue we touched on earlier. For example, how do we measure the quantity of medical care produced during a one-hour therapy session with a psychiatrist?

All these factors combined make it extremely difficult to accurately delineate the relation between the price and the quantity demanded of medical care. In other words, the relation between price and quantity demanded is rather fuzzy (Aaron, 1991). A more accurate depiction of the relation between price and quantity may not be a well-defined line but a gray band similar to the one depicted in Figure 5–6.

FIGURE 5–6
The Fuzzy Demand Curve for Medical Care

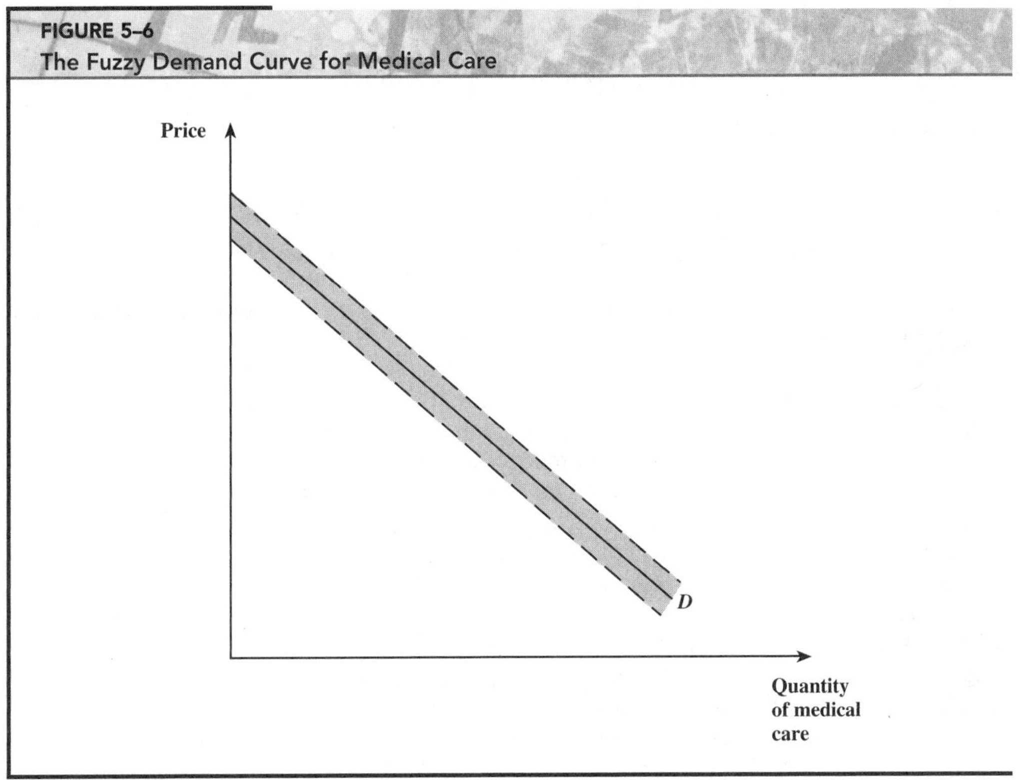

The gray band represents the possible fuzziness of the demand for medical care given uncertainty and the role of the physician.

Two implications are associated with the fuzzy demand curve. First, for a given price, we may observe some variation in the quantity or types of medical services rendered. Indeed, researchers have documented variations in physician practice styles across geographical areas (see, for example, Phelps, 1992); we take up that discussion in Chapter 12. Second, for a given quantity or type of medical service, we are likely to witness price differences. For example, Feldstein (1988) reported a substantial variation in physician fees for similar procedures in the same geographical area. We must stress, however, that the existence of the band is unlikely to detract from the inverse relation between the price and the quantity demanded of medical care as suggested by the empirical evidence that follows.

ELASTICITIES

Economic theory gives us insights into the factors that influence the demand for medical care along with the direction of their influence. For example, we know that if the price of physician services increases by 15 percent, the quantity demanded falls. But by how much does it fall? Is there any way to determine whether the decrease is substantial or negligible? The answer is yes, with the help of a measure economists call an *elasticity*. Elasticity measures that responsiveness of quantity demanded to a change in an independent factor.

Own-Price Elasticity of Demand

The most common elasticity is the **own-price elasticity of demand.** This measure gauges the extent to which consumers alter their consumption of a good or service when its own price changes. The formula looks like this:

(5–6) $$E_D = \%\Delta Q_D / \%\Delta P,$$

where E_D denotes the price elasticity of demand, $\%\Delta Q_D$ represents the percentage change in quantity demanded, and $\%\Delta P$ is the percentage change in price. As you can see from the formula, E_D is a simple ratio that equals the percentage change in quantity demanded divided by the percentage change in price. Because elasticity is specified as a ratio of two percentage changes, it is scale free. This makes it much easier to compare elasticities across different goods. For example, we can compare the price elasticity of demand for physician services with that for nursing home care and not have to concern ourselves with the fact that the demand for physician services is usually measured in terms of the number of visits while the demand for nursing home care is measured in terms of the number of inpatient days.[5]

The value of E_D is negative and reflects the inverse relationship between price and quantity demanded. In economics, the normal practice is to take the absolute value of the price elasticity of demand measure, or $|E_D|$, and eliminate the minus sign. If the price elasticity of demand is greater than 1 in absolute terms ($|E_D|>1$), the demand for the product is referred to as price elastic. In arithmetic terms, $|E_D| > 1$ if the absolute value of the percentage change in price is smaller than the absolute value of the change in the quantity demanded, or $|\%\Delta P| < |\%\Delta Q_D|$. For example, if the price elasticity of demand for dental services equals 1.2, this means the quantity consumed falls by 12 percent if the price of dental care increases by 10 percent, *ceteris paribus*.

The price elasticity of demand is referred to as **inelastic** if $|E_D| < 1$ but greater than zero. In this case, $|\%\Delta P| > |\%\Delta Q_D|$, or the percentage change in price is greater than the percentage in quantity demanded in absolute value terms. For example, if the elasticity of demand for physician services equals 0.6, a 10 percent decrease in price leads to a 6 percent increase in quantity demanded. If $|E_D|$ happens to equal 1 because $|\%\Delta P|$ equals $|\%\Delta Q_D|$, the price elasticity of demand is **unit elastic.** This implies that a 10 percent decrease in the price of the product leads to a 10 percent increase in the quantity demanded.

A demand curve that is vertical is said to be **perfectly inelastic** because no change occurs in the quantity demanded when the price changes. In mathematical terms, E_D equals zero because $\%\Delta Q_D$ equals zero. At the other extreme, if the demand curve is horizontal, it is referred to as being **perfectly elastic** and $|E_D|$ equals infinity (∞). Any change in price leads to an infinite change in the quantity demanded.

It stands to reason that the more elastic the demand for the product, the greater the response of quantity to a given change in price. Compare the effects of a 10 percent decrease in price on two goods—one with a price elasticity of -0.1 and another with a price elasticity of -2.6. In the first case, the quantity demanded increases by only 1 percent, while in the second case, it increases by 26 percent. We can also use the elasticity of demand to make inferences regarding the slope of the demand curve. Generally, the more elastic the demand for the product, the flatter the demand curve at any given price. This also means the curve is relatively steep at any given point for an inelastic demand. Consider the two linear demand curves that intersect at point P_0, Q_0 in Figure 5–7. If the price of the product increases to P_1, the quantity demanded decreases to Q_a off the flat curve

5. The *point elasticity* formula can be used to calculate the elasticity of demand if the changes in the variables are small. The formula equals $(\Delta Q_D/Q_D)/(\Delta P/P)$. For readers with a background in calculus, it equals $(dQ_D/Q_D)/(dP/P)$ if the changes are infinitesimally small.

FIGURE 5–7
The Elasticity of Demand and the Slope of the Demand Curve

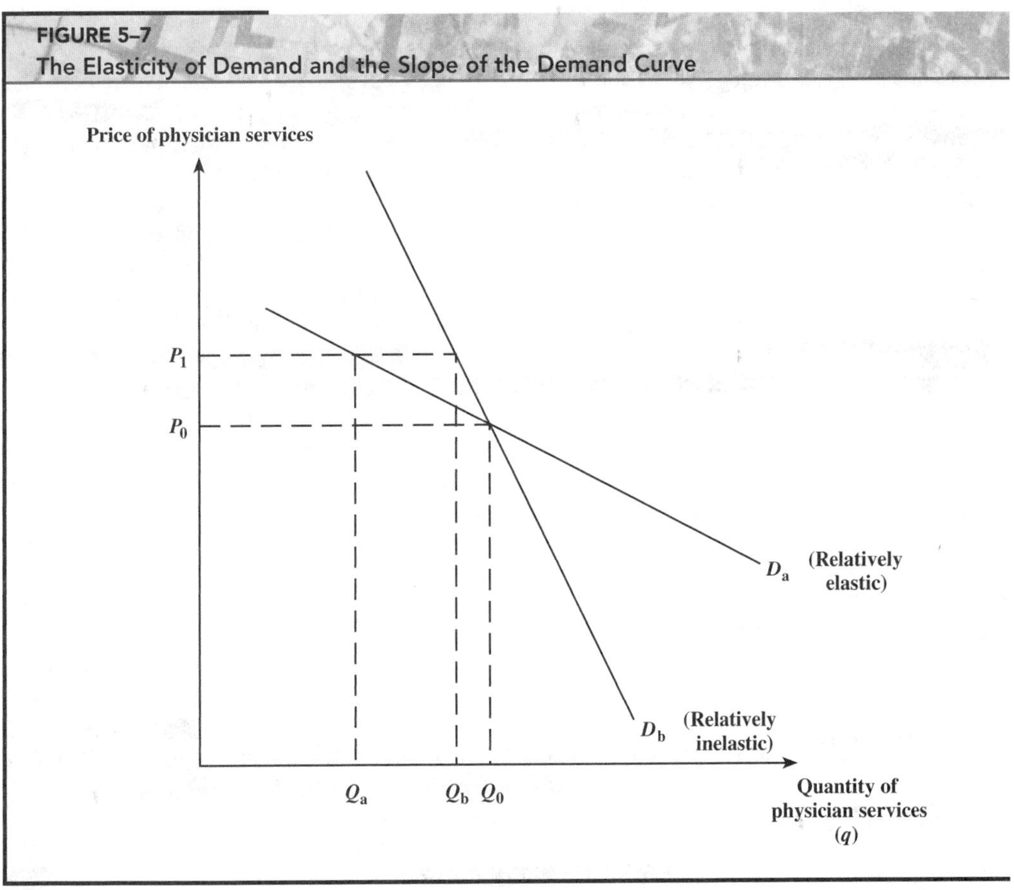

The steep demand curve, D_b, is relatively inelastic and illustrates that an increase in price from P_0 to P_1 generates only a modest decrease in quantity demanded from Q_0 to Q_b. The flatter demand curve, D_a, is relatively elastic and, in this case, the same increase in price for P_0 to P_1 generates a much larger decrease in quantity demanded from Q_0 to Q_a.

TABLE 5–1
A Summary of the Own-Price Elasticity of Demand

Perfectly Inelastic	Inelastic	Unit Elastic	Elastic	Perfectly Elastic
$\lvert E_D \rvert = 0$ $\%\Delta Q_D = 0$	$0 < \lvert E_D \rvert < 1$ $\lvert \%\Delta Q_D \rvert < \lvert \%\Delta P \rvert$	$\lvert E_D \rvert = 1$ $\lvert \%\Delta Q_D \rvert = \lvert \%\Delta P \rvert$	$1 < \lvert E_D \rvert < \infty$ $\lvert \%\Delta Q_D \rvert > \lvert \%\Delta P \rvert$	$\lvert E_D \rvert = \infty$ $\%\Delta Q_D = \infty$

(D_a) and to Q_b off the steep curve (D_b). Therefore, the same percentage increase in price generates a smaller percentage decrease in the quantity demanded for the steeper curve D_b than for the flatter curve D_a at a similar price of P_0. This means demand must be more price elastic for curve D_a than for curve D_b over the range P_0 to P_1. Table 5–1 summarizes our discussion thus far on price elasticity of demand.

The own-price elasticity of demand varies greatly across products, and economists point to several factors that determine its value. Among the factors most often mentioned are the portion of the consumer's budget allocated to the good, the amount of time involved in the purchasing decision, the extent to which the good is a necessity, and the availability of substitutes. Briefly, as the portion of a consumer's budget allocated to a good increases, the consumer is likely to become much more sensitive to price changes. Demand should therefore become more elastic. An increase in the decision-making time frame is also likely to make demand more elastic. If the consumer has more time to make informed choices, he or she is likely to react more strongly to price changes. Because the consumer typically pays a small portion of the cost of medical services because of insurance, and because medical services are sometimes of an urgent nature, these two considerations suggest that in many cases, the demand for medical services is inelastic with respect to price.

If a good is a necessity, such as a basic foodstuff, the own-price elasticity should be relatively inelastic. The product is purchased with little regard for price because it is needed. Basic phone service might be considered another example of a necessity. Because our society depends so heavily on the phone as a form of communication, it is difficult to imagine a household functioning effectively without one. Naturally, basic health care falls into the same category. If an individual needs a particular medical service, such as an operation or a drug, and if not having it greatly affects the quality of life, we can expect that person's demand to be inelastic with respect to price. In addition, when a person needs a particular medical service in a life-or-death situation, demand is likely to be perfectly inelastic because the medical service must be purchased regardless of price if the person has sufficient income.

Given that many medical services are necessities, we expect the overall demand for medical services to be somewhat inelastic. A word of caution, however: This does not mean the amount of health care demanded does not react to changes in price. Rather, it means a given percentage change in price generates a small percentage change in the quantity demanded of medical services. For some types of medical care, however, demand may be more elastic. Elective medical care, such as cosmetic surgery, may fall into this category, because in most instances it is considered a luxury rather than a necessity. As a result, price may play an important role in the decision to have the surgery. To a lesser degree, dentist services and eyewear might fall into this category. In fact, any medical service that can be postponed is likely to display some degree of price elasticity.

The availability of substitutes is another determinant of price elasticity. As we saw earlier, various types of medical services may serve as substitutes for one another. The larger the number of substitutes, the greater the opportunity to do some comparison shopping. As a result, the quantity demanded of any medical service is likely to be more sensitive to price changes when alternative means of acquiring medical care are available. The own-price elasticity of demand for any given product should be directly related to the number of substitutes available. Stated another way, demand should become more price elastic as the number of substitutes expands. One implication is that the demand for an individual medical service or an individual medical care provider is likely to be more elastic than the market demand for medical care.

One more point concerning the elasticity of demand needs to be discussed before we leave this subject. The own-price elasticity of demand can be used to predict what happens to total health expenditures if price increases or decreases. Total revenues (or total expenditures, from the consumer's perspective) equal price times quantity. In mathematical notation,

$$\text{TR} = PQ_{\text{D}}, \tag{5–7}$$

where TR represents total revenue. Demand theory tells us that as the price of a product increases, the quantity demanded decreases, or that P and Q_{D} move in opposite directions. Whether total revenue increases or decreases when the price changes is dictated by the relative rates at which both variables change, or the elasticity of demand. Consider an increase in the price of physician services where demand is inelastic. This means that $|\%\Delta Q_D| < |\%\Delta P|$, or that the percentage increase in price is larger than the percentage decrease in quantity demanded in absolute value terms. In terms of Equation 5–7, P increases faster than Q_D falls. This means total revenue must increase with a higher price. If demand happens to be elastic, the opposite occurs: Quantity demanded falls faster than price increases, and, as a result, total revenue decreases. No change occurs in total revenue when demand is unit elastic because the increase in price is matched by the same percentage decrease in quantity demanded. We leave it to you to work out the implications of a price decrease on total revenue when demand is elastic, inelastic, and unit elastic.

Other Types of Elasticity

The concept of elasticity can be used to measure the sensitivity of quantity demanded to other demand-side factors as well. The **income elasticity of demand** represents the percentage change in quantity demanded divided by the percentage change in income, or $E_Y = \%\Delta Q_D/\%\Delta Y$, where $\%\Delta Y$ equals the percentage change in income. It quantifies the extent to which the demand for a product changes when real income changes. If E_Y is positive, the good is referred to as a *normal good* because any increase in income leads to an increase in quantity demanded. For example, if E_Y equals 0.78, this means a 10 percent increase in income causes the quantity consumed to increase by 7.8 percent. An *inferior good* is one for which E_Y is negative and an increase in income leads to a decrease in the amount consumed. For most types of medical care, the income elasticity of demand should be larger than zero.

The **cross-price elasticity** (E_C) measures the extent to which the demand for a product changes when the price of another good is altered. In mathematical terms, $E_C = \%\Delta Q_X/\%\Delta P_Z$, where the numerator represents the percentage change in the demand for good X and the denominator equals the percentage change in the price of good Z. If E_C is negative, we can infer that the two goods are complements in consumption. Returning to our earlier example, the cross-price elasticity between the demand for optometric services and the price of eyewear should be negative. If the price of eyewear increases, the demand for optometric services should drop. Two goods are substitutes in consumption when the cross-price elasticity is positive. For example, the cross-price elasticity of the demand for physician services with respect to the price of hospital outpatient services may turn out to be positive. Naturally, if E_C equals zero, the demand for the product is independent of the price of the other product.

EMPIRICAL ESTIMATION

Numerous studies have attempted to empirically quantify how various factors influence the demand for medical care. Although the studies varied widely in terms of methodology and scope of analysis, certain broad conclusions emerged. Generally, some form of Equation 5–5 is estimated with the use of regression analysis. Unfortunately, the dependent variable representing the amount of medical services consumed is very difficult to measure. Ideally, quantity demanded should capture both the utilization and the intensity of medical services. Data of these kinds are unavailable, so usually only some utilization measure, such as number of physician visits or hospital patient days, is used to measure the quantity demanded of medical services. Proxy variables are then included as independent variables to control for variations in quality. A failure to properly control for quality biases the results. That is because changes in demand may be attributed to changes in other variables when in fact they are the result of differences in the quality of care provided.

The measurement of the out-of-pocket price of medical care also presents a problem for economists. This problem has become more severe in recent years given the increasing role of third-party payers. In a perfect world, the out-of-pocket price of medical services should equal the amount the consumer pays after the impact of insurance has been considered. Unfortunately, such data are rarely available, and economists often have to resort to using such variables as the average price of medical services rendered. An additional variable is then included in the equation to control for the presence of health insurance. The price variable should negatively affect the demand for medical care, while the presence of insurance should positively influence quantity demanded.

An income variable is included to capture the impact of purchasing power on demand, while time cost variables control for the effects of travel and waiting costs on demand. We expect the income variable to have a positive effect on demand and the time cost variables to have a negative impact. The prices of various substitutes and complements in consumption should also be included in the regression equation. This has become even more important in recent years as medical markets have become more interrelated. For example, if we are trying to assess the quantity demanded of inpatient services at a hospital, we should control for the prices of hospital outpatient services (potentially a substitute service) and physician services (potentially a complementary service). The remaining factors (tastes and preferences, rate of health depreciation, stock of health, and quality of care) are referred to as *control variables* and capture the impact that various noneconomic factors may have on the demand for health care services.

Own-Price, Income, Cross-Price, and Time Cost Elasticity Estimates

Overall, the empirical literature on the elasticity of demand for primary health care is rich and spans the globe. Table 5–2 provides just a sample of the studies on the topic. Although the range of price elasticity estimates is broad, studies tend to find the demand for primary health care to be relatively inelastic. For example, studies using medical expenditures as the dependent variable find the own-price elasticity of demand to vary from −0.04 to −0.7. Other studies that look at the demand for hospital and physician services find similar results. Taken as a whole, the estimates suggest that the own-price elasticity of demand for primary health care hovers from −0.1 to −0.7, which means that a 10 percent increase in the out-of-pocket price of medical services leads to a 1 to 7 percent decrease in the quantity demanded. The inelastic estimates also imply that total expenditures on hospital and physician services increase with a greater out-of-pocket price, *ceteris paribus*.

In general, the research indicates that the demand for other types of medical care is slightly more price elastic than the demand for primary care. That is not at all surprising given that the percentage of out-of-pocket payments tend to be the lowest for hospital and physician services. Everything else held constant, consumers should become more price sensitive as the portion of the bill paid out of pocket increases. For example, Manning and Phelps (1979) found the demand for dental services to be slightly more price elastic and to vary by type of service provided and the sex and age of the patient. The price elasticity of demand for dental services by adult females appears to vary between −0.5 and −0.7, and the demand for dental services by adult males and children seems to be slightly more price elastic. The demand for nursing home services also appears to be more price elastic than primary medical services. Chiswick (1976) found the own-price elasticity for nursing home services to equal −2.3, and Lamberton et al. (1986) estimated that it equals −0.76. Finally, Headen (1993) found the own-price elasticity for the probability of entering a nursing home to be −0.7.

The empirical estimates for the income elasticity of demand vary widely and merit discussion. Studies using household, or individual, data generally find health care to be a normal good with an income elasticity below 1.0. These results are in direct contrast to studies that utilize country-level data to look at the relation between income and health care expenditures either over time or across countries. The goal of these studies is to ascertain how economic growth impacts national health care expenditures. Generally, these studies find the aggregate income elasticity to be slightly above 1. For example,

TABLE 5–2
The Price Elasticity of Demand for Health Care: Selected Studies

Dependent Variable	Study	Elasticity	Country
Medical Expenditures	Eichner (1998)	−0.62 to −0.75	United States
	Newhouse and the Insurance Experiment Group (1993)	−0.17 to −0.22	United States
	Phelps and Newhouse (1974)	−0.04 to −0.12	United States
	Rosett and Huang (1973)	−0.35 to −1.5	United States
	Van Vliet (2001)	−0.079	Netherlands
Hospital Care			
Admissions	Manning et al. (1987)	−0.1 to −0.2	United States
Hospital Inpatient	Davis and Russell (1972)	−0.32 to −0.46	United States
Hospital Outpatient	Davis and Russell (1972)	−1.0	United States
	Bhattacharya et al. (1996)	−0.12 to −0.54	Japan
Patient Days	Feldman and Dowd (1986)	−0.74 to −0.80	United States
Physician Visits	Cockx and Brasseur (2003)	−0.13 to −0.03	Belgium
Total and Elective Surgery	Cromwell and Mitchell (1986)	−0.14 and −0.17	United States
Nursing Home Care			
Probability of Entering a Nursing Home	Headen (1993)	−0.7	United States
Number of Patients	Nyman (1989)	−1.7	United States
Patient Days	Lamberton et al. (1986)	−0.76	United States
Number of Patients	Chiswick (1976)	−2.3	United States
Dental Services	Manning and Phelps (1979)	−0.5 to −0.7	United States
	Mueller and Monheit (1988)	−0.18	United States
Prescription Drugs			
Number	Smith (1993)	−0.10	United States
Expenditures	Contoyannis et al. (2005)	−0.12 to −0.16	Canada

Newhouse (1977) finds the income elasticity to range between 1.13 and 1.31, while Parkin et al. (1987) estimate the rate to be slightly below +1. Finally, Leu (1986), Gerdtham et al. (1992), and Murray et al. (1994) agree with Newhouse and find the aggregate income elasticity to be above 1.

This difference between the micro and macro estimates is interesting and deserves explanation. According to Newhouse, the difference exists because, for example, within the United States at any point in time the average consumer pays only a small portion of the price of medical care (approximately 14 percent in 2003), while over time the country as a whole must pay the full price of health care. As the out-of-pocket price of health care falls for the average consumer, the income elasticity should also fall because the consumer is less conscious of price. For example, if the out-of-pocket price of health care falls to zero, then the average individual is going to consume health care regardless of income. The income elasticity in the extreme equals zero. The country, as a whole, however, must face the entire burden of the cost of health care and, as a result, is going to be much more sensitive to price and income.

One of the more interesting questions concerning this research has to do with whether health care is a luxury good. Economists define a luxury good as one that has an income elasticity above 1.0. In this case, an increase in income leads to an ever larger increase in the quantity consumed of the good. For example, assume that the income elasticity of a good equals 1.5. In this case, a 10 percent increase in income leads to a 15 percent increase in the consumption of the good. Naturally, this means that the portion of one's budget allocated to the consumption of the good also increases with income.

If the aggregate income elasticity of health care is above 1.0, this may provide a demand-side explanation as to why health care expenditures in the United States as a portion of national income have increased over the past few decades. As the U.S. economy grew over the past few decades and income per capita expanded, the nation allocated a greater portion of its income to health care because it is a luxury good. Consequently, the health care sector received a larger slice of the economic pie.

Time costs also appear to have a significant impact on the demand for medical services. In fact, research indicates that the travel time elasticity of demand is approximately equal to the own-price elasticity of demand. According to Acton (1975) and Phelps and Newhouse (1974), the travel time elasticity of demand ranges from −0.14 to −0.51. Using a data set generated in the United Kingdom, Gravelle et al. (2002) found elasticity of admissions with respect to distance to equal −0.35. Taken together, these studies suggest that a 10 percent increase in travel time reduces the quantity demanded for medical services by roughly 3 percent. It also appears that consumers place a value on the time spent waiting for medical services. McCarthy (1985) found the wait time elasticity to range from −0.36 to −1.14, while Martin and Smith (1999) found it to equal −0.20. In addition, Gravelle et al. (2002) estimated the elasticity of admissions with respect to waiting time to equal −0.25. Time costs also influence the decision to acquire medical care; Frank et al. (1995) found the elasticity of travel time costs on the probability of a timely completion of childhood immunization to be roughly −0.08.

The extent to which various types of medical services serve as substitutes or complements in consumption is not clear at this time. For example, there appears to be little consensus as to whether inpatient and outpatient hospital services are substitutes or complements. Davis and Russell (1972) found the cross-price elasticity between the price of inpatient services and number of outpatient visits to vary between 0.85 and 1.46, indicating that they are substitutes. These results were later qualitatively confirmed by Gold (1984). Thus, as the price of inpatient services at a hospital increases, consumers rely more on outpatient services to save money. Freiberg and Scutchfield (1976), on the other hand, found that no substitution occurs between these two types of hospital services. At the other extreme, Manning et al. (1987) suggested that they are complements in consumption. A similar debate in the literature concerns whether physician and hospital inpatient or outpatient services are substitutes or complements.

The Impact of Insurance on the Demand for Medical Care

The growth of health insurance, both public and private, has had a profound impact on the demand for medical care. Instead of reviewing the results from the many studies that analyzed the impact of insurance on the demand for health care, we will focus on a study conducted by the

TABLE 5–3
Sample Means for Annual Use of Medical Care per Capita

Plan*	Face-to-Face Visits	Outpatient Expenses (1984 $)	Inpatient Dollars (1984 $)	Total Expenses (1984 $)	Probability of Using Any Medical Services
Free	4.55	$340	$409	$749	86.8
25%	3.33	260	373	634	78.8
50%	3.03	224	450	674	77.2
95%	2.73	203	315	518	67.7
Individual deductible	3.02	235	373	608	72.3

*The *chi*-square test was used to test the null hypothesis of no difference among the five plan means. In each instance, the *chi*-square statistic was significant to at least the 5 percent level. The only exception was for inpatient dollars.

SOURCE: Willard G. Manning et al. "Health Insurance and the Demand for Medical Care: Evidence from a Randomized Experiment." *American Economic Review* 77 (June 1987), Table 2.

RAND Corporation (Manning et al., 1987). The RAND Health Insurance Study (HIS) is without doubt the most comprehensive study to date. Families from six sites (Dayton, Ohio; Seattle, Washington; Fitchburg, Massachusetts; Charleston, South Carolina; Georgetown County, South Carolina; and Franklin County, Massachusetts) were enrolled in various types of health insurance plans in a controlled experiment to test the impact of differences in insurance coverage on the demand for medical care.[6]

In one phase of the study, families were randomly assigned to fourteen different fee-for-service plans. The plans varied in terms of the consumer coinsurance rate and the upper limit on annual out-of-pocket expenses. Every plan had a *maximum* limit of $1,000 in out-of-pocket expenses per year. Table 5–3 presents selected results for five of the plans: free (0 coinsurance rate), 25 percent coinsurance rate, 50 percent coinsurance rate, 95 percent coinsurance rate, and individual deductible. The individual deductible plan had a 95 percent coinsurance rate for outpatient services, subject to a limit of $150 per person or $450 per family, and free inpatient care. Essentially, an individual or a family with this plan receives free medical care after meeting the deductible for outpatient expenditures. In Table 5–3, face-to-face visits equal the number of visits per year to a medical provider, such as a physician. The category excludes visits for radiology, anesthesiology, or pathology services. The third, fourth, and fifth columns list, respectively, total expenditures per person for outpatient, inpatient, and all medical services, excluding dental care and psychotherapy. The sixth column indicates the probability of using any medical services over the course of the year.

The results largely confirm our expectations concerning the impact of coinsurance on the demand for health care. As the level of coinsurance rises, or the out-of-pocket price of medical care increases, consumers demand less medical care. The number of face-to-face visits decreased from

6. The present discussion focuses on the results published by Manning et al. (1987). However, a number of other articles analyze the data from the RAND HIS study. Among them are Newhouse et al. (1981), Keeler and Rolph (1983), O'Grady et al. (1985), Manning et al. (1985), Leibowitz et al. (1985b), Leibowitz et al. (1985a), and Manning et al. (1986). For a summary of the entire RAND HIS study, consult Newhouse and the Insurance Experiment Group (1993).

4.55 per year when health care was a free good to 2.73 when the consumer paid 95 percent of the bill. This represents a decrease in visits of 40 percent. The largest drop in visits took place between the free plan and the 25 percent coinsurance plan. This overall decrease in visits was matched by an identical drop in outpatient expenses from $340 to $203 per year. According to Manning et al. (1987), this indicates that as the out-of-pocket price of medical care increases, consumers reduce medical expenditures largely by cutting back on the number of visits to health care providers and not on the amount spent on each visit. It is interesting to note that the authors reported no significant differences in the amount spent on inpatient services across plans. This, they concluded, was the result of the $1,000 cap put on out-of-pocket expenditures. In 70 percent of the cases where people were admitted for inpatient services, the cost exceeded the $1,000 limit.

The last two columns in Table 5–3 also largely support our expectations regarding the impact of insurance on the demand for medical services. In every case, as the level of coinsurance increased, the probability of using any medical services, along with total medical expenditures, diminished. The only exception occurred between the 25 and 50 percent coinsurance rates for total medical expenditures.

Finally, the results from the individual deductible plan illustrate the negative impact of deductibles on the consumption of medical care. In every instance, less medical care was consumed with the deductibles than would have been the case if medical care had been a free good. It seems that individuals with this plan consumed medical services at a rate somewhere between the 25 and 95 percent coinsurance rate.

The results also indicate that the own-price elasticity of demand is sensitive to the level of insurance. When the level of coinsurance ranged from 25 to 95 percent, the elasticities of demand for all care and outpatient care were calculated as −0.14 and −0.21. These numbers decreased to −0.10 and −0.13 when the level of coinsurance ranged from 0 to 25 percent. This makes economic sense. As the level of coinsurance drops, consumers become less sensitive to price changes due to lower out-of-pocket payments.

In conclusion, the results from the RAND HIS study point to the significant impact of health insurance on the demand for medical care. It is apparent that if either the rate of coinsurance or the deductible falls, the amount of health care consumed increases.

The Impact of Noneconomic Factors on the Demand for Medical Services

The empirical research also indicates that a host of other factors, such as tastes and preferences or the stock of health, affect the demand for medical care. Researchers generally agree that age and severity of illness directly influence the demand for medical care, while the overall health of the individual inversely affects the demand for care. There does not, however, appear to be a consensus concerning the impact of education on the demand for health care. This may indicate that the direct impact of education on the demand for medical care (a greater willingness to seek care) is offset by the inverse effect (a greater ability to produce health care at home) or that more research needs to be done in this area.

It is interesting to note that a few researchers have focused specifically on the effect of medical knowledge on the demand for medical care. Unlike the results for general education, a positive relationship appears to exist between consumers' medical knowledge and the demand for medical care. This means that consumers with a more extensive background in medicine tend to consume more medical services. For example, Kenkel (1990) found that consumers' medical knowledge is positively related to the probability of visiting a physician for medical care, while Hsieh and Lin (1997) uncovered that those elderly who had a greater understanding of health were more likely to acquire preventive medical care. Both studies suggest that consumers with a lack of medical knowledge tend to underestimate the impact of medical care on overall health and, as a result, fail to consume an appropriate amount. It may also be the case that more medical information enhances the ability of an individual to effectively consume medical care, causing the marginal product of medical care to increase (consult Chapter 2). As a result, the demand for various types of medical care increases with consumer information.

Finally, Hsieh and Lin (1997) found that years of schooling, whether the individual worked in the health care field, medical insurance, and income all positively influenced the level of health information acquired. They also found that age and whether the individual drank or smoked inversely affected the quantity of health information collected. It appears that older people acquire less new knowledge because they have fewer years to live and reap any reward from that knowledge, while individuals who drink or smoke receive less utility from any good health that may result from added medical knowledge.

Health Care Spending in the United States

Continually rising health care costs are certainly one of the most glaring problems associated with the U.S. health care system. According to Table 5–4, nominal national health care expenditures totaled $26.9 billion in 1960 and by 2003 had grown to $1.7 trillion. That represents a little more than a 62-fold increase in 44 years.

The annualized rates of growth, also provided in Table 5–4, indicate that the increase in medical expenditures was sustained throughout the entire period. The average annual rate of increase topped 10 percent between 1960 and 1990. In more recent years the annual rate of growth in national medical care expenditures decreased substantially. During the 1990s, it dropped to 6.6 percent. Recently, however, the rate of growth in national health expenditures has begun to increase modestly, to 7.7 percent in 2003. The rise in total national health care expenditures was

TABLE 5–4
A Historical Look at Health Care Expenditures in the United States, 1960–2003

	1960	1970	1980	1990	2000	2001	2002	2003
National Health Expenditures (billions of dollars)	$26.9	73.2	245.8	696.0	1,309.9	1,426.4	1,559.0	1,678.9
Annual Rate of Growth (average annual percentage change from previous period shown)	—	10.6%	12.9	11.0	6.6	8.9	9.3	7.7
Nominal Health Expenditures per Capita	$141	341	1,067	2,737	4,560	4,914	5,317	5,670
Health Expenditures as a Percentage of GDP	5.1%	7.1	8.9	12.0	13.3	14.1	14.9	15.3

SOURCE: Center for Medicaid & Medicare Services, http://www.cms.hhs.gov. Accessed December 28, 2005.

also accompanied by an increase in national per capita medical expenditures. In 1960 the typical American consumed $141 worth of medical care, and by 2003 annual consumption per capita grew to $5,670. This represents an increase of almost 3,900 percent.

Although these statistics clearly indicate that health care expenditures have risen substantially in the United States over the last four decades, they tell only part of the story, because the U.S. economy also grew over the same period. A more telling statistic is the ratio of medical spending to national income, because it measures the portion of the economic pie allocated to the consumption and production of medical care. These figures appear at the bottom of Table 5–4. In 1960, health care expenditures as a percentage of GDP equaled 5.1 percent; by 1980 this number had grown to 8.9 percent.[7] The ratio continued to grow throughout the 1980s and by the 1990s it topped 12 percent. Throughout the 1990s it remained relatively constant, suggesting that health care expenditures grew at the same rate of the overall economy. Before that, however, health care expenditures in the United States grew at a much faster pace than the economy as a whole. As a result, the portion of GDP allocated to the production of health care increased significantly. In more recent years the ratio has inched up and in 2003 it topped 15.3 percent. As in prior years, the rate of growth in health care expenditures has recently exceeded that of the economy as a whole.

Sources and Uses of Medical Funds in the United States in 2003

Figures 5–8 and 5–9 provide detailed figures regarding the sources and uses of health care funds in the United States in 2003. The sources of funds tell us where the health care dollars came from, while the uses indicate how the funds were spent. In 2003, 54 percent of all funds spent

7. GDP stands for *gross domestic product* and equals the total market value of goods and services produced within a country's borders during a particular time period. GDP is measured on an annual basis in this case.

FIGURE 5–8
Sources of Health Care Funds in the United States 2003

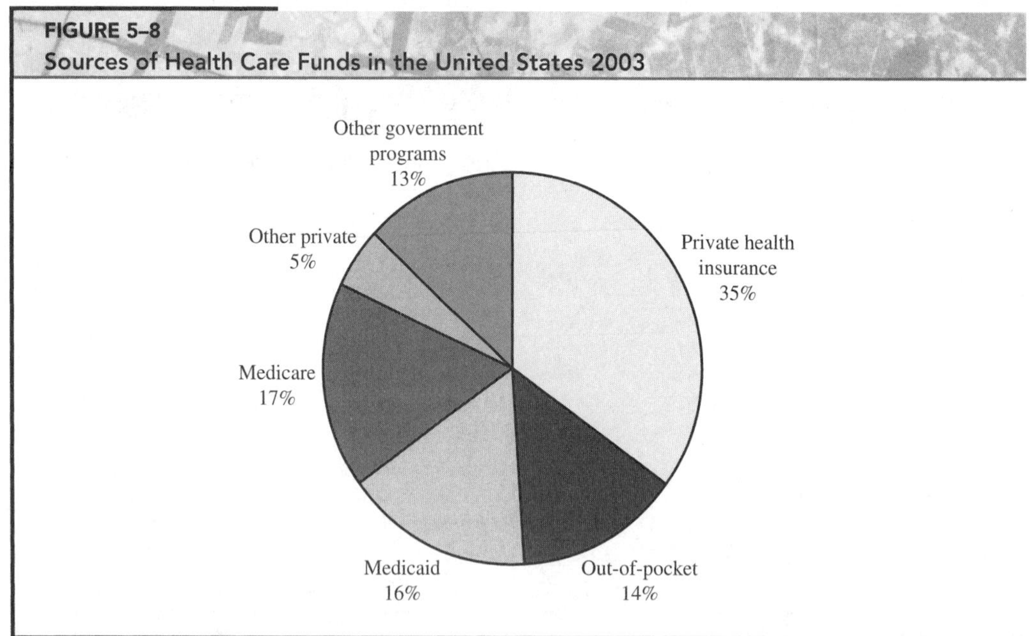

SOURCE: Center for Medicaid & Medicare Services, http://www.cms.hhs.gov. Accessed December 28, 2005.

FIGURE 5–9
Uses of Health Care Funds in the United States 2003

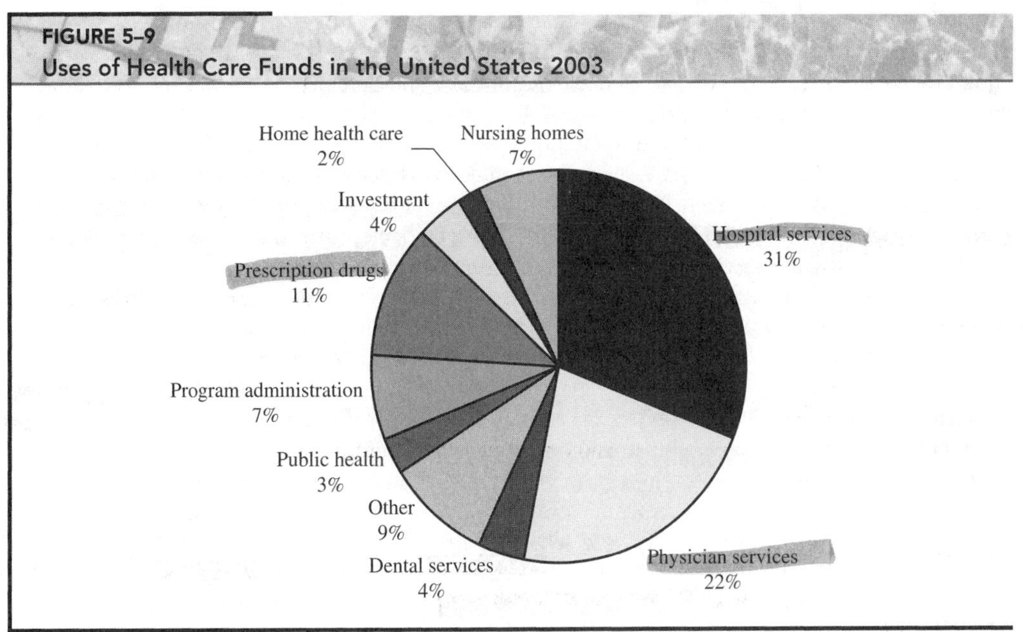

SOURCE: Center for Medicaid & Medicare Services, http://www.cms.hhs.gov. Accessed December 28, 2005.

on national health care came from the private sector, down from approximately 76 percent in 1960. The bulk of this decrease took place in the mid-1960s when the Medicare and Medicaid programs were first introduced. Since 1990, the share of national health expenditures emanating from the private sector has dropped slightly from 59 percent to about 54 percent.

The mix between private insurance and out-of-pocket payments has also changed in recent years. Private insurance expanded its role as a source of funds and substituted partially for out-of-pocket payments. Specifically, in 1980, private health insurance provided the funds for 29 percent of the total national health expenditures, and out-of-pocket payments provided another 17 percent. By 2003 slightly more than one-third of total national health expenditures came from private insurance, while out-of-pocket payments fell to about 14 percent. Other private expenditures, which included funds from businesses to provide health care services directly to employees, philanthropic sources, private construction, and nonpatient revenue sources (such as revenues from hospital gift shops) accounted for 5 percent of the total in 2003.

The largest use of medical funds in 2003 was hospital services, which accounted for 31 percent of the total. The next largest use of funds was physician services (22 percent). Together these two uses of medical dollars make up slightly more than half of all health care spending. It is interesting to note that this percentage has remained relatively constant over the years. In fact, in 1980 the two categories combined to make up 58 percent of total national health care expenditures. The next two largest uses of medical funds in 2003 were prescription drugs and nursing home care, accounting for 11 and 7 percent of total medical expenditures, respectively. The remaining smaller categories are also shown in Figure 5–9.

Before leaving the topic of health care expenditures, it is worthwhile to discuss the work of Woolhandler and Himmelstein (2002) regarding the relative share of health care expenditures financed through government sources. As stated earlier, approximately 45 percent of all health care expenditures emanate from various government programs at the local, state, and federal levels. The other 55 percent comes from the private sector. These percentages suggest that the private sector continues to exert a significant control over healthcare purse strings. Woolhandler and Himmelstein, however, scrutinize the method used by the Centers for Medicare & Medicaid Services (CMS) to measure government spending in the national health accounts and show that government has much more control over health care spending than does the private sector in the United States.

Woolhandler and Himmelstein explain that CMS includes only direct purchasing of medical care for programs such as Medicare, Medicaid, and government-owned hospitals in its measure of government spending. Consequently, public employee benefits, such as those through the Federal Employees Health Benefits Program, are missing from the reported figure by CMS. Although the government supports these public programs with tax financing, private insurers are responsible for writing the actual check because they administer the program on behalf of the government. In addition, Woolhandler and Himmelstein point out that health insurance premiums are exempted from various types of federal, state, and city taxes, so implicitly the government also pays for or finances this portion of health care by granting these tax preferences.

To get a better idea about tax financing of health care, the authors add the direct purchasing of medical care by government, expenditures on public employee health benefits that are tax-financed but administered by the private sector, and the value of the health insurance premium tax preference. In 1999, they showed that direct spending of government equaled 45 percent of all health care spending. Public employees' benefits accounted for another 5.4 percent and the tax subsidy for health insurance premiums amounted to another 9.1 percent. Thus government, at all levels, was responsible for financing nearly 60 percent of all health care costs in the United States, indicating that tax financing accounts for the largest source of health care funds.

On a per capita basis, their estimates for 1999 revealed that the U.S. government spends more on health care than the governments of Switzerland, Canada, Germany, France, Australia, Italy, Japan, Sweden, and the United Kingdom. In these countries the government traditionally has played a much greater role in the financing and reimbursing of health care. Of course, the much higher overall health care spending in the United States partly explains the government's greater per capita spending figure.

These estimates of Woolhandler and Himmelstein are certainly provocative because they show that tax financing represents the major source of funds for health care in the United States. Indeed, tax financing accounts for an even greater share of health care costs considering that not-for-profit health care organizations such as hospitals and nursing homes are also granted tax preferences. It will be interesting to see how these highly credible estimates of Woolhandler and Himmelstein are interpreted and used in future policy discussions concerning health care reform.

Before leaving the topic of health care expenditures, it is worthwhile to discuss changes in out-of-pocket payments in more detail because there appears to be a strong inverse correlation between the amount spent on health care and the percentage financed by out-of-pocket payments. This is true not only over time but also across types of medical expenditures. From 1960 to 2003, when total expenditures on health care grew more than 60-fold, out-of-pocket payments fell from just under 50 percent to 14 percent. Also, the single largest category of medical expenditures in 2003 was hospital care at $515.9 billion, and it had the lowest percentage of out-of-pocket payments at 3.1 percent. Expenditures on physician and clinical services was the next largest category; only 10.1 percent of expenditures were directly financed by consumers. Dental services was one of the smaller categories; out-of-pocket payments equaled 44.3 percent. Thus, cursory evidence is consistent with the hypothesis that a lower out-of-pocket price increases the quantity demanded of medical services. However, it could also reflect just the opposite, that the demand for third-party insurance coverage increases with the magnitude of health care costs. This possibility is discussed in the next chapter.

SUMMARY

Economic theory suggests that the demand for medical care represents a derived demand because it is but one input in the production of health. As a result, the utility received from consuming medical care is in the form of the satisfaction that accrues from improvements in the stock of health. Utility analysis also indicates that the quantity demanded of health care is inversely related to price because improvements in health are subject to diminishing returns. The demand for medical care, like the demand for many other services, depends on the out-of-pocket price, income, the prices of substitutes and complements, and time costs, along with a host of noneconomic factors, such as tastes and preferences, quality of care, and the state of health.

Economists use the concept of elasticity to measure the degree to which an economic agent, such as a consumer, adjusts to a change in the value of an independent variable. The most common elasticity is the own-price elasticity of demand, which measures the extent to which consumers react to a change in the price of a good or service. In mathematical terms, it equals the percentage change in quantity demanded divided by the percentage change in price. If the demand for a product is elastic, the consumer's willingness to purchase the product is very sensitive to a price change. On the other hand, if the demand for the product is inelastic, price changes play a less significant role in determining overall demand. From a graphical perspective, the more elastic the demand for a product, the flatter the demand curve. Additional types of elasticities, such as the income elasticity of demand, have also been employed to assess how demand reacts to changes in variables other than own price.

The empirical evidence indicates that the demand for medical care is inelastic with respect to price. Medical care also appears to be a normal good in that the demand for medical care increases with real income. In addition, time costs along with many noneconomic variables, such as age, gender, severity of illness, education, and consumer knowledge, influence demand. The evidence from the RAND HIS study verifies that health insurance plays a major role in determining the demand for medical care. As economic theory suggests, when the level of health insurance rises, the amount of medical care demanded increases while the price elasticity of demand becomes more inelastic.

Medical expenditures in the United States have grown rapidly in recent decades. In 1960 nominal per capita health expenditures equaled approximately $140, and overall health expenditures accounted for 5.1 percent of GDP. By 2003 per capital expenditures equaled approximately $5,670, while total health expenditures accounted for 15.3 percent of GDP.

CASE STUDIES

5-1 Demand and Moral Hazard[7]

A national pharmacist group has enrolled employers in ten cities in an experiment in treating diabetes aimed at reducing health care costs. Employers who participate in the plan, which began in January 2006, will waive copayments on prescription drugs for diabetes. In waiving the copayments, the program hopes to reduce the shifting of health care costs to employees through higher copayments for medicines. It is expected that in the first year of the plan, employer spending on medications will double as patients become more conscientious with their prescriptions. Additionally, specially trained pharmacists will be paired with patients who have diabetes to

7. Source: Scott Hensley, "Cutting Costs for Diabetes Patients," *The Wall Street Journal,* October 25, 2005.

help them manage their disease. Employers generally spend a lot on employees with diabetes, as complications from the disease can damage the heart, kidneys, eyes, and nerves. GlaxoSmithKline PLC is funding the project and hopes that under the project, workers with diabetes will be more apt to seek care and stick with their medication.

Questions for Discussion

1. *Moral hazard in health care usually refers to the additional consumption of medical care by the insured relative to the uninsured; that is, as the price falls to zero, people consume more services. Should all of the additional "insurance-related" consumption be considered waste? Why or why not?*
2. *The implication is that if we raise prices at the point of service, using deductibles and copayments, we can reduce consumption. Is it possible that we can reduce it too much? Explain how the strategy described in this article addresses this problem.*
3. *To what extent can this strategy—excepting certain kinds of primary care from deductibles and copayment—be adopted for other kinds of health care? Are there "optimal" copayments for all medical procedures and services, ones that can discriminate between welfare-enhancing versus welfare-reducing moral hazard?*

5-2 Law of Many Prices[8]

Now that employees are paying more than ever for health insurance, there is encouragement for consumers to shop around and get the best price for their medical care. However, hospitals, clinics, and labs do not make shopping around for the best price an easy thing to do, and physicians often recommend specific centers for testing without regard for price. Additionally, doctors connected with a hospital usually prefer in-house testing to ensure easier access to the results. Hoping to solve this problem, health insurer Aetna launched online price listings for medical services in Cincinnati. So far no one else has done the same for other areas, which leaves consumers to do the work themselves. To see what it would take for a consumer to get price quotes, *The Wall Street Journal* called nearly a dozen diagnostic testing facilities in the New York City area for price quotes on a lower lumbar spine MRI and a routine mammogram. Included in the facilities were teaching hospitals, freestanding labs, and lab chains; each facility was given the same health insurance information. *The Wall Street Journal* was able to get price quotes without much trouble, but it did not always get accurate information. Prices for the MRI ranged from $1600 to $2000 (most MRIs range in price from $400 to more than $1500), and prices for the mammograms ranged as well (most mammograms range in price from $50 to $300). *The Wall Street Journal* later learned that many of the prices they were quoted were prenegotiated prices, and those with health insurance rarely pay these prices. The hospitals responded by saying that most medical facilities are not equipped to quote the requested prices until a certain procedure has been performed. The comparison of price quotes revealed that a little research could be worth up to several hundred dollars, as prices for procedures from one facility to another vary.

Questions for Discussion

1. *Much of economic theory is predicated on the notion that prices convey lots of useful information, and information about prices needs to be readily available to consumers in order for the positive effects of competition to be realized. Describe the ways in which lack of price information impacts markets.*
2. *What might be some of the practical challenges to reporting prices in health care settings?*

---

8. Source: Loretta Chao, "Shopping for the Best Medical Prices," *The Wall Street Journal*, September 8, 2005.

5-3 How Much for that Colonoscopy in the Window?[9]

In an effort to allow patients to comparison shop and make better decisions with their money, Aetna began providing health care pricing information to those it insures in 2005. It made the prices it negotiated with Cincinnati-area doctors for numerous procedures and tests available online. Aetna was the first major health insurer to publicly disclose its fees and there is hope that Aetna's move will push other insurers to do the same. Unlike most other consumer-driven industries, health care pricing in 2005 was not readily available for customers to examine upfront. With Aetna's new listings, consumers enrolled in any Aetna health plan were able to go online and comparison shop for procedures and tests. Prices vary from doctor to doctor for many reasons, so consumers still need to be cautious when using the price information. Most differences in price between doctors had to do with a doctor's negotiating power and not her quality of care.

Questions for Discussion

1. *Why are prices not a very reliable indicator of quality in the health care industry?*
2. *Prior to the Aetna plan, to what extent did Cincinnati-area Aetna enrollees make health care decisions based on price? To what extent can consumers be expected to make health care decisions based on price? Which other factors might also contribute to health care consumption decisions?*
3. *Describe the physicians' incentives for participating in this program. Can they "game" the system? If so, how?*

Review Questions and Problems

1. In your own words, use utility analysis and production theory to explain why the demand curve for medical care is downward sloping.
2. After reading the chapter on demand theory, a classmate turns to you and says, "I'm rather confused. According to economic theory, people demand a good or service because it yields utility. This obviously does not apply to medical services. Just last week I went to the dentist and had a root canal, and you can't tell me I received any utility or satisfaction from that!" Explain to your classmate how utility analysis can be used to explain why he went to the dentist.
3. Use a graph to illustrate how the following changes would affect the demand curve for inpatient services at a hospital in a large city.
   A. Average real income in the community increases.
   B. In an attempt to cut costs, the largest employer in the area increases the coinsurance rate for employee health care coverage from 10 percent to 20 percent.
   C. The hospital relocates from the center of the city, where a majority of the people live, to a suburb.
   D. A number of physicians in the area join together and open up a discount-price walk-in clinic; the price elasticity of demand between physician services and inpatient hospital services is −0.50.
4. In recent years, many elderly people have purchased Medigap insurance policies to cover a growing Medicare copayment. These policies cover some or all of the medical costs not covered by Medicare. Use economic theory to explain how the growth of these policies is likely to influence the demand for health care by elderly people.

9. Source: Vanessa Fuhrmans, "Insurer Reveals What Doctors Really Charge," *The Wall Street Journal*, August 18, 2005.

5. If you are covered by a private or a public insurance plan, obtain a pamphlet outlining the benefits provided and the cost of the plan. Are there any copayments or deductibles? If so, use economic theory to explain how they may influence your demand for medical care.
6. In your own words, explain what a fuzzy demand curve is. Why does it exist? What are its implications?
7. In reaction to higher input costs, a physician decides to increase the average price of a visit by 5 percent. Will total revenues increase or decrease as a result of this action? Use the concept of price elasticity to substantiate your answer.
8. You have just been put in charge of estimating the demand for hospital services in a major U.S. city. What economic and noneconomic variables would you include in your analysis? Justify why each variable should be included in the study, and explain how a change in each variable would likely affect the overall demand for hospital services.
9. Define *own-price elasticity of demand,* and explain how it is related to the demand curve. Provide four reasons why the demand for medical services is likely to be inelastic with respect to its price.
10. You are employed as an economic consultant to the regional planning office of a large metropolitan area, and your task is to estimate the demand for hospital services in the area. Your estimates indicate that the own-price elasticity of demand equals −0.25, the income elasticity of demand equals 0.45, the cross-price elasticity of demand for hospital services with respect to the price of nursing home services equals −0.1, and the elasticity of travel time equals −0.37. Use this information to project the impact of the following changes on the demand for hospital services.
    A. Average travel time to the hospital diminishes by 5 percent due to overall improvements in the public transportation system.
    B. The price of nursing home care decreases by 10 percent.
    C. Average real income decreases by 10 percent.
    D. The hospital is forced to increase its price for services by 2 percent.
11. According to Whitney et al. (1997), the price of dental services "decreased by $4.86 per day wait for a new-patient appointment and by $5.20 per minute wait in the reception room" (p. 783). Based on these findings, what would happen to the position of the demand curve for dental services if patients had to wait even longer for an appointment with a dentist?
12. A recent study estimates the demand for over-the-counter cough and cold medicines to be:

$$\underset{}{\text{Log } Q} = \underset{(5.52)}{0.885} - \underset{(4.92)}{0.744} \log(P) - \underset{(1.40)}{0.50} \log(INC) + \underset{(6.64)}{0.253} \log(ADV) - \underset{(0.99)}{0.30} \log(PHYSP)$$

Adj. $R^2 = 0.30$

$N = 243$

where Q = Annual dosages demanded of cough and cold medicines

P = Price per dosage of cough and cold medicines

INC = Average income of buyers

ADV = Advertising expenditures on cough and cold medicines

PHYSP = Market price of a physician visit

t-statistics shown in parentheses below the estimated coefficient

All variables expressed in logarithms so the coefficient estimates can be interpreted as elasticities.

A. Which of the estimated coefficients have signs contrary to theoretical expectations? Explain. Be specific in your explanation.

B. Which coefficient estimates are statistically significant from zero at the 5 percent level or better? Explain.

C. What percentage of the variation in dosages demanded remains unexplained? Explain.
D. Suppose the price per dosage increased by 10 percent. By how much would dosages demanded change? Explain. Would total revenues to cold medicine producers increase or decrease? Explain.

CEBS Questions

■ *CEBS Sample Question on Subject Matter from CEBS Course 9 Study Manual*

1. What effect does coinsurance have on the demand curve for medical services? (pages 97–102)

■ *CEBS Sample Exam Questions*

1. When a demand curve for medical care is described as "fuzzy" this refers to the fact that:
   A. Demand is less important than supply.
   B. The concept of a demand curve cannot be applied to medical care.
   C. It is extremely difficult to accurately delineate the relation between the price and the quantity demanded of medical care.
   D. The demand for medical care is a derived demand.
   E. The demand curve for medical care, unlike typical demand curves, does not slope downward to the right.
2. Which of the following statements regarding a demand curve is (are) correct?
   I. In a demand curve illustration, the vertical axis is "quantity."
   II. A demand curve normally slopes downward to the right.
   III. A demand curve shows that a greater quantity will be demanded at a higher income.
      A. II only
      B. III only
      C. I and II only
      D. II and III only
      E. I, II, and III
3. All the following statements regarding elasticity are correct EXCEPT:
   A. If elasticity is negative, the good is called a normal good.
   B. Total revenue decreases when the price increases and the demand is elastic.
   C. When the price elasticity is greater than one, the demand for the product is said to be elastic.
   D. A horizontal demand curve is perfectly elastic.
   E. The availability of substitutes is a determinant of price elasticity.

■ *Answer to Sample Question from Study Manual*

Coinsurance makes the nominal demand curve for medical services rotate clockwise and become steeper. Coinsurance drives a wedge between what the consumer is willing to pay and the actual price paid, or nominal demand, for the medical services. At a zero willingness-to-pay, insurance has no bearing on quantity demanded because medical care is a free good to the individual. In the case where the consumer has full coverage (no out-of-pocket expenses), the nominal demand curve becomes completely vertical.

■ *Answers to Sample Exam Questions*

1. C is the correct answer. The demand curve for medical care is "fuzzy" because the exact relationship between price and quantity demanded is difficult to determine. See pages 106–107 of the text.
2. A is the correct answer. The vertical axis for a demand curve is "price," not quantity. Statement III is incorrect because a demand curve shows the relationship between price and quantity demanded, not income. See pages 95–97 of the text.
3. The correct answer is A. If elasticity is positive, the good is a normal good. All the other statements are correct. See pages 107–111 of the text.

Online Resources

To access Internet links related to the topics in this chapter, please visit our web site at **www.thomsonedu.com/economics/santerre**.

References

Aaron, Henry J. *Serious and Unstable Condition: Financing America's Health Care*. Washington, D.C.: The Brookings Institution, 1991.

Acton, Jan Paul. "Nonmonetary Factors in the Demand for Medical Services: Some Empirical Evidence." *Journal of Political Economy* 83 (June 1975), pp. 595–614.

Bhattacharya, Jayanta, William B. Vogt, Aki Yoshikawa, and Toshitak Nakahara. "The Utilization of Outpatient Medical Services in Japan." *Journal of Human Resources* 31 (1996), pp. 450–76.

Chiswick, Barry. "The Demand for Nursing Home Care." *Journal of Human Resources* 11 (summer 1976), pp. 295–316.

Cockx, Bart, and Carine Brasseur. "The Demand for Physician Services: Evidence from a Natural Experiment." *Journal of Health Economics* 22 (2003), pp. 881–913.

Contoyannis, Paul, Jeremiah Hurley, Paul Grootendorst, Sung-Hee Jeon, and Robyn Tamblyn. "Estimating the Price Elasticity of Expenditure for Prescription Drugs in the Presence of Non-Linear Price Schedules: An Illustration from Quebec, Canada." *Health Economics* 14 (2005), pp. 909–23.

Cromwell, Jerry, and Janet B. Mitchell. "Physician-Induced Demand for Surgery." *Journal of Health Economics* 5 (1986), pp. 293–313.

Davis, Karen, and Louise B. Russell. "The Substitution of Hospital Outpatient Care for Inpatient Care." *Review of Economics and Statistics* 54 (May 1972), pp. 109–20.

Eichner, Matthew J. "The Demand for Medical Care: What People Pay Does Matter." *American Economic Review Papers and Proceedings* 88 (May 1998), pp. 117–21.

Feldman, Roger, and Bryan Dowd. "Is There a Competitive Market for Hospital Services?" *Journal of Health Economics* 5 (1986), pp. 272–92.

Feldstein, Martin S. *Economic Analysis for Health Services Efficiency*. Amsterdam: North-Holland, 1967.

Feldstein, Paul. *Health Care Economics*. New York: Wiley, 1988.

Frank, Richard G., et al. "The Demand for Childhood Immunizations: Results from the Baltimore Immunization Study." *Inquiry* 32 (summer 1995), pp. 164–73.

Freiberg, Lewis, Jr., and F. Douglas Scutchfield. "Insurance and the Demand for Hospital Care: An Examination of the Moral Hazard." *Inquiry* 13 (March 1976), pp. 54–60.

Gerdtham, Ulf-G, et al. "An Econometric Analysis of Health Care Expenditure: A Cross-Section Study of the OECD Countries." *Journal of Health Economics* 11 (1992), pp. 63–84.

Gold, Marsha. "The Demand for Hospital Outpatient Services." *Health Services Research* 19 (August 1984), pp. 384–412.

Gravelle, Hugh, Mark Dusheiko, and Matthew Sutton. "The Demand for Elective Surgery in a Public System: Time and Money Prices in the UK National Health Service." *Journal of Health Economics* 21 (May 2002), pp. 423–49.

Headen, Alvin E. "Economic Disability and Health Determinants of the Hazard of Nursing Home Entry." *Journal of Human Resources* 28 (1993), pp. 80–110.

Hsieh, Chee-ruey, and Shin-jong Lin. "Health Information and the Demand for Preventive Care among the Elderly in Taiwan." *Journal of Human Resources* 32 (1997), pp. 308–33.

Keeler, Emmett B., and John E. Rolph. "How Cost Sharing Reduced Medical Spending of Participants in the Health Insurance Experiment." *Journal of the American Medical Association* 249 (April 22–29, 1983), pp. 2220–22.

Kenkel, Don. "Consumer Health Information and the Demand for Medical Care." *Review of Economics and Statistics* 72 (1990), pp. 587–95.

Lamberton, C. E., W. D. Ellingson, and K. R. Spear. "Factors Determining the Demand for Nursing Home Services." *Quarterly Review of Economics and Business* 26 (winter 1986), pp. 74–90.

Leibowitz, Arleen, et al. "Effects of Cost-Sharing on the Use of Medical Services by Children: Interim Results from a Randomized Controlled Trial." *Pediatrics* 75 (May 1985a), pp. 942–50.

Leibowitz, Arleen, Willard G. Manning, and Joseph P. Newhouse. "The Demand for Prescription Drugs as a Function of Cost-Sharing." *Social Science and Medicine* 21 (1985b), pp. 1063–69.

Leu, Robert E. "The Public-Private Mix and International Health Care Costs." In *Public and Private Health Services,* eds. A. J. Culyer and B. Jonsson. Oxford: Basil Blackwell, 1986.

Manning, Willard, et al. "How Cost Sharing Affects the Use of Ambulatory Mental Health Services." *Journal of the American Medical Association* 256 (October 10, 1986), pp. 1930–34.

Manning, Willard G., et al. "Health Insurance and the Demand for Medical Care: Evidence from a Randomized Experiment." *American Economic Review* 77 (June 1987), pp. 251–77.

Manning, Willard G., Howard L. Bailit, Bernadette Benjamin, and Joseph P. Newhouse. "The Demand for Dental Care: Evidence from a Randomized Trial in Health Insurance." *Journal of the American Dental Association* 110 (June 1985), pp. 895–902.

Manning, Willard G., and Charles E. Phelps. "The Demand for Dental Care." *Bell Journal of Economics* 10 (autumn 1979), pp. 503–25.

Martin, Stephen, and Peter C. Smith. "Rationing by Waiting Lists: An Empirical Investigation." *Journal of Public Economics* 71 (January 1999), pp. 141–64.

McCarthy, Thomas. "The Competitive Nature of the Primary-Care Physicians Service Market." *Journal of Health Economics* 4 (1985), pp. 93–118.

McMenamin, Peter. "What Do Economists Think Patients Want?" *Health Affairs* 9 (winter 1990), pp. 112–19.

Miller, Lisa. "Medical Schools Put Women in Curricula." *The Wall Street Journal*, May 24, 1994, p. B1.

Mueller, Curt D., and Alan C. Monheit. "Insurance Coverage and the Demand for Dental Care." *Journal of Health Economics* 7 (1988), pp. 59–72.

Murray, C. J. L., R. Govindaraj, and P. Musgrove. "National Health Expenditures: A Global Analysis." *Bulletin of the World Health Organization* 74 (1994), pp. 623–37.

Newhouse, Joseph P. "Medical-Care Expenditures: A Cross-National Survey." *Journal of Human Resources* 12 (winter 1977), pp. 115–24.

Newhouse, Joseph P., et al. "Some Interim Results from a Controlled Trial of Cost Sharing in Health Insurance." *New England Journal of Medicine* 305 (December 17, 1981), pp. 1501–7.

Newhouse, Joseph P., and the Insurance Experiment Group. *Free for All? Lessons from the RAND Health Insurance Experiment*. Cambridge, Mass.: Harvard University Press, 1993.

Nyman, John A., "The Private Demand for Nursing Home Care." *Journal of Health Economics* 8 (1989), pp. 209–31.

O'Grady, Kevin F., Willard G. Manning, Joseph P. Newhouse, and Robert H. Brook. "Impact of Cost Sharing on Emergency Department Use." *New England Journal of Medicine* 313 (August 22, 1985), pp. 484–90.

Parkin, David, Alistair Mcquire, and Brian Yule. "Aggregate Health Care Expenditures and National Income: Is Health a Luxury Good?" *Journal of Health Economics* 6 (1987), pp. 109–27.

Phelps, Charles E. "Diffusion of Information in Medical Care." *Journal of Economic Perspectives* 6 (summer 1992), pp. 23–42.

Phelps, Charles E., and Joseph P. Newhouse. "Coinsurance, the Price of Time, and the Demand for Medical Service." *Review of Economics and Statistics* 56 (August 1974), pp. 334–42.

Rosett, Richard N., and Lien-fu Huang. "The Effect of Health Insurance on the Demand for Medical Care." *Journal of Political Economy* 81 (April 1973), pp. 281–305.

Smith, Dean G., "The Effects of Copayments and Generic Substitution on the Use and Costs of Prescription Drugs." *Inquiry* 30 (summer 1993), pp. 189–98.

Van Vliet, Rene C. J. A. "Effects of Price and Deductibles on Medical Care Demand, Estimated from Survey Data." *Applied Economics* 33 (October 10, 2001), pp. 1515–24.

Whitney, Coralyn W., et al. "The Relationship between Price of Services, Quality of Care, and Patient Time Costs for General Dental Practice." *Health Services Research* 31 (February 1997), pp. 773–90.

Winslow, Ron. "In Health Care Low Cost Beats High Quality." *The Wall Street Journal, January* 18, 1994, p. B1.

Woolhandler, Steffie, and David U. Himmelstein. "Paying for National Health Insurance—and Not Getting It." *Health Affairs* 21 (July/August 2002), pp. 88–98.

THE DEMAND FOR MEDICAL INSURANCE: TRADITIONAL AND MANAGED CARE COVERAGE

CHAPTER 6

Remember Joe, who suffered a heart attack at the beginning of Chapter 1? Things turned out quite well, both medically and financially, for our friend Joe. You see, Joe's medical bills were covered by a Blue Cross indemnity insurance plan he had obtained through his employer. Joe could thus afford the best and fastest hospital care money could buy, and the triple bypass surgery he received at the prestigious private teaching hospital was highly successful. Angela, his wife, and the two children are tickled pink now that Joe is back to his former self.

But how might events have differed if Joe had not been covered by medical insurance, or if Joe was enrolled in a managed care plan? Would Joe have been unduly delayed in the busy emergency room of a public hospital? Would Angela have been inordinately stressed out because she was concerned about the unknown financial consequences associated with Joe's illness or worried that the managed care plan might not cover the cost of the care because the hospital did not participate in the plan, or because she did not receive prior authorization for the hospital services? These are among the questions for which we search for answers in this chapter.

Specifically, this chapter:

- presents and compares the conventional and Nyman models of the demand for health insurance
- examines empirical estimates of the price and income elasticities of the demand for health insurance
- discusses the health insurance product, contrasting traditional and managed care coverage
- addresses the regulation of managed care organizations

Introduction

As pointed out briefly in Chapter 4 and further discussed in Chapter 11, employment-related insurance is the dominant type of private health insurance coverage in the United States and only a small percentage of the population purchases health insurance directly from insurance companies. Because most private health insurance is purchased through employers, many people believe that employers pay for their health insurance coverage. But economic theory suggests that nothing could be further from the truth because employees pay for their health insurance coverage in the form of reduced or forgone wages.

Economic theory implies that a trade-off exists between insurance premiums and wages because, during a particular time period, a worker tends to generate a certain value or marginal revenue product (MRP) for a company. The MRP that a worker generates depends on her marginal productivity and the price of the good or service in the marketplace that she helps produce (assuming that output is produced in a competitive market). More precisely, economic theory posits that MRP equals the price of the product times the marginal productivity of the worker. It follows that a higher price and greater productivity both increase a worker's MRP or worth to a company.

Employers are typically pressured by competition in the goods and labor markets to compensate workers based on their market-determined MRP. That is, if an employer compensated its employees at a rate in excess of their MRP, that company would be forced to raise product prices and thereby lose business and profits to competitors in the goods market. At the same time, if the employer did not compensate its employees at a rate that at least matched the market-determined MRP, the company would lose productive employees to competitors in the labor market and thereby also lose business and profits. Consequently, economic theory predicts that workers are compensated for their MRP as long as markets are reasonably competitive. However, compensation comes in the form of both wages and fringe benefits such as life insurance, health insurance, and paid vacations. If you think in terms of total compensation, it follows that more expensive health insurance coverage leads to lower wages or reductions in other fringe benefits for a given level of the MRP. Thus, this trade-off can also be interpreted as meaning that employees actually pay for their health insurance coverage through a reduction in other types of compensation.

Of course, markets are not as frictionless as economic theory sometimes seems to suggest. For example, because of mobility costs, some workers find themselves with more or less health insurance coverage than they truly desire. Also market imperfections, such as wage discrimination, sometimes occur in the real world such that specific workers receive compensation that falls below the competitive rate. However, market forces tend to support long-run outcomes consistent with workers being paid their MRPs as frictions such as mobility costs become less inhibiting and competition for the best workers intensifies.

Representative of several studies, Miller (2004) empirically examines the wage and health insurance trade-off using data for a sample of male workers between ages 25 and 55 during the period 1988–1990. As one might imagine, a wage–health insurance trade-off is difficult to discern statistically because more productive workers tend to receive both higher wages and increased health insurance coverage (as well as greater amounts of other benefits). Thus, it is important that both observable (such as education and experience) and unobservable (such as motivation, dependability, and intelligence) indicators of productivity are held constant in the empirical analysis to isolate the hypothesized inverse relation between wages and the presence of employer-sponsored health insurance. Controlling for observable and unobservable measures of productivity and other factors, Miller finds empirically that health insurance coverage results in 10 to 11 percent less wages. However, Miller warns that his estimate of the trade-off between wages and health insurance may also reflect the presence of other types of fringe benefits such as paid vacations and sick leave, which he was unable to control for because of data limitations. But when health insurance is valued at 11 percent of average wages, the resulting figure of $2,000 compares very closely to the average annual cost of employer-sponsored insurance plans at that time. Thus, Miller's study lends empirical support for the wage and health insurance trade-off and the idea that employees pay for their own health insurance benefits in terms of forgone wages.

The notion that employers do not pay for the health insurance benefits of their employees and therefore only sponsor the insurance is important for the discussion that follows. Both models of the demand for health insurance that are presented assume that workers pay for and choose their own coverage. The first model, the so-called conventional theory or standard gamble model, assumes that people purchase health insurance to avoid or transfer risk. In this case, insurance serves as a pooling arrangement to replace the high risk or variability of individual losses with the reduced risk or variability associated with aggregated losses. The second model, the Nyman model, views people as desiring financial access to medical care that health insurance offers. In this case, a pooling arrangement allows individuals, in the event they become ill, to receive a transfer of income from those who remain healthy. The transfer helps solve an affordability constraint that people face when their net worth falls below the cost of medical treatments. Both of these models offer important insights into the reasons why people demand health insurance and valuable lessons regarding the proper role of public policy with respect to health insurance markets.

The Conventional Theory of the Demand for Private Health Insurance

Because of imperfect information, many of the choices individuals make as health care consumers or providers involve a substantial amount of uncertainty. For example, for an individual consumer, many medical illnesses occur randomly, and therefore the timing and amount of medical expenditures are uncertain. Likewise, from the health care provider's perspective, patient load and types of treatment are unknown before they actually occur. Because these events are unpredictable, they involve a substantial degree of risk. Because most people generally dislike risk, they are willing to pay some amount of money to avoid it.

Consumers actually purchase a pooling arrangement when they buy a policy from an insurance company. Pooling arrangements help mitigate some of the risk associated with potential losses. We will illustrate this point through an example. Suppose, two individuals, Joe and Leo, face the same distribution of losses. We can think of a loss distribution as showing the probability of a number of different outcomes occurring, with the sum of the probabilities equaling 1 or 100 percent. More specifically, assume that both Joe and Leo each face a 20 percent probability of losing $20 and an 80 percent probability of losing nothing.[1] Also assume that the losses of Joe and Leo are perfectly uncorrelated, or independent of one another. That is, Leo does not incur a loss just because Joe incurs a loss, and vice versa.

1. Most individual loss distributions are characterized by a low probability of losing a large sum of money and a high probability of losing very little. The dollar losses are kept to a minimum to ease the calculations that follow. The ensuing discussion may be more meaningful if you think in terms of thousands or millions of dollars, however.

Standard statistics theory suggests that the expected value, μ, of a distribution of outcomes such as losses can be computed as the sum of the weighted values of the outcomes, L_i, with the probabilities, π, serving as the weights. The expected value serves as a summary measure of the distribution of outcomes. For our example, the expected loss equals:

(6–1) $$\mu = \pi_1 L_1 + \pi_2 L_2 = .2 \times \$20 + .8 \times \$0 = \$4.$$

Equation 6–1 can be interpreted as meaning that Joe and Leo can each expect to lose \$4 on average.

But people are also concerned about the variability of the expected loss. It stands to reason that a distribution of likely outcomes involves greater risk when more variability exists around the expected value. For example, Joe and Leo are likely to feel financially more secure knowing that they can expect to lose somewhere between \$3 and \$5 than between \$1 and \$7. Statistics theory suggests that we can measure the variability or variance of a distribution of outcomes such as losses using the following formula:

(6–2) $$\begin{aligned}\text{Variance} &= \sum \pi_i (L_i - \mu)^2 = .2(\$20 - \$4)^2 + .8(\$0 - \$4)^2 \\ &= \$51.20 + \$12.80 = \$64\end{aligned}$$

Along with the expected value, the variance also serves as a summary measure of a distribution. Notice that the variance increases when the actual outcomes, L_i, are further away from the expected outcome, μ. It can also be shown that the variance increases when the probability of extreme outcomes increases. That is, the variance increases when extreme outcomes are more likely to occur than the intermediate outcomes along a distribution. Typically, the variability of a distribution of outcomes is represented by its standard deviation rather than its variance. The standard deviation, which is found mathematically by taking the square root of the variance, equals \$8 in this case.

Both the expected loss of \$4 and its standard deviation of \$8, in this example, can be thought of as measures of risk. Generally speaking, more risk is associated with a higher expected loss and when the distribution of the expected loss, or standard deviation, exhibits wider variability. If both Joe and Leo are risk averse to some degree we can show that they might be better off by pooling their losses. Risk aversion occurs when people receive disutility from taking on additional risk and are willing to pay to avoid it or must be paid to accept it.

Let's now show how Joe and Leo might mutually gain from entering into a pooling-of-losses arrangement. The idea is that both Joe and Leo will share in covering the losses of the other if a loss occurs. If Joe and Leo enter into a pooling arrangement, four possible outcomes are likely. One likely outcome is that both Joe and Leo lose no money at all. The joint probability of both Joe and Leo facing zero losses is found by multiplying the individual probabilities of zero losses occurring, or $.8 \times .8 = .64$. Notice that the probability of an extreme outcome is lowered by the pooling arrangement from .80 on an individual basis to .64 on a group basis.[2] This result already provides a favorable sign that Joe and Leo may be better off by entering into a pooling arrangement.

The second likely outcome is that Joe loses \$20 but Leo suffers no losses and the third likely outcome is that Leo loses \$20 but Joe does not. Each of these separate outcomes must be weighted by their respective probabilities of occurring, .2 and .8, respectively. The final likely outcome is that both Joe and Leo simultaneously suffer a loss of \$20. The joint probability of this

2. This is similar to the joint probability of flipping a coin and obtaining two consecutive heads. The probability of a head toss equals .50, so the probability of two consecutive head tosses equals .25.

TABLE 6–1
The Expected Loss from Entering into a Pooling Arrangement

Outcome	Combined Probability	Combined Loss	Probable Loss from That Outcome
Both Joe and Leo face zero losses	.8 × .8 = .64	$0	$0
Joe loses $20 but Leo does not	.2 × .8 = .16	$20	$3.20
Leo loses $20 but Joe does not	.2 × .8 = .16	$20	$3.20
Both Joe and Leo lose $20	.2 × .2 = .04	$40	$1.60
		Expected total loss	$8.00
		Joe's and Leo's share of the expected loss	$4.00

outcome occurring is found by multiplying the individual probabilities of occurrence, .2 × .2, which amounts to .04. Notice once again that the probability of an extreme outcome occurring is reduced by the pooling arrangement. Table 6–1 summarizes the four likely outcomes and their probable values. Notice that the probabilities of the four outcomes sum to 1 or 100 percent, as they should.

The calculations in Table 6–1 suggest that the pooling arrangement does not make either Joe or Leo better off in terms of the expected loss. Each person faces an expected loss of $4 with or without the pooling arrangement. But when people face the same distribution of outcomes, a pooling arrangement is not about reducing the expected loss; the pooling arrangement is all about reducing the standard deviation or variability of the loss. If we apply the formula for the variance in Equation 6–2, we can obtain the variability of the share of the losses faced by either Joe or Leo as

$$\text{(6–3)}\quad \text{Variance} = .64(\$0 - \$4)^2 + .16(\$1.60 - \$4)^2 + .16(\$1.60 - \$4)^2 + .04(\$0.80 - \$4)^2$$
$$= \$10.24 + \$0.92 + \$0.92 + \$0.41 = \$12.49.$$

It follows that the standard deviation associated with the expected loss equals the square root of the variance, or $3.53.

Notice that the standard deviation of the loss distribution declines from $8 without the pooling arrangement to $3.53 with the pooling arrangement. Both Joe and Leo clearly gain from the reduced variability associated with their expected losses of $4. What may be unclear at this point, however, is the intuition behind the reduction in the variability of the losses that each individual faces because of the pooling arrangement. Entering into a pooling arrangement essentially replaces each person's individual loss distribution with the average loss distribution of the group. The average loss distribution of the group involves a lower probability of extreme outcomes occurring because it is much less likely that both Joe and Leo will simultaneously lose nothing or lose $20. In other words, what happens to one individual will typically be offset by its not simultaneously happening to the other individual.

In addition, the variability of the expected loss decreases as more individuals with similar individual loss distributions join a pooling arrangement. Assuming that losses are not perfectly correlated, more individuals joining the pooling arrangement help reduce the probability of the extreme outcomes occurring and thereby make the expected loss less variable and more predictable. It also can be shown that the group loss distribution becomes more symmetrical and bell-shaped, unlike an individual loss distribution, which is heavily skewed toward the left.[3] A loss distribution heavily skewed toward the left means that small dollar losses occur more frequently than large dollar losses.

The preceding discussion suggests that consumers typically gain from entering into pooling arrangements because the pooling helps reduce the variability of the expected losses. Certainly, consumers benefit when they enter into a medical expense pool. The individual loss function associated with medical expenses is heavily skewed toward the left, indicating that only a very few people will actually incur large medical expenses in the absence of insurance. Indeed for the United States as a whole, a mere 5 percent of all patients accounted for more than half of all health care spending in 1996 (Berk and Monheit, 2001). From an individual consumer's perspective, a pooling arrangement can reduce the variability associated with medical expenses to some degree.

We have not yet established why insurance companies become involved in pooling arrangements. Certainly, people enter into simple forms of pooling arrangements on their own. For example, large families often provide informal sharing of losses, and businesses with a large number of employees sometimes self-insure. However, in cases involving people with no informal or formal relationships, personal pooling arrangements involve an unnecessarily large number of contracts written.[4] In contrast, when the pooling arrangement is developed by an insurance company, only one contract is written between each policyholder and the insurer. Also, if those in the personal pooling arrangement decide to increase the size of the group they must engage in marketing and underwriting (that is, determining whom and on what terms to cover) activities, among others. Most people lack expertise in these areas, but insurance companies can hire the necessary personnel and monitor their activities. Hence, insurance companies often serve as intermediaries and develop and sell pooling arrangements to individuals.

Thus, consumers pay an insurer a certain amount of income (that is, a premium), and the insurer covers some or all of the medical costs in the event an illness actually occurs. During any given period the actual benefits paid out by an insurer to any single consumer may be higher or lower than the premiums received from that consumer. By operating on a large scale, an insurer pools or spreads the risk among many subscribers so that, on average, the total premiums received *at least* compensate for the total cost of paying for medical services, particularly in the long run. In addition, given some amount of competition in the health insurance market, the difference between total premiums and total benefits paid out to all subscribers (or the loading fee) should approximate a "normal" amount.

Consumers differ in terms of the amounts and types of health insurance coverage they buy, and these differences are reflected in such items as the deductible amount, the coinsurance rate, and the number of events covered. (We will examine the health insurance product more closely later on in the chapter.) In general, a high deductible and a high coinsurance rate reflect less extensive or less complete health insurance coverage. For example, some consumers purchase health insurance plans that offer first-dollar coverage for all types of medical services, including

3. See Harrington and Niehaus (2004) for an excellent treatment of basic insurance principles.

4. The number of contracts would equal $[n(n-1)]/2$, where n equals the number of individuals in the pool.

routine care. Others purchase health insurance plans with large deductibles and copayments that cover only catastrophic illnesses. Differences in health care coverage can be explained by a host of factors, including the price of obtaining health insurance, the individual's degree of risk aversion, the perceived magnitude of the loss relative to income, and information concerning the likelihood that an illness will actually occur. The following section offers a model to address how each of these factors individually affects the demand for health insurance.

Deriving the Demand for Private Health Insurance

We can better understand how these factors influence the quantity demanded of health insurance by focusing on Figure 6–1, where the actual utility, U, associated with different levels of income, Y, is shown for a representative consumer (ignore the chord AB for now). The slope of this utility function at any point is $\Delta U/\Delta Y$ and represents the marginal utility of income. The declining slope, or marginal utility of income, is based on the premise that the individual is risk averse. This means the risk-averse person is opposed to a fair gamble where there is a 50–50 chance of losing or gaining one dollar because a dollar loss is valued more highly than a dollar gain. That is, for any given level of income, the pain of losing an incremental dollar exceeds the pleasure associated with gaining an additional dollar.

Suppose a person has an income of Y_0 equaling $40,000. As indicated in the figure, this income level yields actual utility of U_0, which amounts to 90 utils.[5] Further, suppose the person faces a choice concerning whether to purchase health insurance. The decision is based partly on a belief that if an illness occurs, the medical services will cost $20,000. Consequently, if the illness occurs and the consumer pays the entire medical bill, income declines to $20,000 and the level of actual utility falls to U_1, or 70 utils.

The two outcomes that can occur if the consumer does not purchase health insurance are represented by points A and B. At point A, no illness occurs and income remains at $40,000 such that actual utility equals U_0. At point B, an illness occurs and (net) income falls to $20,000 such that actual utility equals U_1. Because the resulting outcome is unknown before it actually occurs, the individual forms expectations concerning the probability of each outcome occurring. With these subjective probabilities, the expected (rather than actual) levels of utility and income can be determined. Specifically, the individual's expected level of utility, $E(U)$, can be determined by weighing the actual utility levels associated with the two possible outcomes by their subjective probabilities of occurrence, π_0 and π_1:

$$\text{(6–4)} \qquad E(U) = \pi_0 \times U_0(Y_0 = \$40{,}000) + \pi_1 \times U_1(Y_1 = \$20{,}000),$$

or

$$\text{(6–5)} \qquad E(U) = \pi_0 \times 90 + \pi_1 \times 70,$$

where π_0 and π_1 sum to 1. Based on Equation 6–5, the chord AB in Figure 6–1 shows the level of expected utility for various probabilities that the illness will occur. As the probability of getting ill increases, expected utility declines, and this outcome is associated with a point closer to B on the chord. The precise probability value that the individual attaches to the illness occurring is based on his best personal estimate. It is likely to depend on such factors as the individual's stock of health, age, and lifestyle.

5. For expository purposes, we assume utility can be measured directly in units called *utils.*

FIGURE 6–1
Expected Utility Model

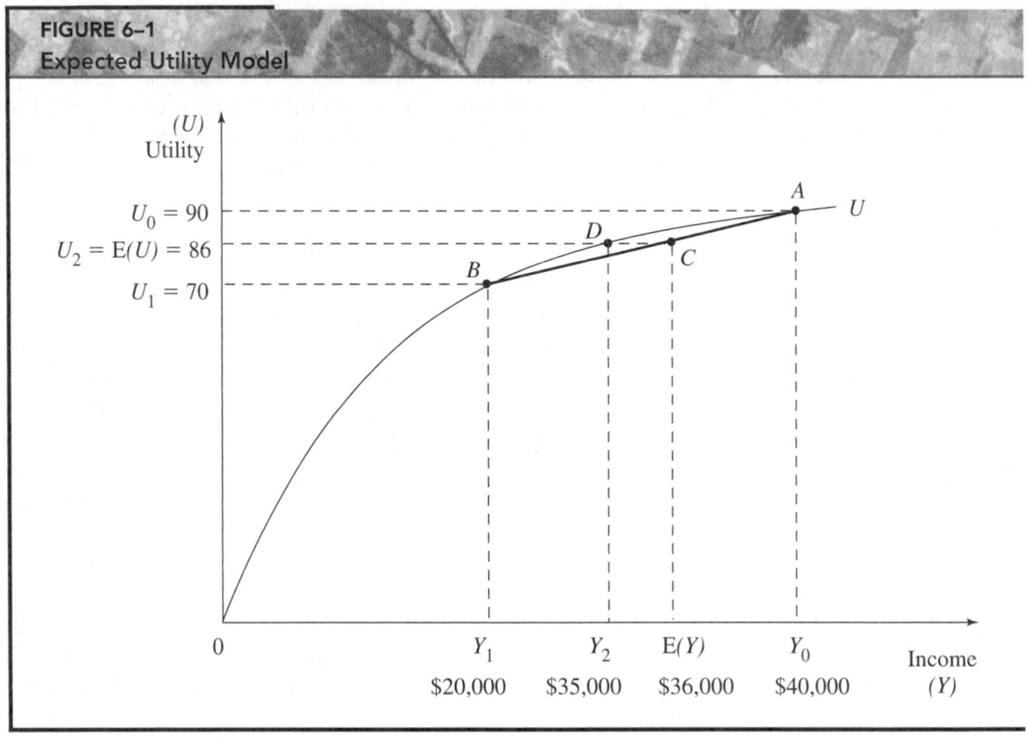

The curve shows the actual utility associated with different levels of income (not drawn to scale). The concavity of the curve illustrates risk aversion. Suppose a person has $40,000 of income and a medical illness costs $20,000. Assuming no health insurance, chord *AB* represents the expected utility associated with different probability values (π) between 0 and 1 of an illness occurring. Points *A* and *B* represent two extreme outcomes for which the illness is not expected to occur ($\pi = 0$) and the illness is perfectly certain ($\pi = 1$). Point *C* reflects an example of an intermediate position where there is a 20 percent chance ($\pi = .20$) of an illness occurring such that expected income after the loss equals $36,000 and expected utility equals 86. Notice that a risk-averse person is indifferent in terms of utility levels between losing a known amount of $5,000 at point *D* and an expected amount of $4,000 at point *C*. Thus, the expected utility model suggests that a risk-averse person can be made better off by paying an insurer some amount above the expected loss to be relieved of the associated risk.

Suppose the consumer attaches a subjective probability of 20 percent to an illness actually occurring. Following Equation 6–5, the expected utility is

(6–6) $$E(U) = .8 \times 90 + .2 \times 70 = 86$$

and the expected level of income, E(*Y*), is

(6–7) $$E(Y) = \pi_0 \times Y_0 + \pi_1 \times Y_1 = .8 \times 40{,}000 + .2 \times 20{,}000 = 36{,}000.$$

Equation 6–7 represents the weighted sum of the two income levels with the probability values as the weights. Thus, expected income equals $36,000 and the expected level of utility is 86 utils if insurance is not purchased (and full risk is assumed) given a perceived probability of illness equal to .2 and a magnitude of the loss equal to $20,000. The levels of expected income and expected utility are also shown in Figure 6–1.

Notice in the figure (not drawn to scale) that the person is just as well off in terms of actual utility by paying a third party a "certain" amount of $5,000 to insure against the expected loss of $4,000. The certain loss of $5,000 reduces net income to $35,000 and provides the consumer with an actual utility level of 86 utils, which equals the expected utility level without insurance. To the consumer, the $1,000 discrepancy, or distance *CD*, represents the maximum amount he is willing to pay for health insurance above the expected loss. It reflects the notion that a risk-averse consumer always prefers a known amount of income rather than an expected amount of equal value. This preference reflects the value the consumer places on financial security. It is for this reason that the typical person faces an incentive to purchase health insurance.

It is easy to see from this analysis why an insurance company is willing to insure against the risk. Assuming this person is the average subscriber in the insured group and the probability of an illness occurring is correct from an objective statistical perspective, the insurance company could potentially receive premium revenues of $5,000 to pay the expected medical benefits of $4,000 with enough left over to cover administrative expenses, taxes, and profits. The expected medical benefits can also be referred to as the actuarial fair value or "pure premium." To the insurer, the difference between the total premium and medical benefits paid out, or pure premium, is referred to as the **loading fee.** In the economics of insurance literature, the loading fee is also typically referred to as the *price of insurance*.

Factors Affecting the Quantity Demanded of Health Insurance

The model in Figure 6–1 can be used to explain how the price of insurance affects the quantity demanded of health insurance. Under normal circumstances, the consumer purchases health insurance if the actual utility with health insurance exceeds the expected utility without it.[6] In Figure 6–1, that happens whenever the loading fee leads to an income level associated with a point between *D* and *C* on the actual utility curve for the given set of circumstances (that is, probability values, degree of risk aversion, and magnitude of loss). In terms of the present example, the consumer demands health insurance if the loading fee is less than $1,000 because actual utility exceeds expected utility at that dollar amount. If expected utility exceeds actual utility, the consumer does not purchase health insurance coverage because the price is too high (a loading fee producing actual utility between points *D* and *B*). This happens if the loading fee exceeds $1,000 in our example. Finally, if actual and expected utility are equal due to the loading fee, the individual is indifferent between buying and not buying health insurance (point *D* or a loading fee of $1,000). Both options make the consumer equally well off. Therefore, it follows that the loading fee, or the price of health insurance, helps establish the completeness of insurance coverage and the number of people who insure against medical illnesses. Specifically, as the price of insurance declines, actual utility increases relative to expected utility and the quantity demanded of health insurance increases, *ceteris paribus*.

At this point, it is useful to note that employment-related health insurance premiums, unlike cash income, are presently exempt from federal and state income taxes even though they are a form of in-kind income. For example, if an employer pays cash wages of $800 and provides health insurance benefits equal to $200 per month to an employee, only the $800 is subject to taxes even though total compensation equals $1,000. Assuming a 20 percent marginal tax rate, the individual pays $160 in taxes on $800 of cash income rather than $200 on $1,000 of total compensation.

---

6. The theoretically correct comparison is between the expected utility with health insurance and the expected utility without health insurance. Because the amount of the premium payment is perfectly certain with a probability of occurrence equal to 1, however, the expected and actual utility with health insurance are equal. We use actual utility here to avoid confusion.

Thus, relative to cash income (or all other goods purchased out of cash income), health insurance is effectively subsidized by the government because of its tax-exempt status. We can view this tax subsidy on health insurance benefits in another way. Each time the employer raises the employee's wage by $1, the employee receives only $100 - t$ percent of that $1 as after-tax income, where t percent is the marginal tax rate. However, if employer health insurance contributions increase by $1, the employee receives the entire dollar as benefits. In effect, the government picks up t percent of the price of the health insurance in forgone taxes and the employee pays the remaining $(100 - t)$ percent in forgone wage income (since both wages and in-kind benefits are substitute forms of compensation). Given $t = 20$, the government implicitly pays 20 cents and the employee pays 80 cents of the marginal dollar spent on health insurance. If we allow for the possibility that not all health insurance premiums are tax exempt (such as the health insurance premiums of some individuals who purchase individual policies), the user price of health insurance can be written as $(1 - et/100)P$, where e is the fraction of health insurance premiums exempted from taxes and P is the price of health insurance (the loading fee). The user price of health insurance obviously decreases with a higher marginal income tax rate and tax-exempt fraction.

Figure 6–2 provides a graphical illustration of the impact of the tax exemption of insurance premiums on the quantity demanded of health insurance. In the figure, the vertical axis captures

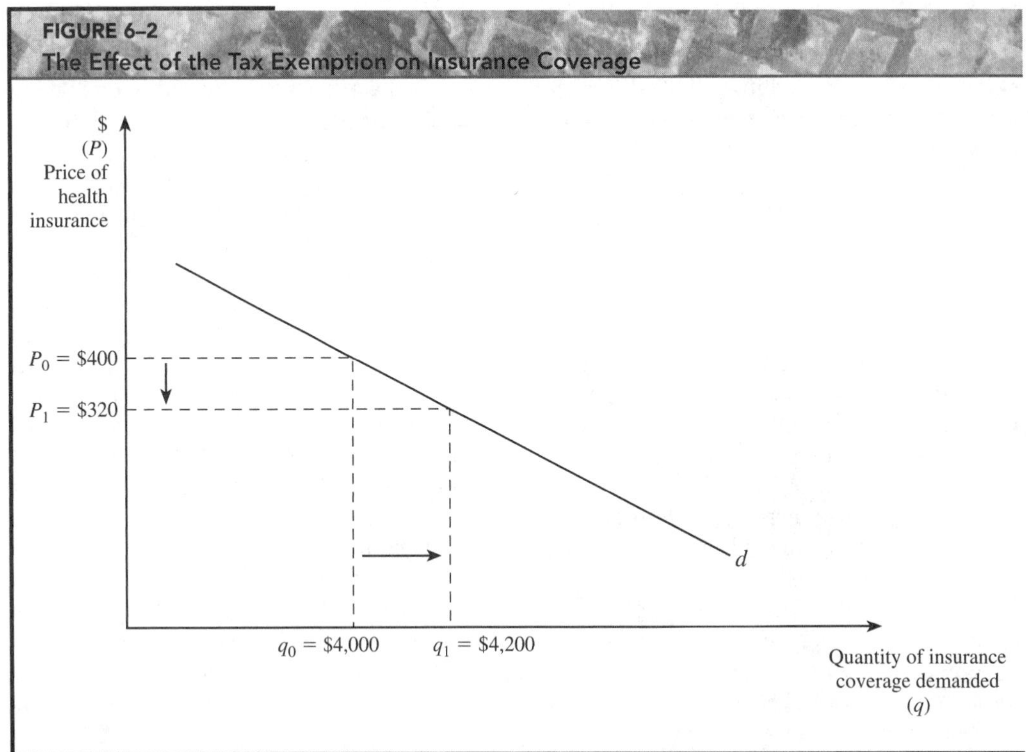

Given the 20 percent tax rate, the tax exemption on health insurance premiums lowers the opportunity cost of purchasing health insurance from $400 to $320 and thereby leads to more insurance coverage purchased as long as demand is not perfectly inelastic with respect to price.

the loading fee or price, P, and the horizontal axis indicates the amount of insurance coverage demanded, q. A rightward movement along the horizontal axis indicates policies with lower deductibles and copayments or more risky events covered by the plan, and consequently, a higher premium payment. An individual's demand for insurance coverage is drawn as a downward-sloping curve to reflect the law of diminishing marginal utility. In addition, a downward-sloping demand for insurance might signify that people typically face relatively few high-risk situations but many more low-risk events. As price declines, people are therefore more willing to have more of these less-risky events covered by insurance.

Let's simplify the discussion by taking the employer out of the picture and suppose that the demand in Figure 6–2 represents a self-employed worker's demand for health insurance. Before 1996, self-employed workers were allowed to exempt only 25 percent of their premiums from taxable earnings. However, for discussion purposes let's suppose that initially the self-employed worker is not allowed a tax exemption on any type of spending and that her income is taxed at 20 percent. Let's also assume that the self-employed worker earns $60,000 of annual income and the loading fee for an insurance policy is set in the marketplace at $400. The government therefore collects $12,000 in taxes ($60,000 times 0.2) from this self-employed worker.

Thus, price P_0 in Figure 6–2 equals $400. The individual matches up market price with marginal benefit, as indicated by demand, and purchases q_0 amount of insurance in the process of maximizing utility. We assume that q_0 equals $4,000 worth of insurance coverage. Notice in this case that an additional dollar spent on health insurance comes at the same cost of an additional dollar spent on any other type of good or service because taxes are applied equally to all types of spending out of income. That is, an additional dollar of pretax income purchases only 80 cents of insurance and any other good or service the individual might buy because of the 20 percent tax rate on wage income. Alternatively stated, the opportunity cost of $1 of additional insurance coverage is $1 spent on all other goods and services.

Now suppose the government exempts all insurance premiums of the self-employed from income taxation, which reflects what actually occurred in 2003. Now, because of the differential tax treatment, an additional dollar out of pretax income purchases $1 of insurance but only 80 cents of all other goods and services. Thus, the opportunity cost of an additional dollar spent on insurance declines from $1 to 80 cents. In terms of our example, this means that the opportunity cost of purchasing health insurance is no longer $400 but now equals $320 or $(1 - t)P_0$.

Figure 6–2 shows the impact of the lower after-tax price of health insurance on the quantity demanded of health insurance. As long as demand is not perfectly inelastic, the self-employed worker responds to the lower after-tax price by purchasing more health insurance, which for discussion purposes is set at $4,200. The government now collects $11,160 of taxes from the self-employed worker.

Thus, economic theory suggests that people purchase more health insurance because of the preferential tax treatment of health insurance premiums. The tax exemption effectively serves as a subsidy for the purchase of health insurance coverage. As we saw in our example, the government effectively pays 20 percent of the loading fee and thereby reduces the individual's out-of-pocket price when purchasing health insurance. Also, it should be noted that the government gives up tax revenues because of the preferential tax treatment of health insurance premiums. These lost tax revenues could have been used to finance various public goods and services. In this example, the government lost $840 of tax revenues. In the aggregate, estimates suggest that the government lost roughly $150 billion of tax revenues in 2004 because of the tax exemption (Sheils and Haught, 2004).

The expected utility model in Figure 6–1 can also help explain other factors affecting the demand for health insurance. First, the subjective probability of an illness occurring affects the amount of health insurance demanded. In terms of the figure, as the probability of an illness increases from 0 to 1, the relevant point on chord *AB* moves from *A* toward *B*. Given the shapes of the two curves, the horizontal distance between the actual utility curve and the expected utility line, which measures the willingness to pay for health insurance beyond the expected level of medical benefits, at first gets larger, reaches a maximum, and then approaches 0 with a movement from *A* to *B*. Therefore, all else held constant, including the loading fee, the quantity demanded of health insurance first increases, reaches a maximum amount, and then decreases with respect to a higher probability of an illness occurring. The implication is that individuals insure less against medical events that are either highly unlikely (closer to *A*) or most probable (closer to *B*). In the latter case, it is cheaper for the individual to self-insure (that is, save money for a "rainy day") and avoid paying the loading fee. For example, assume the probability of illness is 1. In this case, the expected and actual levels of utility are equal at point *B* in Figure 6–1. In this situation, it is cheaper for the individual to self-insure than to pay a loading fee above the medical benefits actually paid out. Alternatively stated, there is no need for insurance since the outcome is certain. The probability of an illness occurring is one reason more people insure against random medical events than against routine medical events, such as periodic physical and dental exams, which are expected.

Another factor affecting the amount of insurance coverage is the magnitude of the loss relative to income. Assuming the same probabilities as before, the expected utility line (chord *AB*) in Figure 6–1 rotates down and pivots off point *A* if the magnitude of the loss increases. In this case, the new expected utility line meets the actual utility curve somewhere below point *B*. For the same probability values as before, the horizontal distance between the expected and actual utility curves increases. Thus, the willingness to purchase health insurance increases with greater magnitude of a loss. This implies that a greater number of people insure against illnesses associated with a large loss, at least relative to income. Insurance coverage is also more complete. The potential for a greater loss is one reason more people have hospital insurance than dental or eye care insurance coverage.

The final factor affecting the amount of health insurance demanded is the degree of risk aversion. Obviously, people who are more risk averse have more insurance coverage than otherwise identical people who are less risk averse. Greater risk aversion makes the utility curve more concave. In fact, if the person is risk neutral, the marginal pain of a dollar loss equals the marginal pleasure of a dollar gain and the slope of the utility curve is constant (a straight line through the origin). In this case, a person would be indifferent with respect to purchasing or not purchasing insurance because the expected and actual utilities are equal at different levels of income. For a risk lover, the pleasure of an additional dollar gained exceeds the pain of an incremental dollar loss and the slope of the utility curve increases in value. In the case of a risk lover, no insurance is purchased because expected utility is greater than actual utility at any level of income.

In sum, according to conventional theory, we can specify the quantity demanded of health insurance, Q, as a function of the following factors:

$$Q = f[(1 - et/100) \times P, \text{Degree of risk aversion, Probability of an illness occurring, Magnitude of loss, Income}]. \quad (6\text{–}8)$$

Note that a change in the first explanatory factor results in a movement along a given demand curve, whereas an adjustment in any of the other four factors results in a shifting of the curve.

With suitable data, Equation 6–8 can be estimated to determine the user price and income elasticities of the demand for health insurance. In practice, however, it is very difficult to measure

TABLE 6–2
Price and Income Elasticities of the Demand for Health Insurance

Study	Price Elasticity	Income Elasticity
Taylor and Wilensky (1983)	–0.21	0.02
Farley and Wilensky (1984)	–0.41	0.04
Holmer (1984)	–0.16	0.01
Short and Taylor (1989)	–0.32	0.13
Manning and Marquis (1989)	–0.54	0.07
Marquis and Long (1995)	–0.03	0.15
Liu and Christianson (1998)	–0.33	0.12

the user price and quantity demanded of health insurance. Therefore, various proxies are used depending on data availability. For example, the price of health insurance, P, is sometimes proxied by the size of the insured group. The expectation is that the loading fee, or the price of health insurance, falls with a larger group size due to administrative and risk-spreading economies. Some studies assume that the price of health insurance is the same for all individuals and allow only marginal tax rates, t, and the tax-exempt fraction, e, to vary.

Proxy measures for the quantity of health insurance must also be employed. The quantity of health insurance is usually measured by either total insurance premiums, some measure of insurance coverage completeness, or a coverage option (for example, less versus more restrictive health insurance plans). Table 6–2 displays some of the estimated price and income elasticities of the demand for health insurance reported in various studies. The studies reveal that individuals possess a price-inelastic demand for health insurance. Furthermore, while health insurance is considered a normal good (that is, it has an income elasticity greater than zero), the studies found a relatively small income effect. Even the demand for long-term care insurance is found to be inelastic, with price and income elasticities of about −0.39 and 0.18, respectively (Kumar et al., 1995).

However, these studies generally assume the individual is able to make marginal changes in the insurance policy. But employer-sponsored group insurance policies are largely beyond the control of the single individual employee. Typically, the employer or union representatives make decisions concerning the insurance package by considering the welfare of the overall group rather than that of any one individual employee.[7] See Goldstein and Pauly (1976) or Pauly (1986) for further discussion on this point. When employees can select from multiple similar plans offered by the employer and must pay more out-of-pocket for more expensive plans, demand is found to be much more responsive to price. For example, Dowd and Feldman (1994/95) found that the demand for a health plan is highly elastic with respect to price at about –7.9 when multiple similar plans are offered. Strombom et al. (2002) estimate elasticities ranging from –2.0 to –8.4 depending on the cost of switching plans as measured by age, job tenure, and medical risk category.

7. Nevertheless, most studies find that the demand for individual health insurance is also inelastic with respect to price. For example, see Marquis et al. (2004).

Nyman's Access Theory of the Demand for Private Health Insurance

As we discussed previously, standard insurance theory suggests that risk-averse individuals purchase health insurance as a way of transferring or avoiding some of the risk associated with the variability of medical care expenses. They avoid or transfer some of the risk by entering into a pooling arrangement to replace their individual loss distributions with the average loss distribution of the group. Compared to the individual loss distributions, the average loss distribution involves less variability around the expected loss and thereby results in less risk faced by an individual when engaged in a pooling arrangement.

John Nyman (2003) recently advanced an alternative reason why people desire medical insurance. Nyman begins by pointing out that many medical interventions, such as a liver transplant or coronary artery bypass surgery, cost more than most people hold in terms of their net worth (value of assets less the value of liabilities). For example, a liver transplant can cost around $300,000, yet most households hold as little as $50,000 in net worth. In addition, banks are reluctant to loan out money for a potentially lifesaving medical intervention when they are unsure whether the ill person will be able to repay the loan. Thus, in the absence of medical insurance coverage, many people might be denied access to lifesaving medical interventions because they lack the financial means to pay for them.

Because many people lack the wherewithal to purchase the medical care required by a major medical intervention, Nyman argues that people value medical insurance because they desire an income transfer from those who remain healthy in the event they become seriously ill. Notice that, unlike in the standard model, income rather than risk is being transferred in the Nyman model. As an illustration, suppose that actuarial data indicate that 1 out of 75,000 people will require a liver transplant in a given year. Also suppose that 75,000 people join an insurance pool and the liver transplant costs $300,000. Thus, for an actuarial fair premium of $4 ($300,000/75,000), a person with a relatively low net worth has access to a potentially lifesaving medical intervention because she will receive an income transfer of $299,996 from the other 74,999 individuals in the pool if she requires a liver transplant. Insurance offers a solution to an affordability problem brought about by the need for a major medical intervention. According to Nyman, medical insurance creates value by providing financial access to medical care that people could not otherwise afford.

Conventional Insurance Theory According to Nyman

Most economists agree that a model should be judged by the plausibility of its assumptions and its ability to accurately predict behavior in the real world. For example, students typically learn in principles of macroeconomics that John Maynard Keynes (1936) refuted classical theory by showing that several of its assumptions, such as perfect wage and price flexibility, do not always hold in practice. Keynes also pointed out that classical theory predicts full employment, yet 25 percent of the workforce was unemployed at one point during the Great Depression of the 1930s. Hence classical theory was not a useful model at that period of time, according to Keynes, because of its weak assumptions and failure to predict correctly.

In a similar vein, Nyman points to several inconsistencies associated with the assumptions and predictions of the conventional insurance model as a way of judging its usefulness as a theory of the demand for health insurance. Most of these inconsistencies are fairly technical in nature so we only highlight a few of the more crucial ones, especially those whose scrutiny offers direct insights into the Nyman model.

Moral Hazard Is Always Welfare Decreasing. Conventional theory treats medical insurance coverage as reducing the representative consumer's out-of-pocket price of medical care. The lower out-of-pocket price, in turn, creates a movement down along the demand curve and leads to additional units of medical care demanded for which their marginal costs exceed marginal benefits. In Chapter 5, we referred to this situation as the moral hazard problem. Figure 6–3 helps to describe the economic reasoning behind the conventional treatment of moral hazard.

In the figure, the horizontal axis represents the quantity of medical services demanded by a representative consumer. The typical consumer's demand for medical care, *d*, is shown as being downward sloping; MC, reflecting the marginal cost of delivery of medical care, is assumed to be constant with respect to the amount of medical care produced and determined in the marketplace. Consumer equilibrium, for the uninsured individual, occurs where MC and demand intersect at a price of P_1 and quantity of q_1. The amount of medical care consumed is considered efficient because for every unit between the origin and q_1, willingness to pay or marginal benefit, as revealed by demand, never falls below MC.

Now suppose that the representative consumer purchases full insurance coverage. According to conventional theory, complete insurance coverage can be treated as simply lowering the fully

FIGURE 6–3
The Conventional View of Moral Hazard

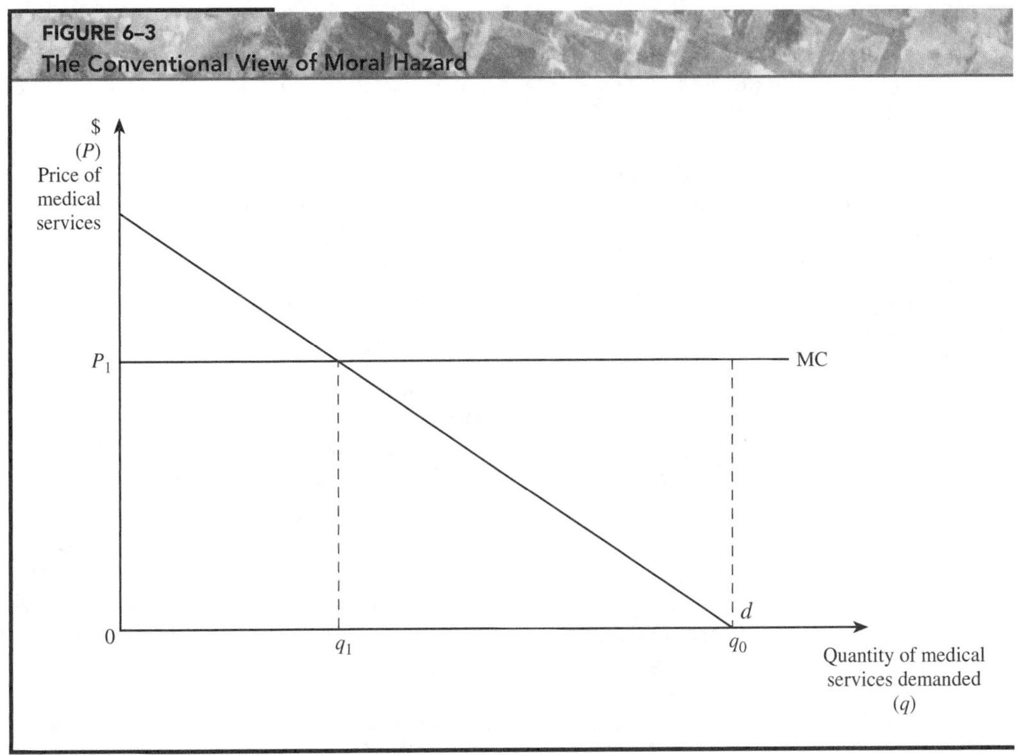

Complete coverage causes the consumer's out-of-pocket price to fall from P_1 to 0. As a result, quantity increases from q_1 to q_0. The additional units are treated as creating a welfare loss because MC exceeds willingness to pay.

insured consumer's out-of-pocket price down along the demand curve from P_1 to 0. At the new fully insured consumer equilibrium, q_0 amount of medical care is now consumed and a welfare loss occurs because each additional unit of medical care between q_1 and q_0 generates more costs than benefits at the margin. These additional units may reflect spending on discretionary items such as prescription sunglasses and cosmetic surgery—things that people purchase with insurance coverage that they would not have otherwise purchased if they had to pay the full price. These additional units of medical care may also reflect extra visits to doctors or longer stays in hospitals than medically necessary. Thus, conventional theory treats the transition from uninsured to insured status as resulting in the consumption of frivolous or unnecessary medical care.

Nyman believes that this prediction of the conventional model offers an inconsistency because several empirical studies have found that the transition from uninsured to insured status results in vast improvements in people's health, especially among vulnerable populations such as infants and the elderly. Nyman also refers to empirical studies indicating that the uninsured often fail to receive standard care and delay or defer seeking medical care. Given that health improves when people transition from uninsured to insured status, Nyman argues that the additional medical care consumed cannot be as frivolous or clinically unnecessary as conventional theory tends to suggest it is.

Nyman claims that conventional theory makes this false prediction because it treats the medical insurance payoff as resulting solely in a lower out-of-pocket price and not producing a corresponding income transfer. If the insurance payoff is treated as an income transfer at time of sickness, as Nyman proposes, then the demand for medical care effectively shifts to the right and results in much less inefficiency. Figure 6–4 shows what happens when the insurance payoff is treated as an income payoff.[8]

Assuming the consumer purchases full insurance coverage, the demand for medical care shifts from D_U, the uninsured demand, to D_I, the insured demand. The greater demand represents the income transfer that the consumer receives at the time of illness from those who remain healthy. Obviously, the consumer possesses a greater willingness to pay for medical care when she is sick and has the income to pay for it. Consequently an important distinction between the two models is that conventional theory assumes that willingness to pay is determined before the payout takes place, whereas Nyman treats willingness to pay as being determined at the time the payout is made.

If the insurance payoff were accomplished through a lump-sum transfer and price remained at P_1, the new equilibrium quantity of medical care would be represented by q_N. Notice that this equilibrium is characterized by additional units of medical care for which willingness to pay or marginal benefit exceeds MC. However, the new equilibrium actually occurs at q_2, with a **price-payoff contract** accounting for the additional units of medical care between q_N and q_2. A price-payoff contract pays out by reducing price rather than offering a lump-sum reimbursement. For example, a medical expense contract may specify that the insured will be reimbursed for the actual cost of physician services less any stipulated coinsurance each time he makes an office visit. In our hypothetical case, as depicted in Figure 6–4, we assume that the price-payoff contract

8. In Figure 6–4, q_0 exceeds q_2 because the premium payment reduces the amount of income available to purchase additional medical care. Our purpose here is to compare the Nyman model to the conventional model for a situation in which the consumer possesses complete insurance coverage. It should be pointed out, however, that a different demand curve exists for each coinsurance rate. The demand curve shown in Figure 6–4 is the one for a zero coinsurance rate. If the coinsurance rate is 0.5, for example, the demand curve shifts half of the distance to the right from D_U and point q_2 moves half of the distance closer to q_0 because the premium payment is now proportionately lower. The total amount of medical care demanded, in the case, is determined at the point on the demand curve where the coinsurance rate equals $0.5P_1$.

FIGURE 6–4
Nyman's View of Moral Hazard

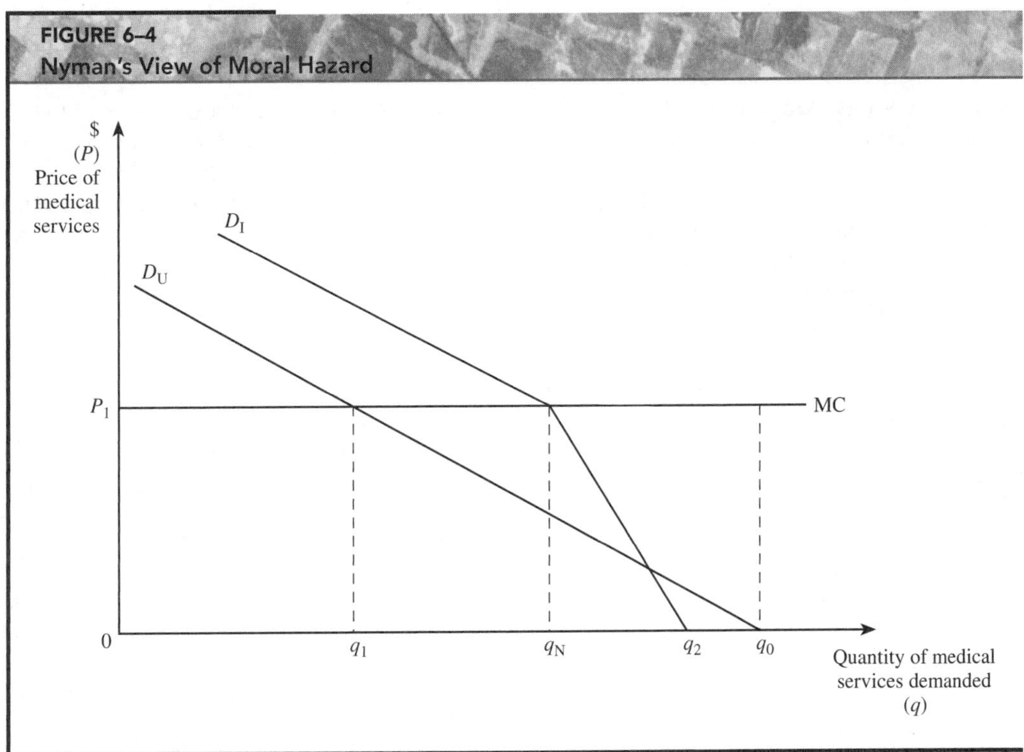

Complete insurance leads to both an income transfer and a substitution effect. The income transfer shifts the demand from D_U to D_I and quantity demanded increases from q_1 to q_N as a result. The insurance, because it is designed as a price-payoff contract, also results in a substitution effect from q_N to q_2. The range between q_1 and q_N represents efficient moral hazard, whereas the range between q_N and q_2 represents inefficient moral hazard.

reduces price to zero. In both cases, the price reduction feature of the price-payoff contract potentially triggers a substitution effect (as well as the income effect discussed previously).

Recall that a substitution effect occurs when people switch away from higher- to lower-priced goods. In this specific case, people may switch away from other goods and purchase more medical care than they otherwise would have because of the substitution effect brought on by the insurance coverage. As a result, the price-payoff contract is associated with some inefficient moral hazard similar to what we learned from the conventional analysis of moral hazard. This inefficient moral hazard represents the cost of using a price reduction to pay off the insurance contract. The benefit of a price-payoff contract is that health care providers monitor and verify illnesses on behalf of the insurance companies and thereby prevent consumer fraud. That is, if the insurance company paid their insured a lump sum amount for an illness, rather than a reduced price when seeking treatment through health care providers, many people might falsely claim to be ill to receive a payout.

Thus, another significant distinction between the two models is that both efficient and inefficient moral hazard may occur in the Nyman model. That is, insurance coverage causes people's behavior to change but some behavioral changes result in efficiencies whereas others do not. The conventional theory considers only inefficient moral hazard. In Figure 6–4, the efficient moral hazard is represented by the quantity of medical care between q_1 and q_N because marginal benefit exceeds MC and the inefficient medical care falls between q_N and q_2.

Voluntary Purchasing of Health Insurance Makes People Worse Off. Conventional theory assumes that people purchase health insurance to avoid risk. Thus, health insurance offers the benefits of risk reduction. As we just saw, conventional theory also argues that health insurance creates corresponding costs by resulting in excessive spending levels associated with (inefficient) moral hazard. Interestingly, conventional theory suggests that the benefits of risk reduction and moral hazard costs tend to move in opposite directions with changes in the coinsurance rate. For example, raising the coinsurance rate increases the consumer's risk exposure but lowers the moral hazard costs.

Within this perspective, people make trade-offs between risk exposure and moral hazard costs when they purchase health insurance just as they make trade-offs when choosing among cars with different amounts of economy, safety, style, and other characteristics. For instance, highly risk-averse individuals who are drawn to plans with less exposure to risk (that is, a lower coinsurance rate) must accept potentially greater moral hazard costs and pay a greater premium. Consequently, one would think that the characteristics of real-world insurance contracts reflect what consumers personally find ideal or utility maximizing given the trade-offs they face. In particular, the coinsurance rate selected by individuals should reflect their rational choice between risk reduction benefits and moral hazard costs.

Based upon conventional theory, several researchers have calculated estimates of the optimal coinsurance rate and compared them to the coinsurance rates specified in real-world insurance policies. Feldstein (1973) shows that the optimal coinsurance rate depends on values for the price elasticity of demand for medical services and the consumer's degree of risk aversion. He finds that raising the coinsurance rate to 66 percent would improve consumer welfare. More recently, Manning and Marquis (1996) estimate the demand for health insurance to measure the degree of risk aversion and the demand for health care services to measure the price elasticity of demand. They use data from the RAND health insurance study of the 1970s that was discussed in Chapter 5 and find an optimal coinsurance rate of 40 to 50 percent.

Nyman points out that these estimates of the optimal coinsurance rate are much higher than the ones specified in actual health insurance policies (typically well below 30 percent). This discrepancy leads Nyman to wonder why people would voluntarily purchase a policy that made them worse off. In other words, why would the typical consumer pay a higher premium and receive more coverage than she truly finds optimal? As we discussed in Chapter 1, rational economic behavior predicts that people never purposely and knowingly make themselves worse off. As a result, this inconsistency led Nyman to conclude that something must be wrong with conventional theory if it predicts irrational behavior. It also provided him with the motivation to develop an alternative theory of the demand for health insurance—one that is not driven by risk avoidance.

A Simple Exposition of the Nyman Model

Similar to the conventional model, the Nyman model is based on a comparison of the expected utility from being insured (EU_I) with the expected utility from remaining uninsured (EU_U). Insurance is purchased if $EU_I > EU_U$. However, the Nyman model does not depend on consumers being risk averse. The basic idea behind the Nyman model is that purchasing insurance reduces one's income when healthy by the amount of the premium (opportunity cost) but potentially raises one's income through a transfer when sick (the benefit). This means that one factor affecting the

FIGURE 6–5
Nyman's Expected Utility Model

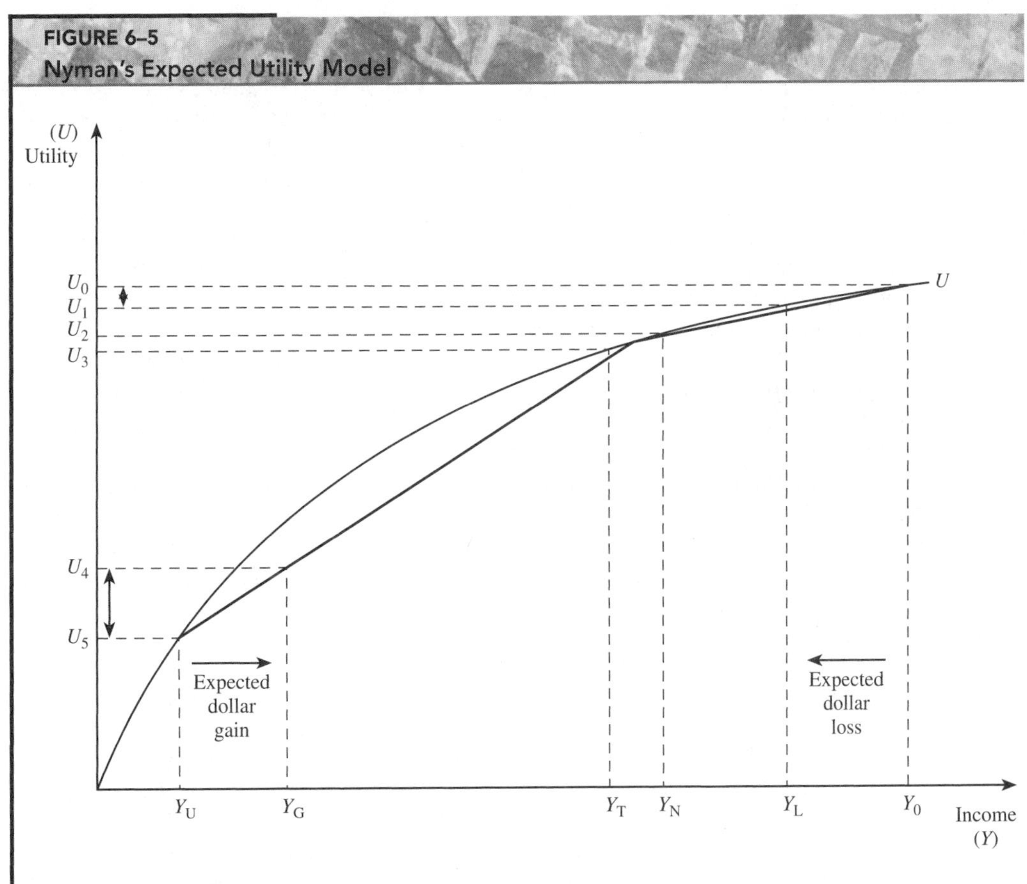

The premium payment results in an expected dollar loss of $Y_0 - Y_L$. The insurance payoff results in an expected dollar gain of $Y_G - Y_U$. Since the expected utility gain of $U_4 - U_5$ exceeds the expected utility loss of $U_1 - U_0$, insurance will be purchased. In this case the expected gain from the income transfer when ill exceeds the expected cost of the insurance policy from remaining healthy.

purchasing of medical expense insurance is a person's preference regarding when he would rather have more income. Would a person prefer a gain of income when sick or a similar gain of income when well? Most people are willing to give up some income when well to receive an income transfer when sick. In effect, the payment of the premium when well reduces utility less than an equal expected income transfer raises utility when sick. The main reason is that additional income is more valuable to an individual when he has less of it, and the cost of medical care causes uninsured people, when sick, to have less income to spend on other goods and services.

Figure 6–5 shows a simplified graphical model offered by Nyman.[9] We suppose that the consumer initially possesses Y_0 amount of income. If she remains healthy, she stays at this level of income and enjoys U_0 amount of utility. However, if she is without medical insurance, becomes

9. This simplified approach assumes that the utility function for income is independent of health status, the quantity of medical care does not enter the utility function, and insurance is not associated with any substitution or income effects. Basically we want to compare this approach with the conventional approach under fairly similar circumstances to illustrate their differences.

sick, and spends M dollars on medical care, only $Y_0 - M$ dollars would be left over to spend on other things, so income falls to Y_U $(= Y_0 - M)$ and utility falls to U_5.

Now suppose the person purchases insurance and remains healthy. In that case she has to pay the actuarially fair insurance premium of $\neq(1 - c)M$, where $\neq$ represents the probability of an illness occurring and c stands for the coinsurance rate. Income net of the premium falls to Y_N. However, if the individual pays the premium only when healthy, the expected cost of paying the premium equals the probability of remaining healthy, $(1 - \neq)$, times the actuarial fair premium such that the expected loss of income when healthy and insured corresponds to the horizontal distance between Y_0 and Y_L. Income less the expected loss of income when healthy and insured is associated with an expected utility of U_1. Hence, the expected utility loss of purchasing health insurance is represented by the vertical distance $U_0 - U_1$.

Now, if the individual purchases insurance and becomes ill, she potentially gains an income transfer equal to $(1 - \neq)(1 - c)M$ from those who remain healthy. When this income transfer is added to the amount of income left over to spend on all other goods when uninsured, Y_U, it results in an income level of Y_T and utility level of U_3. Y_T and U_3 reflect the level of income and utility that actually result if she becomes sick and receives the stipulated medical insurance coverage. Given the probability of becoming sick, she can expect to receive $\neq$ times the income transfer, or $\neq(1 - \neq)(1 - c)M$, which, when added to Y_U, corresponds to the level of expected income represented by point Y_G and expected utility of U_4 in Figure 6–5. Thus, the expected utility gain from purchasing medical insurance is represented by the vertical distance $U_4 - U_5$, the difference between the uninsured utility level and the expected utility level with insurance coverage.

Notice that the expected cost of paying the premium when healthy, as measured by the horizontal distance $Y_0 - Y_L$, equals the expected gain when sick, as measured by the horizontal distance $Y_G - Y_U$, as it should, given that an actuarial fair premium was assumed. Also notice that the expected utility gain from the transfer when sick, $U_4 - U_5$ exceeds the expected utility loss from paying the premium when healthy, $U_1 - U_0$. As Nyman (2003) notes (p. 52), "With this specification of the expected utility model, it is simply necessary that the income transfer gain be evaluated on a steeper portion of the utility function than the premium loss, for insurance to be purchased." It is important to recognize that the law of diminishing marginal utility with respect to income, and not risk aversion, is all that is necessary to draw this implication from the Nyman model. It is because of the law of diminishing marginal utility that the expected utility gain from health insurance is typically valued more highly than its expected utility loss.

In sum, Nyman offers a model of the demand for health insurance that is not based on risk aversion. When deciding whether to purchase health insurance, a person compares the expected utility forgone by paying a premium and remaining healthy to the expected utility received from an income transfer in the event that he or she becomes ill. For most people the expected loss in utility of paying a premium when healthy is less than the expected gain in utility from receiving the income transfer when sick because uninsured medical expenses would seriously reduce their wealth or income. Hence the expected utility from the income transfer is evaluated at a steeper point on the utility curve than the expected utility loss from the premium payment.

Insights and Policy Implications of the Nyman Model

The Nyman model appears to offer an exciting and internally consistent alternative to the conventional model and provides a number of important insights. First, people demand medical expense insurance because they desire an income transfer in the event they become ill and purchase insurance when the expected utility gain from receiving the income transfer when sick exceeds the expected utility loss of paying the premium when healthy.[10] Second, insurance that pays off by paying medical expenses generates both efficient and inefficient moral hazard. Previously, economists focused exclusively on the inefficiencies associated with medical insurance. Third, inefficient moral hazard results from the price-payoff feature of health insurance contracts, which is necessary for transaction cost reasons. Fourth, the demand for medical insurance essentially represents a derived demand because its value derives from the ability of medical care to restore, maintain, and improve the quality and quantity of lives. As such, medical insurance offers value to consumers by improving their access to medical care.

The policy implications associated with the Nyman model are equally significant and worth mentioning. For one, Nyman points out that rising health care costs since the mid-1960s reflect, in part, the increasing number of people covered over the years by medical insurance. As income has been redistributed from the healthy to the sick because of insurance coverage, the sick have been able to exercise their greater willingness to pay for medical care, causing medical expenditures to rise over time. Consequently, rising health care costs and insurance premiums capture the growing social benefits of medical care, and public policies designed to contain health care costs may come at a sizable trade-off in terms of the quality and quantity of lives lost.

Two, many economists have advocated greater consumer cost sharing as a means to prevent (inefficient) moral hazard. But increased consumer cost sharing may also squeeze out efficient moral hazard. As Nyman asks, who would regard as optimal an insurance policy that requires a $150,000 out-of-pocket payment on a $300,000 liver transplant? Third, subsidizing insurance premiums is efficient. Nyman stresses that people value the additional income they receive from insurance when they become ill more than they value the income they lose when they pay a premium and remain healthy. Because everyone has an equal chance of becoming ill, the redistribution of income from the healthy to the ill is efficient because it increases the welfare of society.

Fourth, some health care analysts have considered that high medical prices might encourage efficiency by discouraging consumption of medical care and preventing (inefficient) moral hazard. For example, within that perspective, an efficiency justification might be made for allowing a horizontal merger between two local hospitals that would knowingly lead to high hospital prices. Nyman points out, however, that policies should promote low medical prices to increase access to medical care and encourage more efficient moral hazard. Finally, Nyman warns that managed care organizations may be socially beneficial if they help prevent inefficient moral hazard but may be harmful if they reduce access to needed medical care through restrictive policies.

The Health Insurance Product: Traditional versus Managed Care Insurance

Before the 1980s, the health insurance product was fairly easy to define because the consumer, insurer, and health care provider relationship was much less complicated. Most consumers, through their employers, purchased conventional insurance that allowed for free choice of health care provider. Insurance premiums were largely determined by community rating, in which the premium is based on the risk characteristics of the entire membership. In contrast,

10. Recall that conventional theory treats the loading fee as the price of health insurance. In contrast, the premium payment reflects the price of health insurance in the Nyman model because it represents the opportunity cost of purchasing health insurance (that is, the additional goods and services that might have been consumed when healthy).

when premiums are determined using **experience rating,** insurers place individuals, or groups of individuals, into different risk categories based on various identifiable personal characteristics, such as age, gender, industrial occupation, and prior illnesses. The main difference among health insurance plans before the 1980s was simply the amount of the deductible and copayment, if any, that the subscriber had to pay for medical services and the specific benefits covered under the plan.

Because physicians typically operated in solo practices, enrollees dealt directly with individual physicians or local hospitals for care rather than with a network of providers before the 1980s. Health care providers had full autonomy and practiced medicine as they deemed appropriate. The main function of the insurer was to manage the financial risk associated with medical care and to pay the usual, customary, or reasonable (UCR) charge for any medical services rendered by physicians. UCR means that the fee is limited to the lowest of three charges: the actual charge of the physician, the customary charge of the physician, or the prevailing charge in the local area.

Since 1980, however, managed care organizations (MCOs) have exploded on the health care scene. The phrase *managed care* has been assigned to these organizations because, by design, they are supposed to emphasize cost-effective methods of providing comprehensive services to enrollees. MCOs integrate the financing and delivery of medical care. The integration often involves such practices as a network of providers, reimbursement methods other than UCR charges, and various review mechanisms. MCOs also rely to a greater degree on experience rating of enrollees because of the price competition that results.

The main types of MCOs are the health maintenance organization, the preferred provider organization, and the point of service plan. A **health maintenance organization (HMO)** combines the financing and delivery of care into one organization. A distinguishing feature of an HMO is that the assigned or chosen primary care provider acts as a gatekeeper and refers the patient for specialty and inpatient care. Four distinct types of HMOs are generally recognized:

Staff model: In this type of HMO, physicians are directly employed by the organization on a salary basis. In terms of Figure 4–1, a staff HMO completely merges the insurer and provider functions. Because medical care is not reimbursed on a fee-for-service basis, physicians have little if any personal financial incentive to overutilize medical services.

Group model: This type of HMO provides physician services by contracting with a group practice. Normally the group is compensated on a capitation basis. As a result, physicians in the group face a strong disincentive to overutilize medical services.

Network model: The only difference between the group model and the network model is that in the latter case, the HMO contracts with more than one group practice for physician services. As is the case with the group model, compensation is generally on a capitation basis.

Individual Practice Association (IPA) model: This form of HMO contracts with a number of independent physicians from various types of practice settings for medical services. In this situation, physicians generally provide care in a traditional office setting and are normally compensated on a fee-for-service basis, but at a discounted rate. In return, the HMO promises a large and continuous volume of patients.

A **preferred provider organization (PPO)** is a different type of insurer and health care provider arrangement. A PPO exists when a third-party payer provides financial incentives to enrollees to acquire health care from a predetermined network of physicians and hospitals. The incentive can be in terms of a higher coinsurance or a higher deductible when someone acquires medical care outside the network of health care providers. To participate in a PPO network, physicians agree to accept a lower fee for services rendered. In return for a lower fee, physicians are promised a steady supply of patients. Normally, patients can directly seek out specialty or inpatient care if they belong to a PPO. Because of their less restrictive policies, Robinson (2002) labels PPOs as *managed-care-lite organizations.*

Like PPOs, **point-of-service (POS) plans** provide generous coverage when enrollees use in-network services and cover out-of-network services at reduced reimbursement rates. Unlike PPOs but similar to HMOs, POS plans assign each enrollee a primary caregiver who acts as a gatekeeper and authorizes specialty and inpatient care.

Estimates indicate that 97 percent of all privately insured workers in 2005 were covered by MCOs, reflecting a continual decline in conventional insurance coverage, which stood at 73 percent as recently as 1988. Most of the enrollment increase has taken place in the least restrictive managed care plans over the last five years. HMOs witnessed a decline in market share from a high of 31 percent in 1996 to 21 percent in 2005. PPOs, the least restrictive of the MCOs, enjoyed the largest surge in enrollment, from 11 percent in 1988 to 61 percent by 2005. Enrollments in POS plans also witnessed a decline in market share, from 24 percent in 1998 to 15 percent in 2005.[11]

Landon et al. (1998), among others, argue that the traditional distinction among health insurance products, such as conventional insurance and MCOs, or even the distinction among MCOs, has become blurred in practice. For example, even the so-called conventional insurance plans now involve some type of utilization review program. Given that the traditional taxonomy of insurance plans may no longer adequately describe the differences among organizations, it is better to differentiate among health insurance products based on the types and restrictiveness of the financial incentives and management strategies facing patients and health care providers. Let us elaborate.

Financial Incentives and Management Strategies Facing Consumers/Patients

Depending on the precise nature of the health insurance product, consumers/patients face different financial incentives to use medical care. As examined theoretically in Chapter 5, the consumer's out-of-pocket price, as captured by the size of the deductible and coinsurance, inversely affects the quantity demanded of medical care. Some health insurance plans contain high deductibles and coinsurance as a way of containing medical prices. In addition, some plans set their premiums on an experience-rated basis as an incentive for subscribers to adopt more healthy lifestyles.

In addition to indirect financial incentives, insurers may also adopt various management strategies to directly affect the consumer's utilization of medical care. First, the insurer may require prior medical screening to avoid insuring high-risk patients or exclude coverage for preexisting conditions. Insurers may also restrict the choice of provider by building provider networks in which the consumer must participate. In addition, the insurer may employ a primary care gatekeeper to determine whether further services are medically warranted. Pre-authorization of medical services, a type of utilization review practice, is another management strategy affecting the consumer's direct use of medical care.

By combining the financial incentives and management strategies facing patients, we can get a better understanding of the underlying health insurance product. For example, a health insurance

11. The Kaiser Family Foundation and Health Research and Educational Trust. "Employee Health Benefits, 2005 Annual Survey." http://www.kff.org/insurance/7315/index.cfm. Accessed October 12, 2005.

plan with a high deductible and coinsurance and experience-rated premiums, combined with limits on choice of physician and pre-authorization, offers much less insurance than one with no out-of-pocket costs or pre-authorization, community-rated premiums, and full choice of provider. The latter situation aptly describes the conventional insurance offered by Blue Cross plans back in the 1970s. A POS plan comes close to an example of the former situation as far as management strategies facing consumers are concerned.

Financial Incentives and Management Strategies Facing Health Care Providers

The health insurance product may also contain financial incentives and/or management strategies to affect the delivery of medical care by health care providers. As a result, the health insurance product can also be differentiated based on the types and restrictiveness of the financial incentives and management strategies facing health care providers. In terms of financial incentives, the health insurance product may adopt different provider reimbursement practices, such as fee-for-service, capitation, bonuses, and/or withholds. Withholds occur when the insurer withholds part of the health care provider's reimbursement until after a stipulated period at which the appropriate use of medical care has been evaluated. Inappropriate use of medical care results in the physician not receiving all or part of the withheld money. The prospect of incomplete reimbursement payments presumably acts as an incentive for health care providers to offer truly medically necessary care.

As we saw in Chapter 4, fixed payment systems, such as capitation, can discourage the delivery of high-cost, low-benefit medicine. Capitation places health care providers financially at risk for any cost overruns. When properly designed, performance-based measures, such as bonuses and withholds, can accomplish that same goal.

Insurers can also directly influence the delivery of medical care through various management strategies. Selective contracting, deselection of providers, physician profiling, utilization review, practice guidelines, and formularies are among the more common management strategies facing health care providers. Selective contracting occurs when managed care plans contract solely with an exclusive set of providers. The selection and **deselection** of providers involves the establishment of the criteria and process by which health care providers will be included in or terminated from the network. For example, insurers may include physicians in their network who are of high quality and/or utilize cost-effective practice patterns. **Physician profiling** may be used to monitor performance in the selection or deselection process. The profiling may include only information, for example, on the primary care physician's track record regarding referrals to specialty and inpatient care as a way to identify high-cost providers, or it may include information on quality of care or patient satisfaction.

Utilization review programs "seek to determine whether specific services are medically necessary and whether they are delivered at an appropriate level of intensity and cost" (Ermann, 1988, p. 683). **Practice guidelines** provide information to health care providers about the appropriate medical practice in certain situations. A **formulary** contains a list of pharmaceutical products that physicians must prescribe whenever necessary. All these management strategies are designed to directly affect how a physician behaves in a specific clinical circumstance.

Consequently, the health insurance product also differs based on the type of provider reimbursement method and the existence and restrictiveness of various management strategies. For example, a capitation reimbursement scheme in conjunction with utilization review and practice guidelines means a much different insurance product than one with a fee-for-service payment system in which the health care provider has full autonomy over patient care. The former situation resembles the staff HMO whereas the latter reflects the traditional BC/BS or commercial insurance of the 1970s.

The first column in Table 6–3 provides a summary of the four basic features of any health insurance product: patient financial incentives, consumer management strategies, provider financial incentives, and provider management strategies. Below each feature is a list of specific policies aimed at altering the behavior of either consumers or health care providers. As you can see, health insurance is a complex and multidimensional product. At one extreme lies the perfectly unrestricted health insurance plan, the basic characteristics of which are provided in the second column of Table 6–3. With this type of insurance consumers pay no out-of-pocket prices; health care providers are reimbursed based on the usual, customary, and reasonable fee for service; and there are no consumer or provider management strategies. At the other extreme, the basic characteristics of a perfectly restrictive insurance plan are shown in the third column of Table 6–3. In this case, significant financial incentives and management strategies face both consumers and health care providers. In terms of examples, the traditional Blue Cross/Blue Shield insurance plan of the 1970s compares quite closely to the unrestricted plan described in Table 6–3, while the staff HMO, except for the significant out-of-pocket price, fits the insurance plan described in the last column of Table 6–3.

TABLE 6–3
Spectrum of Health Insurance Products

Basic Features (Examples)	Unrestricted or Complete Insurance Plan	Restrictive Insurance Plan
Patient Financial Incentives Deductibles Coinsurance	No or low deductible with no coinsurance	Significant deductible with a high coinsurance
Premiums	Community rated	Experience rated
Consumer Management Strategies Prior medical screening Restrictions on choice Gatekeeper Pre-authorization	No restrictions	Consumers must receive care exclusively from the network of providers
Provider Financial Incentives Risk-sharing and/or bonus arrangements	None—UCR charges	Capitation with bonuses or withholds
Provider Management Strategies Selective contracting Deselection Physician profiling Utilization review Practice guidelines Formularies	None	An array of management strategies are employed to control costs

Although Table 6–3 provides a good framework for defining and conceptualizing the health insurance product, some caveats are in order. It is important to realize that any one health insurer may offer multiple health insurance products. For example, a health insurer may offer both a staff HMO and a traditional indemnity plan. Of course, the prices of the two plans should differ significantly. It is also important to realize that any one health care provider may deal with various health insurance products. A large physician practice may treat some patients who belong to a PPO plan and others who subscribe to HMO plans, for example. An additional complexity is that a group physician practice may be reimbursed on a capitation basis by the insurer whereas the individual physician within the practice is compensated on a salary basis. It is also important to mention that financial incentives and management strategies may serve as complementary or substitute methods of controlling the behavior of consumers and providers. As Gold et al. (1995, p. 315) point out:

> *For example, plans that capitate primary care physicians and place them at risk for specialty referrals and inpatient care through a withholding account may be expected to place particular emphasis on monitoring physicians to ensure that the financial incentives do not result in underservice. On the other hand, plans operating in areas where physicians are resistant to accepting much financial risk may rely particularly heavily on nonfinancial mechanisms such as utilization management to influence practice patterns.*

The Regulation of MCOs

There has been considerable debate in the academic literature and the popular press concerning the effect of managed care plans on the cost and quality of medical care. By design, MCOs are supposed to employ cost-effective methods of delivering a comprehensive set of services to enrollees. The original proponents of managed care thought that MCOs would encourage preventive and coordinated primary care as a way of reducing the need for more expensive specialty and inpatient care. Also, advocates thought that MCOs would eliminate the high-cost, low-benefit medicine associated with traditional fee-for-service indemnity insurance (that is, the moral hazard problem). As a result, high quality of care and low operating costs were expected from MCOs.

Because lower quality of care translates into lower costs and higher profits, critics claim that MCOs face an incentive to reduce the quality of care, perhaps by denying or skimping on costly but necessary medical treatments. Health care providers have no recourse but to follow the wishes of the MCOs given the restrictive financial incentives and management strategies they face, according to the critics.

Given this controversy, which we discuss more fully in later chapters, many states and the federal government have introduced or enacted various regulations to influence the behavior of MCOs. Miller (1997, p. 1102) notes that the regulatory actions taken to control managed care practices have been "referred to as 'patient protection' or 'patient bill of rights' acts by proponents and as 'anti-managed' bills by those opposed." The legislation has attempted to extend the rights of patients and physicians and also improve the patient/physician relationship under managed care. According to Miller, in just six months from January to July 1996, more than four hundred bills were introduced in the various states to control managed care practices. Most of the laws concern such issues as anti-gag rules, limits on financial incentives, continuity of care, and expanding the rights of health care professionals. Let's examine each of these issues more closely.

Gag rules prohibit doctors in a managed care plan from discussing treatment options not covered under the plan, from providing information on plan limitations, or from commenting unfavorably on the plan. Opponents of managed care argue that gag rules cause physicians to deny care by suppressing useful information on alternative treatments that the managed care plan may not find cost effective to provide. Managed care representatives claim that the so-called gag rules are designed to prevent physicians from disparaging the plan or releasing proprietary information concerning compensation and similar issues.

Critics further argue that managed care payment systems, such as capitation or performance-based systems like bonuses or withholds, create a financial incentive for physicians to deny medically appropriate or useful treatments. Indeed, much mention has been made in the popular press of "drive-through medicine," involving short maternity stays in hospitals or mastectomies taking place in outpatient rather than inpatient facilities because of managed care financial arrangements. Laws limiting financial incentives are designed to prevent denial of care from taking place. Managed care representatives, on the other hand, argue that the financial incentives of MCOs are necessary to control the moral hazard problem.

Miller notes that state policies offer little concrete guidance about how the general prohibition against financial incentives applies to the myriad financial arrangements set by MCOs. As a result, she claims that without additional clarification, regulatory actions against managed care financial arrangements will have to be argued on a case-by-case basis, creating much uncertainty for the various parties involved.

Medical experts argue that continuity of care is an important consideration for the patient/physician relationship and for patient well-being, especially for certain groups, such as pregnant women or the severely ill. Critics of MCOs claim that continuity of care is at stake because some employers subscribe to only one managed care plan, because a managed care plan may change its networks of physicians, or because physicians may be deselected. In all these cases, consumers have to pay more to visit a physician of their own choice and the continuity of care is compromised. Although proponents argue that MCOs can only provide the desired health care cost savings for society by directing patients to selected physicians, laws have been introduced in many states to extend the option of continued care from primary caregivers.

In addition, numerous laws have been introduced across the states that aim to expand the rights of health care professionals. With the growth of MCOs, many health care professionals feel the pressure from market demands and also the loss of autonomy brought on by contracts with managed care plans. For example, some physicians find themselves unable to participate in or deselected from managed care plans without being provided with the rationale.

The first laws introduced concerned any willing provider (AWP) or freedom of choice (FOC) laws. According to Hellinger (1995, p. 297), "AWP laws require managed care plans to accept any qualified provider who is willing to accept the terms and conditions of a managed care plan." According to the law, MCOs do not have to contract with all providers but must explicitly state evaluation criteria and ensure "due process" for providers wishing to contract with the plan. Due process rights provide professionals with access to information regarding MCO standards, termination decisions, and physician profiling. FOC laws allow a patient to be reimbursed for medical services received from qualified physicians from outside the network. FOC laws do not guarantee that the patient will incur the same out-of-pocket cost, however. Proponents of AWP and FOC laws argue that they increase the continuity of care by offering a fuller choice of providers. Opponents argue that without selective contracting, managed care plans are unable to obtain volume discounts because they are powerless to channel patients to selected providers. In addition, it is alleged that these laws lead to a diminished quality of care because of the higher monitoring costs brought on by a greater number of health care providers.

In sum, anti-gag laws, laws restricting the financial incentives of MCOs, laws promoting continuity of care, and laws extending the rights of health care professionals are among the various regulations advanced by various states to control the practices of MCOs. The basic hypothesis is that MCOs face an incentive to restrict the quality of care because increased profits can be made. Critics claim that various financial incentives and management strategies help MCOs achieve their objective of maximum profits. Interestingly, all these laws essentially attempt to transform MCOs into indemnity plans. The superiority of indemnity and managed care plans remains a controversial issue and is the subject of ongoing theoretical and empirical debates.

SUMMARY

To someone schooled in economics, it should be quite obvious that people demand private health insurance, just as they voluntarily demand any other consumer good or service, because it provides utility or satisfaction for them. Less obvious is the exact mechanism by which insurance coverage translates into utility gains. To clear up some of the ambiguity, two models of private health insurance demand are introduced in this chapter to more carefully explore the linkage between insurance coverage and utility.

The first model, conventional theory, argues that risk-averse people gain from the risk reduction offered by insurance coverage. More precisely, people can reduce the variability of their financial losses, potentially resulting from irregular and unpredictable medical expenditures, by joining a sharing-of-losses arrangement. The reduced variability of losses or risk avoidance provides utility to risk-averse individuals, according to conventional theory. Within an expected utility maximization model, the conventional demand for medical expense insurance is a function of the user price of health insurance, degree of risk aversion, probability of a loss, magnitude of the expected loss, and income. In general, empirical studies based on conventional theory suggest that the demand for private health insurance is relatively inelastic with respect to both user price and income.

The second model, Nyman's access theory, treats insurance coverage as offering people an income transfer from those who remain healthy to themselves in the event they become ill. Given that most uninsured people lack sufficient funds, insurance coverage helps provide financial access to medical care at time of illness. The income transfer at time of illness or access value provides utility, according to Nyman. Within an expected utility framework, people purchase health insurance when the expected utility gain from the income transfer when ill exceeds the expected utility loss of paying the premium and remaining healthy.

A comparison of the conventional and Nyman models yields a number of insights. One insight of particular importance to economists concerns the interpretation of moral hazard. Conventional theory treats insurance as simply lowering the out-of-pocket price the insured consumer pays for medical care. Accordingly, the lowered price triggers a substitution effect that results in an increased quantity of medical care demanded for which marginal costs exceed marginal benefits. Thus, the additional units of medical care reflect a welfare loss and suggest that all moral hazard is inefficient.

In contrast, the Nyman model points out that the insurance payout also possesses an income effect. The income effect leads to a greater demand for medical care at time of illness and leads to efficient moral hazard. Consequently, not all moral hazard is inefficient, according to the Nyman model.

Finally we discussed the health insurance product. We learned that the health insurance product is multidimensional and complex because many attributes, such as benefits covered, out-of-pocket expenses, choice of provider, and the provider payment scheme, must be considered. Nearly all of the privately insured in the United States are covered by some type of managed care plan. Managed care plans differ with respect to the restrictiveness of the financial incentives and management strategies facing both consumers and health care providers. We learned that many states have enacted various regulations to control the restrictiveness of the financial incentives and management strategies adopted by managed care plans. The efficiency properties of these regulations continue to be explored and debated by economists and policy makers.

CASE STUDIES

6-1 Employee-Based Health Benefits[12]

General Motors stock skidded to its lowest level since 1993 after the head of the United Auto Workers (UAW) said the union would not reopen its contract to reduce the automaker's health care burden. UAW president Ron Gettelfinger said GM and the union routinely work to find ways to trim costs from GM's massive health care system, but the union had no plans to allow GM to change the basic health care package it agreed to offer UAW-represented hourly workers under a four-year master contract that was set to expire in 2007. GM estimated that total health care costs could rise to $5.6 billion in 2005. The corporation suggested that hourly workers should have the same, less generous health plan as GM salaried employees. UAW members paid about 7 percent of their health care costs, while salaried employees paid about 27 percent. According to industry officials, American workers paid on average about 32 percent of their health care costs that year. GM faced considerable challenges in its efforts to reduce its health care burden substantially in the short term. In April 2005, GM and the UAW had taken small steps toward cost cutting in its health plans but more was needed. At that time GM had some leeway in its contract with the union to increase certain medical deductibles and copayments if costs were to rise, but broader changes could not be made unilaterally.

Questions for Discussion

1. *Some economists argue that health care benefit costs should be treated by the employer as labor costs; that is, rising health care premiums will ultimately be passed on to employees. In this context, was the UAW bargaining for health care coverage or protection from wage reductions?*
2. *Assuming that the UAW shares the view of economists and perceives health care benefits as a noncash form of wages, what kinds of labor market conditions may encourage the UAW to accept less generous health care benefit packages?*
3. *One argument is that higher health care prices are to be expected because the aggregate level of medical care quality has risen substantially over the past several years. Do you agree or disagree with this statement? If we assume the statement is correct, what are some of the likely consequences of spreading the costs of those quality increases across those possibly less willing to pay for them?*

12. Source: Lee Hawkins, Jr., "UAW's Stand Pummels GM Stock: Shares Hit a 12-Year Low; Union Won't Open Contract to Cut Health-Care Burden," *The Wall Street Journal,* April 15, 2005.

6-2 Consumer-Directed Plans[13]

UnitedHealth Group is the leader in the trend toward consumer-driven health care. The idea behind consumer-driven health plans is that people will shop around for health care if they have to pay the majority of the cost themselves. With traditional health insurance no longer growing and premiums continuing to climb, more companies are starting to say no to traditional plans. Consumer-directed plans hopefully address this problem by each year having employees put cash into a health savings account to spend on health care or to carry over tax-free to the next year. The plans have higher deductibles but lower premiums, but the idea behind the plans is to make people think about what they spend on health care. There are also risks to the new plans in that they could potentially discourage people from getting the care they need because of the high cost. While UnitedHealth did not expect to gain as much profit from the consumer-driven plans, the company hoped the plans would appeal to new markets, such as America's 45 million uninsured. In a show of commitment to the new plans, UnitedHealth required its own 41,000 employees to switch to the plans in 2005 and hopes that people will deposit their medical savings in its bank, Exante, because by 2010 UnitedHealth expected consumers to accumulate $10 to $26 billion in health savings accounts.

Questions for Discussion

1. *Sounds promising, but are there downsides to high-deductible health plans?*
2. *If given a choice of enrollment in a high-deductible plan versus a more traditional (and more expensive) plan, what kinds of employees will choose one over the other? What are the potential problems associated with this kind of selection?*
3. *Assume that enrollees use less medical care while covered by a high-deductible plan than they use with a traditional plan. Describe the difference in utilization between the two plans. Is the difference waste? Is it "moral hazard"?*

6-3 High-Deductible Plans[14]

Health savings accounts (HSAs) were initially designed as a way for business owners to cut down on the rising cost of health insurance for their employees. HSAs allow consumers to save money in special savings accounts and then pay part of their medical expenses with that money; they can be opened only in conjunction with an insurance policy that is HSA-qualified. If the money saved in an HSA is used for nonmedical expenses, then it is taxed as income. Particularly with small businesses, care must be taken to aid employees in understanding and accepting the unfamiliar accounts. The transition can prove difficult for employees with burdensome medical expenses, and it can be hard to get employees to embrace the accounts when they have not built up funds and are not seeing the accounts as a way to save. At the onset, it is important for employers to put company money in the HSAs so it is less difficult for employees to adjust to the high deductibles that accompany the accounts. Many employers have attempted to make the transition easier by offering educational sessions and compiling lists of what certain services and medications will cost with local doctors and hospitals.

---

13. Source: Vanessa Fuhrmans, "A Big Insurer Bets on Hot Trend: Shopping Around for Health Care," *The Wall Street Journal,* October 24, 2005.

14. Source: Sarah Rubenstein, "Using Health Savings Accounts Cuts Costs, but It's Not Easy," *The Wall Street Journal,* July 5, 2005.

Questions for Discussion

1. *Critics of HSAs argue that health care consumers have difficulty synthesizing health care information. Discuss examples of other industries in which consumers make decisions with imperfect information.*
2. *Discuss some strategies that employers might use to help their employees obtain useful health care information.*
3. *Although the stock and flow of health care information has increased markedly in the past decade, a uniform, easy-to-read* Consumer Reports *type of source for choosing doctors and hospitals does not exist. Why? What are the barriers to creating such a universal source?*

REVIEW QUESTIONS AND PROBLEMS

1. Suppose Joe and Leo both face the following individual loss distribution:

Probability of Loss	Amount of Loss
.7	$0
.2	$40
.1	$60

   A. Determine the expected loss and standard deviation of the expected loss faced by Joe and Leo on an individual basis.
   B. Suppose that Joe and Leo enter into a pooling-of-losses arrangement. Show what happens to the expected loss and variability of the expected loss as a result of the pooling arrangement.
2. Given their benefits, why don't most people simply form their own pooling-of-losses arrangements rather than involve insurance companies?
3. Joe is currently unemployed and without health insurance coverage. He derives utility (U) from his interest income on his savings (Y) according to the following function:

$$U = 5Y^{1/2}.$$

   Joe presently makes about $40,000 of interest income per year. He realizes that there is about a 5 percent probability that he may suffer a heart attack. The cost of treatment will be about $20,000 if a heart attack occurs.
   A. Calculate Joe's expected utility level without any health insurance coverage.
   B. Calculate Joe's expected income without any health insurance coverage.
   C. Suppose Joe must pay a premium of $1,500 for health insurance coverage with ACME insurance. Would he buy the health insurance? Why or why not?
   D. Suppose now that the government passes a law that allows all people—not just the self-employed or employed—to have their entire insurance premium exempted from taxes. Joe is in the 33 percent tax bracket. Would he buy the health insurance at a premium cost of $1,500? Why or why not? What implication can be drawn from the analysis?
   E. Suppose Joe purchases the health insurance coverage and represents the average subscriber, and his expectations are correct. Calculate the loading fee the insurance company will receive.

4. During the Reagan administration, the marginal tax rate on wage income fell dramatically. For example, the top rate was sliced from 70 to 33 percent. Use the demand theory of health insurance to predict the effect of this change on the quantity demanded of employer-sponsored health insurance.
5. Explain the effect of the following changes on the quantity demanded of health insurance.
   A. A reduction in the tax-exempt fraction of health insurance premiums
   B. An increase in buyer income
   C. An increase in per capita medical expenditures
   D. New technologies that enable medical illnesses to be predicted more accurately
   E. A tendency among buyers to become less risk averse, on average
6. What are the primary differences between the HMO, PPO, and POS plans?
7. Explain the following terms:
   A. Community rating
   B. Experience rating
   C. Selective contracting
   D. Utilization review
   E. Physician profiling
   F. Practice guidelines
   G. Formulary
   H. Gatekeeper
   I. Gag rules
   J. Any willing provider law
   K. Freedom of choice law
8. Suppose that an individual's demand for the number of physician visits per year, Q, can be represented by the following equation: $Q = 5 - 0.04P$, where P, the market price of an office visit, equals the marginal cost of $100. Determine the efficient number of office visits according to conventional theory. Now assume that the person purchases complete health insurance coverage and the demand for (but not quantity demanded of) physician care remains unchanged. How many times would this fully insured person visit the physician? Calculate the welfare loss or moral hazard cost associated with the insurance coverage.
9. Graphically and in words, explain how the analysis in question 8 might change if we adopt the conceptual framework provided by Nyman.
10. Use all of the information in question 1 to calculate the expected utility loss of paying the premium and remaining healthy and compare it to the expected utility gain of the income transfer if ill (ignore the tax exemption feature of premium payments). Would Joe purchase health insurance according to the Nyman model? How does that prediction compare to the prediction of the conventional model under similar circumstances?
11. According to Nyman, conventional theory predicts that people behave irrationally. How does he justify this criticism? Explain.
12. Briefly summarize the two ways that managed care might affect the cost and quality of medical care.
13. If you had a choice between a traditional unrestricted indemnity plan with a 10 percent copayment and a staff HMO with no copayment, at what percentage difference in premiums (that is, 10 percent, 20 percent, 30 percent) would you be indifferent between the plans? Do you think your choice of the percentage difference is a function of your age and/or health status? If you were elderly and/or sickly, which plan would you prefer if they cost you the same amount? Why?

Online Resources

To access Internet links related to the topics in this chapter, please visit our web site at **www.thomsonedu.com/economics/santerre**.

References

Berk, Marc L., and Alan C. Monheit. "The Concentration of Health Care Expenditures, Revisited." *Health Affairs* 20 (March/April 2001), pp. 9–18.

Dowd, Bryan, and Roger Feldman. "Premium Elasticities of Health Plan Choice." *Inquiry* 31 (winter 1994/95), pp. 438–44.

Ermann, Dan. "Hospital Utilization Review. Past Experience, Future Directions." *Journal of Health Politics, Policy, and Law* 13 (winter 1988), pp. 683–704.

Farley, Pamela J., and Gail Wilensky. "Household Wealth and Health Insurance as Protection against Medical Risks." In *Horizontal Equity, Uncertainty, and Economic Well-Being,* eds. David Martin and Timothy Smeeding. Chicago: University of Chicago Press for the NBER, 1984, pp. 323–54.

Feldstein, Martin S. "The Welfare Loss of Excess Health Insurance" *Journal of Political Economy* (March-April 1973), pp. 257–80.

Gold, Marsha, Lyle Nelson, Timothy Lake, Robert Hurley, and Robert Berenson. "Behind the Curve: A Critical Assessment of How Little Is Known about Arrangements between Managed Care Plans and Physicians." *Medical Care Research and Review* 52 (September 1995), pp. 307–41.

Goldstein, Gerald S., and Mark V. Pauly. "Group Health Insurance as a Local Public Good." In *The Role of Health Insurance in the Health Services Sector,* ed. Richard Rossett. New York: NBER, 1976, pp. 73–110.

Harrington, Scott E., and Gregory R. Niehaus. *Risk Management and Insurance.* Boston: McGraw-Hill/Irwin, 2004.

Hellinger, Fred J. "Update: Any-Willing-Provider and Freedom-of-Choice Laws: An Economic Assessment." *Health Affairs* 14 (winter 1995), pp. 297–302.

Holmer, Martin. "Tax Policy and the Demand for Health Insurance." *Journal of Health Economics* 3, no. 3 (1984), pp. 203–21.

Keynes, John Maynard. *The General Theory of Employment Interest and Money.* New York: Harcourt Brace and Company, 1936.

Kumar, Nanda, Marc A. Cohen, Christine E. Bishop, and Stanley S. Wallack. "Understanding the Factors behind the Decision to Purchase Varying Coverage Amounts of Long-Term Care Insurance." *Health Services Research* 29 (February 1995), pp. 653–78.

Landon, Bruce E., Ira B. Wilson, and Paul D. Cleary. "A Conceptual Model of the Effects of Health Care Organizations on the Quality of Medical Care." *Journal of the American Medical Association* 279 (May 6, 1998), pp. 1377–82.

Liu, Chuan-Fen, and Jon B. Christianson. "The Demand for Health Insurance by Employees in a Voluntary Small Group Insurance Program." *Medical Care* 36 (1998), pp. 437–43.

Manning, Willard and M. Susan Marquis. "Health Insurance: The Trade Off Between Risk Pooling and moral Hazzard." *Journal of Health Economics* 15 (1996), pp. 609–59.

Manning, William G., and M. Susan Marquis. "Health Insurance: The Trade-Off between Risk Pooling and Moral Hazard." (R-3729-NCHSR) Santa Monica, Calif.: RAND, 1989.

Marquis, M. Susan, Melinda B. Bunting, Jose J. Escarce, Kanika Kapur, and Jill M. Yegian. "Subsidies and The Demand for Individual Health Insurance in California." *Health Services Research* 39 (October, 2004), pp. 1547–70.

Marquis, M. Susan, and Stephen H. Long. "Worker Demand for Health Insurance in the Non-Group Market." *Journal of Health Economics* 14 (1995), pp. 47–63.

Miller, Richard D. "Estimating the Compensating Differential for Employer-Provided Health Insurance." *International Journal of Health Care Finance and Economics* 4 (2004), pp. 27–41.

Miller, Tracy E. "Managed Care Regulation: In the Laboratory of the States." *Journal of the American Medical Association* 278 (October 1, 1997), pp. 1102–9.

Nyman, John A. *The Theory of Demand for Health Insurance.* Stanford University Press, 2003.

Pauly, Mark V. "Taxation, Health Insurance, and Market Failure in the Medical Economy." *Journal of Economic Literature* 24 (June 1986), pp. 629–75.

Sheils, John, and Randall Haught. "The Cost of Tax-Exempt Health Benefits in 2004." *Health Affairs*, http://www.healthaffairs.org, February 25, 2004.

Short, Pamela F., and Amy K. Taylor. "Premiums, Benefits, and Employee Choice of Health Insurance Options." *Journal of Health Economics* 8 (1989), pp. 293–311.

Strombom, Bruce A., Thomas C. Buchmueller, and Paul J. Feldstein. "Switching Costs, Price Sensitivity and Health Plan Choice." *Journal of Health Economics* 21 (2002), pp. 89–116.

Taylor, Amy K., and Gail R. Wilensky. "The Effect of Tax Policies on Expenditures for Private Health Insurance." In *Market Reforms in Health Care,* ed. Jack Meyer. Washington, D.C.: American Enterprise Institute, 1983.

CHAPTER 7

MEDICAL CARE PRODUCTION AND COSTS

In December 2000 it was announced that Northeast Georgia Health System, a 338-bed not-for-profit hospital in Gainesville, Georgia, proposed to buy Lanier Park Hospital, a 119-bed for-profit hospital also in Gainesville, for $40 million. The acquisition would result in only one hospital in Gainesville. Executives at the hospitals claim the acquisition would save $2 million annually (Kirchheimer, 2000). Similarly, in July 2005 it was announced that United Health Group, the nation's second-largest health insurer, planned to join with PacifiCare Health Systems, the second-largest private administrator of Medicare health plans. The combination would create one of the nation's largest private health plan providers with about 26 million subscribers. A spokeperson for the two insurers claimed that the merger would cut operating costs by an estimated $100 million in the first year alone (Jablon, 2005).

These are just two examples of the many mergers that take place in the health care sector. Recent combinations among firms in other health care markets, such as the physician, pharmaceutical, and nursing home industries, also testify to the assertion that larger firm size confers significant cost advantages. But are there any plausible economic reasons to support the claim that cost savings are associated with larger organizational size? If so, sound economic reasoning can justify a merger among two or more firms in the same industry. On the other hand, might operating costs actually increase as a firm gets too large? If that is the case, a merger among firms is not desirable if cost savings are the overriding concern.

This chapter introduces various microeconomic principles and concepts that can be used to analyze the cost structure of medical firms and thereby determine the true relation between firm size and costs of production. In addition, the chapter:

- discusses various production characteristics, including marginal and average productivity and the elasticity of substitution among inputs
- uses the resulting production theory to derive short-run and long-run costs of production
- examines economies and diseconomies of scale and scope

The Short-Run Production Function of the Representative Medical Firm

All medical firms, including hospitals, physician clinics, nursing homes, and pharmaceutical companies, earn revenues from producing and selling some type of medical output. Production and retailing activities occur regardless of the form of ownership (that is, for-profit, public, or not-for-profit). Because these activities take place in a world of scarce resources, microeconomics can provide valuable insights into the operation and planning processes of medical firms. In this chapter, we focus on various economic principles that guide the production behavior of all types of firms, including medical firms. We begin by analyzing the short-run production process of a hypothetical medical firm.

To simplify our discussion of short-run production, we make five assumptions. First, we assume the medical firm produces a single output of medical services, q. Second, we initially assume only two medical inputs exist: nurse-hours, n, and a composite capital good, k. We can think of the composite capital good as an amalgamation of all types of capital, including any medical equipment and the physical space in the medical establishment. Third, since the short run is defined as a period of time over which the level of *at least* one input cannot be changed, we assume the quantity of capital is fixed at some amount. This assumption makes intuitive sense, because it is usually more difficult to change the stock of capital than the number of nurse-hours in the short run. Fourth, we assume for now that the medical firm faces an incentive to produce as efficiently as possible. Finally, we assume the medical firm possesses perfect information regarding the demands for its product. We relax the last two assumptions at the end of the chapter.

As we know from Chapter 2, a production function identifies how various inputs can be combined and transformed into a final output. In the present example, the short-run production function for medical services can be mathematically generalized as

(7–1) $$q = f(n, \bar{k}).$$

The short-run production function for medical services in Equation 7–1 indicates that the level of medical services is a function of a variable nurse input and a fixed (denoted with a bar) capital input. The production function identifies the different ways nurse-hours and capital can be combined to produce various levels of medical services. The production function allows for the possibility that each level of output may be produced by several different combinations of the nurse and capital inputs. Each combination is assumed to be **technically efficient,** since it results in the maximum amount of output that is feasible given the state of technology. Later we will see that both technical and economic considerations determine a unique least-cost, or economically efficient, method of production.

We begin our analysis by examining how the level of medical services, q, relates to a greater quantity of the variable nurse input, n, given that the capital input, $\bar{k}$, is assumed to be fixed. Various microeconomic principles and concepts relating to production theory are used to determine the precise relation between the employment of the variable input and the level of total output. As mentioned in Chapter 2, one important microeconomic principle from production theory is the law of diminishing marginal productivity. This is not really a law; rather, it is a generalization about production behavior and states that total output at first increases at an *increasing* rate, but after some point increases at a *decreasing* rate, with respect to a greater quantity of a variable input, holding all other inputs constant.[1]

1. In Chapter 2, we assumed for simplicity that the law of diminishing marginal returns sets in immediately; that is, the marginal product of medical services was always declining. In this chapter, we take a less restrictive approach to allow for the theoretical possibility that the marginal product of the variable input may increase initially. The fundamental idea remains the same, however. Eventually a point is reached where additional units of an input generate smaller marginal returns.

FIGURE 7–1
The Total Product Curve

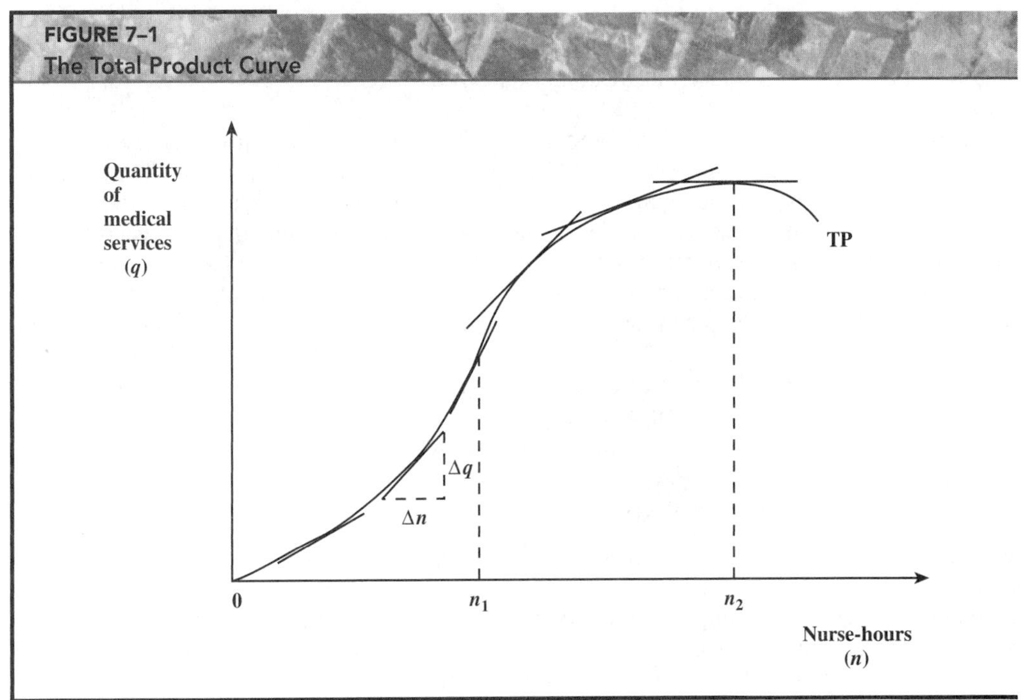

The total product curve shows that output initially increases at an increasing rate from 0 to n_1 nurse-hours, then increases at a decreasing rate from n_1 to n_2 nurse-hours, and finally declines after n_2 nurse-hours as the medical firm employs more nurse-hours. Diminishing marginal productivity provides the reason why output fails to expand at an increasing rate after n_1 nurse-hours.

Figure 7–1 applies the law of diminishing productivity. It shows a graphical relation between the quantity of medical services on the vertical axis and the number of nurse-hours on the horizontal axis. The curve is referred to as the *total product curve*, TP, because it depicts the total output produced by different levels of the variable input, holding all other inputs constant. Notice that the quantity of services first increases at an increasing rate over the range of nurse-hours from 0 to n_1. The rate of increase is identified by the slope of the curve at each point. As you can see, the slope of the total product curve increases in value as the tangent lines become steeper over this range of nurse-hours.

Beyond point n_1, however, further increases in nurse-hours cause medical services to increase, but at a decreasing rate. That is the point at which diminishing productivity sets in. Notice that the slope of the total product curve gets smaller as output increases in the range from n_1 to n_2 (as indicated by the flatter tangent lines). At n_2, the slope of the total product curve is zero, as reflected in the horizontal tangent line. Finally, beyond n_2, we allow for the possibility that too many nurse-hours will lead to a reduction in the quantity of medical services. The slope of the total product curve is negative beyond n_2.

In terms of the production decision at the firm level, we have not yet accounted for the specific reasoning underlying the law of diminishing marginal productivity. Economists point to the fixed short-run inputs as the basis for diminishing productivity. For example, when nurse-hours are increased at first, there is initially a considerable amount of capital, the fixed input, with which to produce medical services. The abundance of capital enables increasingly greater amounts of medical services to be generated from the employment of additional nurses. In addition, a synergy effect may dominate initially. The synergy effect means that nurses, working cooperatively as a team, are able to produce more output collectively than separately because of labor specialization, for example.

At some point, however, the fixed capital becomes limited relative to the variable input (for example, too little medical equipment and not enough medical space), and additional nurse-hours generate successively fewer incremental units of medical services. In the extreme, as more nurses are crowded into a medical establishment of a fixed size, the quantity of services may actually begin to decline as congestion sets in and creates unwanted production problems.

In general, any physical constraint in production, such as the fixed size of the facility or a limited amount of medical equipment, can cause diminishing productivity to set in at some point. In fact, if it weren't for diminishing productivity, the world's food supply could be grown in a single flowerpot and the demand for medical services could be completely satisfied by a single large medical organization. What a wonderful world it would be! Unfortunately, however, diminishing productivity is the rule rather than the exception.

Marginal and Average Products

We can also use marginal and average product curves rather than the total product curve to illustrate the fundamental characteristics associated with the production process. In general, the marginal product is the change in total output associated with a one-unit change in the variable input. In terms of our example, the marginal product or quantity of medical services associated with an additional nurse-hour, MP_n, can be stated as follows:

(7–2) $$MP_n = \Delta q/\Delta n.$$

The magnitude of the marginal product of a nurse-hour reveals the additional quantity of medical services produced by each additional nurse-hour. It is a measure of the marginal contribution of a nurse-hour in the production of medical services.

In Figure 7–1, the slope of the total product curve at every point represents the marginal product of a nurse-hour, since it measures the rise (vertical distance) over the run (horizontal distance), or $\Delta q/\Delta n$. Consequently, we can determine the marginal product of an additional nurse-hour by examining the slope of the total product curve at each level of nurse-hours. Figure 7–2 graphically illustrates the marginal product of a nurse-hour. Initially, MP_n is positive and increases over the range from 0 to n_1 due to increasing marginal productivity. In the range from n_1 to n_2, the marginal product is positive but decreasing, because diminishing marginal productivity has set in. At n_2, the marginal product of a nurse-hour is zero and becomes negative thereafter. The marginal product curve suggests that each additional nurse-hour cannot be expected to generate the same marginal contribution to total output as the previous one. The law of diminishing marginal productivity dictates that in the short run, a level of output is eventually reached where an incremental increase in the number of nurse-hours leads to successively fewer additions to total output (because some other inputs are fixed).

In addition to MP_n, the average product of a nurse-hour can provide insight into the production process. In general, the average product equals the total quantity of output divided by the level of the variable input. In terms of the present example, the average product of a nurse-hour, AP_n, is calculated by dividing the total quantity of medical services by the total number of nurse-hours:

(7–3) $$AP_n = q/n.$$

The average product of a nurse-hour measures the average quantity of medical services produced within an hour. For example, suppose we (crudely) measure total medical services by the

FIGURE 7–2
The Marginal Product Curve

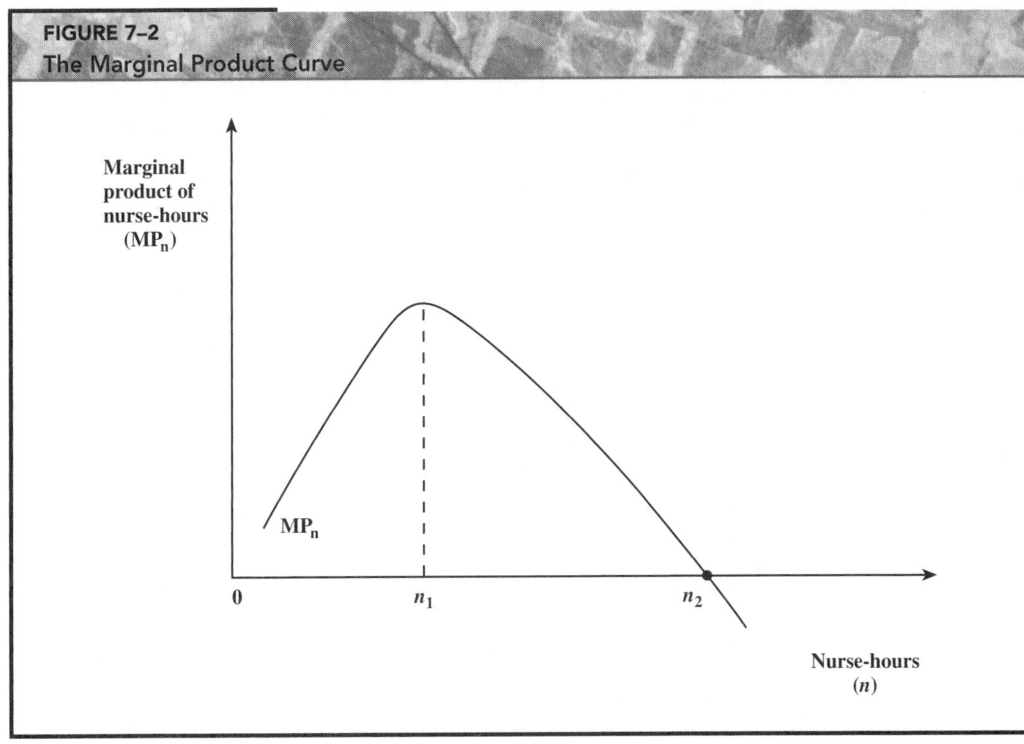

The marginal product of an additional nurse-hour is found by dividing the change in output by the change in the number of nurse-hours and is measured by the slope of the total product curve. Marginal productivity first increases with the number of nurse-hours because of synergy and labor specialization and then falls because of the fixed input that exists in the short run.

number of daily patient-hours at a medical facility. In addition, suppose 200 nurse-hours are employed to service 300 daily patient-hours. In this example, the average product of a nurse-hour equals 300/200 or 1½ patients per hour.

We can also derive the average product of a nurse-hour from the total product curve, as shown in Figure 7–3*a*. To derive AP_n, a ray from the origin is extended to each point on the total product curve. The slope of the ray measures AP_n for any given level of nurse-hours, since it equals the rise over the run, or q/n. In Figure 7–3*a* three rays, labeled 0*A*, 0*B*, and 0*C*, emanate from the origin to the total product curve. The slope of ray 0*A* is flatter than that of 0*B* and therefore is of a lower magnitude. In fact, as it is drawn, ray 0*B* has a greater slope than any other ray emanating from the origin. At this level of nurse-hours, the average product is maximized. The slope of ray 0*C* is flatter and of a lower magnitude than that of 0*B*. The implication is that average product initially increases over the range from 0 to n_3 reaches a maximum at n_3, and then decreases, as shown in Figure 7–3*b*. It is the law of diminishing marginal productivity that accounts for the shape of AP_n.

In Figure 7–4, the marginal and average product curves are superimposed to illustrate how they are related. Some characteristics of the relation between these two curves are worth mentioning. First, the marginal product curve cuts the average product curve at its maximum point. In fact, it is a common mathematical principle that the marginal equals the average when the

FIGURE 7–3
Deriving the Average Product Curve from the Total Product Curve

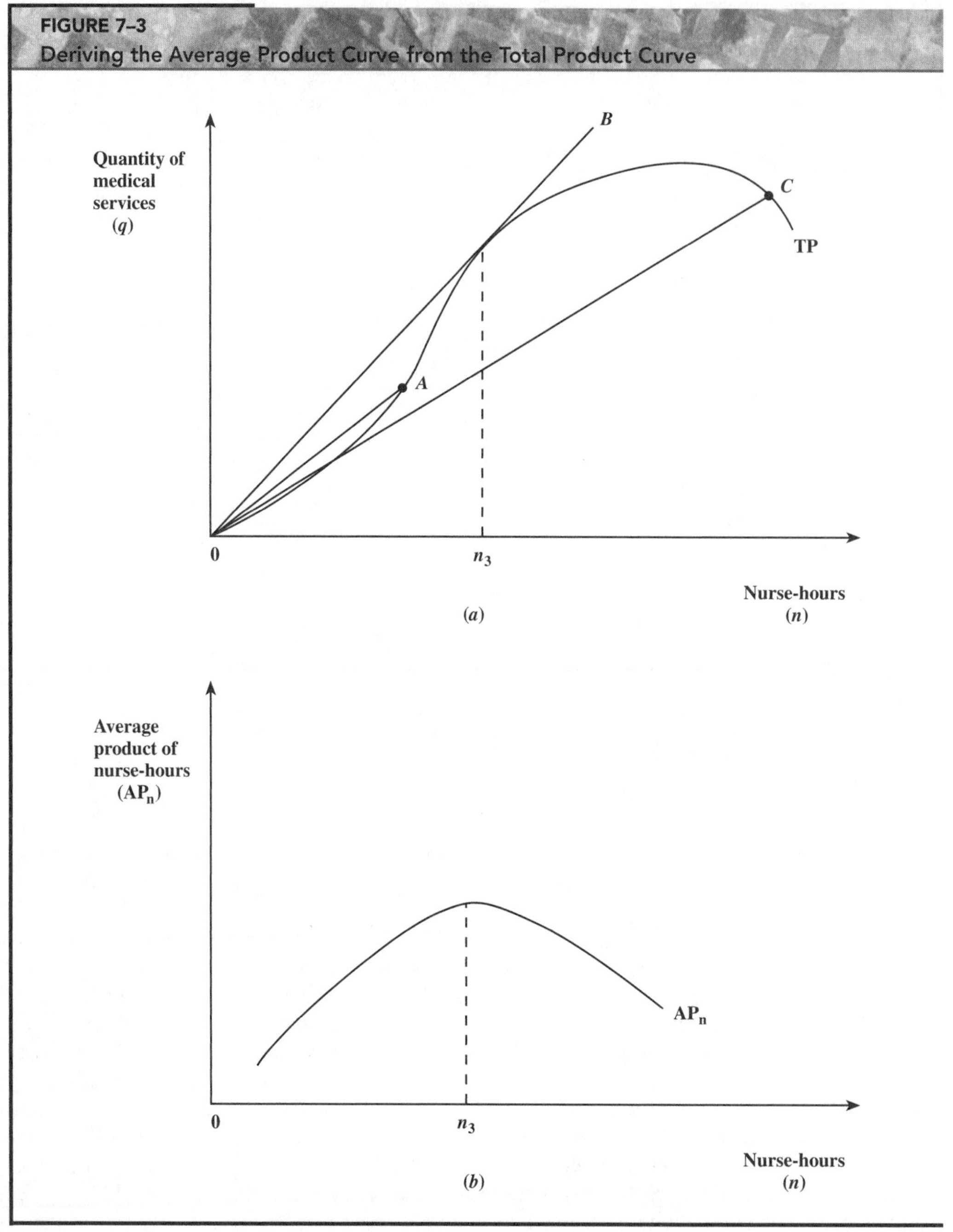

The average product of a nurse-hour is found by dividing total output by the total number of nurse-hours and can be derived by measuring the slope of a ray emanating from the origin to each point on the total product curve. Average productivity first increases with the number of nurse-hours and then declines because of increasing and then diminishing marginal productivity.

FIGURE 7–4
Relation between the Marginal and Average Product Curves

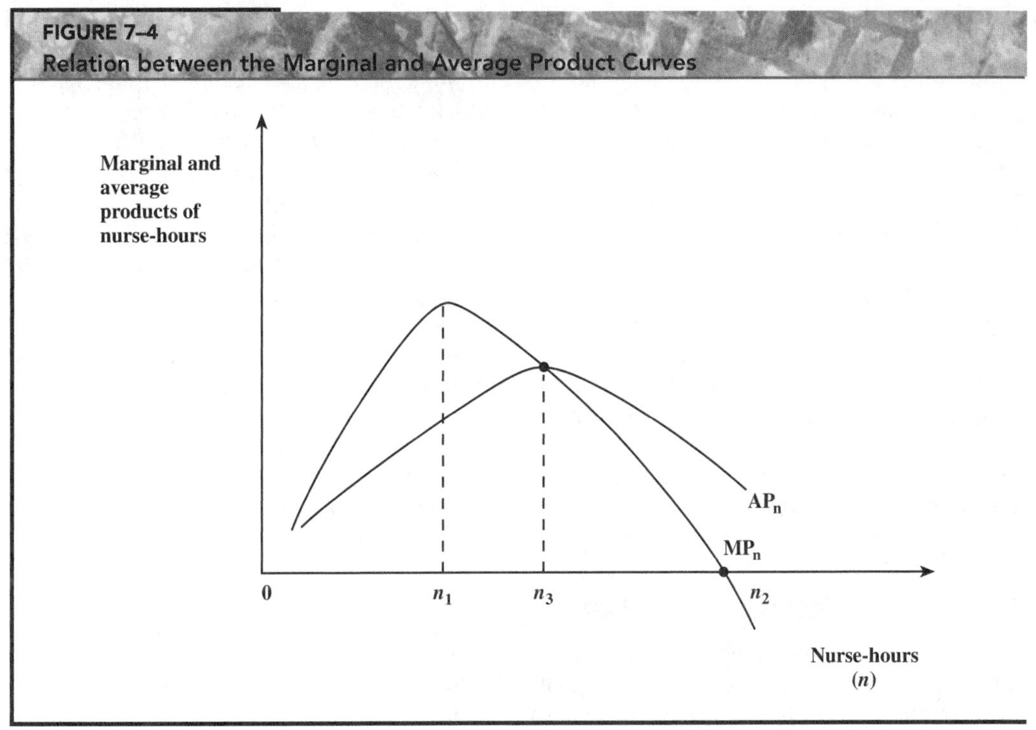

Average productivity rises when marginal productivity exceeds average productivity. Average productivity falls when marginal productivity lies below average productivity. Marginal productivity equals average productivity when average productivity is maximized.

average is at its extreme value.[2] Second, MP_n lies above AP_n whenever AP_n is increasing. This too reflects a common mathematical principle and should come as little surprise to the reader. For example, if your average grade in a course is a B+ until the final and you receive an A on the final exam, this incremental higher grade pulls up your final average grade. Third, MP_n lies below AP_n whenever AP_n is declining. This relation between marginal and average values also should not be surprising. As you know, your course grade slips if you receive a lower grade on the final exam relative to your previous course average.

Putting the grades aside (because learning is more important than grades—right?), we can discuss the relation between the marginal and average product curves in terms of our example concerning nurse-hours and the production of medical services. For this discussion, it helps to think of the marginal product curve as the amount of medical services generated hourly by the next

2. *Proof:* For simplicity, suppose the production function relates the quantity of output, q, to a single input of nurse-hours, n, such that $q = f(n)$. The average product of nurse-hours, AP_n, can be written as $f(n)/n$. To determine where AP_n reaches a maximum point, we can take the first derivative of AP_n and set it equal to zero. Following the rule for taking the derivative of a quotient of two functions (see Chiang, 1984), it follows that

(7–1*a*) $$f'(n) = \frac{f(n)}{n}.$$

since $f'(n)$ equals MP_n and $f(n)/n$ equals AP_n, $MP_n = AP_n$ when AP_n is maximized.

nurse hired. Also, we can think of the average product curve as the average quantity of medical services generated by the existing team of nurses within an hour—that is, the "team" average.

Looking back at Figure 7–4, notice that the next nurse hired always generates more services per hour than the team average up to point n_3. Consequently, up to this point, each additional nurse helps pull up the team's average level of output. Beyond n_3, however, the incremental nurse hired generates less services per hour than the team average; as a result, the team average falls. It is important to realize that any increase or decrease in the marginal product has nothing to do with the individual talents of each additional nurse employed. Rather, it involves the law of diminishing marginal productivity. At some point in the production process, the incremental nurse becomes less productive due to the constraint imposed by the fixed input. The marginal productivity, in turn, influences the average productivity of the team of nurses.

At first glance, it seems logical to assume that a medical firm desires to produce at a point like n_1 or n_3 in Figure 7–4. After all, they represent the points at which either the marginal or the average product is maximized. In most cases, however, a medical firm finds it more desirable to achieve some financial target, such as a maximum or break-even level of profits. As a result, we need more information concerning the revenue and cost structures the medical firm faces before we can pinpoint the desired level of production. In later chapters we will see that under normal conditions, the relevant range of production in Figure 7–4 is between n_3 and n_2.

Elasticity of Input Substitution

Up to now, we have assumed only one variable input. Realistically, however, the medical firm operates with more than one variable input in the short run. Thus, there may be some possibilities for substitution between any two variable inputs. For example, licensed practical nurses often substitute for registered nurses in the production of inpatient services, and physician assistants sometimes substitute for physicians in the production of ambulatory services. The actual degree of substitutability between any two inputs depends on technical and legal considerations. For example, physician assistants are prohibited by law from prescribing medicines in most states. In addition, licensed practical nurses normally lack the technical knowledge needed to perform all the duties of registered nurses.

In general terms, the elasticity of substitution between any two inputs equals the percentage change in the input ratio divided by the percentage change in the ratio of the inputs' marginal productivities, holding constant the level of output, or

(7–4)
$$\sigma = \frac{\Delta(I_1/I_2)}{I_1/I_2} \div \frac{\Delta(\mathrm{MP}_2/\mathrm{MP}_1)}{\mathrm{MP}_2/\mathrm{MP}_1}$$

I_i ($i = 1,2$) stands for the quantity employed of each input. The ratio of marginal productivities, $\mathrm{MP}_2/\mathrm{MP}_1$, referred to as the *marginal rate of technical substitution*, illustrates the rate at which one input substitutes for the other in the production process, at the margin. For example, suppose the marginal product of a registered nurse-hour is four patients and the marginal product of a licensed practical nurse-hour is two patients. It follows that two licensed practical nurse-hours are needed to substitute completely for one registered nurse-hour.

Theoretically, σ (Greek letter sigma) takes on values between 0 and $+\infty$ and identifies the percentage change in the input ratio that results from a 1 percent change in the marginal rate of technical substitution. The magnitude of σ identifies the degree of substitution between the two inputs. For example, if $\sigma = 0$, the variable inputs cannot be substituted in production. In contrast, when $\sigma = \infty$, the two variable inputs are perfect substitutes in production. In practice, it is more common for σ to take on values between these two extremes, implying that limited substitution possibilities exist.

A Production Function for Hospital Admissions

Jensen and Morrisey (1986) provide one of the more interesting empirical studies on the production characteristics of hospital services. In keeping with Equation 7–1, Jensen and Morrisey estimated a production function for admissions at 3,540 nonteaching hospitals in the United States as of 1983 in the following general form:[3]

(7–5) Case-mix-adjusted hospital admissions = f(Physicians, nurses, other nonphysician staff, hospital beds, X)

Notice that hospital admissions serve as the measure of output. Given the heterogeneous nature of hospital services, however, this output measure was adjusted for case-mix differences across hospitals by multiplying it by the Medicare patient index. This index is the weighted sum of the proportions of the hospital's Medicare patients in different diagnostic categories where the weights reflect the average costs per case in each diagnostic group. The number of physicians, nurses (full-time equivalent [FTE] units), and other nonphysician staff (FTE) represented the labor inputs; the number of beds constituted the capital input; and X stood for a number of other production factors not central to the discussion.

To put Equation 7–5 in a form that can be estimated with a multiple regression technique, Jensen and Morrisey specified a translog production function. The form and properties of this particular mathematical function are too complex to describe briefly; it suffices to note that the translog is a flexible functional form that imposes very few restrictions on the estimated parameters.[4]

From the empirical estimation, Jensen and Morrisey were able to derive estimates of each input's marginal product. As expected, the marginal products were all positive. Jensen and Morrisey noted that the marginal product of each input declined in magnitude with greater usage, as the law of diminishing marginal product suggests. The estimated marginal product of a physician implied that an additional doctor generated 6.05 additional case-mix-adjusted annual admissions. The nurse input was by far the most productive input. In particular, the marginal nurse was responsible for producing about 20.3 additional case-mix-adjusted annual admissions. The marginal products of other nonphysician staff and beds were found to be 6.97 and 3.04 case-mix-adjusted annual admissions, respectively.

The estimation procedure also generated sufficient information to enable Jensen and Morrisey to measure the input substitution possibilities available to hospitals. Each input was found to be a substitute for the others in production. In particular, the substitution elasticities between physicians and nurses, physicians and beds, and nurses and beds were reported to be .547, .175, and .124, respectively. The relatively large elasticity of .547 between physicians and nurses tells us that the average hospital can more easily substitute between these two inputs. This particular input elasticity estimate can be interpreted to mean that a 10 percent increase in the marginal productivity of a doctor causes a 5.47 percent increase in the ratio of nurses to doctors, *ceteris paribus*. These positive substitution elasticities suggest that hospital policy makers can avoid some of the price (wage) increase in any one input by substituting with the others. For example, to maintain a given level of admissions, a wage increase for nurses might be partially absorbed by increasing the number of hospital beds.

---

3. For the sake of brevity, we do not discuss their results for the sample of teaching hospitals.

4. In a translog function, (the natural log of) each independent variable enters the equation in both linear and quadratic form. In addition, a cross-product linear term is created between any two independent variables and specified in the function. Similar cross-product terms are eliminated from the specification. To ensure a well-behaved function, restrictions are normally imposed on the parameter estimates.

SHORT-RUN COST THEORY OF THE REPRESENTATIVE MEDICAL FIRM

Before we begin our discussion of the medical firm's cost curves, we need to address the difference between the ways economists and accountants refer to costs. In particular, accountants consider only the *explicit costs* of doing business when determining the accounting profits of a medical firm. Explicit costs are easily quantified because a recent market transaction is available to provide an accurate measure of cost. Wage payments to the hourly medical staff, electric utility bills, and medical supply expenses are all examples of the explicit costs medical firms incur because disbursement records can be consulted to determine the magnitudes of these expenditures.

Economists, unlike accountants, consider both the explicit and implicit costs of production. *Implicit costs* reflect the opportunity costs of using any resources the medical firm owns. For example, a general practitioner (GP) may own the physical assets (such as the clinic and medical equipment) used in producing physician services. In this case, a recent market transaction is unavailable to determine the cost of using these assets. Yet an opportunity cost is incurred when using them because the physical assets could have been rented out for an alternative use. For example, the clinic could be remodeled and rented as a beauty salon, and the medical equipment could be rented out to another physician. Thus, the forgone rental payments reflect the opportunity cost of using the physical assets owned by the GP.[5]

Consequently, when determining the economic (rather than accounting) profits of a firm, economists consider the total costs of doing business, including both the explicit and implicit costs. Economists believe it is important to determine whether sufficient revenues are available to cover the cost of using all inputs, including those rented and owned. For example, if the rental return on the physical assets is greater than the return on use, the GP might do better by renting out the assets rather than retaining them for personal use.

The Short-Run Cost Curves of the Representative Medical Firm

Cost theory is based on the production theory of the medical firm previously outlined and relates the quantity of output to the cost of production. As such, it identifies how (total and marginal) costs respond to changes in output. If we continue to assume the two inputs of nurse-hours, n, and capital, $\bar{k}$, the short-run total cost, STC, of producing a given level of medical output, q, can be written as

$$\text{STC}(q) = w \times n + r \times \bar{k}, \tag{7–6}$$

where w and r represent the hourly wage for a nurse and the rental or opportunity cost of capital, respectively. Input prices are assumed to be fixed, which means the single medical firm can purchase these inputs without affecting their market prices. This is a valid assumption as long as the firm is a small buyer of inputs relative to the total number of buyers in the marketplace.[6]

5. The general practitioner's labor time should also be treated as an implicit cost of doing business if she independently owns the clinic. As an entrepreneur, the GP does not receive an explicit payment but instead receives any residual profits that are left over after all other costs are paid. If the physician does not receive an appropriate rate of return, she may leave the area or the profession to get a better rate of return.

6. If the single firm were a large or an influential buyer, it might possess some "monopsony" power and could affect the market prices of the inputs.

Equation 7–6 implies that the short-run total costs of production are dependent on the quantities and prices of inputs employed. The wage rate times the number of nurse-hours equals the total wage bill and represents the total variable costs of production. Variable costs respond to changes in the level of output.[7] The product of the rental price and the quantity of capital represent the total fixed costs of production. Obviously, this cost component does not respond to changes in output, since the quantity of capital is fixed in the short run.

The total product curve not only identifies the quantity of medical output produced by a particular number of nurse-hours but also shows, reciprocally, the number of nurse-hours necessary to produce a given level of medical output. With this information, we can determine the short-run total cost of producing different levels of medical output by following a three-step procedure. First, we identify, through the production function, the necessary number of nurse-hours, n, for each level of medical output. Second, we multiply the quantity of nurse-hours by the hourly wage, w, to determine the short-run total variable costs, STVC, of production, or $w \times n$. Third, we add the short-run total fixed costs, STFC, or $r \times \bar{k}$, to STVC to derive the short-run total costs, STC, of production. If we conduct this three-step procedure for each level of medical output, we can derive a short-run total cost curve like the one in Figure 7–5.

7. For simplicity, we assume the wage rate represents total hourly compensation, including any fringe benefits.

FIGURE 7–5
The Short-Run Total Cost Curve

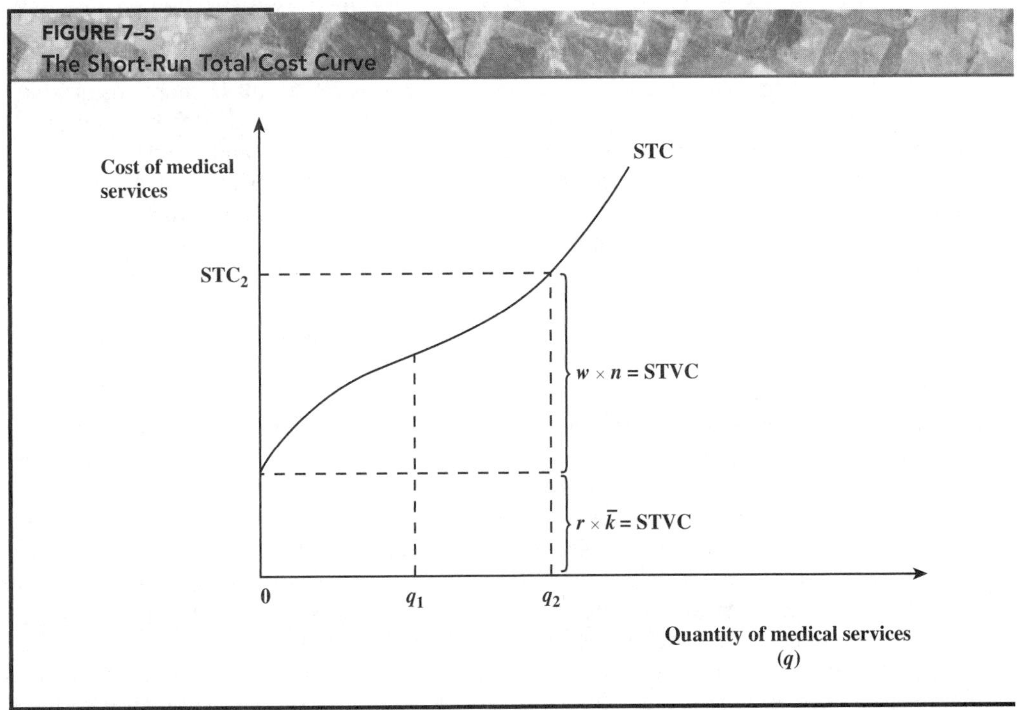

The short-run total cost, STC, of producing medical services equals the sum of the total variable, STVC, and fixed costs, STFC. STC first increases at a decreasing rate up to point q_1 and then increases at an increasing rate with respect to producing more output. STC increases at an increasing rate after q_1 because of diminishing marginal productivity.

Notice the reciprocal relation between the short-run total cost function in Figure 7–5 and the short-run total product curve in Figure 7–1. For example, when total product is increasing at an *increasing* rate up to point n_1 in Figure 7–1, short-run total costs are increasing at a *decreasing* rate up to point q_1 in Figure 7–5. This is because the increasing productivity in this range causes the total costs of production to rise slowly. Output increases at a *decreasing* rate immediately beyond point n_1 in Figure 7–1 (as shown by the slope of the total product curve), and, as a result, short-run total costs increase at an *increasing* rate beyond q_1 in Figure 7–5. Also notice that total costs increase solely because additional nurses are employed as output expands. Figure 7–5 also shows how short-run total cost can be decomposed into its variable and fixed components for the level of output q_2.

In practice, distinguishing between fixed and variable costs can be particularly challenging. Recall that variable costs change proportionately, whereas fixed costs do not change, in response to any adjustment in the quantity of output actually produced. Fixed costs occur in the short run, during the so-called *operating period,* when the levels of some inputs are fixed. In contrast, all inputs are variable during the long run or *planning period,* when, for instance, future budgets are being designed. The physical size of a production facility is often treated as a fixed input because a significant amount of time is needed to construct or relocate to a larger building. Hourly workers are typically treated as a variable input because they can be promptly hired or laid off, depending on the desired adjustment in output. As you can see, time plays a crucial role in determining the fixity of inputs and costs. It follows that long-term contracts, although potentially providing offsetting benefits, impose more fixed costs into a firm's budget.

In an article in the *Journal of the American Medical Association,* Roberts et al. (1999) were interested in distinguishing between the fixed and variable costs at a hospital because they wanted to know whether a significant amount of hospital costs could be saved by discouraging unnecessary hospital services. Reductions in hospital services can result in more cost savings when variable costs comprise a greater percentage of overall costs. But as Roberts et al. note, "a computed tomographic (CT) scan is thought of as an expensive test and a source of significant cost savings if it is not performed. However, the scanner and space have already been rented or paid for, and the technician receives a salary that must be paid whether any individual receives a CT scan or not. If the radiologist who interprets the test is also receiving a salary, the additional cost to the hospital of doing the test is minimal—the price of radiographic film, paper and contrast."

Roberts et al. examine the distribution of variable and fixed costs at Cook County Hospital in Chicago, Illinois, which was an 886-bed urban public teaching hospital when the study was done in 1993. The authors included capital, employee salaries, benefits, building maintenance, and utilities in the fixed-cost category. Note that employee salaries were included in the fixed-cost category, with the assumption being that Cook County was contractually obligated to pay these salaries during the budget period. Variable costs were specified to include health care worker supplies, such as gloves, patient care supplies, paper, food, radiographic film, laboratory reagents, glassware, and medications with their delivery systems such as intravenous catheters or bottles.

The authors found that the fixed costs comprised 84 percent of Cook County's total budget at that time. However, they caution that their results may not be applicable to cases in which hospitals hire more hourly or fee-for-service workers. At Cook County Hospital, most employees were salaried. But even in the case of nonsalaried personnel, Roberts et al. note that the intense employee specialization may make it more difficult for hospitals to downsize than traditional firms. For example, pediatric nurses may not be able to promptly adapt to adult cardiac care units. Given that a majority of costs were fixed, their study implies that a reduction in hospital services would have very little impact on Cook County's costs in the short run.

Short-Run Per-Unit Costs of Production

Another way to look at the reciprocal relation between production and costs is to focus on the short-run marginal and average variable costs of production. The short-run marginal costs, SMC, of production are equal to the change in total costs associated with a one-unit change in output, or

(7–7) $$\text{SMC} = \Delta\text{STC}/\Delta q.$$

In terms of Equations 7–6 and 7–7, the short-run marginal costs of production look like the following:

(7–8) $$\text{SMC} = \Delta(w \times n + r \times \bar{k})/\Delta q.$$

Because the wage rate and short-run fixed costs are constant with respect to output, Equation 7–8 can be rewritten in the following manner:

(7–9) $$\text{SMC} = w \times (\Delta n/\Delta q) = w \times (1/\text{MP}_\text{n}) = w/\text{MP}_\text{n}.$$

Notice on the right-hand side of Equation 7–9 that short-run marginal costs equal the wage rate divided by the marginal product of nurse-hours.

The short-run average variable costs, SAVC, of production equal the short-run total variable costs, STVC, divided by the quantity of medical output. Because STVC is the total wage bill (that is, $w \times n$),

(7–10) $$\text{SAVC} = \text{STVC}/q = (w \times n)/q = w \times (1/\text{AP}_\text{n}) = w/\text{AP}_\text{n}$$

such that SAVC equals the wage rate divided by the average product of a nurse-hour. Notice that the short-run marginal and average variable costs are inversely related to the marginal and average products of labor, respectively. Thus, marginal and average variable costs increase as the marginal and average products fall, and vice versa. Figure 7–6 shows the graphical relation between the per-unit product and cost curves.

The two graphs in Figure 7–6 clearly point out the reciprocal relation between production and costs. For example, after point n_1 in Figure 7–6*a*, diminishing productivity sets in and the marginal product begins to decline. As a result, the short-run marginal costs ($= w/\text{MP}_\text{n}$) increase beyond output level q_1 given a fixed wage. Similarly, the average product of a nurse-hour declines beyond n_3, so the average variable costs of production increase beyond q_3. Obviously, the shapes of the marginal cost and average variable cost curves reflect the law of diminishing marginal productivity. Because of this reciprocal relation, production and costs represent dual ways of observing various characteristics associated with the production process.

It is apparent from Equations 7–9 and 7–10 that the maximum points on the marginal and average product curves correspond directly to the minimum points on the marginal and average variable cost curves. Note in Figure 7–6*b* that the short-run marginal cost curve passes through the minimum point of the short-run average variable cost curve. In addition, the SMC curve lies below the SAVC curve when the latter is decreasing and above the SAVC curve when it is increasing.

In simple terms, the graph in Figure 7–6*b* identifies how costs behave as the medical firm alters output in the short run. Initially, as the medical firm expands output and employs more nurse-hours, both the marginal and average variable costs of production decline. Eventually, diminishing productivity sets in due to the fixed inputs, and both marginal and average variable

FIGURE 7–6
Relation between the Per-Unit Product and Cost Curves

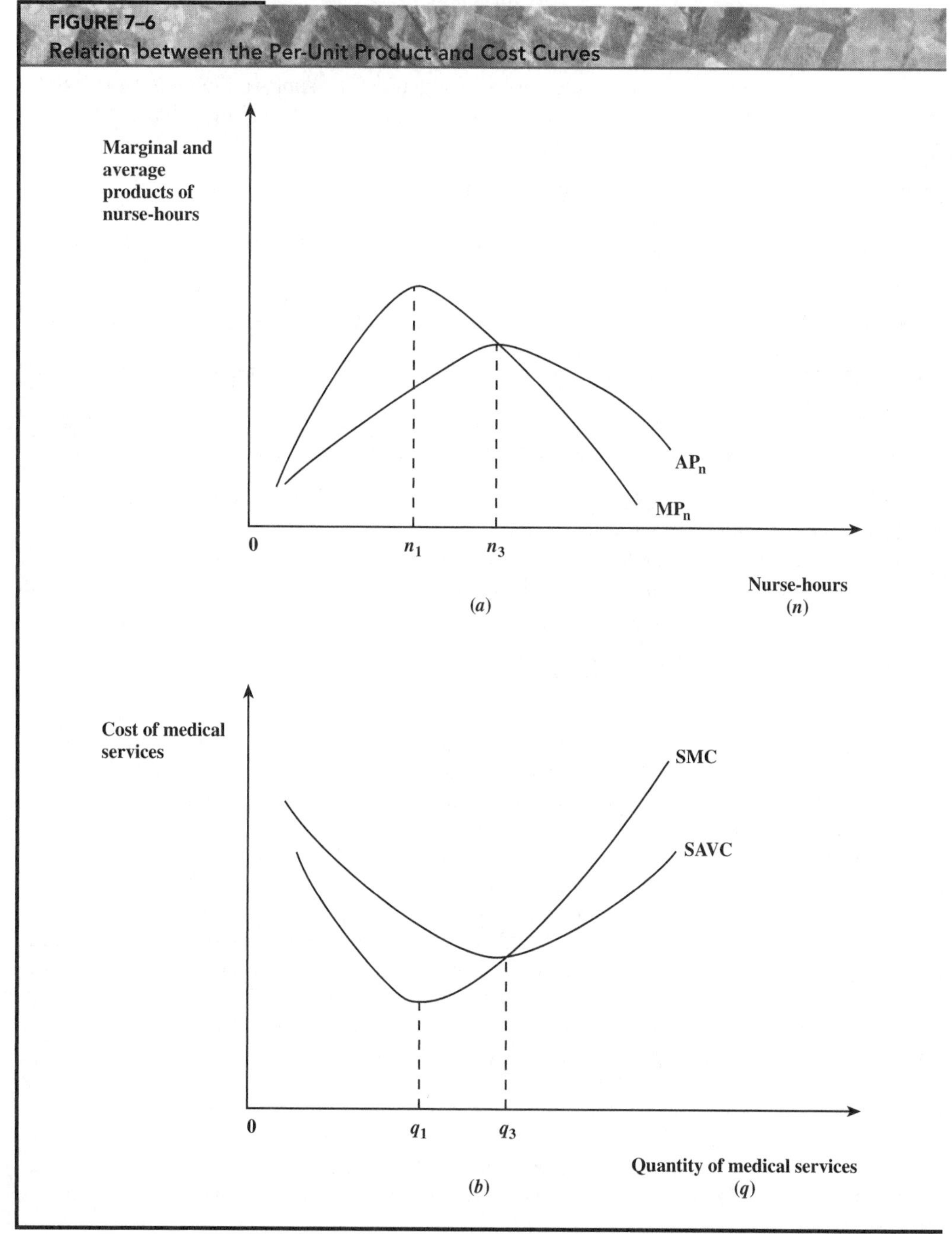

Short-run marginal cost, SMC, equals the change in total costs brought on by a one-unit change in output. Short-run average variable cost, SAVC, equals short-run total variable cost divided by total output. SMC and SAVC are inversely related to marginal and average productivity. For example, marginal costs decline as marginal productivity increases.

costs increase. It follows that the marginal and average variable costs of production depend in part on the amount of output a medical firm produces in the short run.

Besides the marginal and average variable costs of production, decision makers are interested in the short-run average total costs of operating the medical firm. Following Equation 7–6, we can find the short-run average total costs of production by summing the average variable costs and average fixed costs.[8] Short-run average fixed costs (SAFC) are simply total fixed costs (STFC) divided by the level of output, or

(7–11) $$\text{SAFC} = \text{STFC}/q.$$

Because by definition the numerator in Equation 7–11 is fixed in the short run, the SAFC declines as the denominator, medical services, increases in value. Consequently, the average fixed costs of production decline with greater amounts of output because total fixed costs (or overhead costs) are spread out over more and more units.

Figure 7–7 shows the graphical relation among SMC, SAVC, and SATC. Note that the marginal cost curve cuts the average total cost curve at its minimum point. (The minimum SATC lies to the right of the minimum SAVC. Why?) Also, note that the vertical distance between the average total and variable cost curves at each level of output represents the average fixed costs of production. This should not be surprising, since total costs include both variable and fixed costs. The vertical distance between the two curves gets smaller as output increases because the SAFC approaches zero with increases in output. One implication of the model is that average total costs increase at some level of output because eventually the cost-enhancing impact of diminishing productivity outweighs the cost-reducing tendency of the average fixed costs.

The unwitting reader may think that the medical firm should choose to produce at the minimum point on the SATC curve because average costs are minimized. As mentioned earlier, however, the level of output the medical firm chooses depends on the firm's objective (for example, to achieve maximum or break-even level of profits). Hence, a proper analysis requires some knowledge of the revenue structure in addition to the cost structure. In later chapters, we entertain some alternative objectives that may motivate the production behavior of medical firms. For now, however, assume for pedagogical purposes that the firm has chosen to produce the level of medical output, q_0, in Figure 7–7. Let's identify the various costs associated with producing q_0 units of medical output.

The identification of the per-unit cost of producing a given level of output is a fairly easy matter. We can determine the per-unit cost by extending a vertical line from the appropriate level of output until it crosses the cost curves. For example, the average total cost of producing q_0 units of output is SATC_0, while the average variable cost is SAVC_0. The average fixed cost of producing q_0 units of output is represented by the vertical distance between SATC_0 and SAVC_0, or distance *ab*.

---

8. Equation 7–6 can be rewritten as

(7–6*a*) $$\text{STC} = \text{STVC} + \text{STFC}.$$

Dividing both sides of Equation 7–6*a* by the level of output gives

(7–6*b*) $$\text{STC}/q = \text{STVC}/q + \text{STFC}/q.$$

Thus, by definition;

(7–6*c*) $$\text{SATC} = \text{SAVC} + \text{SAFC}.$$

FIGURE 7–7
Relation among Short-Run Marginal, Average Variable, and Average Total Costs

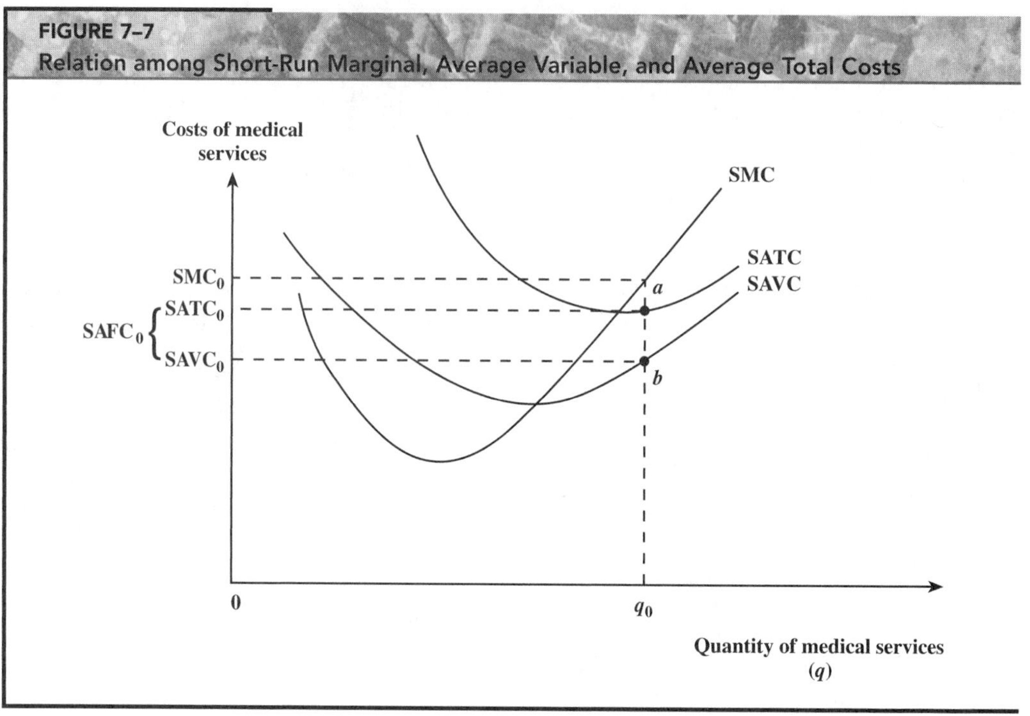

Short-run average total cost, SATC, equals the sum of short-run average variable cost, SAVC, and short-run average fixed cost, SAFC. Hence, SAFC is reflected in the vertical distance between the SATC and SAVC curves at each level of output. SMC cuts both of the average cost curves at their minimum points. SMC lies above the SAVC and SATC curves when they are rising and below them when they are falling.

In addition, SMC_0 identifies the marginal cost of producing one more unit assuming the medical firm is already producing q_0 units of medical services.

Now suppose that instead of the per-unit costs, we want to identify the various total costs (that is, STC, STVC, and STFC) associated with producing q_0 units of output. We can do this by multiplying the level of output by the per-unit costs of production. For example, the rectangle $SAVC_0$–b–q_0–0 in Figure 7–7 measures the total variable costs of producing q_0 units of output, since it corresponds to the area found by multiplying the base of 0–q_0 by the height of 0–$SAVC_0$. Following similar logic, the total fixed costs are represented by rectangle $SATC_0$–a–b–$SAVC_0$, and total costs can be measured by area $SATC_0$–a–q_0–0. The ability to interpret and read these cost curves is useful for the discussion that follows.

Factors Affecting the Position of the Short-Run Cost Curves

A variety of short-run circumstances affect the positions of the per-unit and total cost curves.[9] Among them are the prices of the variable inputs, the quality of care, the patient case-mix, and the amounts of the fixed inputs. Whenever any one of these variables changes, the positions of

9. The position of the average and total fixed cost curves is influenced by the price of the fixed input. Fixed costs do not affect the typical marginal decision in the short run. Therefore, we do not discuss the factors affecting the position of the fixed cost curves.

the cost curves change through either an upward or a downward shift depending on whether costs increase or decrease. For example, if input prices increase in the short run, the cost curves shift upward to reflect the higher costs of production (especially since SAVC = w/AP_n and SMC = w/MP_n). If input prices fall in the short run, the cost curves shift downward to indicate the lower production costs.

Furthermore, if the medical firm increases the quality of care or adopts a more severe patient case-mix, the cost curves respond by shifting upward. That is because a higher quality of care or a more severe patient case-mix means that a unit of labor is less able to produce as much output in a given amount of time. In terms of our formal analysis, a higher quality of care or a more severe patient case-mix reduces the average and marginal productivity of the labor input and thereby raises the costs of production. For example, a nurse can care for many more patients within an hour when these patients are less severely ill and quality of care is of secondary importance. Conversely, a reduction in the quality of care or a less severe patient case-mix is associated with lower cost curves.

Finally, a change in the amount of the fixed inputs can alter the costs of production. For example, it can be shown that excessive amounts of the fixed inputs lead to higher short-run costs (Cowing and Holtmann, 1983). We discuss the specific reasoning underlying the relation between fixed inputs and short-run costs when we examine the long-run costs of production later in this chapter.

In sum, a properly specified short-run total variable cost function for medical services should include the following variables:

(7–12) STVC = f(output level, input prices, quality of care, patient case-mix, quantity of the fixed inputs).

We suspect that these factors can explain cost differentials among medical firms in the same industry. Specifically, output influences short-run variable costs by determining where the medical firm operates along the cost curve, whereas the other factors affect the location of the curve. Most likely, high-cost medical firms are associated with more output, higher wages, increased quality, more severe patient case-mixes, and/or an excessive quantity of fixed inputs.

Estimating a Short-Run Cost Function for Hospital Services

Cowing and Holtmann (1983) empirically estimated a short-run total variable cost function for a sample of 138 short-term general care hospitals in New York using 1975 data. Along the lines of Equation 7–12, they specified the short-run total variable cost (STVC) function in the following general form:

(7–13) $$\text{STVC} = f(q_1, q_2, q_3, q_4, q_5, w_1, w_2, w_3, w_4, w_5, w_6, K, A).$$

Each q_i $(i = 1{,}5)$ represents the quantity of one of five different patient services—emergency room care, medical-surgical care, pediatric care, maternity care, and other inpatient care—measured in total patient days; each w_j $(j = 1{,}6)$ stands for one of six different variable input prices for nursing labor, auxiliary labor, professional labor, administrative labor, general labor, and material and supplies; K is a single measure of the capital stock (measured by the market value of a hospital); and A is the fixed number of admitting physicians in the hospital.[10]

Compared to Equation 7–12, Cowing and Holtmann's specification of the cost function is more complex and introduces a greater degree of realism into the empirical analysis. First, the hospital is realistically treated as a multiproduct firm, simultaneously producing and selling five different

10. Cowing and Holtmann also specify two dummy variables reflecting for-profit versus not-for-profit ownership status and teaching versus nonteaching institution as a way to control for differences in quality and case-mix severity across hospitals. The inadequate control for quality and severity of case-mix is one of the few faults we can find with this paper.

types of patient services. Second, instead of our single variable input price (that is, hourly nurse wage), six different variable input prices are specified. Finally, Cowing and Holtmann include the number of admitting physicians in the model because they play such a key role in the hospital services production process.

The authors assumed a multiproduct translog cost function for Equation 7–13. We do not discuss the properties associated with this specific functional form; it suffices to note that this flexible form enables us to assess a large number of real-world characteristics associated with the production process.

First, this functional form allows for an interaction among the various outputs so that economies of scope can be examined. **Economies of scope** result from the joint sharing among related outputs of resources, such as nurses, auxiliary workers, and administrative labor. Scope economies exist if the joint cost of producing two outputs is less than the sum of the costs of producing the two outputs separately. For example, many colleges and universities produce both an undergraduate and a graduate education jointly due to perceived cost savings from economies of scope. The same professors, library personnel, and buildings can be used in producing both educational outputs simultaneously.

Cowing and Holtmann found some very intriguing results. First, their study reveals evidence of **short-run economies of scale,** meaning that an increase in output results in a less than proportionate increase in short-run total variable costs. Evidence of short-run economies indicates that the representative hospital operates to the left of the minimum point on the short-run average variable cost curve and implies that larger hospitals produce at a lower cost than smaller ones in the short run. They point out that this result is consistent with the view that aggregate hospital costs could be reduced by closing some small hospitals and merging the services among the remaining ones.

Second, in contrast to scale economies, Cowing and Holtmann discovered only limited evidence for economies of scope with respect to pediatric care and other services. They also found limited evidence to support diseconomies of scope with respect to emergency services and other services. In fact, they argued that the results for both scope and scale economies indicate that larger but more specialized hospitals may be more effective given the significance of the scale effects and the general lack of any substantial economies of scope.

Third, Cowing and Holtmann also noted that the short-run marginal cost of each output, $\Delta STVC/\Delta q_i$, declined and then became constant over the levels of output observed in their study. For example, the marginal cost of an emergency room visit was found to be approximately $32 for 54,000 visits per year and about $20 for 100,000 visits per year. For medical-surgical care, marginal cost was found to fall from $255 per patient day for 6,000 annual patient days to around $100 for 300,000 annual total patient days. For maternity care, the evidence suggests that the marginal costs of $540 per patient day for hospitals with 1,500 total annual patient days declined to $75 for hospitals with 20,000 total annual patient days. Eventually each of the marginal costs leveled off.

Finally, Cowing and Holtmann estimated the short-run elasticities of input substitution between all pairs of variable inputs. They reported that the results indicate a substantial degree of substitutability between nursing and professional workers, nursing and general workers, nursing and administrative workers, and professional and administrative labor.

The Cost-Minimizing Input Choice

A medical firm makes choices concerning which variable inputs to employ. Recognizing that there is usually more than one way to produce a specific output, medical firms typically desire to produce with the least-cost or cost-minimizing input mix. For example, suppose administrators desire to produce some given amount of medical services, q_0, at minimum total cost, TC, using two variable inputs: registered nurses, RN, and licensed practical nurses, LPN. (For ease of exposition, we ignore the capital input in this example.) These two inputs are paid hourly wages of w_R and w_L, respectively. The medical firm wants to minimize

(7–14) $$TC(q_0) = w_R \times RN + w_L \times LPN$$

subject to

(7–15) $$q_0 = f(RN, LPN)$$

by choosing the proper mix of registered nurses and licensed practical nurses.

Taken together, Equations 7–14 and 7–15 mean that administrators want to minimize the total cost of producing q_0 units of medical services by choosing the "right," or efficient, mix of RNs and LPNs so that $TC(q_0)$ is as low as possible and sufficient amounts of the two inputs are available to produce q_0. The efficient combination depends on the marginal products and relative prices of the two inputs. By using a mathematical technique called *constrained optimization*, we can show that the efficient mix of RNs and LPNs is chosen when the following condition holds:[11]

(7–16) $$MP_{RN}/w_R = MP_{LPN}/w_L.$$

Equation 7–16 means that the marginal product to price ratio is equal for both registered nurses and licensed practical nurses in equilibrium. The equality implies that the last dollar spent on registered nurses generates the same increment to output as the last dollar spent on licensed practical nurses. As a result, a rearranging of expenditures on the two inputs cannot generate any increase in medical services, since both inputs generate the same output per dollar at the margin.[12]

To more fully appreciate this point, suppose this condition does not hold such that

(7–17) $$MP_{RN}/w_R < MP_{LPN}/w_L.$$

In that case, the last dollar spent on a licensed practical nurse generates more output than the last dollar spent on a registered nurse. A licensed practical nurse is more profitable for the hospital at the margin, because the medical organization receives a "bigger bang for the buck." But as the organization hires more LPNs and fewer RNs, the marginal productivities adjust until the equilibrium condition in Equation 7–16 results. Specifically, the marginal productivity of the LPNs decreases, while the marginal productivity of the RNs increases due to diminishing marginal productivity.

For example, suppose a newly hired RN can service six patients per hour and a newly hired LPN can service only four patients per hour. At first blush, with no consideration of the price of each input, the RN might appear to be the "better buy" because productivity is 50 percent higher. But suppose further that the market wage for an RN is $20 per hour, while an LPN requires only $10 per hour to work at the medical facility. Given relative input prices, the 50 percent higher productivity of the RN costs the medical facility 100 percent more. Obviously, the LPN is the better buy. That is, the last dollar spent on an LPN results in the servicing of 0.4 additional patients per hour, while a dollar spent on an RN allows the servicing of only 0.3 more patients per hour.

As another example, most physicians are not hospital employees and paid an explicit salary; instead they are granted admitting privileges by the hospitals. The granting of admitting privileges

11. The interested reader can consult Chiang (1984).

12. The astute reader most likely recognizes that Equation 7–16 is similar to the utility-maximizing condition noted in Chapter 5.

comes at a cost to the hospital, however. For example, the hospital incurs costs when it reviews and processes the physician's application, monitors the physician's performance to ensure quality control, and allows the physician to use its resources. Based on their empirical procedure discussed earlier, Jensen and Morrisey (1986) were able to estimate the shadow price, or implicit cost, of a physician with admitting privileges at a representative hospital. They imputed the shadow price of a physician by using the condition for optimal input use. Following the format of Equation 7–16, the optimal combination of doctors, doc, and nurses, n, is chosen when

$$MP_{doc}/w_{doc} = MP_n/w_n. \quad (7\text{–}18)$$

By substituting in the estimated marginal products for doctors (6.05) and nurses (20.3) from their study, and the sample average for the annual nurses' salary ($23,526), Jensen and Morrisey solved for the shadow price of a doctor, w_{doc}. The resulting figure implies that the typical hospital in the sample incurred implicit costs of approximately $7,012 per year from granting admitting privileges to the marginal physician.

Long-Run Costs of Production

Up to now, we have focused on the short-run costs of operation and assumed that one input is fixed. The fixed input leads to diminishing returns in production and to U-shaped average variable and total cost curves. In the long run, however, when the medical firm is planning for future resource requirements, all inputs, including capital, can be changed. Therefore, it is also important to analyze the relation between output and costs when all inputs are changed simultaneously in the long run.

Long-Run Cost Curves

The long-run average total cost curve can be derived from a series of short-run cost curves, as shown in Figure 7–8. The three short-run average total cost curves in the figure reflect different amounts of capital. For example, each curve might reflect the short-run average total costs of producing units of medical services in physically larger facilities of sizes k_1, k_2, and k_3. If decision makers know the relation among different-size facilities and the short-run average total costs, they can easily choose the SATC or size that minimizes the average cost of producing each level of medical services in the long run.

For example, over the range 0 to q_a, facility size k_1 results in lower costs of production than either size k_2 or k_3. Specifically, notice that at output level q_1, $SATC_2$ exceeds $SATC_1$ by a significant amount. Therefore, the administrators choose size k_1 if they desire to produce q_1 units of medical services at least cost in the long run. Similarly, from q_a to q_b, facility size k_2, associated with $SATC_2$, results in lower costs than either size k_1 or k_3. Beyond q_b units of medical services (say, q_2), a size of k_3 enables lower costs of production in the long run.

The three short-run cost curves in Figure 7–8 paint a simplistic picture, since conceptually each unit of medical services can be linked to a uniquely sized cost-minimizing facility (assuming capital is divisible). If we assume a large number of possible sizes, we can draw a curve that connects all the cost-minimizing points on the various short-run average total cost curves. Each point indicates the least costly way to produce the corresponding level of medical services in the long run when all inputs can be altered. Every short-run cost curve is tangent to the connecting or envelope curve, which is referred to as the *long-run average total cost (LATC) curve*. The curve drawn below the short-run average cost curves in Figure 7–8 represents a long-run average total cost curve.

FIGURE 7–8
The Short-Run Average Cost Curves and the Long-Run Planning Curve

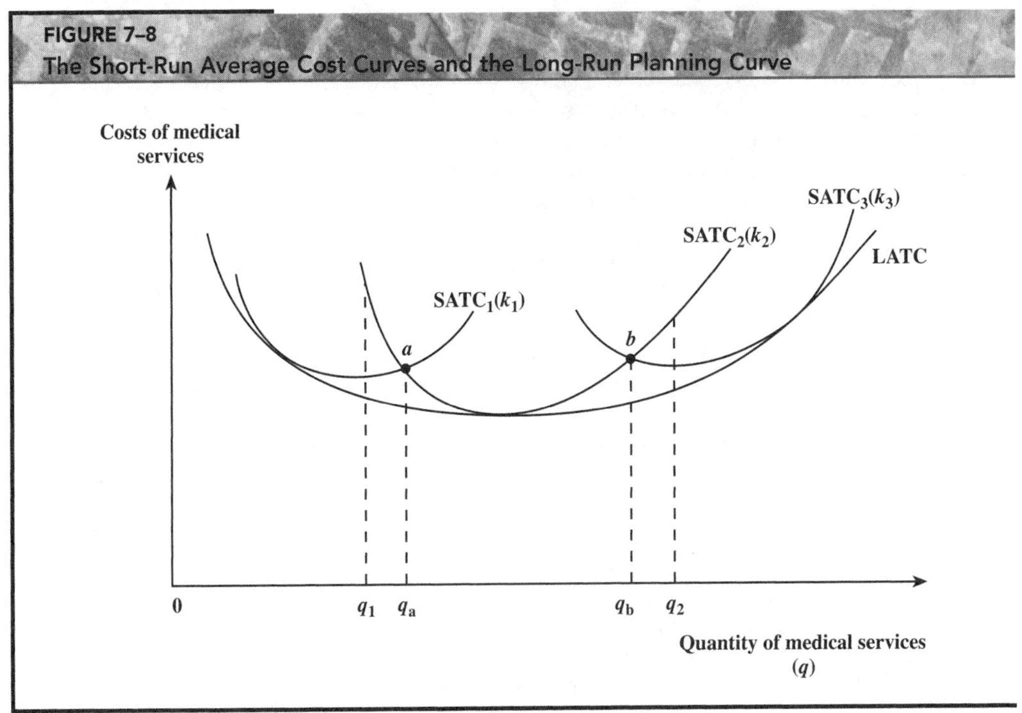

All inputs are variable in the long run. $SATC_1$, $SATC_2$, and $SATC_3$ represent the cost curves for small, medium, and large facilities, respectively. If decision makers choose the efficiently sized firm for producing output in the long run, a long-run average total cost, LATC, can be derived from a series of short-run average total cost curves brought on by an increase in the stock of capital. The U shape of the LATC reflects economies and diseconomies of scale.

Notice that the U-shaped long-run average cost curve initially declines, reaches a minimum, and eventually increases. Interestingly, both the short-run and long-run average cost curves have the same shape, but for different reasons. The shape of the short-run average total cost curve is based on the law of diminishing productivity setting in at some point. In the long run, however, all inputs are variable, so by definition a fixed input cannot account for the U-shaped long-run average cost curve. Instead, the reason for the U-shaped LATC curve is based on the concepts of *long-run economies* and *diseconomies of scale*.

Long-run economies of scale refer to the notion that average costs fall as a medical firm gets physically larger due to specialization of labor and capital. Larger medical firms are able to utilize larger and more specialized equipment and to more fully specialize the various labor tasks involved in the production process. For example, people generally get very proficient at a specific task when they perform it repeatedly. Therefore, specialization allows larger firms to produce increased amounts of output at lower per-unit costs. The downward-sloping portion of the LATC curve in Figure 7–8 reflects economies of scale.

Another way to conceptualize long-run economies of scale is through the direct relation between inputs and output, or returns to scale, rather than output and costs. Consistent with long-run economies of scale is increasing returns to scale. **Increasing returns to scale** result when an increase in all inputs results in a more than proportionate increase in output. For example, a doubling of all inputs that results in three times as much output is a sign of increasing returns to scale. Similarly, if a doubling of output can be achieved without a doubling of all inputs, the production process exhibits long-run increasing returns, or economies of scale.

Most economists believe that economies of scale are exhausted at some point and diseconomies of scale set in. **Diseconomies of scale** result when the medical firm becomes too large. Bureaucratic red tape becomes common, and top-to-bottom communication flows break down. The breakdown in communication flows means management at the top of the hierarchy has lost sight of what is taking place at the floor level. As a result, poor decisions are sometimes made when the firm is too large. Consequently, as the firm gets too large, long-run average costs increase. Diseconomies of scale are reflected in the upward-sloping segment of the LATC curve in Figure 7–8.

Diseconomies of scale can also be interpreted as meaning that an increase in all inputs results in a less than proportionate increase in output, or **decreasing returns to scale.** For example, if the number of patient-hours doubles at a dental office and the decision maker is forced to triple the size of each input (staff, office space, equipment, and so on), the production process at the dental office is characterized by decreasing returns, or diseconomies of scale.

Another possibility, not shown in Figure 7–8, is that the production process exhibits constant returns to scale. **Constant returns to scale** occur when, for example, a doubling of inputs results in a doubling of output. In terms of long-run costs, constant returns imply a horizontal LATC curve, in turn implying that long-run average total cost is independent of output.

Shifts in the Long-Run Average Cost Curve

The position of the long-run average cost curve is determined by a set of long-run circumstances that includes the prices of all inputs (remember, capital is a variable input in the long run), quality (including technological change), and patient case-mix. When these circumstances change on a long-run basis, the long-run average cost curve shifts up or down depending on whether the change involves higher or lower long-run costs of production. For example, an increase in the long-run price of medical inputs leads to an upward shift in the long-run average cost curve. A cost-saving technology tends to shift the long-run average cost curve downward. Conversely, a cost-enhancing technology increases the average costs of production in the long run and shifts the LATC curve upward. Higher quality of care and more severe patient case-mixes also shift the LATC curve upward.

Long-Run Cost Minimization and the Indivisibility of Fixed Inputs

Long-run cost minimization assumes that all inputs can be costlessly adjusted upward or downward. For an input such as an hourly laborer, employment adjustments are fairly simple because hours worked or number of workers can be changed relatively easily. Capital inputs cannot always be as easily changed, however, because they are less divisible. As a result, a medical firm facing a sharp decline in demand may be unable to reduce the physical size of its facility. For example, Salkever (1972) found that hospitals realize less than 10 percent of the desired cost savings per year.[13] Therefore, medical firms may adjust slowly to external changes, not produce in long-run equilibrium, and operate with excess capital relative to a long-run equilibrium point.

Figure 7–9 clarifies this point. Suppose that initially a dental clinic produces q_0 amount of output (say, dental patient-hours) with a facility size of 1,200 square feet, as represented by the

13. As cited in Cowing et al. (1983, p. 265).

FIGURE 7–9
Long-Run Disequilibrium of the Medical Firm

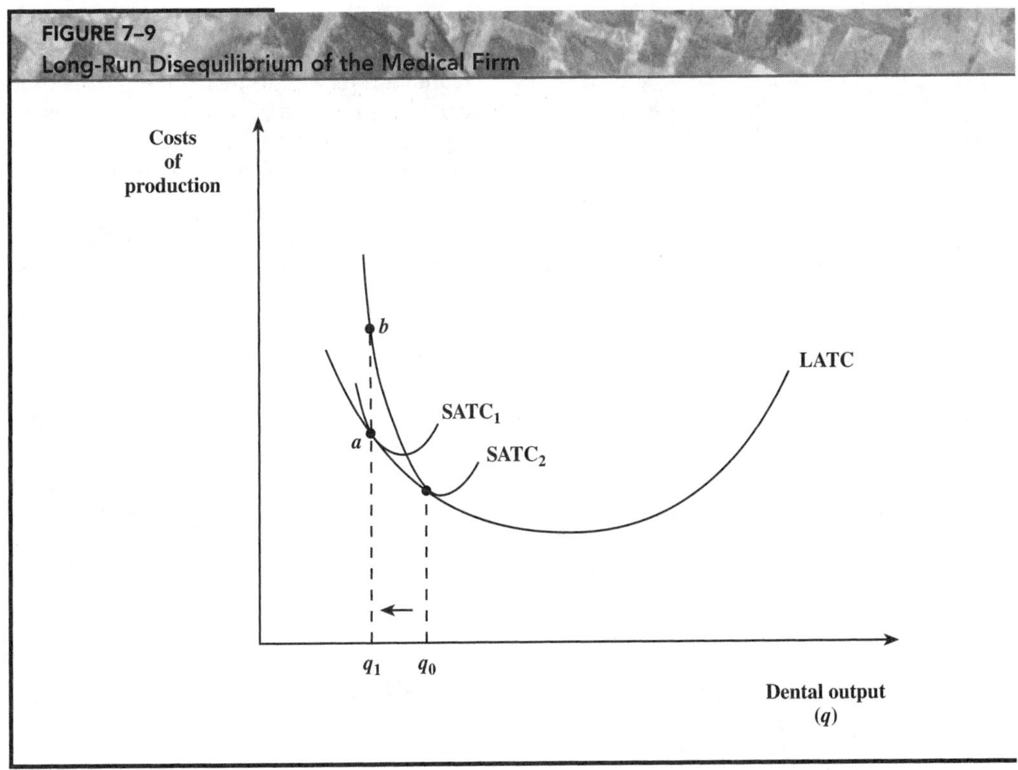

A firm may not operate in long-run equilibrium because of the sizeable costs of adjusting to a sharp change in demand. For example, assuming that the dental clinic is initially producing in long-run equilibrium at q_0 and output sharply falls to q_1, it may take time for the dental clinic to downsize its capital facility. As a result, the dental clinic may operate with costs, point *b*, that are higher than that predicted by long-run equilibrium, point *a*.

curve $SATC_2$. This represents a long-run equilibrium point because the efficient plant size is chosen such that $SATC_2$ is tangent to the LATC curve at q_0; that is, q_0 is produced at the lowest possible long-run cost and 1,200 square feet is the efficiently sized facility. Now suppose output sharply falls to q_1 due to a decline in demand. Long-run cost minimization suggests that the dental firm will reduce the size of its facility to that represented by $SATC_1$ and operate at point *a* on the LATC curve. It might do this by selling the old facility and moving into a smaller one. Because it may take time to adjust to the decline in demand, the dental clinic may not operate on the long-run curve at q_1 (point *a*) but instead continue to operate with the larger facility as represented by point *b* on $SATC_2$. The dental clinic incurs higher costs of production as indicated by the vertical distance between points *b* and *a* in the figure.

Cowing and Holtmann (1983) derived a test to determine whether firms are operating in long-run equilibrium. Using a simplified version of Equation 7–12, we can write a long-run total cost (LTC) function as

(7–19) $$\text{LTC} = \text{STVC}(q, w, k) + r \times k,$$

where all variables are as defined earlier. According to Equation 7–19, long-run total costs equal the sum of (minimum) short-run total variable costs and capital costs. The level of short-run total variable costs is a function of, or depends on, the quantity of output, the wage rate, and the quantity of capital (and other things excluded from the equation for simplification).

According to Cowing and Holtmann, a necessary condition for long-run cost minimization is that $\Delta STVC/\Delta k = -r$.[14] The equality implies that the variable cost savings realized from substituting one more unit of capital must equal the rental price of capital in long-run equilibrium. That is, the marginal benefits and costs of capital substitution should be equal when the firm is minimizing the long-run costs of production. A nonnegative estimate for $\Delta STVC/\Delta k$ is a sufficient condition for medical firms to be overemploying capital. A nonnegative estimate implies that the cost of capital substitution outweighs its benefit in terms of short-run variable cost savings.

In their study, Cowing and Holtmann specified two fixed inputs: capital and the number of admitting physicians. As with capital, hospitals may operate with an excessive number of admitting physicians relative to a long-run equilibrium position. That is because the loss of one admitting physician can mean the loss of many more patients in the future. Cowing and Holtmann estimated the change in short-run total variable costs resulting from a one-unit change in capital and number of admitting physicians. Both estimates were found to be positive rather than negative. Thus, the authors found that the "average" hospital in their New York sample operated with too much capital and too many physicians. Their empirical results suggest that hospitals could reduce their costs by limiting the amount of capital and controlling the number of physicians.

Neoclassical Cost Theory and the Production of Medical Services

The cost theory introduced in this chapter, typically referred to as *neoclassical cost theory* under conditions of perfect certainty, assumes firms produce as efficiently as possible and possess perfect information regarding the demands for their services. Based on the underlying theory, the short-run or long-run costs of producing a given level of output can be determined by observing the relevant point on the appropriate cost curve. However, when applied to medical firms, this kind of cost analysis may be misleading for two reasons.

First, some medical firms, such as hospitals or nursing homes, are not-for-profit entities or are reimbursed on a cost-plus basis or both. Therefore, they may not face the appropriate incentives to produce as cheaply as possible and, consequently, may operate above rather than on a given cost curve. Second, medical firms may face an uncertain demand for their services. Medical illnesses occur irregularly and unpredictably, and therefore medical firms such as hospitals may never truly know the demand for their services until the actual events take place. Accordingly, medical firms may produce with some amount of reserve capacity just in case an unexpected large increase in demand occurs.

Although these two considerations may pose problems when conducting a cost analysis of medical firms, do not be misled into thinking that the material in this chapter is without value. That is clearly not the case. These two considerations are modifications that can and should be incorporated into the cost analysis when possible. Indeed, a strong grounding in neoclassical cost analysis under conditions of perfect certainty is necessary before any sophisticated analyses or model extensions can be properly conducted and understood.

14. This equality can be derived by taking the first derivative of Equation 7–19 with respect to k and setting the resulting expression equal to zero.

SUMMARY

In this chapter, we focused on characteristics and concepts pertaining to the costs of producing medical services. First, we examined the underlying production behavior of a single medical firm. The short-run production function that resulted from this examination relates productivity to input usage. Among the more important principles we examined was the law of diminishing marginal productivity, the notion that the marginal and average productivities of a variable input first increase but eventually fall with greater input usage because a fixed input places a constraint on production.

Second, we discussed the inverse relation between productivity and costs. Simply stated, increasing marginal and average productivities translate into decreasing marginal and average variable costs. Conversely, declining productivities imply higher per-unit costs of production. As a result, the average variable cost curve is U-shaped, implying that the average variable cost of production first decreases with greater production but at some point begins to increase as output expands. Taking the property of fixed costs into consideration, we also derived a U-shaped short-run average cost curve, which relates average operating costs to the amount of medical services produced.

Finally, we examined some concepts relating to long-run costs of production, including economies and diseconomies of scale. We also discussed the determinants of the optimal input mix.

CASE STUDIES

7-1 Digital Operating Suites[15]

California's Sutter Delta Medical Center paid $250,000 for a fiber-optic digital operating suite that it hopes will reduce the costs of performing minimally invasive surgeries. The new technology produces exceptionally clear digital images from a tiny camera placed inside the patient and close to the site of surgery, allowing surgeons to conduct the surgery while looking only at video monitors. The cameras transmit images to monitors that hang above the operating table, thereby reducing the amount of operating room clutter. After installing the new equipment, Sutter observed a 15 minute reduction in average operating room time, reductions in the average time under anesthesia, and quicker patient recovery times. Sutter has performed about 50 operations with the equipment thus far.

Questions for Discussion

1. *Discuss how operating room total costs, average costs, and marginal costs might change following the adoption of the fiber-optic digital imaging equipment.*
2. *Thinking back to Chapter 3, discuss how you might go about evaluating the rate of return for the new equipment.*

7-2 Fixed versus Variable Costs in Hospitals

What proportion of the typical U.S. community hospital's total costs is fixed? High fixed costs have implications for economies of scale and scope, and may also determine the extent to which other firms can realistically enter the market. Roberts et al. (1999) examine data from Cook

15. Source: Susan L. Thomas, "Sutter Delta Jumps Ahead: Digital OR Images Speed Surgeries, Save Money," *East Bay Business Times*, December 19, 2005.

County Hospital in Chicago (from which TV's fictional *ER* draws its inspiration) and find that a surprising 84 percent of total costs were fixed over the short term. The authors determine that fixed costs consist mainly of costs related to physical structures, equipment, salaried labor, and overhead.

Questions for Discussion

1. *Most hospitals are paid a prospectively determined price for services. Discuss the unique challenges prospective fee schedules might pose for firms with relatively high fixed costs.*
2. *What are the implications for occupancy rates?*

Review Questions and Problems

1. Suppose you are to specify a short-run production function for dental services. What inputs might you include in the production function? Which would be the variable inputs and which the fixed inputs?
2. In your own words, explain the law of diminishing marginal productivity. Be sure to mention the reason this law tends to hold in the short run.
3. Explain the difference between technical efficiency and economic efficiency.
4. Discuss the relation between the marginal and average productivity curves and the marginal and average variable cost curves.
5. What does the elasticity of substitution illustrate? How is it expressed mathematically? What two factors affect its magnitude?
6. Explain the difference between the explicit and implicit costs of production. Cite an example of each.
7. Suppose that with 400 patients per year, the SAFC, SATC, and SMC of operating a physician clinic are $10, $35, and $30 per patient, respectively. Furthermore, suppose the physician decides to increase the annual patient load by one more patient. Using short-run cost theory, explain the impact of this additional patient on the SAVC and SATC. Do they increase or decrease? Why?
8. What factors shift the short-run average variable and total cost curves? Explain why these curves would shift up or down in response to changes in these factors.
9. Suppose you are to specify a short-run total variable cost function for a nursing home. Explain the variables you would include in the function. What is the expected relation between a change in each of these variables and short-run total variable costs?
10. What does *economies of scope* mean? Provide an example.
11. Explain the reasoning behind the U shape of the long-run average total cost curve. Why might this cost curve shift upward?
12. You are responsible for hiring one of two hygienists for a dental office. The first dental hygienist has 25 years of experience. Given her record, she is likely to satisfactorily service 16 patients per day. Her hourly wage would be approximately $16 per hour. The other hygienist is new to the industry. He is expected to satisfactorily service 10 patients per day at an hourly wage of $8. Which dental hygienist would be the better hire? Why?
13. Santerre and Bennett (1992) estimated the short-run total variable cost function for a sample of 55 for-profit hospitals in Texas (*t*-statistics are in parentheses below the estimated coefficients).

$$\ln \text{STVC} = \underset{(0.69)}{1.31} + \underset{(3.31)}{0.47\ln q} + \underset{(4.42)}{0.80\ln w} + \underset{(2.58)}{0.73\ln \text{QUALITY}}$$

$$+ \underset{(1.48)}{0.11\ln \text{CASEMIX}} + \underset{(3.16)}{0.29\ln k} + \underset{(0.88)}{0.07\ln \text{DOC}}$$

$$+ \text{Other factors}$$

Adj. $R^2 = .95$
$N = 55$

where STVC = short-run total variable cost, q = a measure of output (total inpatient days), w = average wage rate or price of labor, QUALITY = a measure of quality (number of accreditations), CASEMIX = an indicator of patient case-mix (number of services), k = a measure of capital (beds), and DOC = number of admitting physicians. All variables are expressed as natural logarithms (ln), so the estimated coefficients can be interpreted as elasticities.

A. How much of the variation in STVC is explained by the explanatory variables? How do you know that?
B. Which of the estimated coefficients are not statistically significant? Explain.
C. Does the estimated coefficient on output represent short-run economies or diseconomies of scale? Explain.
D. What are the expected signs of the coefficient estimates on w, QUALITY, and CASEMIX? Explain.
E. Provide an economic interpretation of the magnitude of the estimated coefficient on w.
F. What do the estimated coefficient on k and DOC suggest about the amount of capital and physicians at the representative hospital?

14. Draw a U-shaped LATC curve. Then draw the related long-run marginal cost (LMC) curve, keeping in mind the geometric relation between marginal cost and average cost (see the discussion on short-run cost curves). What is the relation between LATC and LMC when increasing returns to scale are present? Between LATC and LMC when the production process exhibits decreasing returns to scale? What type of returns to scale holds when LMC equals LATC?
15. Describe the two limitations associated with the cost theory provided in this chapter when it is applied to explain the behavior of medical firms.
16. Suppose that you are interested in comparing the costs of producing inpatient services at Saving Grace Hospital with those at ACME Hospital. Further suppose that the two hospitals annually admit about 24,000 and 32,000 patients, respectively, at average short-run total costs per admission of roughly \$11,000 and \$12,000.
    A. Why may these two dollar figures not represent the economic cost of providing inpatient services at these two hospitals? Explain fully.
    B. Suppose that these cost figures accurately reflect the economic costs of providing inpatient services at these two hospitals and that the two hospitals face the same average total cost curve. Draw a graphical representation of the average total cost curve (only) and graphically show and verbally explain why ACME Hospital produces at a higher cost than Saving Grace Hospital.
    C. Using cost theory as presented in class and the text, identify and fully explain four other factors that might explain why ACME Hospital has higher average costs of production than Saving Grace Hospital.
    D. Fully explain how the comparative analysis becomes muddled if one considers that one (or both) of the two hospitals is not organized on a for-profit basis.

CEBS Questions

■ *CEBS Sample Question on Subject Matter from CEBS Course 9 Study Manual*

1. Explain, in words—not a mathematical formula—the condition that must exist for the most efficient mix of RNs and LPNs. (pages 180–182)

■ *CEBS Sample Exam Questions*

1. Economists and accountants treat production costs differently. The difference is that economists consider:
   A. Only the explicit costs
   B. Only verifiable costs
   C. Historical costs
   D. Opportunity costs
   E. Actual costs
2. A medical firm increased all inputs 10 percent and output increased 12 percent. Which of the following statements is (are) correct?
   I. This is an example of an exception to the law of diminishing productivity.
   II. This is an example of increasing returns to scale.
   III. This example must involve the long run, not the short run.
      A. II only
      B. III only
      C. I and III only
      D. II and III only
      E. I, II, and III
3. All the following statements regarding the neoclassical cost theory are correct EXCEPT:
   A. The theory assumes that all firms are operating under conditions of perfect certainty.
   B. The theory assumes that all firms produce as efficiently as possible.
   C. The theory has limited usefulness to medical firms because these organizations usually have short-run cost curves that are not U shaped.
   D. The theory may be difficult to apply to medical firms because some firms may not have the incentive to produce as cheaply as possible.
   E. The theory poses problems for medical firms because the demand for medical services is unpredictable.

■ *Answer to Sample Question from Study Manual*

The condition that must exist for the most efficient mix of RNs and LPNs is that the last dollar spent on registered nurses (the marginal cost of nurses) must generate the same increment to output as the last dollar spent on licensed practical nurses. In other words, both inputs will generate the same output per dollar at the margin.

■ *Answers to Sample Exam Questions*

1. D is the correct answer. Economists, unlike accountants, consider both the explicit and implicit costs of production. Implicit costs include opportunity costs. See page 172 of the text.

2. The correct answer is D. Increasing returns to scale involve the long run when all inputs are increased. Statement I is incorrect because at least one factor must be held constant to apply the concept of diminishing productivity. See pages 164–165 and 183 of the text.
3. C is the correct answer. The short-run cost curves for medical firms must have a U shape under the assumptions of the theory. See pages 172–178 and 184–186 of the text.

ONLINE RESOURCES

To access Internet links related to the topics in this chapter, please visit our web site at **www.thomsonedu.com/economics/santerre**.

REFERENCES

Chiang, Alpha C. *Fundamental Methods of Mathematical Economics*. New York: McGraw-Hill, 1984.

Cowing, Thomas G., and Alphonse G. Holtmann. "Multiproduct Short-Run Hospital Cost Functions: Empirical Evidence and Policy Implications from Cross-Section Data." *Southern Economics Journal* 49 (January 1983), pp. 637–53.

Cowing, Thomas G., Alphonse G. Holtmann, and S. Powers. "Hospital Cost Analysis: A Survey and Evaluation of Recent Studies." In *Advances in Health Economics and Health Services Research*, Vol. 4, eds. Richard M. Scheffler and Louis F. Rossiter. Greenwich, Conn.: JAI Press, 1983, pp. 257–303.

Jablon, Robert. "Health Merger Worries Consumer, Doctor Groups." *The Providence Journal*, July 9, 2005, p. B3.

Jensen, Gail A., and Michael A. Morrisey. "The Role of Physicians in Hospital Production." *Review of Economics and Statistics* 68 (1986), pp. 432–42.

Kirchheimer, Barbara. "Ga. Hospitals to Combine." *Modern Healthcare*, December 11, 2000.

Roberts, Rebecca R., et al. "Distribution of Variable vs. Fixed Costs of Hospital Care." *Journal of the American Medical Association* 281 (February 17, 1999), pp. 644–49.

Roberts, R. R. et al. "Distribution of Variable vs. Fixed Costs of Hospital Care." *Journal of the American Medical Association* 281, no. 7 (1999), pp. 644–49.

Salkever, David. "A Microeconomic Study of Hospital Cost Inflation." *Journal of Political Economy* 80 (November 1972), pp. 1144–66.

Santerre, Rexford E., and Dana C. Bennett. "Hospital Market Structure and Cost Performance: A Case Study." *Eastern Economic Journal* 18 (spring 1992), pp. 209–19.

STRUCTURE, CONDUCT, PERFORMANCE, AND MARKET ANALYSIS

CHAPTER 8

"Genentech's Activase Faces Competition from New Set of Blood-Clot Dissolvers" (The Wall Street Journal).

"Market Forces Are Starting to Produce Significant Cuts in Health-Care Costs" (The Wall Street Journal).

"Price Competition Hits Hospitals" (Hartford Courant).

"Yes, the Market Can Curb Health Costs" (Fortune).

In Chapter 3 we discussed the efficient allocation of resources in the context of a benevolent surgeon general in a hypothetical economy. We learned, from a theoretical perspective, that an efficient allocation of resources occurs when each good and service is produced at the point where marginal social cost equals marginal social benefit. Taking the discussion a step further, Chapter 4 pointed out that actual decisions in the real world concerning resource allocation may be conducted at a centralized or decentralized level.

Continuing with this line of reasoning, this chapter develops a theoretical framework to examine how resource allocation takes place in a decentralized medical marketplace. That is, instead of a benevolent dictator, the decisions of individual consumers and producers allocate society's scarce resources among various goods and services. The analysis allows the marketplace to take on varying degrees of competition.

At the top of this page are various headlines from the popular press extolling the existence and virtues of competitive markets for medical services. The belief many people hold in the ability of competitive markets to efficiently allocate resources should not surprise anyone schooled in economics. According to traditional microeconomic theory, perfect competition creates a "survival of the fittest" market mentality and thereby forces firms to satisfy consumer wants and produce with least-cost methods of production. If competition has the power to weave this same magic in medical markets, incentives exist for medical firms to offer high-quality, cost-effective medical products at the lowest possible prices. With health care costs comprising such a significant percentage of national income, competitive behavior among medical firms might be a welcome sight in today's health economy.

But are the various features normally associated with perfect competition applicable to medical care industries? Do the characteristics necessary for a perfectly competitive framework hold in medical markets? If some particular medical industries closely resemble the perfectly competitive model, how are markets expected to behave according to economic theory? What happens to market outcomes if markets are not perfectly competitive? This chapter answers these questions. Specifically, the chapter:

- introduces the structure, conduct, and performance paradigm of industrial organization
- discusses the structural characteristics of perfect competition, monopolistic competition, oligopoly, and monopoly
- shows how a perfectly competitive market determines the price and quantity of a good or service, allocates resources, and corrects for shortages and surpluses
- examines the characteristics of pure monopoly
- compares and contrasts perfect competition and pure monopoly with respect to resource allocation
- discusses intermediate market outcomes between the polar extremes of perfect competition and pure monopoly
- provides a conceptual and empirical framework for defining the relevant market and defining market concentration

Structure, Conduct, and Performance Paradigm

When conducting an industry study, many economists rely on the structure, conduct, and performance (SCP) paradigm developed in industrial organization (IO), a field of economics interested in the behavior of firms and markets. Figure 8–1 illustrates the major elements that constitute the SCP paradigm. The first of the three important elements in the IO triad, **market structure,** establishes the overall environment or playing field within which each firm operates. Essential market structure characteristics include the number and size distribution of the sellers and buyers, the type of product offered for sale, barriers to entry, and whether any asymmetry of information exists between buyers and sellers. Entry barriers reflect any increased costs that new firms must incur relative to existing firms when entering a particular market. As we will see in this chapter, high costs may deter entry. Product type considers whether firms in the same industry produce standardized or differentiated products. As we will learn, differentiated products are less substitutable and may thereby reduce the level of actual competition observed in an industry. Also notice in Figure 8–1 that market structure often differs across industries because of variations in basic conditions, including the underlying technological base, the legal environment, demand conditions, and economies of scale. All of these basic conditions tend to affect the number and size distribution of firms observed in an industry.

Market conduct, the second element, shows up in pricing, promotion, and research and development activities. Whether a firm decides its policies independently or in conjunction with other firms in the market has a crucial impact on the conduct of the industry. The third element, **market performance,** feeds off conduct and is reflected in the degree of production and allocative efficiencies, equity, and technological progress.

Overall, the IO triad predicts that the structure of an industry, in conjunction with the objectives of firms (see Figure 8–1), determines the conduct of the firms, which in turn influences market performance. While significant feedback effects exist among the three elements, the overriding implication of the model is that the structure of the market indirectly affects industrial performance through its impact on the market conduct of individual firms. An underlying belief of the SCP analysis is that society values greater efficiency and technological progress, and fairness in the distribution of income. If unfettered markets do not produce desired levels of performance, the general idea is that public policies should be aimed at correcting this failure of the market. For example, public policies may involve restructuring or regulating an industry. For this reason, public policies also show up in the SCP paradigm of Figure 8–1.

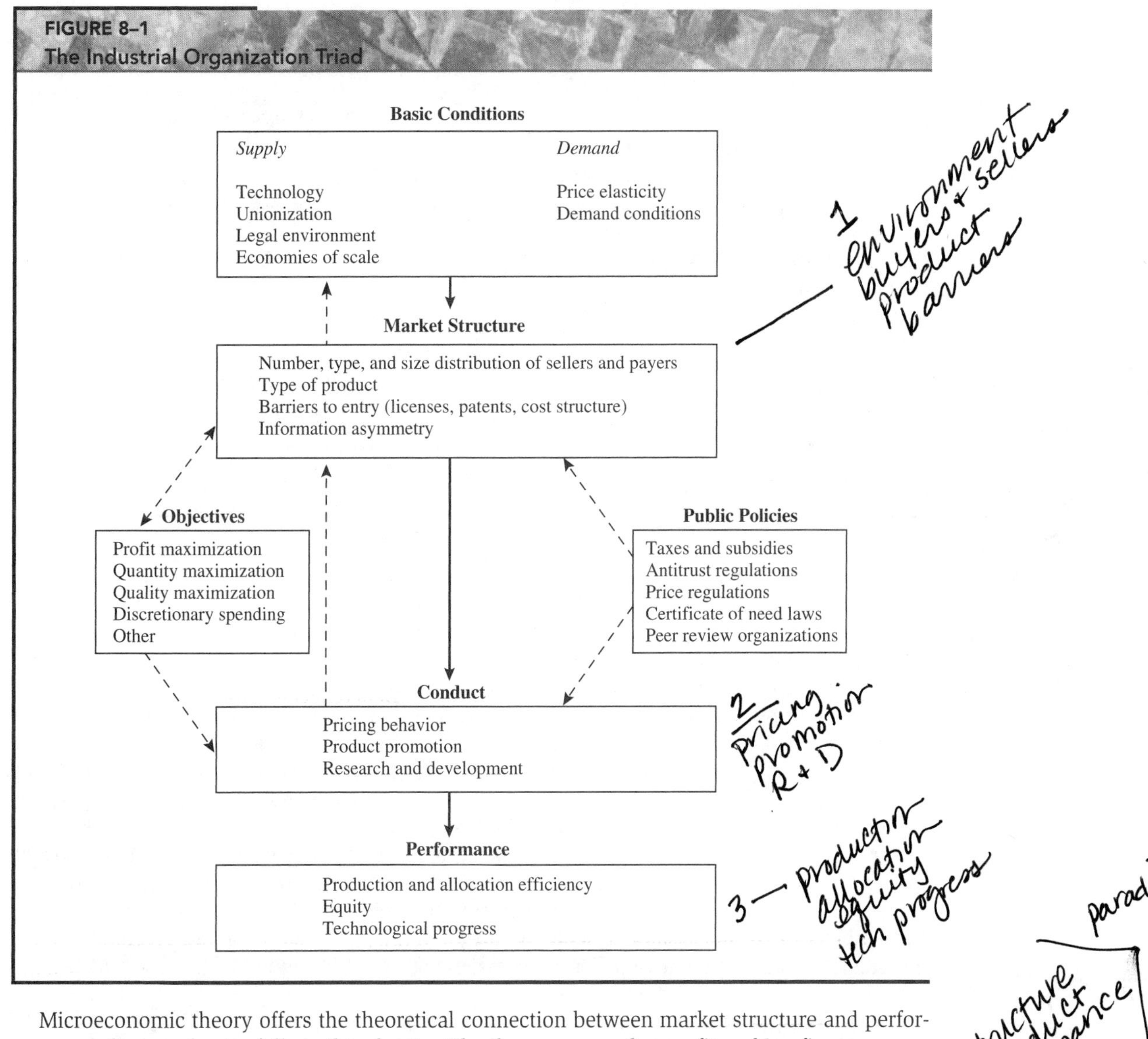

Microeconomic theory offers the theoretical connection between market structure and performance as discussed more fully in this chapter. The theory argues that profit-seeking firms are usually driven by competitive market forces to serve the interests of society by efficiently allocating scarce resources—the so-called invisible hand of Adam Smith. When competitive market forces are absent or weak because firms acquire **market power,** profit seeking may lead to a misallocation of society's resources. Market power refers to the firm's ability to restrict output (or quality) and thereby raise price. The amount of market power held by an individual firm or a collection of firms is a matter of degree and is dictated by the various characteristics that make up market structure. Table 8–1 presents the various structural characteristics that interact to affect the degree of market power possessed by firms. Across the top of the table, the degree of market power is measured from zero to 100 percent. The next row gives four market structure classifications commonly identified by economists, from the most (perfect competition) to the least (pure monopoly) competitive. The body of the table lists the major characteristics of each type of market structure.

TABLE 8–1
Market Structure and Market Power

	Degree of Market Power			
	0%	. . .		100%
Characteristics	**Perfect Competition**	**Monopolistic Competition**	**Oligopoly**	**Pure Monopoly**
Number of sellers	Many	Many	Few, dominant	One
Individual firm's market share	Tiny	Small	Large	100%
Type of product	Homogeneous	Differentiated	Homogeneous or differentiated	Homogeneous by definition
Barriers to entry	None	None	Substantial	Complete
Consumer information	Perfect	Slightly imperfect	Perfect or imperfect	Perfect or imperfect

According to Table 8–1, the characteristics of **perfect competition** are many sellers possessing tiny market shares, a homogeneous product, no barriers to entry, and perfect consumer information. The characteristics of many sellers with tiny market shares and homogeneous products, taken together, mean that a considerable amount of **actual competition** exists in the industry because many substitute firms offer identical products. No barriers to entry suggest that the threat of **potential competition** is high because nothing prevents new firms from entering the industry. For example, a single supplier of frozen pizzas may be reluctant to increase price if the resulting higher profits entice new firms offering frozen pizzas to enter the market. The high degree of both actual and potential competition in a perfectly competitive market indicates that a single perfectly competitive firm lacks any market power.

Monopolistic competition refers to a market that has many sellers possessing relatively small market shares, a product that is somewhat differentiated across firms, no barriers to entry, and some slight imperfections concerning consumer information. Numerous sellers and no entry barriers imply that a single monopolistically competitive firm may also lack market power. However, a monopolistically competitive firm may gain some power over output and price in a niche market because of its differentiated product.

A few dominant firms and substantial barriers to entry characterize an **oligopoly.** Given the relatively large size of each firm and protection from new firms because of high barriers to entry, oligopolistic firms either individually or collectively may be able to exercise market power. However, competition among the few dominant firms, provided collusion does not take place, has the potential of harnessing each firm's behavior. Finally, the least competitive market structure is a **pure monopoly,** in which one firm is the sole provider of a product in a well-defined market with complete or perfect barriers to entry. These circumstances offer the greatest potential for a single firm to exploit its market power in a socially undesirable manner.

To gain a better appreciation of the differences among these four market classifications and their impact on performance, we next examine the polar cases of perfect competition and monopoly. After this discussion, the intermediate cases of monopolistic competition and oligopoly are studied.

Is a Perfectly Competitive Market Relevant to Medical Care?

People who have had little exposure to the study of economics tend to have different ideas about what perfect competition entails. To some, perfect competition means that each firm in the marketplace strives to attain the greatest market share by charging low, cutthroat prices. Others believe that perfectly competitive firms compete for customers through advertisements or preferred locations. Perfect competition, however, is an abstract concept—a model—and therefore involves the four conditions specified in Table 8–1. It also involves the assumptions of utility and profit maximization that underlie conventional microeconomic analysis. That is, standard or neoclassical microeconomics assumes that consumers maximize utility and that firms maximize profits. If any one of these characteristics or assumptions is violated, firms and markets are unlikely to behave as the perfectly competitive model predicts.

When applied to medical care industries, many of the assumptions behind conventional microeconomic analysis and characteristics of perfect competition often do not fit well. Several examples highlight this point. First, the not-for-profit status of many medical enterprises means that health care providers may not pursue maximum economic profits. Second, physician licensure creates an occupational barrier to entry and may shield highly salaried physicians from new competition. Finally, consumers typically lack perfect information about the prices and technical aspects of many medical services. Lack of information places health care providers in a strong position to practice opportunistic behavior.

While deviations from the assumptions of microeconomics and characteristics of perfect competition occur in practice, we believe the model serves a number of important functions. First, the supply and demand model, which is based on perfect competition, often provides a useful framework for explaining or predicting changes in the price and quantity of some good or service at the market level, particularly when the markets are "reasonably" competitive. In fact, we will see that rising health care costs over time in the United States (and elsewhere) can be explained quite well by a supply and demand model of medical care. Second, the perfectly competitive market outcome serves as a valuable benchmark with which to compare market outcomes under noncompetitive conditions. For example, in this chapter we compare the monopoly outcome to the perfectly competitive outcome in terms of the price charged and quantity of output produced. In later chapters, we relax other assumptions associated with the perfectly competitive model, even the profit maximization assumption, and compare that outcome to the perfectly competitive one.

A Model of Supply and Demand

As mentioned previously, perfect competition is based on a model in which a large number of consumers maximize their personal utilities and many producers individually maximize their economic profits. The massive number of consumers and producers results in each individual consumer and producer acting as a **price taker.** By definition, a price taker can buy or sell as much quantity as it wants without affecting market price. To maximize (personal) utility, the typical consumer continues to buy units of a good or service up to the point where marginal private benefit, MPB, as revealed by demand, equals market price. Similarly, the representative profit-maximizing firm continues to produce and sell units of a good or service up to the point where market price equals marginal private cost, MPC. Consequently, a perfectly competitive market clears at the level of output where the marginal private benefit to consumers equals the marginal

FIGURE 8–2
The Perfectly Competitive Outcome

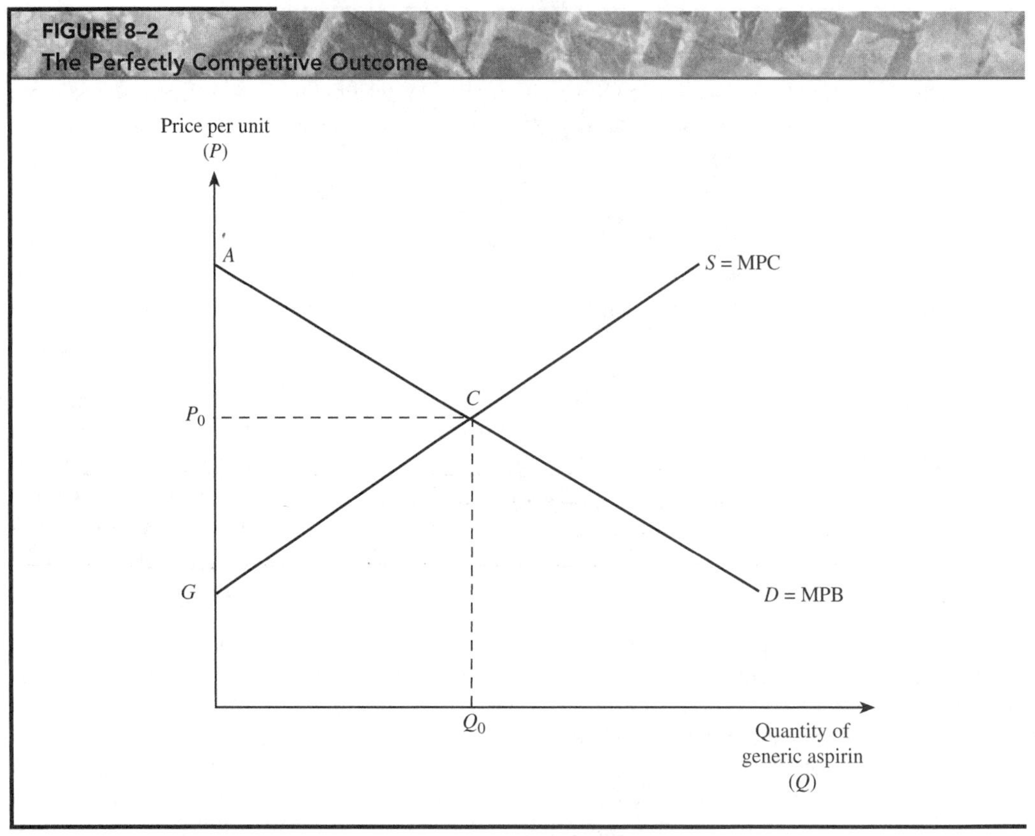

Market demand, *D*, represents the marginal private benefit, MPB, associated with the consumption of various units of a good. MPB is downward sloping to reflect the law of diminishing marginal utility. Market supply, *S*, reflects the marginal private cost, MPC, of production and is upward sloping to reflect the law of diminishing marginal productivity. Equilibrium in a perfectly competitive market occurs at the intersection of supply and demand. The triangular area P_0AC represents consumer surplus and the triangular area P_0CG captures producer surplus. Total social surplus equals the triangle *ACG* and shows that both buyers and sellers mutually gain from free trade.

private costs to producers, with market price serving as a coordinating device. We can use a graphical version of a supply and demand model to illustrate the market-clearing process.

Suppose the supply and demand model in Figure 8–2 represents the market for generic aspirin. The per-unit price of generic aspirin, *P*, is specified on the vertical axis, and the quantity of generic aspirin, *Q*, is shown on the horizontal axis. The market demand curve, *D*, is downward sloping, reflecting the substitution and income effects normally associated with a lower relative price for a product, as discussed in Chapter 5. The demand curve also shows the diminishing marginal private benefit that consumers receive from additional tablets of aspirin. The supply curve, *S*, is upward sloping, indicating that marginal private cost increases with respect to the production of additional tablets of aspirin. Marginal private cost reflects the variable costs of production that individual firms incur from hiring labor and purchasing materials. As noted in Chapter 7, marginal private cost typically increases in the short run because of a capacity constraint caused by a fixed input (such as the size of the production facility or amount of equipment). Because of the rising marginal cost, a higher price is necessary to encourage producers to produce and sell more aspirin.[1]

The equilibrium, or market-clearing, price and output of aspirin are at the point where demand intersects with supply or where quantity demanded equals quantity supplied. By definition, equilibrium occurs when there is no tendency for further change. At the equilibrium price of P_0, consumers are willing and able to purchase Q_0 tablets of aspirin because that represents the utility-maximizing amount. In addition, manufacturers of aspirin wish to provide Q_0 tablets on the market at this price because that represents the profit-maximizing amount. Thus, both consumers and producers are perfectly satisfied with the exchange because both can purchase or sell their desired quantities at a price of P_0. The area under the demand curve but above price (triangle P_0AC) measures **consumer surplus,** reflecting the net benefit to consumers from engaging in free exchange. Consumer surplus shows the difference between what the consumer would be willing to pay and what the consumer actually has to pay over the relevant range of output. Similarly, the area below market price but above the supply curve (triangle P_0CG) represents **producer surplus,** signaling the net benefit to producers from participating in free trade. Producer surplus measures the difference between the actual price received by the seller and the required price as reflected in the marginal costs of production. The sum of consumer and producer surplus captures the total net gains from trade to both consumers and producers (triangle ACG).

Notice the similarity between the market supply and demand curves in Figure 8–2 and the marginal social benefit and marginal social cost curves of Figure 3–2, where we learned that an efficient allocation of resources occurs in an economy when MSB equals MSC for each and every good. The similarity between the two figures should not be surprising because consumers and producers constitute an important part of society in a market economy. If demand and supply represent the full marginal social benefit and cost of the exchange, that is, if MPB = MSB and MPC = MSC, a perfectly competitive market results in allocative efficiency in the process of individual consumers maximizing their private utilities and individual producers maximizing economic profits. That is, decentralized decision making in the marketplace automatically results in allocative efficiency when markets are perfectly competitive.

However, an inefficient allocation of resources may result in a perfectly competitive market when others, in addition to market participates, are affected either beneficially or adversely by a market exchange. Inefficiency results because utility-maximizing consumers and profit-maximizing producers consider only their marginal private benefits and costs and not the full social impact of their choices. It is likely that allocative efficiency results for our generic aspirin example because others besides the consumers and producers of aspirin are normally unaffected by that exchange. We take up externalities and public goods, two situations where a perfectly competitive market may fail to allocate resources efficiently, in Chapter 9. We also learn later in this chapter that a monopoly fails to efficiently allocate resources.

Comparative Static Analysis

The supply and demand model can be used to examine how surpluses and shortages of goods temporarily develop, as well as to study changes in the price and quantity of goods and services in the marketplace. Using the model to study changes in price and quantity is referred to as **comparative static analysis.** Comparative static analysis examines how changes in market

1. Recall from Economics 101 that each perfectly competitive firm, as a price taker, faces an infinitely elastic or horizontal demand for its product. Also recall that market supply is derived by horizontally summing across all firms the portion of the marginal cost curve that lies above the minimum point on the average variable cost curve.

conditions influence the positions of the demand and supply curves and cause the equilibrium levels of price and output to adjust. As the demand and supply curves shift, we can trace out price and output effects by comparing the different equilibrium points. Comparative static analysis can be used to explain the effects of market changes in the past or to forecast future market outcomes.

As discussed in Chapter 5, several factors, such as the number of buyers, consumer tastes, income, and the prices of substitutes and complements, affect the position of the market demand curve. Similarly, various factors, including input prices and technology, determine the position of the supply curve by affecting the costs of production (see Chapter 7). A change in any one of these factors shifts the corresponding curve and alters the price and output of goods and services in the marketplace.

For example, suppose consumer income increases by a significant amount. Assuming aspirin represents a normal good, the higher income causes the demand curve to shift to the right. In Figure 8–3, notice that as the demand curve shifts to the right, a temporary shortage of *EF* is created in the market for aspirin if price remains constant. A shortage develops because at the

FIGURE 8–3
Effect of an Increase in Demand

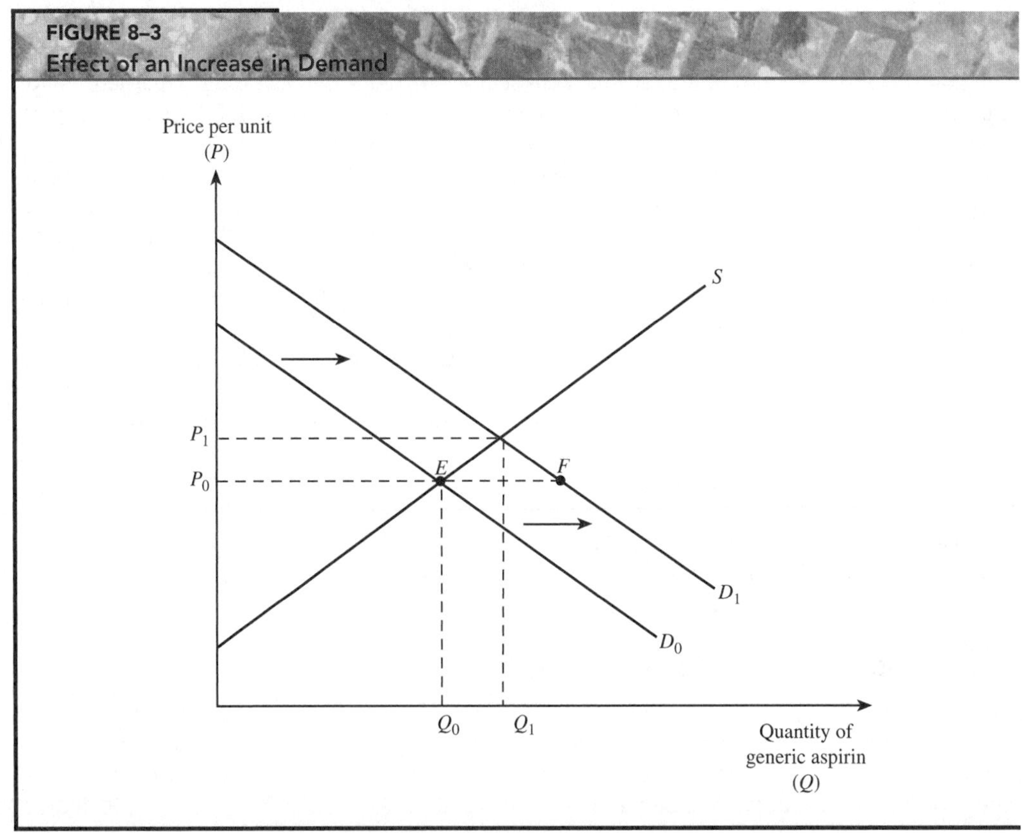

A change in demand causes a change in the equilibrium price and quantity of a good. Here the demand increases from D_0 to D_1 because of an increase in consumer income, assuming that generic aspirin is a normal good. As a result, a temporary shortage equal to the horizontal distance *EF* is created in the market at the existing price of P_0. Eventually price increases in the market from P_0 to P_1 in response to the increase in demand. Quantity also increases from Q_0 to Q_1.

initial price, the quantity demanded on the new demand curve, D_1, exceeds the quantity supplied of aspirin. However, price does not remain constant in a competitive market and is eventually bid up from P_0 to P_1. The higher price creates an incentive for manufacturers to offer more aspirin in the marketplace, and quantity supplied increases from Q_0 to Q_1. The higher prices also create an incentive for consumers to purchase less aspirin than originally planned at point F, perhaps by switching to alternative painkillers, consuming only half of a tablet per use, or postponing their consumption. Thus, under normal conditions, supply and demand analysis predicts that a higher price and quantity of aspirin are associated with greater consumer income, *ceteris paribus*.

As another example, suppose aspirin manufacturers adopt a cost-saving technology that increases supply. Therefore, the supply of aspirin shifts to the right, as shown in Figure 8–4. If the price of aspirin remains at P_0, a surplus of AB results because quantity supplied exceeds quantity demanded. In a competitive market, however, the surplus creates an incentive for the price of aspirin to decline from P_0 to P_1. Consequently, the quantity demanded of aspirin increases from Q_0 to Q_1 as price declines and consumers face an incentive to purchase more aspirin. At the same time, the quantity that producers are willing to supply falls when price declines toward

FIGURE 8–4
Effects of an Increase in Supply

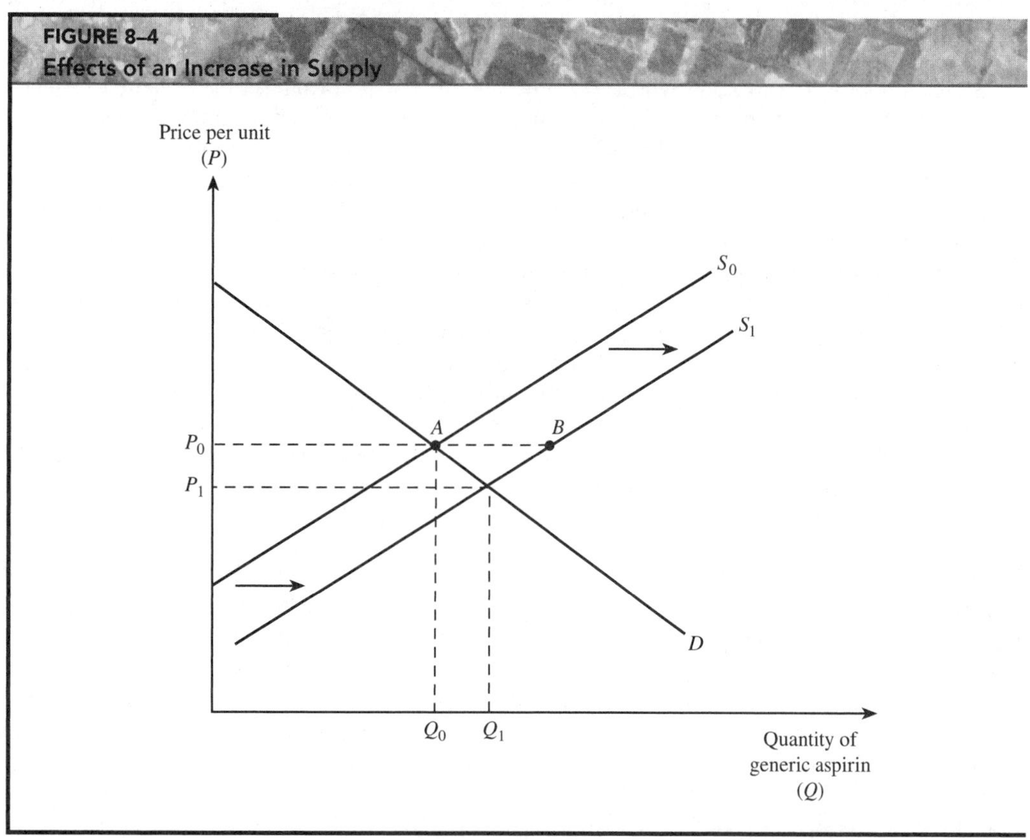

A change in supply causes a change in the equilibrium price and quantity of a good. Here the supply increases from S_0 to S_1 because of the introduction of a cost-saving technology. As a result, a temporary surplus of horizontal distance AB is created in the market at the existing price of P_0. Eventually price decreases in the market from P_0 to P_1 in response to the increase in demand. Quantity increases from Q_0 to Q_1.

equilibrium. These actions result in a new equilibrium and market-clearing price and quantity. Thus, supply and demand analysis predicts that the adoption of a cost-saving technology causes price to decline and quantity to increase, assuming all else remains constant.

Notice in the previous discussion that price serves several important functions. First, price provides useful information to both consumers and producers regarding the relative availability and value of a good or service in the marketplace. Second, price serves as a coordination device, bringing the actions of consumers and producers into harmony and helping to clear markets. Third, price serves as a rationing device, distributing the goods or services to the consumers who value them the most. Fourth, price acts as an incentive mechanism, encouraging more resources to markets with shortages and less resources to markets with surpluses of goods.

A Note on Long-Run Entry and Exit in a Perfectly Competitive Market

The analyses thus far have concerned short-run adjustments because the number of firms has remained unchanged. But entry and exit of firms may take place in the long run as sellers take advantage of changing profit opportunities in various markets. For example, since there are no barriers to entry in a perfectly competitive marketplace, excess profits create an incentive for new firms to enter an industry as they strive to make a higher than normal rate of return. Conversely, economic losses create an incentive for firms to leave an industry as they try to avoid an unusually low rate of return on their investment. Finally, when normal profits exist in a perfectly competitive industry, the market is in long-run equilibrium and firms have no incentive to either enter or exit the industry. **Normal profits** result when there are just enough revenues to cover the opportunity cost of each and every input, including a normal return to capital.

Long-run entry in response to excess profits can be treated as shifting the short-run market supply curve to the right. Similarly, long-run exit causes the short-run market supply curve to shift to the left. Given a stable demand curve, these adjustments in the short-run supply curve create a change in the price of the good and eventually restore a normal profit situation. In particular, long-run entry lowers price and eliminates excess profits, whereas exit leads to higher prices and eliminates the economic losses of the firms that remain in the industry. Because of entry and exit, we can expect that the typical perfectly competitive firm earns a normal profit in the long run.

The importance of long-run adjustments in a market is illustrated in the following example. In the mid-1980s, physicians, dentists, and other health care providers became concerned about contracting the AIDS and hepatitis B viruses in the work environment. This concern caused a considerable increase in the demand for form-fitting disposable latex gloves, which are preferred over vinyl gloves because they allow flexibility for detail work and are impermeable to blood and body fluids. From 1986 to 1990, annual sales of latex gloves increased by approximately 58 percent (Borzo, 1991). Initially, as the demand for latex gloves increased, a tremendous shortage of latex gloves developed. As the shortage gave way to higher prices in the short run, medical supply manufacturers operated their plants around the clock in an attempt to make higher profits. Consequently, the shortage declined as price increased and created an incentive for increased production. Greater profit opportunities in this market created incentives for medical suppliers to construct new manufacturing plants to produce more disposable latex gloves. According to the popular press, at one point in 1988, 116 permits were pending in Malaysia for the construction of disposable latex glove factories (Zikos, 1988). These new plants provided for new entry and an increased supply of latex gloves in the long run.

This example helps highlight the importance of entry and exit in a marketplace. Entry of new firms leads to a greater allocation of resources in response to favorable profit opportunities. Likewise, exiting of firms helps eliminate relatively inefficient resources and producers from a market. Profit, in both cases, serves as an important incentive mechanism and brings about an efficient allocation of resources in the long run. Of course, entry and exit of firms can take place only in perfectly competitive markets because entry and exit barriers are nonexistent. In the following discussion of monopoly, we will see that barriers prevent new firms from entering markets, resulting in an inefficient allocation of resources.

Using Supply and Demand to Explain Rising Health Care Costs

Supply and demand analysis offers many reasons why national health care expenditures in the United States exploded from 5.1 percent in 1960 to more than 15 percent of the nation's income more recently. Specifically, the demand for medical care increased because of rising income, an aging population, and a falling out-of-pocket price since 1960. In terms of the supply and demand model, all of these factors simultaneously created a shift in the demand curve to the right, causing a higher price and quantity of medical care over time. Expenditures on medical care, the product of price and quantity, also increased as a result.

On the supply side, Baumol (1967) points out that wages in service industries, like medical care, tend to increase with higher wages in the manufacturing sector. Higher wages in the manufacturing sector result from increased worker productivity caused by technological advances. Because wage increases in various medical care industries are tied to the growing manufacturing wage but are not necessarily matched with commensurate increases in productivity, per-unit costs of medical care are driven upward. In terms of supply and demand analysis, the supply curve for medical care has shifted to the left over time because of wages outpacing productivity. As a result, the price of medical care increased. And because the demand for medical care tends to be price inelastic, the increase in price caused health care expenditures to increase.

Cost-enhancing technologies provide another explanation for rising health care costs on both the supply and demand sides of the market. Over the years, a number of new medical technologies, such as computer tomography (CAT) scans, magnetic resonance imaging (MRI), and organ transplant technology, have raised the quality and costs of providing health care services. New technologies tend to supplement rather than supplant old technologies in the medical field. The widespread adoption of these cost-enhancing (rather than cost-saving) technologies shifted the supply curve to the left, causing health care expenditures to rise given the price-inelastic demand curve. In addition, since these technologies often simultaneously create a demand for new treatments because they can help extend lives and are less risky, the demand curve also shifted to the right. Consequently, medical care expenditures increased due to the lower supply and greater demand caused by cost-enhancing technology.

In conclusion, rising income, an aging population, a declining out-of-pocket price, and the demand for new treatments helped fuel higher health care costs from the demand side of the market for medical care. From the supply side, the adoption of new technologies and higher wages also may have contributed to rising medical costs. Thus, supply and demand analysis can serve as a useful tool for explaining market changes even though the underlying assumptions do not perfectly conform to market realities.

The Monopoly Model of Market Behavior and Performance

If a firm has some market power, the competitive model is an inappropriate tool of analysis and a noncompetitive model should be employed. The difference between the two models concerns how the individual firm treats market price. In a perfectly competitive market, the individual firm is a price taker. That is, price is beyond the control of a single firm so each time a perfectly competitive firm sells an additional unit of output, market price measures the additional revenues received. Economists refer to **marginal revenue** (MR) as the additional revenues received from selling one more unit of a good. Thus P = MR for a price taker. A noncompetitive firm with some degree of market power, in contrast, faces a downward-sloping demand curve and thereby has some ability to influence the market price by reducing or restricting the quantity produced. To illustrate how a noncompetitive model can be used to examine firm behavior, we will first consider a pure monopoly in which there is only one producer of a good or service in the entire market. A pure monopoly is the logical opposite of a perfectly competitive market. We will compare the equilibrium outcome for a monopoly to that of a perfectly competitive market.

Monopoly versus Perfect Competition

In precise terms, a monopoly is the sole provider of a product in a well-defined market with no close substitutes. Because it is the only firm in the market, a monopolist faces the market demand curve, which is always downward sloping because of the substitution and income effects associated with a price change. Given the downward-sloping demand, the only way the monopolist can increase quantity sold is to lower the price of the product. Assuming price is the same for all units sold at a point in time, price must be lowered not only for the additional unit but for the previous units as well. As a result, marginal revenue will be less than price at each level of output. In fact, it can be shown for a linear demand that marginal revenue has the same intercept but twice the slope.[2]

Figure 8–5 can be used to show how the equilibrium price and quantity for a monopolist compare to the market price and quantity in an otherwise equivalent perfectly competitive market. As before, our example is the market for generic aspirin. The market demand for aspirin is labeled *AD*. The supply curve is labeled *GS* and reflects the marginal private cost of producing aspirin. (Ignore the curve *A*MR for now.) Point *C* represents equilibrium in a perfectly competitive market where the supply and demand curves intersect. The market price and output of aspirin equal P_C and Q_C, respectively. Consumer surplus equals the triangular area $P_C AC$ and producer surplus equals the triangular area $P_C CG$. The entire triangular area *ACG* reflects the net gain from trade in a perfectly competitive market.

Now suppose only one firm produces and sells aspirin in that same market. Perhaps the award of a government franchise provides the aspirin manufacturer with the monopoly position. Further suppose that an entry barrier, such as the government franchise, prevents other firms from entering the market. Relevant to the monopolist's choice of price and quantity is the marginal revenue curve labeled *A*MR. Notice that marginal revenue shares the same intercept as the linear demand but has twice its slope. The monopolist chooses market price and quantity such that profits are maximized. Profit maximization occurs at the level of output, Q_M, where MR = MC because producing and selling additional tablets of aspirin always add more to revenues than costs up to that point. Beyond the Q_M level of output, additional production does not add to total profits because marginal cost exceeds marginal revenue. Consequently, the monopoly outcome is represented by point *M* and the price charged equals P_M.

Notice that a monopoly charges a higher price and produces less aspirin than a perfectly competitive market. Also notice that the monopolist receives some of the surplus that consumers receive in a perfectly competitive market. More precisely, consumer surplus shrinks from triangular

2. Suppose the (inverse) demand is captured by the equation $P = a - bQ$. Total revenues equal P times Q or $(a - bQ)Q = aQ - bQ^2$. Taking the first derivative of this revenue function with respect to Q to get $d\text{TR}/dQ$ gives $\text{MR} = a - 2bQ$. Notice that MR has the same intercept but twice the slope of the demand.

FIGURE 8–5
The Monopoly Outcome

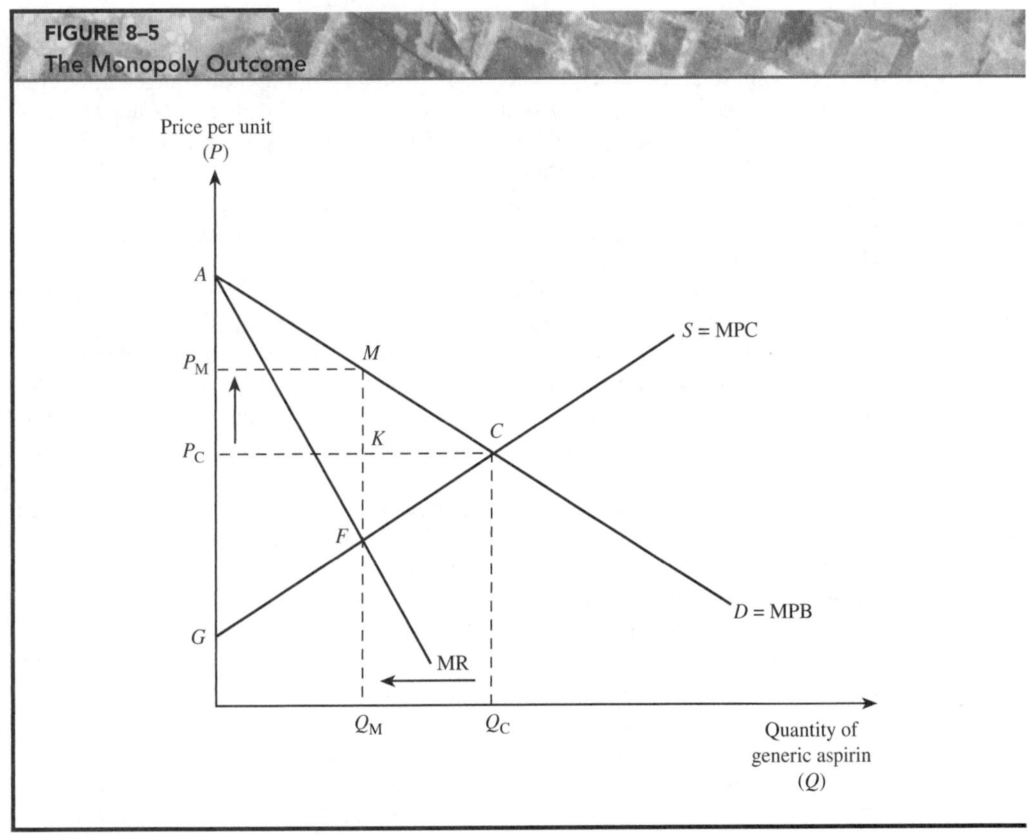

This illustration compares the perfectly competitive and monopoly outcomes. The perfectly competitive outcome is represented by point *C*. A monopoly produces at Q_M where MR = MC and charges price P_M. Because a monopoly exists in the market, consumer surplus shrinks to the triangle P_MAM and the producer surplus increases to the area outlined by P_MMFG. Reflecting that society's scarce resources are misallocated, a deadweight loss of area *MCF* is created by the monopolist.

area $P_C AC$ in a perfectly competitive market to triangular area $P_M AM$ in a market dominated by a monopoly. Producer surplus increases from area $P_C CG$ to area $P_M MFG$. The rectangular area $P_M MKP_C$ reflects the surplus that is transferred from consumers to producers in a market controlled by a monopoly. In addition to this redistribution of income is the deadweight loss created by a monopoly. Notice that the net gain from trade is much smaller in a monopoly market than in a perfectly competitive market. The difference is the triangular area *MCF* that reflects the deadweight loss created by a monopoly. The deadweight loss shows that the value of the units no longer produced is greater than the opportunity costs of the resources used to produce them. It follows that a monopoly underproduces output and thereby misallocates society's scarce resources. The cost of monopoly shows up in the size of the deadweight loss.

Barriers to Entry

For a firm to maintain its market power for an extended period of time, some type of barrier to entry must exist to prevent other firms from entering the industry. As Haas-Wilson (2003, pp. 127–28) explains, “entry of new competitors will most likely occur in at least one of three ways: (1) Established firms in the local market, not currently selling X (for example, a physician organization of internists in the local market) may begin to sell X even though they had not done so in the past; (2) established firms currently selling X, but not in the local market (for example, a physician organization of pediatricians located in a distant city) may open a local office and begin to sell X in the local market; and (3) new business may start (for example, pediatricians establishing their first practices after completing their medical education). This entry of additional competitors and the associated increase in the availability of product X defeats the incumbent’s attempt to exercise market power.”

Barriers to entry make it costly for new firms to enter markets in a timely manner and may exist for technical or legal reasons. Exclusive control over a necessary input, sunk costs, an absolute cost advantage, and scale economies represent some technical reasons to suspect that entry barriers may exist in some market environments. If a firm has exclusive control over a necessary input, competitors are without the required resources to produce substitute products. Exclusive control over bauxite, a necessary input in the production of aluminum, provided Alcoa with a monopoly position in the 1940s. After losing its antitrust suit, Alcoa was required to sell some of its bauxite to two new competitors, Reynolds and Kaiser Aluminum, created by the government. Likewise, incumbent health insurers may have already developed exclusive contracts with various health care provider networks in an area. The difficulty of establishing a network of health care providers may make it difficult for a new insurer to sell its health plans in an area.

Sunk or irretrievable costs can result in a barrier to entry into an industry. Irretrievable costs involve initial investments or assets that cannot be easily salvaged when a firm exits an industry. These initial investments may take the form of specialized buildings and equipment, advertising, or the establishment of a reputation or brand name. Contestability theory suggests that markets are more contestable or potentially competitive when sunk costs are low because new entrants realize they can leave an industry relatively costlessly if economic circumstances do not turn out as initially suspected. Conversely, if sunk costs are significant, firms may be reluctant to enter new markets, *ceteris paribus*. Hence, the prospect of high exit costs can discourage firms from entering an industry. All other factors held constant, incumbent firms have less market power in “hit and run” industries in which sunk costs are low.

An absolute cost advantage arises when the incumbent firm can produce at a lower cost than potential competitors. Incumbents may be able to produce at a lower cost because suppliers offer them a price discount for materials as a result of the favorable reputation they have built up over the years. Incumbents can also benefit from **learning by doing.** Firms gain from learning by doing when they produce more output over time and thereby learn from their experience. That is, practice makes perfect. The greater cumulative output and experience translates into lower average costs of production for a given level of quality or a higher level of quality for a given level of costs. Absolute cost advantages can make it difficult or more costly for new firms to enter the market and effectively compete against incumbent firms.

Scale economies may also serve as an entry barrier. When production exhibits economies of scale, a firm operates on the downward-sloping portion of the long-run average total cost curve, ATC, and the average cost of production decreases as output expands, as shown in Figure 8–6. An existing firm in that situation has a cost advantage that results from the scale of production. Potential competitors could not effectively compete with the established firm on a cost basis. In fact, the larger existing firm with average costs of C_X could set its price slightly below the average cost of the potential entrant, C_E; earn profits; and discourage the potential entry from actually entering the market. Pricing to deter entry is called **limit pricing.** Thus, economies of scale can serve as a barrier to entry that insulates an existing firm from potential competitors. Price

FIGURE 8–6
Scale Economies as an Entry Barrier

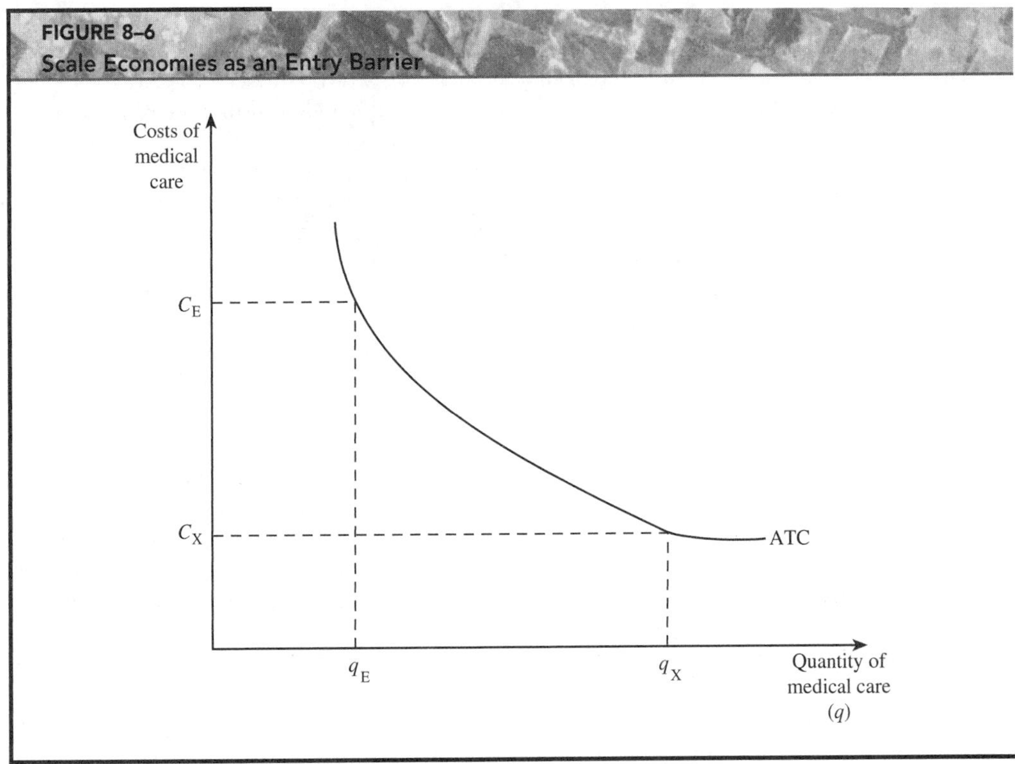

The declining average total cost curve, ATC, reflects scale economies in production. An existing firm producing a large volume of output at q_X produces at a cost of C_X. An entrant with a relatively small volume of output of q_E produces at a cost of C_E. Because of the scale economies, an existing firm can charge a price slightly below C_E and discourage the entry from actually entering the market. This practice is referred to as limit pricing.

regulations are often necessary when a firm holds a monopoly position of this kind (for example, TV cable service).[3]

Legal restrictions that prevent other firms from entering markets and providing services similar to those of existing firms can also serve as a barrier to entry. Legal patent protection provides a firm with a 20-year monopoly right to a product. As another example, prior to the late 1970s, the U.S. government purposely limited the number of firms in many industries, such as air transportation and long distance telephone services. However, deregulation took place in the late 1970s because many people were dissatisfied with the performance of these industries.

Drug patents, occupational licenses, and certificate of need (CON) laws are sometimes treated as examples of legal entry barriers into medical care markets. A CON law requires health care providers to obtain government approval before constructing new buildings or purchasing expensive capital equipment. Some feel that CON laws are necessary to prevent health care organizations from unnecessarily duplicating resources within an area. For example, a number of

3. Not all economists agree that scale economies serve as an entry barrier. Bain (1956) defines an entry barrier as any factor that allows sellers to elevate price above marginal costs. Stigler (1968) defines an entry barrier as costs that new entrants face but not incumbents. Therefore Bain treats scale economies as an entry barrier but Stigler does not.

hospitals may simultaneously purchase and offer the same new, expensive piece of capital equipment to treat patients in an area. Because each of the various hospitals may be unable to sufficiently spread the large fixed costs given a limited number of patients in the area, the average cost per patient of using the expensive equipment is higher than if only one hospital purchased and offered services from the capital item.

Others argue, however, that CON laws unduly inhibit entry into medical care markets. Because of the restricted entry in a market area, health insurance plans are less able to negotiate competitive prices from the limited number of health care providers. The higher prices paid by health insurers reflect in part that incumbent firms can exploit their market power by reducing output and driving up medical prices because they feel less threatened by the prospect of potential competitors.

Not too many studies have empirically examined the impact of CON laws on the entry of medical firms. Among the few, Ford and Kaserman (1993) analyzed the impact of CON laws on the entry of new firms into the dialysis industry. Specifically, the authors used multiple regression analysis to explain entry into the dialysis industry across the 50 states of the United States over the period from 1982 to 1989. As independent variables, they specified a 0/1 dummy variable indicating whether a particular state possessed CON regulations regarding dialysis clinics in a particular year, along with a number of control variables. The control variables essentially captured the potential profitability of firms entering the dialysis industry in the 50 states and included various costs and demand-side factors. Recall that economic theory suggests that increased entry takes place when profits are higher and entry barriers are lower. Among their results, Ford and Kaserman found empirically that the presence of CON laws significantly reduced the entry and expansion of dialysis firms. This finding led them to conclude that "CON regulation of the dialysis industry has sustained the monopoly power of incumbent clinics and thereby provided the wherewithal to increase profits by reducing service quality" (p. 790).

Monopolistic Competition and Product Differentiation

Now that we have discussed the models of perfect competition and monopoly, we need to turn our attention to the other two models listed in Table 8–1. In a monopolistically competitive market structure, there are many firms and low or no barriers to entry. The distinguishing characteristic of monopolistic competition is that firms within the same industry sell a slightly differentiated product. The product differentiation may result from a preferred location, different levels of quality (either real or perceived), or advertising and other promotional strategies. Because of product differentiation, each firm faces a downward-sloping demand curve that is highly but not perfectly elastic. Since the demand curve is downward sloping, the monopolistically competitive firm has some limited ability to raise price without losing all of its sales. Product differentiation leads to a certain degree of brand loyalty and that is why the individual firm can raise price and continue to sell output. Everything held equal, a more differentiated product translates into a less elastic demand curve facing the monopolistically competitive firm.

Figure 8–7 illustrates a model of a profit-maximizing, monopolistically competitive firm. Notice the highly elastic demand facing the individual firm, reflecting the relatively large number but imperfect substitutes for its product. Bayer Aspirin may be a good example of a branded product that faces a downward-sloping demand. Bayer competes against many generic producers of aspirin but has a brand name that allows it to charge a higher price. Given the linear demand, the marginal revenue is drawn with the same intercept but has twice the slope. The long-run average total cost, ATC, and marginal cost, MC, curves allow economies and then diseconomies of scale.

FIGURE 8–7
Long-Run Equilibrium for a Monopolistically Competitive Firm

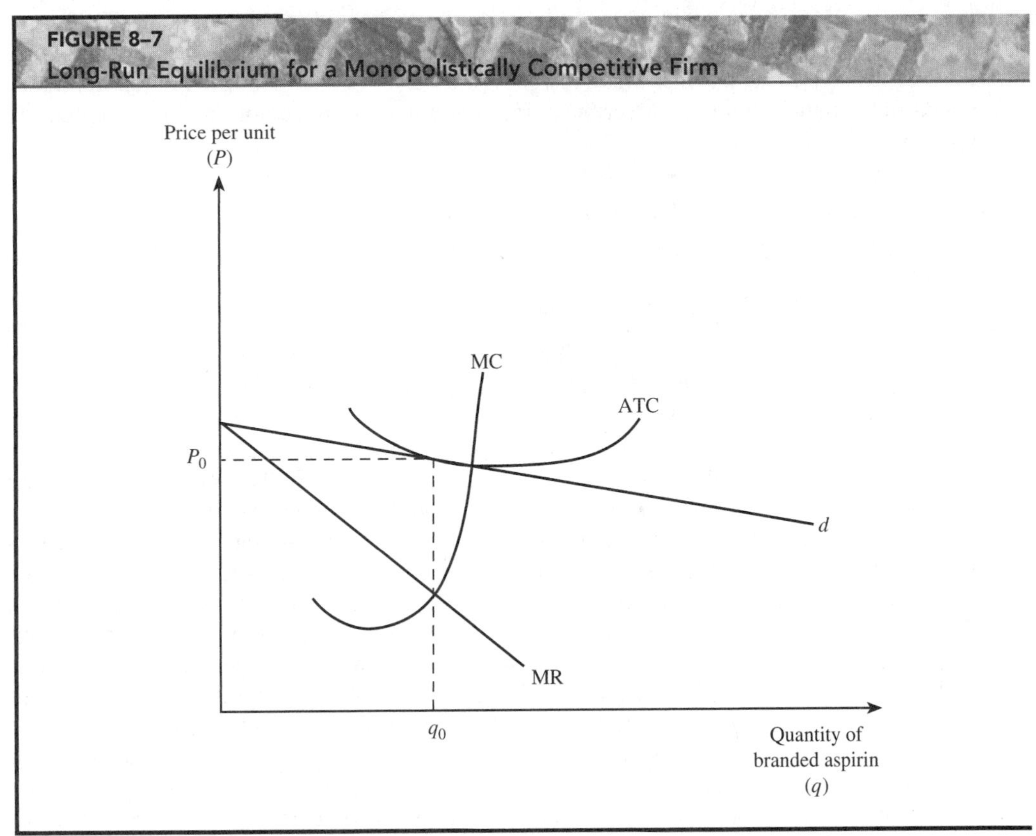

A monopolistically competitive firm faces a downward-sloping demand curve because of product differentiation. Because there are no meaningful entry barriers, firms continue to enter the market until the representative firm earns only a normal profit. Hence, in the long run, the representative monopolistically competitive firm produces at q_0 where MR = MC and charges a price equal to average total costs.

Given the downward-sloping demand, the individual firm may earn an economic profit in the short run if the price charged is greater than average total cost at the level of output where marginal cost equals marginal revenue. However, the absence of any barriers to entry prevents excess profits from continuing in the long run in a monopolistically competitive industry. Over time other firms are attracted to the industry by the possibility of earning economic profits. As more firms enter the market, each firm sees its market share slowly diminish, which translates into a decrease in the demand for its product. The demand curve faced by each firm continues to shift to the left until the market price for the product is driven down to the point where economic profits are zero, or price equals average total cost. Demand becomes more elastic as well. At that point firms are no longer attracted to the industry and the market settles into a long-run equilibrium situation where economic profits are zero.

Figure 8–7 shows long-run equilibrium in a monopolistically competitive industry. Notice that the demand curve is tangent to the average total cost at the level of output where MR = MC. The monopolistically competitive firm earns zero profits in the long run because price or average revenue equals average total costs. Notice that the monopolistically competitive firm does not produce at the point where price equals marginal cost as does a perfectly competitive firm. As a result, one might argue that this type of industry inefficiently allocates resources. But before that conclusion can be drawn, we must first consider the costs and benefits of production differentiation and whether such things as advertising and brand names impede or enhance competition among firms.

Procompetitive and Anticompetitive Aspects of Product Differentiation

In the perfectly competitive model, consumers are treated as being perfectly informed about the prices and quality of all goods and services in the marketplace. The assumption that all consumers possess perfect information about prices implies that all identical products sell at the same lowest possible price. Otherwise, high-priced businesses lose sales to low-priced businesses when consumers are perfectly informed.

But, realistically, there are both costs and benefits to acquiring information. Therefore, in many situations, people choose to be less than perfectly informed, or **rationally ignorant,** because the marginal costs of additional information outweigh the additional benefits. Positive information and search costs mean that consumers may find it uneconomical to seek out all available suppliers. As a result, any one individual supplier faces a less than perfectly elastic demand and is able to restrict output and raise price to some degree. As a result, the price of a product in the real world is likely to be dispersed and higher, on average, than the competitive ideal (since theoretically prices cannot be lower than the competitive level). The average price and degree of price dispersion depend on the marginal benefits and costs of acquiring price information. Higher benefits and lower costs of acquiring information imply lower and less dispersed prices.

Imperfect consumer information may also affect the level of quality observed in a market, but the relation between information and product quality is more involved. It stands to reason that high-quality goods cost more to produce than low-quality goods. If consumers are perfectly informed, high-quality goods sell at a higher price than low-quality goods in a competitive market. In the real world with imperfect information, however, consumers are not fully knowledgeable about product quality. Consequently, if consumers base their willingness to pay on the average quality in the market and pay the average price, low-quality products drive out high-quality products, and the process continues until no products remain. The implication is that the level of product quality is higher when consumer information is more readily available.

Given imperfect information about various products in the real world, some economists argue that various features of production differentiation, such as advertising, trademarks, and brand names, convey important information regarding the value of a good or service. For example, they argue that advertising provides relatively cheap information to consumers about the price and quality of a good and thereby promotes lower prices and higher quality. In fact, studies by Benham (1972), Cady (1976), and Kwoka (1984) found that the prices of eyeglasses and prescription drugs were higher, on average, in areas where price advertising was prohibited. Even when price and quality information is not directly conveyed, a large advertisement in the Yellow Pages or the local newspaper, for example, may signal consumers that the firm is willing to incur a sizeable expense because it is confident that it is offering a quality product at a reasonable price. Through repeat buying, the firm hopes to get a sufficient return on its advertising investment. In this case, the mere presence of an expensive advertising message generates information about the value of a product.

Other economists such as Klein and Leffler (1981) argue that brand names and trademarks serve a similar purpose for promoting competition. Because the quality of many products cannot be properly evaluated until after purchase (or repeat purchase), brand names and trademarks help identify businesses that have enough confidence in the quality of their products to invest in establishing a reputation. Given the sunk-cost nature of the investment, the argument is that a business will not sacrifice its established reputation by offering shoddy products on the market and take the chance of losing repeat buyers. A firm that expends considerable sums of money to polish its image and establish a brand name can lose a valuable investment by selling inferior products and tarnishing that image.

However, not all economists agree that advertising, trademarks, and brand names are always procompetitive. Some economists are concerned that promotional activities are used to establish brand loyalty, mislead consumers, and thereby cause "habit buying" rather than "informed buying." In this view, promotional activities are anticompetitive and advertising is treated as persuasive rather than informative. Persuasive advertising attempts to convince consumers that the attributes of product A are better than those of product B. Sometimes the advertising message points out real differences, but often the advertising is used to create imaginary or perceived differences across goods or services. For example, both Bayer and generic brands contain the same aspirin ingredient, yet many people are willing to pay a higher price for the Bayer product. Some argue that people pay a premium for branded products because past advertising successfully convinced people that Bayer aspirin, for example, is a superior product. Instead of creating a new market demand, persuasive advertising attempts to attract consumers from competitor firms. Considering advertising, trademarks, and brand names as quality signals, Robinson (1988) points out "a signal can be heard as long as it stands out over and against the background level of noise. As each seller amplifies his or her signal, the background noise level rises, necessitating further amplification on the part of individual sellers. This is clearly undesirable from a social perspective because the signaling mechanism imposes costs" (p. 469).

According to the anticompetitive view, product differentiation manipulates the demand for a product. For example, a successful advertising campaign can influence consumer tastes and preferences and thereby affect the position of the demand curve for the product. Advertising may affect the position of the demand curve in two ways. First, the demand curve may shift upward as a result of successful advertising because consumers are now willing to pay a higher price for the firm's product. Second, advertising may cause the demand curve to become less elastic with respect to price and, as a result, give the firm some ability to reduce output and raise the price of the good or service.

As an example, many public health officials claim that the purpose behind cigarette advertising is to manipulate the demand for cigarettes. Of major concern is advertising aimed at influencing teenager demand for cigarettes. A report by the Centers for Disease Control found that among smokers aged 12 to 18, preferences were greater for Marlboro, Newport, and Camel, three brands that are heavily advertised (Ruffenach, 1992). RJR Nabisco's Old Joe advertising campaign for Camel cigarettes was of particular concern to health officials. As George Will (1992) writes:

> *A study of children aged 3 to 6 showed that Old Joe was not quite as familiar as the McDonald's and Coca-Cola emblems but was more familiar than the Cheerios emblem. An astonishing 91 percent of 6-year-olds recognized Old Joe, about as many as recognized Mickey Mouse.*

Existing firms may also use advertising or other types of product differentiation to create barriers to entry. If existing firms can control consumers through advertising, for example, new firms have a difficult time entering a market because they are unable to sell a sufficient amount of output to break even financially. It follows that product differentiation directed toward creating artificial wants, habit buying, or barriers to entry results in a misallocation of society's scarce resources. Resources are misused if they are employed to create illusory rather than real value.

When evaluating the social desirability of product differentiation, it is useful to remember that all products are homogeneous within the abstract model of the competitive industry and that most people agree that variety is the spice of life. People like diversity and enjoy choosing among a wide assortment of services selling at different money and time prices. People also receive utility when buying goods of different colors, shapes, and sizes. In this vein, the higher-than-competitive price that is paid for product differentiation may simply reflect the premium consumers place on variety. Nevertheless, economic theory suggests that firms may use product differentiation as a way to increase demand in some situations. If supply creates demand in this manner, some of society's scarce resources may be wasted.

OLIGOPOLY

Oligopoly involves a market structure with a few large or dominant firms and relatively high barriers to entry. While there may be a large number of firms in the industry, those other than the few dominant firms have relatively small market shares and act as price takers. The important aspect of oligopoly is that the dominant firms must be sufficiently sized and limited so the behavior of any one firm influences the pricing and output decisions of the other major firms in the market. It is this **mutual interdependence** among firms that distinguishes oligopoly from the other market structures. Because the nature of the interdependence varies, economists have been unable to develop a single model of oligopoly behavior. As a result, many formal and informal models of oligopoly have been developed that depict firm behavior under a variety of different scenarios. It is beyond the scope of this text to delve into all of these models so we have limited the discussion to two broad models of firm behavior: the collusive and competitive models of oligopoly.

Collusive Oligopoly

According to the **collusive oligopoly** model, all the firms in the industry cooperate rather than compete on price and output and jointly maximize profits by collectively acting as a monopolist. To illustrate, assume that there are only three identical firms in a given market with similar demand curves and that these firms have decided to collude and jointly maximize profits. Under these circumstances, the firms collectively act like a monopolist and jointly set the price and output indicated by point *M* on the market demand curve in Figure 8–5. It follows that a deadweight loss and a misallocation of society's scarce resources results from the collusive oligopoly.

The collusion among the oligopolistic firms may be of an overt or a tacit nature. Overt collusion refers to a situation in which representatives of the firms formally meet, perhaps in a clandestine location such as a smoke-filled room, and coordinate prices and divide up markets. Tacit collusion occurs when firms informally coordinate their prices. The price leadership model represents an example of tacit collusion in which the firms in an industry agree that one firm will serve as a price leader. The rest of the firms in the industry simply match or parallel the price of the leader. The resulting conscious parallelism can theoretically produce the same monopoly outcome as overt collusion and deadweight losses result (point *M* in Figure 8–5).

While it appears that firms in an oligopoly have a strong incentive to collude and form a cartel, a number of factors make collusion difficult. First and foremost are legal and practical considerations. The Sherman Antitrust Act prohibits overt collusion. Firms found in violation of overt price fixing can be subjected to severe financial penalties and the CEOs of these companies can be imprisoned.

However, antitrust officials, largely because of the difficulty of establishing proof, do not pursue cases involving tacit collusion. Firms in an industry may parallel their actions simply because they react to the same swings of demand and costs in the marketplace. But a tacit collusive arrangement has its practical difficulties. The informality of a tacit price-fixing arrangement can lead to problems because other firms in the industry may have a difficult time interpreting why the industry leader adjusts price. For example, suppose that the price leader decreases its price. Other firms in the industry can interpret this either as a simple reaction to an overall decrease in market demand or as an aggressive attempt on the part of the price leader to improve market share. In the first case, the other firms would simply lower prices and go about their business. In the second case, however, they may aggressively counteract this move by decreasing their prices even further in an attempt to initiate a price war.

Second, cost differences make it more difficult for firms to cooperate and agree on a common price. High-cost firms will desire a higher price than low-cost firms. But the success of a cartel depends on all of the firms adhering to a common price. Third, collusion is less successful when entry barriers are low. New firms offering lower prices will seize market share away from the cartel members when entry barriers are low. Fourth, for several reasons, collusion is more likely when few firms exist in an industry. One reason is that the ability to collude becomes more difficult as more firms enter into collusive agreement. Low negotiation costs make it much easier for two firms to collude than a dozen. Another reason is that more firms increase the probability that any one firm will act as a maverick and act independently by charging a lower price than others. Finally, more firms increase the probability that one firm may cheat or chisel on the agreement. For example, one firm may grant a secret price concession to a large buyer to improve sales. Naturally, when the other firms in the industry learn of this behavior they will abandon the collusive agreement and strike out on their own. The potential for cheating behavior is greater when more firms exist in the industry because of high monitoring and detection costs. For these four reasons, collusive agreements are more difficult to negotiate and maintain than most people imagine.

Competitive Oligopoly

Competitive oligopoly lies at the opposite extreme of collusive oligopoly. **Competitive oligopoly** considers that rivals in an oligopolistic industry may not coordinate their behavior but instead aggressively seek to individually maximize their own profits. If the firms in an oligopolistic market sell relatively homogeneous products, and thus one firm's product is a strong substitute for the others, each firm may realize that consumers will choose to buy the product offering the lowest price. If so, each firm faces an incentive to lower its price to marginal cost because at that level it will at least share part of the market with the others and not be undersold. If oligopolistic firms act in a competitive manner like this, market output is produced at the point where price equals marginal cost and resources are efficiently allocated (point *C* in Figure 8–5) even though a few dominant firms exit in the industry.

Whether firms act as a collusive or competitive oligopoly, or somewhere in between, depends on how each firm forms its beliefs or **conjectural variations** about how its rivals will react to its own price and output decisions. Conjectural variations consider how, say, firm A believes its rivals will react to its output decision. For example, firm A might believe that rivals will offset its behavior by producing more if it reduces output. Firm A has no incentive to restrict output given that market output and price remain the same because of offsetting behavior. On the other hand, Firm A might believe that its rivals will react by matching its behavior and producing less. The matching behavior results in less market output and a higher price for the product. Thus, if firms form similar conjectural variations and each expects matching behavior, a point closer to point *M* in Figure 8–5 and the associated deadweight losses result. In contrast, if firms form similar conjectural variations and each expects offsetting behavior, a point closer to point *C* in Figure 8–5 and the related efficiency gains occur.

Economic theory indicates that firm characteristics and market conditions influence the conjectural variations held by oligopolistic rivals. Many involve the same characteristics and conditions mentioned earlier that affect the success of a collusive oligopoly. First, firms are more likely to expect matching behavior when fewer firms exist and entry barriers are high because each firm realizes the greater profit potential from engaging in matching behavior. For example, each firm receives 50 percent of the monopoly profits when only two firms exist in the industry, so greater expectations can be attached to matching behavior.

Rivals are more likely to expect matching behavior when they share social and historical ties. Social and historical ties consider such things as industry trade associations, maturity and growth of an industry, and the proximity of firms in an industry. Specifically, rivals are more likely to anticipate matching behavior in industries in which trade associations play an important role. Trade associations foster cooperative behavior by establishing common bonds and the sharing of information among firms. Anticipation of matching behavior is greater among rivals in older industries that are growing slowly. Less entry takes place and fewer new owners exist in older, slow-growing industries. New owners are more likely to act as independent mavericks and reduce the likelihood of matching behavior.

The proximity of firms in an industry considers how close firms are on a number of dimensions including location, products, technologies, and sources of capital. Rivals in closer proximity more likely share similar expectations. The organizational structure of the firms in an industry may also affect conjectural variations. More centralized firms respond slowly to market changes and thus may be biased toward cooperation and expecting matching behavior. Also, prices tend to be determined at the top of the hierarchy while output decisions are made at the lower levels in more centralized organizations. If firms within an industry possess similar centralized organizational structures, the hierarchical arrangement may lead to price rigidity but output flexibility. Lastly, bounded rationality may favor expectations of matching behavior among rivals. **Bounded rationality** refers to the limited ability of human behavior to solve complex problems. Bounded rationality may lead to rules of thumb for pricing in an industry and act as facilitating device for firms to match or coordinate their behavior.

Oligopolistic Behavior in Medical Care Markets

The two different models just discussed indicate that oligopolistic firms are more likely to compete among themselves, rather than tacitly or overtly coordinate their policies, when firms are more numerous and entry barriers are lower, among other factors. Consequently we may witness only two firms in an industry yet aggressive price competition because entry barriers are low, for instance. In contrast, another industry may be characterized by five firms that coordinate their policies because entry barriers are high and the firms share similar histories and common bonds. Sorting out the behavior of real-world oligopolistic firms typically requires a careful study that simultaneously controls for a host of conditions that impact how firms may react to each other's decisions.

With that caveat in mind, we illustrate a couple of real-world situations that portray two different medical care industries as reflecting the behavior of a competitive oligopoly. That is, the existence of rivals resulted in lower prices. The first example relates to the $2 billion blood banking industry during the late twentieth century. Interestingly, this case involves two dominant not-for-profit firms.

In the mid-1990s, American Red Cross held a 46 percent share of the nation's blood banking business. Its closest national rival, America's Blood Centers (ABC), an affiliation of local independent blood banks, controlled another 47 percent. Individual hospital blood banks across the nation collectively held the remaining 7 percent of the market. Despite their relatively equivalent national market shares, either American Red Cross or a local member of ABC enjoyed a monopoly position in many regional markets at that time because federal policy since the 1970s had sanctioned local blood monopolies.

However, in 1998, American Red Cross made a bold move to increase its national market share to 65 percent by entering various regional markets such as Kansas City, Dallas, and Phoenix, originally monopolized by one of the local members of ABC. Based on this aggressive behavior, a competitive oligopoly model appears to do a better job of predicting the behavior of these two dominant firms than does a collusive oligopoly model. Evidence indicates that a lower price of blood resulted in local markets where a member of ABC coexisted with American Red Cross than in markets where an independent operated alone. For example, the price of a unit of blood cells was about $60 in Florida, one the nation's most cutthroat markets, and $105 in upstate New York, where competition was minimal (Hensley, 1998).

Our other example pertains to Johnson and Johnson (J&J), the well-known drug and medical device manufacturer. The relevant product in this case is a stent.[4] At the beginning of 1997, J&J was a dominant firm controlling 95 percent of the $600 million stent market through its patent protection. By the middle of 1998, the stent market had grown to yearly sales of $1 billion but J&J only held a meager 8 percent market share at that time (Winslow, 1998)! How could a company lose nearly 90 percent of its market share with a patented product over an eighteen-month span? It appears that J&J made a major blunder by failing to consider potential competition.

To be more specific, J&J angered key customers with rigid pricing for its $1,600 stent, refusing discounts even for hospitals that purchased more than $1 million worth of stents per year. With no comparable stent options, the buyers of stents had little alternative but to pay the high price. The high prices eventually caused cardiologists to pressure the Food and Drug Administration to approve new stents as quickly as possible. Physicians helped quicken the approval process by willingly testing the stents offered by new firms. Guidant Corporation took advantage of this new approval process and, 45 days after its patent was approved, controlled 70 percent of sales in the stent industry.[5]

While both of our examples provide evidence to support the competitive oligopoly model, it is important to note that a collusive oligopoly model may be more relevant in other situations, depending on the precise market conditions. Because overt price-fixing is per se illegal in the United States (see Chapter 9), it doesn't reveal itself as competitive behavior does. Tacit collusion is also hard to detect in practice given that the prices charged by firms in the same industries, even competitive ones, tend to move together. Nevertheless, industrial organization theory suggests that firms may collude when certain structural conditions hold in a market. When firms collude to make additional profits, economic theory tells us that they restrict output (and quality), raise price and thereby harm consumers. Chapter 9 provides some examples of noncompetitive oligopoly in the context of antitrust enforcement.

4. A stent resembles a small metal mesh tube, no thicker than a pencil lead, which is squeezed onto a tiny balloon and threaded into the heart's arteries. At the blockage site, the balloon is inflated to expand and deposit the stent, creating a scaffolding device resembling a ballpoint pen spring that remains in place to keep the vessel open after the balloon is withdrawn. Blood can then flow through the previously blocked artery.

5. Interestingly, J&J developed new types of stents and began merger proceedings with Guidant Corporation over the next several years.

Defining the Relevant Market and Measuring Concentration

This chapter has focused on the theoretical relationship between market structure, conduct, and performance. We learned that the structural characteristics of a market influence how firms conduct themselves with respect to pricing and other business practices, which in turn affects the performance of the industry. Little regard, however, has been given to delineating the precise boundaries of a market. Hypothetically, we know that a market reflects a place where the buyers and sellers of a product, through their collective negotiations, determine the price and quantity of a good or service that is bought and sold. While a hypothetical definition may be fine for theoretically studying the welfare implications of various market structures such as monopoly, a more practical definition of the market is necessary when conducting real-world analysis for private and public policy purposes. If a market is defined too broadly (narrowly) in practice, firms will appear to possess less (more) market power than they actually hold.

Consequently, if we intend to apply the SCP model to better understand and predict market behavior and performance, determining the precise boundaries of a market becomes an important exercise. To begin with, we have to determine the precise product that is being bought and sold. We also have to figure out how many sellers of that particular product are located in the market area. We discuss next some of the theoretical issues and practical limitations involved when defining markets. We also consider how market concentration is often measured in practice.

The Relevant Product and Geographical Markets

While hypothetically easy to imagine, a market is very hard to define in practice. Economists note that a market has two dimensions. The first dimension, the **relevant product market (RPM)** considers all of the various goods and services that a set of buyers might switch to if the price of any one good or service is raised by a nontrivial amount for more than a brief amount of time. Obviously, these goods and services must share some similarity or substitutability in terms of satisfying demand. For instance, general and family practitioners are likely to substitute for one another whereas urologists and pediatricians are not, because the latter two types of physicians fulfill different demands. As another example, suppose clinic-based physicians raise their fees by 5 percent or more and hold them at that level for at least a year. If a reasonable number of insurers, as the buyers of physician services, respond to this nontrivial and nontransient price increase by adding the outpatient facilities of hospitals to their network of ambulatory care providers, then services of clinic-based and hospital-based doctors can be considered as offering goods and services in the same RPM. If insurers do not switch, then hospital outpatient facilities most likely cannot be considered to be in the same RPM as clinic-based services.

The relevant geographical market (RGM) represents the second dimension of the market. The RGM establishes the spatial boundaries in which a set of buyers purchase their products. A RGM may be local (physician, nursing home care, acute hospital care, and dialysis services), regional (tertiary care in hospitals, health insurance), national, or international (pharmaceuticals, medical devices) in scope. For example, a hospital in Utica, New York, is unlikely to compete with a hospital in Hartford, Connecticut (about 205 miles away) for the same patients or insurers, but it may compete with a hospital in Rome, New York (about 16 miles away). Similar to determining the RPM, the conceptual exercise is to imagine all of the sellers of the same good or service that a set of buyers might switch to as a result of a nontrivial, nontransient price increase (or quality decrease). The RGM is then defined to include all of the seller locations to which buyers have switched. For example, suppose dental practices in Ivy Towers raise their prices by 5 percent or more and the price increase is expected to last indefinitely. If consumers and insurers are observed switching to dental practices in communities other than Ivy Towers, then all of the dental practices in all of those communities to which the buyers switch should be included in the RGM.

Although its practical relevance is limited, this conceptual exercise of a nontrivial, nontransient price increase is helpful because it tells us that we cannot necessarily rely on current purchasing practices when defining the relevant market for different types of medical care. For example, suppose several health insurers have contracts for all of their ambulatory care needs with three independent group physician practices in an area. Now suppose that these three independent group practices announce that they plan to merge their organizations in the upcoming year. If only current purchasing arrangements are relied on, we might be led into believing that the consolidated physician practice would result in monopoly pricing. However, that may not be the case if the insurers can switch to other providers of ambulatory care in that same immediate area or switch to providers outside the immediate area. The availability of substitutes can be expected to inhibit the newly consolidated practice from raising price. In fact, the consolidation of the three physician clinics might actually benefit the community if scale economies exist and lower rather than higher prices result.

In any case, it should be evident that determining the scope of the RGM and the RPM remains more of an art than a science. Typically, analysts refer to current purchasing practices and expert opinion when determining the current willingness of buyers to substitute among products and among sellers at different locations. They also must consider that other substitute products and sellers at different locations may be available but are not yet economical at existing prices. Their mere existence, however, prevents current sellers from raising price. We must also remember that new suppliers help maintain reasonable prices when entry barriers are low and they can easily and quickly enter markets.

Measuring Market Concentration

Suppose we are reasonably comfortable with our definition of the relevant market for a good or service after considering both its product and geographical dimensions. Further suppose that we want to measure the degree of **market concentration** as reflected in the number and size distribution of the firms within an industry. For instance, we learned that perfectly competitive markets are characterized by a large number of firms with tiny market shares whereas a few dominant firms characterize an oligopolistic industry. We want to capture the structural aspect of an industry with a relatively simple statistic, with the general idea that a market can be viewed as being more highly concentrated when fewer firms produce a larger share of industry output.

Economists typically offer the concentration ratio and the Herfindahl-Hirschman index as measures of market concentration. The concentration ratio identifies the percentage of industry output produced by the largest firms in an industry. The four-firm concentration ratio, CR_4, which is the most common, equals the sum of the market shares of the four largest firms. Industry output is often measured in terms of sales, volume of output, or employment. The CR_4 ranges between 0 and 100 percent, with a higher value reflecting that the largest four firms account for a larger share of industry output or, alternatively stated, that the industry is more highly concentrated. For example, a CR_4 of 60 percent indicates that the four largest firms account for 60 percent of all industry output.

Over the years, economists have assigned labels to industries depending on their four-firm concentration ratios. An industry with a CR_4 of 60 percent or more is considered to be tightly oligopolistic whereas an industry with a CR_4 between 40 and 60 percent is labeled as a loose oligopoly. Industries with a CR_4 of 40 percent or less are treated as being reasonably competitive. However, some words of caution: these industry classifications consider only the number and size distribution of firms. As we learned earlier, other market conditions, such as the height of any entry barriers, should also be considered when evaluating the relative structural competitiveness of an industry.

When data are available only for total industry output and the output produced by the few largest firms but not for the rest of the firms in an industry, a concentration ratio must be used to gauge the degree of industrial concentration. But concentration ratios possess a shortcoming because they do not identify the distribution of industry output among the largest firms. For example, if the CR_4 in some market equals 60 percent, it is unclear whether the largest four firms each produce 15 percent of industry output or the largest firm produces 57 percent and the others each produce 1 percent. The distribution of output among the largest firms can make a difference in terms of the market conduct of firms. Economists tend to agree that firms are more likely to engage in active price competition when they are more similarly sized compared to a market environment where one firm dominates the industry and the others are much smaller. In the latter case, the smaller firms are likely to act as followers and simply mirror the pricing behavior of the dominant firm. We talked earlier about this type of tacit collusion in the context of the price leadership model.

Because a concentration ratio fails to reveal the distribution of industry output among the largest firms, most economists prefer to use the Herfindahl-Hirschman index (HHI), when the necessary data are available, to measure the degree of industry concentration.[6] The HHI is derived by summing the squared market shares of all the firms in the relevant market, or

$$\text{HHI} = \sum_{i=1}^{N} S_i^2 = S_1^2 + S_2^2 + \cdots + S_N^2, \qquad (8\text{–}1)$$

where S_i stands for the percentage market share or percentage of industry output produced by the ith firm and $0 < \text{HHI} \leq 10{,}000$.

When a market is dominated by one firm, the HHI equals its maximum value of 10,000 or 100^2. The HHI takes on a value closer to zero when a greater number of firms, N, exist in the market and/or when the existing firms are more equally sized. As the value of the HHI approaches zero, an industry is considered to be less concentrated or more structurally competitive.

For example, in 2003 the five largest manufacturers of soft contact lenses were Vistakon (Johnson & Johnson), Ciba Vision, Bausch & Lomb, Cooper Vision, and Occular Sciences, with market share based on total patient visits when dispensed of 36.2%, 23.1%, 14.0%, 13.1%, and 12.4%, respectively.[7] Supposing that soft contact lenses represent the RPM, the CR_4 can be

6. The disadvantage of the HHI is that market share data are needed for all of the firms in the industry with shares of more than 1 percent. The four-firm concentration ratio requires only market share data for the largest four companies.

7. See http://www.ftc.gov/reports/contactlens/050214contactlensrpt.pdf (accessed October 18, 2005). The figures sum to 98.8 percent because the smallest firms have been omitted.

calculated by summing the four largest market shares. The resulting figure of 86.4 percent suggests that the four major producers of soft contact lenses in the United States account for slightly more than 86 percent of all soft contact lenses dispensed. In terms of market concentration, the soft contact lens industry clearly resembles a tight oligopoly given that the CR_4 greatly exceeds 60 percent. But notice that the CR_4, by itself, does not reveal the distribution of output among the four largest firms. For example, the CR_4 would also equal 86.4 percent if Vistakon's market share were 80 percent and the three other firms accounted for the remaining amount of industry output.

The distribution of market shares among the largest firms in the soft contact lens industry can be considered by applying Equation 8–1 and computing the HHI as 2,370.2. To gain some insight into the meaning of this figure, suppose that the two smallest contact lens suppliers, Occular Sciences and Cooper Vision, decide to consolidate their companies. The postmerger HHI would be $(36.2^2 + 23.1^2 + 14^2 + 25.5^2)$ or 2,690.3. Notice that a smaller number of firms leads to a higher value for the HHI and reflects the greater concentration of output among a smaller number of firms in the industry. Now suppose the market shares of the four remaining soft contact lens suppliers become equal over time. If so, the HHI declines to 2,500 (25^2 times 4). In general, it can be shown that the HHI takes on a lower value when a larger number of equally sized firms exist in an industry.

Although the SCP model predicts that firms are more likely to unilaterally or collectively exploit their market power by restricting output and raising price (and reducing quality) when firms are fewer in number, that same theory is unable to predict the precise value of HHI at which behavior of this kind takes place. The HHI reflects only the structural competitiveness of the market; it reveals nothing explicit about the behavioral intensity of competition among firms. Consequently, economic theory alone is unable to identify a specific competition-monopoly cutoff level for the HHI.

However, the Department of Justice (DOJ) has established some guidelines concerning the level of the HHI that the agency believes triggers a concern about the potential exploitation of market power. That is, the DOJ generally challenges a merger when the postmerger HHI exceeds 1,800 and the merger increases the premerger HHI by 50 points or more. The DOJ may also challenge a merger that results in a postmerger HHI above 1,000 and raises the the premerger HHI by more than 100 points. A merger that results in a postmerger HHI of less than 1,000 is seldom challenged by the DOJ.

The DOJ therefore believes that reasonably competitive conditions hold when the HHI is less than 1,000. In addition, the industry is treated by the DOJ as being mildly concentrated when the HHI falls between 1,000 and 1,800. Finally, the DOJ regards the industry as being highly concentrated when the HHI exceeds 1,800. Interestingly, these cutoffs for the HHI correspond fairly closely to the benchmarks for the CR_4 mentioned previously with regard to an industry being labeled as reasonably competitive and loosely or tightly oligopolistic. If all of the firms in an industry are equally sized, the HHI equals 1,000 when the CR_4 equals 40 percent and roughly 1,800 when the CR_4 equals 60 percent.[8]

8. There is also a measure referred to as the *numbers equivalent HHI,* which is found by dividing 10,000, the maximum value of the HHI, by the actual HHI for an industry. This measure provides a picture of an industry regarding the number of equally sized firms potentially represented by a given HHI. For example, an HHI of 1,800 reflects a market environment where roughly 5.6 (10,000/1,800) similarly sized firms exist in an industry. Rounding this number up to 6 and supposing each firm holds an equal market share of 16 percent results in a CR_4 of 64 percent. Notice that the 60 percent cutoff for the CR_4 compares closely to the 1,800 cutoff for the HHI. A similar argument can be made for the 40 percent CR_4 cutoff.

SUMMARY

In this chapter, the structure, conduct, and performance (SCP) paradigm was offered as a way of conceptualizing how market structure affects both industry conduct and market performance. We saw that markets range from being perfectly competitive to pure monopoly depending on factors such as the number and size distribution of firms, height of any barriers to entry, and the type of product offered for sale by firms in an industry. In general, a greater degree of both actual and potential competition leads to greater efficiency because individual firms have less market power.

Perfect competition was the first market structure that we analyzed in some detail. Perfect competition means that individual firms are price takers and maximize profits, consumers maximize utility, no barriers to entry exist, and consumers possess perfect information. Based on these characteristics, it was shown that perfectly competitive markets allocate resources efficiently when all social benefits and costs are internalized by those engaged in the market exchange. Perfect competition also results in the maximum sum of consumer and producer surplus, another sign of allocative efficiency.

The model of pure monopoly was then offered as a logical extreme to the perfectly competitive model. One seller of a good or service and perfect barriers to entry characterize monopoly. Because a monopoly has market power and faces a downward-sloping demand, it was shown theoretically that a monopoly results in a restriction of output and a misallocation of society's resources. A deadweight loss and redistribution of income also occur when a monopolist exists in a market.

Monopolistic competition was introduced as an intermediate market structure. The distinguishing feature of monopolistic competition is a differentiated product. A differentiated product means that the individual firm possesses some slight market power because it can raise price without losing all sales. Because entry barriers are nonexistent in the long run, the typical monopolistically competitive firm makes normal profits in the long run. Given that variety is highly valued by consumers, the only legitimate criticism against a monopolistically competitive firm may be its use of product differentiation. While elements of product differentiation such as advertising, trademarks, and brand names may provide cheap information and promote competition, it was also argued that these same features might impede competition through habit buying and creating entry barriers.

Oligopoly, another intermediate market structure, was examined next. A few large dominant firms and, thus, mutual interdependence among firms distinguish oligopoly from the other market structures. The efficiency of an oligopolistic industry depends on whether the individual firms in the industry compete or cooperate with one another. Cooperation or collusion leads to monopoly-like behavior and a restriction of output and a misallocation of society's scarce resources. It was pointed out that the conjectural variations formed by firms influence their behavior if they expect offsetting or matching behavior by rivals in the industry. Expecting offsetting (matching) behavior leads to the competitive (monopoly) outcome. It was further discussed that matching behavior is more likely to be expected when the number of firms is fewer, entry barriers are higher, trade associations exist, the industry is mature and slow growing, organizational structures are more centralized, and firm decision makers possess bounded rationality.

Finally, the chapter ended with a discussion concerning how to define the relevant market and measure the degree of market concentration. We learned that the relevant market possesses both a product and spatial dimension. In particular, when addressing the relevant market in which a firm operates, one must consider all of the other products and companies that consumers might turn to if that firm raised the price or lowered the quality of a specific product by a nontrivial amount for a non-temporary period of time. All of the other products and companies that consumers switch to would be considered as being in the same relevant market as the firm and product for which the price has increased or quality has declined.

To measure the degree of market concentration, the four-firm concentration ratio (CR_4) and Herfindahl-Hirschmann Index (HHI) are typically calculated. The CR_4 is calculated by adding up the market shares of the four largest firms in a market. As the CR_4 increases in value, the market is treated as being more highly concentrated. The HHI is found by squaring and summing the market shares of all firms in the same relevant market. The HHI varies between 0 to 10,000 with higher values indicating a more highly concentration industry and takes on a greater value when fewer, dissimilarly sized firms exist in an industry. The HHI is typically preferred over the CR_4 because it captures the distribution of output among the largest firms in an industry. An industry is considered to be tightly concentrated when the CR_4 and HHI are greater than 60 percent and 1,800, respectively.

Before concluding this chapter, it should be pointed out that the SCP analysis might become muddled when applied to medical markets for two reasons. First, conventional microeconomic theory is based on a profit maximization assumption, whereas many medical organizations are organized on a not-for-profit basis. Second, the industrial organization triad may not be appropriate for the medical care industry because quality usually matters more than price to consumers and government takes a more active role in the production, regulation, and distribution of output. These considerations diminish the role that profits and price play in the allocation of health resources and rationing of medical goods and services.

Despite these considerations, we believe that the SCP paradigm remains a useful tool for analyzing health care markets. Even the conduct of not-for-profit organizations is influenced by market structure to some degree. For example, market structure places a restraint on the maximum price not-for-profit firms can charge, and even not-for-profit organizations are subject to a financial solvency constraint. Also, for-profit firms are strongly represented in the health care sector. Many community hospitals, home health and hospice care agencies, mental health facilities, and nursing homes are organized on a for-profit basis. All pharmaceutical and commercial health insurance companies and nearly all physician, dental, and optometric clinics are also organized on a for-profit basis. Thus, while the quest for profits may have a smaller impact on the behavior of firms in the health care sector than on that of firms in other industries, profits still play an important role. Certainly, the investigator should conduct the industry analysis very carefully and be cognizant of the peculiarities of health care industries when drawing any inferences from the SCP paradigm.

Case Studies

8-1 Physicians and Health Plans[9]

In July 2005, WellPoint reached an agreement with more than 700,000 physicians to settle claims of unfair reimbursement to the physicians. WellPoint agreed to pay $135 million to physicians and donate $5 million to a not-for-profit foundation. Before becoming final, this deal required the approval of a U.S. district judge and the resolution of two national lawsuits against WellPoint and Anthem, which acquired WellPoint for $20.88 billion in December 2004. At the time of the agreement, WellPoint had 28.5 million members and was expected to incur a pretax expense of $103 million, or 10 cents a share after tax, in the second quarter of 2005.

9. Source: Vanessa Fuhrmans, "WellPoint Reaches Pact with 700,000 Physicians," *The Wall Street Journal*, July 12, 2005.

Questions for Discussion

1. *Describe the attributes of health care markets that make it possible for voluntary transactions ex ante (before the fact) to result in one party making legal claims of unfair payment ex post (after the fact).*
2. *How can we determine which argument—physicians' or health plans'—is closest to what is really transpiring in the market? In other words, are physician fees too high or reimbursements too low? Comment on how you might explore this question.*
3. *One implication of the lawsuits might be that some large health insurers systematically underpay physicians with which they contract, presumably due to some nontrivial degree of market power on the part of health plans. (a) Describe how you would assess the role of market power in payment levels, and (b) describe some possible solutions, apart from ongoing litigation, to address asymmetrical market power.*

8-2 Does Size Matter?[10]

In 2005, UnitedHealth Group agreed to acquire PacifiCare Health Systems for $8.1 million in cash and stock, further increasing the size of the nation's second-largest health insurer. The acquisition increased UnitedHealth's enrollment total by 13 percent, bringing the insurer's total ranks to 26 million. As a result of the acquisition, UnitedHealth gained a big presence in the Medicare HMO market and a stronger presence in California, where UnitedHealth had an agreement with Blue Shield to use a network of doctors and hospitals. Many of UnitedHealth's previous acquisitions were designed to help the company compete in the consumer-directed health plan market. As of July 2005, UnitedHealth had more than one million people enrolled in consumer-directed plans, considerably more than any other company at that time. UnitedHealth said the acquisition was done to increase efficiency, lower costs, and expand offerings to consumers, rather than to simply make UnitedHealth larger.

Questions for Discussion

1. *UnitedHealth indicates that the merger is expected to increase efficiency and lower costs. Discuss how these economies might come about after the merger.*
2. *Is the new merged entity likely to obtain additional economies of scale in increasing size from 23 million to 26 million enrollees? Why or why not?*
3. *UnitedHealth appears to be diversifying into consumer-directed products (for example, high-deductible plans for use with health savings accounts). An alternative to merger would be to develop the products internally. Discuss some possible reasons for UnitedHealth's decision to "buy" rather than "make."*

Review Questions and Problems

1. Suppose the supply curve of medical services is perfectly inelastic. Analyze the impact of an increase in consumer income on the market price and quantity of medical services. Next, assume the demand for medical services is perfectly inelastic while the supply curve is upward sloping. Explain the impact of an increase in input prices on the market price and quantity of medical services.

10. Source: Vanessa Fuhrmans, Dennis K. Berman, and Rhonda A. Rundle, "Two Health Plans Agree on a Deal for $8.1 Billion," *The Wall Street Journal*, July 7, 2005.

2. In the country of Drazah Larom (moral hazard spelled backward), health insurance is nonexistent and all medical markets are perfectly competitive. Use supply and demand analysis to explain the impact of the following changes on the price and output of physician services.
   A. A decrease in the wage of clinic-based nurses.
   B. The adoption of cost-enhancing medical technologies.
   C. An aging population and a correspondingly more severe patient case-mix.
   D. Declining consumer income.
   E. A lower market price for physician services (be careful here!).
3. In the 1980s, a shortage of registered nurses in the United States led to an increase of almost 21 percent in the real average hourly earnings of RNs from 1981 to 1989 (Pope and Menke, 1990). This increase was the highest of any occupational group. Use supply and demand theory to show the shortage and explain why a dramatic rise in the wage rate occurred. Was there still a shortage of registered nurses by 1994?
4. Using supply and demand analysis, show graphically and explain verbally some of the factors that may have led to rising health care costs in the United States from 1960 to the present day.
5. In the mid-1980s, female nurses became increasingly aware that a relatively large number of attractive job opportunities existed outside the medical services industry. In fact, a large number of colleges offered life and transfer credits for nurses so that they could change careers at less cost. Using an equilibrium model of the market for nurses, show what impact this market change had on the wage rate and employment of nurses. Work through the comparative statics and explain whether a temporary shortage or surplus occurred and the various market adjustments that took place as a result of the temporary imbalance.
6. Assume the sale of human organs is legalized and a free market develops. Furthermore, assume the market is in equilibrium. Trace through the price and output effects of the following:
   A. An increase in the incomes of potential buyers of human kidneys.
   B. A decrease in the price of kidney dialysis.
   C. The development of a new drug that leaves the immune system intact while preventing transplant rejection (Waldholz, 1992).
   D. A greater willingness by individuals to supply human kidneys.
7. A June 10, 1996, *Wall Street Journal* article titled "Americans Eat Up Vitamin E Supplies" discusses the shortage that existed for vitamin E at that time. According to the article, the shortage was created by two changes in the marketplace. First, the supply of soybeans, from which vitamin E is extracted, declined sharply. Second, a stream of scientific research from mainstream institutions shows that vitamin E helps to ward off such ailments as heart disease and cancer and some symptoms of aging.
   A. Using two separate supply and demand graphs, graphically show and verbally explain how a shortage is created by each of the two changes.
   B. Explain what eventually happens to price because of a shortage in a free market.
   C. Explain how suppliers and buyers adjust their behavior as the shortage is eliminated in each of the two cases.
   D. Explain what adjustment may take in the long run because of these changes.
8. Show graphically and explain verbally how a monopoly results in a deadweight loss. Also point out the redistribution that takes place in society because of monopoly.
9. Explain why economic profits are zero under monopolistic competition in the long run.
10. Explain the difference between the collusive and competitive oligopoly models and explain the role that the number of firms and barriers to entry play in determining how real-world oligopolistic industries behave.

11. Use the four market structures provided in the chapter to explain the critical role played by barriers to entry in determining the level of competition in any given market.
12. Critically evaluate the following statement made by a marketing executive: "Advertising is good because it always promotes competition."
13. What beneficial role do trademarks and brand names serve when information imperfections otherwise exist?
14. Explain the economic reasoning underlying the following statement: "People often fail to acquire information about the price they pay for medical services because of health insurance."
15. Discuss the two ways product differentiation affects the demand for a product.
16. Explain how lack of information affects the price and quality of a medical good relative to a perfectly competitive situation.
17. Suppose XER Inc. is a monopoly and produces a drug that cures the common cold. The weekly (inverse) market demand for its product takes the form $P = 660 - 4Q$, where Q is measured as number of tablets. The marginal costs (MC) and average total costs (ATC) are equal at $100 per tablet (that is, a horizontal marginal cost curve).
    A. Given this information, solve for the level of output that will be produced by XER Inc. if it maximizes profits (you may need to consult footnote 2 in the chapter).
    B. Solve for the price charged and amount of profits earned by XER Inc.
    C. From a societal point of view, does the profit-maximizing level of output represent an efficient level of output? Why or why not? Calculate the social damages created by XER Inc. (*Hint:* You will have to know how to calculate the area of a triangle.)
    D. Suppose the source of the entry barrier was removed so XER Inc. is no longer a monopoly. How would equilibrium change? Explain fully.
18. Suppose that the annual number of admissions can be used as a measure of output for a group of hospitals operating in the same RGM. Categorize the type of market based on the degree of structural competition as measured by the four-firm concentration ratio and the Herfindahl-Hirschman index.

Hospital	Number of Admissions (in thousands)
Saving Grace Hospital	4,000
Mercy Me Hospital	3,000
Price Plus Hospital	1,500
HealthMart Hospital	750
Health Depot Hospital	1,000
Health R Us Hospital	1,500

CEBS Questions

■ *CEBS Sample Question on Subject Matter from CEBS Course 9 Study Manual*

1. Explain the concept of rationally ignorant. (page 210)

■ *CEBS Sample Exam Questions*

1. A monopolist will maximize profits if it produces an output where:
   A. Average total costs are minimized
   B. Marginal costs equal marginal revenue
   C. Marginal costs equal demand
   D. Marginal revenue is zero
   E. Marginal revenue exceeds demand
2. Which of the following statements regarding a collusive oligopoly market is (are) correct?
   I. Production cost differences make it difficult for firms to cooperate
   II. The beliefs each firm forms about its rivals affects market output and price
   III. The presence of trade associations in the market reduces the likelihood of collusive behavior
      A. I only
      B. II only
      C. I and II only
      D. I and III only
      E. I, II, and III only
3. All the following are correct statements regarding the types of economic markets EXCEPT:
   A. The major difference between perfect competition and monopolistic competition is that the latter has differentiated products.
   B. Imperfect consumer information is the dominant characteristic of an oligopoly.
   C. The exiting of firms in the long run in a perfectly competitive industry eliminates the economic losses of firms that remain in the industry.
   D. Oligopolistic markets often have substantial barriers to entry.
   E. The demand curve for a pure monopolist is downward sloping.

■ *Answer to Sample Question from Study Manual*

There are both costs and benefits to acquiring information. Therefore, in many situations, people choose to be less than perfectly informed, or rationally ignorant, because the marginal costs of additional information outweigh the additional benefits.

■ *Answers to Sample Exam Questions*

1. The correct answer is B. See page 204 of the text.
2. C is the correct answer. Statements I and II are correct. Statement III is incorrect because trade associations facilitate collusion. See pages 212–214 of the text.
3. B is the correct answer. It is a few dominant firms and substantial barriers to entry that characterize an oligopoly. Either perfect or imperfect consumer information may exist in an oligopolistic market. See pages 194–196 and 212 of the text.

ONLINE RESOURCES

To access Internet links related to the topics in this chapter, please visit our web site at **www.thomsonedu.com/economics/santerre**.

References

Bain, Joe S. *Barriers to New Competition*. Cambridge, Mass.: Harvard University Press, 1956.

Baumol, William J. "Macroeconomics of Unbalanced Growth: The Anatomy of Urban Crisis." *American Economic Review* 57 (June 1967), pp. 415–26.

Benham, Lee. "The Effect of Advertising on the Price of Eyeglasses." *Journal of Law and Economics* 15 (October 1972), pp. 337–52.

Borzo, Greg. "Glove Shortage Creates Anxiety." *Health Industry Today* 54 (November 1991), p. 1.

Cady, John F. "An Estimate of the Price Effects of Restrictions on Drug Price Advertising." *Economic Inquiry* 14 (December 1976), pp. 493–510.

Ford, Jon M., and David L. Kaserman. "Certificate-of-Need Regulation and Entry: Evidence from the Dialysis Industry." *Southern Economics Journal* 59 (April 1993), pp. 783–91.

Haas-Wilson, Deborah. *Managed Care and Monopoly Power: The Antitrust Challenge*. Cambridge, Mass.: Harvard University Press. 2003.

Hensley, Scott. "Out for Blood." *Modern Healthcare*, June 22, 1998, pp. 26–32.

Klein, Benjamin, and Keith B. Leffler. "The Role of Market Forces in Assuring Contractual Performance." *Journal of Political Economy* 89 (August 1981), pp. 615–41.

Kwoka, John E. "Advertising and the Price and Quality of Optometric Services." *American Economic Review* (March 1984), pp. 211–16.

Pope, Gregory C., and Terri Menke. "DataWatch: Hospital Labor Markets in the 1980s." *Health Affairs* 9 (winter 1990), pp. 127–37.

Robinson, James C. "Hospital Quality Competition and the Economics of Imperfect Information." *Milbank Memorial Quarterly* 66 (1988), pp. 465–81.

Ruffenach, Glenn. "Study Says Teen-Agers' Smoking Habits Seem to Be Linked to Heavy Advertising." *The Wall Street Journal*, March 13, 1992, p. B8.

Stigler, George. *The Organization of Industry*. Homewood, Ill.: Richard D. Irwin, 1968.

Waldholz, Michael. "New Drug Leaves Immune System Intact While Preventing Transplant Rejection." *The Wall Street Journal*, August 7, 1992, p. B8.

Will, George. "Where There's Smoke There's Cancer and Death, Too." *Norwich Bulletin*, February 16, 1992.

Zikos, Joanna. "It's Tough to Get Grip on Rubber Gloves." *The Worcester Evening Gazette*, August 10, 1988, p. 1.

PART 2

THE ROLE OF GOVERNMENT

GOVERNMENT, HEALTH, AND MEDICAL CARE

CHAPTER 9

"Needham, Mass., Biotech Company Executive Criticizes FDA" (Knight Ridder Tribune Business News).

"FTC Soon to Clear $6 B Bayer-Aventis Merger" (The Daily Deal).

"State Looks at Tax on Hospitals" (Crain's Detroit Business).

"Doctors Resolve Antitrust Charges" (USA Today).

"Unwanted HMOs, Hundreds of Massachusetts Doctors, Citing Low Fees, Refuse Medicare Plans" (Boston Globe).

Up to this point, we have given little attention to the role and effects of government intervention in the U.S. health care system. Yet, as the preceding headlines suggest,[1] government plays an important role in the various medical markets and either directly or indirectly influences the health of the population in a number of ways. For example, regulatory and taxing policies affect the production or consumption of certain products (such as prescription drugs, narcotics, alcohol, and tobacco) and thereby beneficially or adversely affect the population's health. Regulations also have the potential to alter the price, quantity, or quality of medical services and can thereby inhibit or promote efficiency in the allocation of resources. The degree of government intervention varies considerably across the country. Some state governments choose to actively regulate the production and reimbursement of nursing home, hospital, and psychotherapy services. Other state governments take more of a laissez-faire attitude toward the health care industry.

We have already seen several examples of government intervention in the health care sector. For example, earlier chapters pointed out that government-created legal barriers to entry, such as professional licensure requirements and CON laws, often confer monopoly status on the established health care providers in a market. In addition, we know that the Medicare and Medicaid programs provide public health insurance to elderly people, people with disabilities, and selected economically disadvantaged groups. These are just a few of an immeasurable number of government policies that affect the conduct and performance of medical care markets and the health status of American consumers.

This chapter provides an overview of the impact of public sector policies on the allocation of medical resources and the distribution of medical output. Although the design, complexity, and nature of health care policies differ across states, and federal health care policies are multidimensional in scope, a common body of economic theory is drawn upon to analyze such policies.

1. FDA and FTC stand for the Food and Drug Administration and the Federal Trade Commission, respectively.

This chapter:

- examines the reasons for government intervention in a market-based health care system
- discusses the implications of various types of public sector involvement, such as price and quality regulations and antitrust laws
- explores the methods used by government to redistribute income in society and the reason for such redistribution

Reasons for Government Intervention

Two general alternative views or models describe why government intervenes in a market-based health care system. These are the public interest and special interest group theories of government behavior. According to the **public interest theory,** government promotes the general interests of society as a whole and chooses policies that enhance efficiency and equity. Recall from Chapter 3 that an efficient allocation of resources is achieved when, for a given distribution of income, each good and service is produced at the point where marginal social benefit equals marginal social cost. In the presence of market imperfections, such as imperfect consumer information or monopoly, markets fail to allocate resources efficiently. We will see shortly that market failure also occurs when public goods such as national defense or externalities such as air pollution are involved, or when distributive justice is a concern.

The public interest is served when government corrects instances where the market fails to allocate resources efficiently or to distribute income equitably. When the market fails, government attempts to restore efficiency and promote equity by encouraging competition, providing consumer information, reducing harmful externalities, or redistributing income in society. Consequently, the public interest model of government behavior predicts that the laws, regulations, and other actions of government enhance efficiency and equity.

According to the **special interest group theory** (Stigler, 1971; Peltzman, 1976; and Becker, 1983), the political forum can be treated like any private market for goods and services; that is, the amounts and types of legislation are determined by the forces of supply and demand. Vote-maximizing politicians represent the suppliers of legislation, while wealth-maximizing special interest groups are the buyers of legislation. In this model, incumbent politicians attempt to increase their probability of being reelected by supplying legislation that promises to redistribute wealth away from the general public and toward various special interest groups. In return, politicians expect votes, political support, and campaign contributions. Professional lobbies representing the special interest groups negotiate with politicians and arrive at the market-clearing prices and quantities of different kinds of legislation. Special interest group legislation changes over time when relative power shifts among different interest groups. Power or political pressure is determined by the amount of resources the group controls, the size of the group, and the efficiency with which the group transforms resources into pressure.

The successful politician stays in office by combining the legislative programs of various special interest groups into an overall fiscal package to be advanced in the political arena. The beneficiaries are the special interest groups, while the costs fall disproportionately on the general public. For example, individual pieces of legislation that provide protection from imported automobiles, milk price supports, and a larger education budget individually benefit those associated with the Automobile Workers Union, the American Dairy Association, and the National Education Association, respectively. The same politician can offer wealth transfers to each of these three groups and in return receive their combined votes, political support, and contributions. Naturally, special interest groups and politicians are made better off by the political exchanges; otherwise, these exchanges would not occur. Politicians retain or acquire elected positions, while the special interest groups receive wealth-enhancing legislation.

The general public, however, is unknowingly made worse off by the political exchanges. Individuals are typically rationally ignorant about the wealth implications of government activities because the personal cost of acquiring information about the true effect of legislation is high, whereas the corresponding private benefit is low. For example, suppose a certain piece of legislation redistributes $250 million a year away from the general public to a special interest group. Although this wealth transfer is a large amount of money in absolute terms, it is insignificant when expressed in per capita terms. In the United States, the cost of this wealth transfer is only about $1 per person. Raising the per capita cost of special interest group legislation to $100 increases the total wealth transfer to $25 billion. Yet even at a potential per-person savings of $100, few people are likely to become involved due to the money and time costs associated with political activity. To challenge special interest group legislation, a group or an individual must organize a legitimate counter political movement, inform others, circulate a petition, and engage in lobbying. All these activities entail sizeable personal time and money costs.

Ross Perot's grassroots bid for the presidency in 1992 exemplifies this point on a grandiose scale. Perot attempted to challenge the political establishment by running for president as a third-party candidate. After spending millions of his own money, he garnered a respectable 19 percent of the overall vote, but not enough to win the presidential election. Imagine all the other potential "Perots" who never get involved in the political process at even the local or state level because of the staggering costs involved.

The special interest group model of government behavior implies that the typical individual consumer is "nickeled and dimed" by wealth-transferring legislation. Even worse, the wealth transfer is not simply a dollar-for-dollar transfer from the general public to the special interest groups. The political negotiations leading to the wealth transfer involve scarce resources such as the politicians' time and professional lobbies. As more resources are diverted to political negotiations, fewer are available for productive purposes. In addition, any additional taxes imposed on the general public create a disincentive for individuals to commit resources to production. Consequently, inefficiencies are normally associated with special interest group legislation.

Therefore, according to the special interest group theory of government behavior, public regulations and laws exist because some special interest group benefits at the expense of the general public. Individuals in a special interest group are collectively powerful because they share a common concentrated interest. Consumers as a group, however, are generally diverse, fragmented, and powerless. Organization costs typically prohibit general consumers from taking action even when wealth transfers are known.

As an example, Ohsfeldt and Gohmann (1992) analyze whether various state regulations concerning AIDS-related health insurance underwriting practices are influenced by the pressure of special interest groups. They focus on state regulations prohibiting (1) questions during the insurance application process about past HIV testing, (2) insurers from requiring insurance applicants to submit to HIV antibody tests, (3) questions on the application regarding sexual orientation, and (4) the exclusion of any AIDS-related costs from the services covered by the health insurance contract.

The authors argue that the losers from these insurance regulations are private health insurance companies (due to lower profits) and private insurance holders with a low average risk for AIDS (higher premium costs). Individuals who gain include those at high risk for AIDS (lower premium costs) and private providers of health care services (higher profits from more generous private insurance coverage). In general, the empirical findings of their regression analysis support the hypothesis that the presence of state regulations restricting AIDS-related health insurance underwriting practices is related to special interest group pressure. Specifically, Ohsfeldt and Gohmann find that underwriting regulations are more likely in states where the AIDS prevalence rate (as a proxy for the AIDS group) is high and insurance industry strength is low.

The public interest and special interest group models are two contrasting theories regarding the reasons government intervenes in a market-based system. In the real world, government most likely intervenes for both reasons. In some instances, government actions correct for market failure and thereby promote efficiency and equity. In other situations, government policies enhance the well-being of specific groups at an overall cost to society and thereby cause an inefficient allocation of resources and an inequitable distribution of income. Indeed, a careful cost-benefit analysis would have to be conducted before the winners and losers could be identified and the efficiency and equity implications determined for each piece of legislation. It is important to remember that both the government and the marketplace are imperfect institutions and, as a result, both fail to some extent; that is, government failure and market failure can coexist. Our job as policy makers or informed consumers is to determine which institution can accomplish which objective in the more efficient and equitable manner.

Types of Government Intervention

Government can alter the performance of markets in terms of efficiency and equity by providing public goods, levying taxes, correcting for externalities, imposing regulations, enforcing antitrust laws, operating public enterprises, and sponsoring redistribution programs. As an example of a public good, a government health officer inspects the sanitary conditions at local restaurants to protect the public's health. To correct for an externality, the government taxes the emissions of firms to reduce the level of air or water pollution in an area. A certificate of need (CON) law is essentially a health care regulation that restricts entry into hospital and nursing home markets, whereas the Sherman Antitrust Act of 1890 prohibits independent physicians from discussing their pricing policies to prevent monopolistic practices, such as price fixing. A hospital operated by the Veterans Administration provides an example of a government medical enterprise. Finally, the Medicare and Medicaid programs are examples of public medical care redistribution programs. Each of these government policies either directly or indirectly influences the allocation of medical resources and the distribution of medical output in the U.S. health economy. The following sections discuss the effects of these types of government intervention in more detail.

Public Goods

One legitimate function of government is to provide public goods. A public good must satisfy two criteria. First, unlike a private good, more than one individual can simultaneously receive benefits from a public good. That is, a public good exhibits nonrivalry in consumption, thus allowing one person to increase his or her consumption of the good without diminishing the quantity available for others. Second, it is costly to exclude nonpaying individuals from receiving the benefits of a public good.

National defense is a good example of a public good. Everyone simultaneously benefits, and it is impossible to exclude nonpayers from receiving the benefits of national defense.

The preservation of water quality in public swimming areas by the local public health department is another example of a public good. A large number of people can simultaneously enjoy the benefits of improved water quality (at least until the beaches become overcrowded). In addition, it is costly to exclude nonpayers from receiving the benefits of improved water quality at the local pond (unless the entire pond can be fenced off).

Because of the high cost of excluding nonpaying individuals, private firms are unwilling to produce and sell public goods; thus, the private sector fails to provide public goods, and government intervention is necessary. Government ensures that public goods are produced in either the private or public sector and collects the necessary funding through taxation.[2]

Some people incorrectly consider medical services to be public goods because they are so essential for life. From a theoretical standpoint, however, the benefits of medical services are almost completely internalized by the individual buyer, and the cost of excluding nonpayers from receiving medical care is very low. Simply put, prospective patients can be required to pay the necessary fee at the door of the medical facility or be denied access to medical services. Thus, medical services are not public goods.[3]

Externalities

Ordinarily, all costs and benefits are fully internalized by the parties directly involved in a market transaction, and others not involved in the exchange are unaffected. For example, consider an individual who wakes up one morning with a bad toothache and decides to visit the dentist. After some probing, the dentist informs the patient that a wisdom tooth is causing the problem and recommends that the tooth be extracted immediately. The (uninsured) patient consents, the task is expertly performed, and the $100 fee is paid at the desk. In a competitive market, the $100 fee reflects the marginal benefit the individual receives from being relieved of pain and the dentist's marginal cost of providing the service. Notice that in this example, only the individual consumer and dentist internalize the benefits and costs of the market transaction. This transaction is efficient because both parties are made better off; otherwise the transaction would not have taken place.

Sometimes, however, a market transaction affects parties other than the individual consumer and producer. In this situation, an externality occurs. An **externality** is an unpriced by-product of production or consumption that adversely or beneficially affects another party not directly involved in the market transaction. When an externality occurs, the buyers and sellers do not fully internalize all the costs and benefits of the transaction. As a result, external costs or benefits are generated, and the product is usually under- or overproduced from a societal perspective. In the following discussion, we examine the impact and implications of demand-side and supply-side externalities.

Demand-Side Externalities. A demand-side externality occurs when the marginal social benefit diverges from the marginal private benefit associated with a good or service. A **positive demand-side externality** means that marginal social benefit is greater than marginal private benefit; a **negative demand-side externality** implies that marginal social benefit is less than marginal private benefit. Cigarette smoking provides a contemporary example of a negative demand-side externality.

According to Manning et al. (1989), external costs are associated with cigarette smoking, meaning smokers impose costs on nonsmokers. The external costs are generated in three ways.

2. The aggregate demand for a public good is derived through a vertical summation of individual demands. See Chapter 6 in Rosen (1995).

3. Closely related to a public good is the notion of a *merit good.* Musgrave and Musgrave (1989) point out that people are often bound by similar historical experiences or cultural traditions. The common bond gives rise to common interests, values, and wants, "wants which individuals feel obliged to support as members of the community" (p. 57). For example, people in the community may believe that everyone needs at least some minimal amount of food, housing, or medical services and therefore may be willing to support the provision of those merit goods through redistribution of income.

FIGURE 9–1
External Costs of Cigarette Smoking

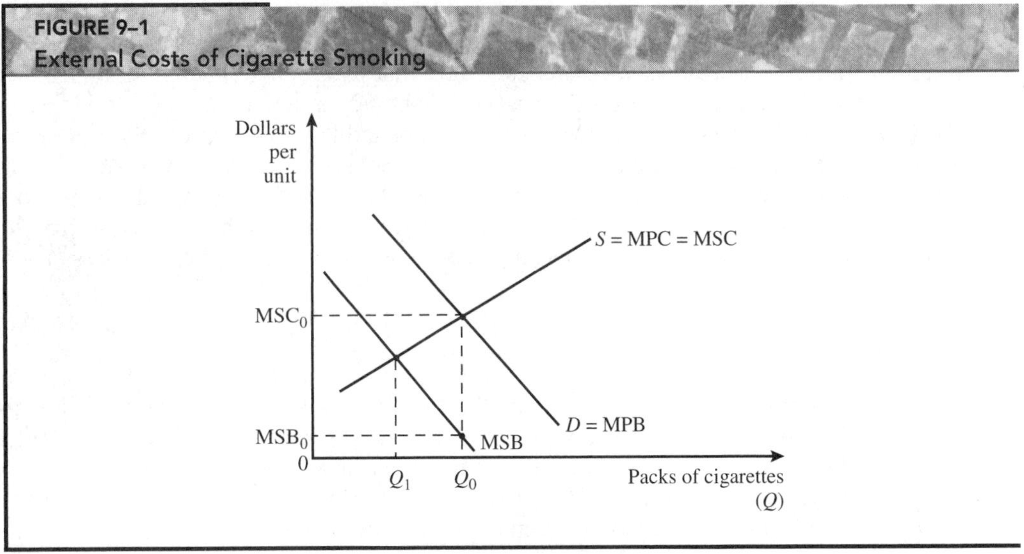

The graph captures the market for cigarettes. In the process of consumers maximizing utility and producers maximizing profits, market equilibrium results in the outcome at Q_0 where marginal private benefit, MPB, equals marginal private cost, MPC. However, the market outcome is inefficient because at that point, marginal social cost, MSC, exceeds marginal social benefit, MSB, because of the external damages caused by cigarette smoking. An efficient allocation of resources occurs at Q_1 because MSB = MSC. Left alone, the market tends to overproduce goods that generate negative externalities in consumption.

First, collectively financed programs, such as health insurance, pensions, sick leave, disability insurance, and group life insurance, are financed by taxes or group premiums and do not differentiate between smokers and nonsmokers. Because smokers have shorter life expectancies, they pay less taxes and premiums into the system. Second, smokers usually incur higher health care costs than nonsmokers.[4] Third, external costs arise when nonsmokers die prematurely from both passive smoking and smoking-related fires. The implication is that nonsmokers subsidize smokers and incur costs for which they are not compensated in the private marketplace.

Figure 9–1 shows the effect of cigarette smoking on resource allocation. The supply curve, *S*, corresponds to both marginal private and social costs and represents the marginal costs of using various inputs to manufacture and retail cigarettes. Thus, it is assumed that all resource costs of production are internalized on the supply side of the market. On the demand side, we must allow for the fact that the marginal private benefit, MPB, is likely to be greater than the marginal social benefit, MSB, of cigarette consumption. The MPB curve in the figure represents the marginal private benefit received from smoking, or the private demand curve for cigarettes. The MSB curve considers the additional costs inflicted on society and therefore lies below the MPB curve. The external costs underlie the difference between the two benefit curves.

For discussion purposes, we assume external costs per pack are the same at each level of cigarette consumption so that the two benefit curves are parallel to each other. We also assume the marginal social benefit is positive at every level, although it might be negative if the external

4. Since smokers may die earlier and fail to live to the more medically intensive years of life, it is unclear theoretically whether smokers always incur higher overall health costs than nonsmokers.

costs exceed the marginal private benefits of cigarette consumption. As an illustration, Manning et al. (1989) estimates the external costs of cigarette smoking at approximately 15 cents per pack, exclusive of the costs due to passive smoking (2,400 deaths annually) and smoking-related fires (1,600 deaths annually). If we consider the value of lives lost from passive smoking and smoking-related fires, the total external costs increase to approximately 38 cents per pack.[5]

Consumers compare their marginal private benefit only to price (that is, their internal costs) when deciding how many packs of cigarettes to purchase. Thus, in the process of maximizing personal utilities, consumers purchase Q_0 packs of cigarettes. This amount of cigarette consumption is inefficient from a societal perspective because at Q_0 the marginal social cost, MSC_0, exceeds the marginal social benefit, MSB_0, of cigarettes; that is, some nonsmokers are adversely affected by the consumption of cigarettes, and these external costs are not considered by smokers in the private marketplace. Since the individual consumers and producers do not fully internalize all the costs and benefits of their actions, the quantity of cigarettes is overproduced and overconsumed. An efficient quantity of cigarettes exists at Q_1, where marginal social benefit equals marginal social cost. Because individual consumers and producers are unlikely to voluntarily alter their consumption and production behavior, some type of government intervention, such as a tax on cigarettes, may be necessary to curb this harmful type of consumption activity.[6]

This example represents a negative consumption externality because others not directly involved are made worse off by the exchange. A positive consumption externality can also occur when a consumption activity generates external benefits. A vaccination to prevent an infectious disease, such as rabies, is an example of a positive consumption externality. Figure 9–2 illustrates the logic underlying this example.

In the figure, the number of dogs receiving a rabies vaccine is shown on the horizontal axis. The marginal private benefit curve, MPB, reflects the value dog owners place on the rabies vaccination. The marginal social benefit curve, MSB, reflects the MPB plus all external benefits. The external benefits include the dollar benefit others receive when a dog gets the rabies vaccine and prevents the spread of the infection to humans or other animals. The supply curve, S, reflects the resource cost of providing the rabies vaccine.

In a free market, consumers compare their marginal private benefit to price when deciding whether to get the rabies vaccine for their dogs. As a result, Q_0 represents the total number of vaccinations in a free market where demand and supply intersect. But notice that at Q_0 the marginal social benefit, MSB_0, is greater than the marginal social cost, MSC_0, of providing the rabies vaccine. An inefficient outcome occurs because some individuals place very little value on the rabies vaccination (when maximizing personal utility) since they do not consider its external benefits. From a societal perspective, therefore, there are too few rabies vaccinations in a free market. An efficient number of vaccinations occurs at Q_1. This implies that government intervention of some kind, such as a mandatory requirement and a fine, may be needed to ensure the efficient number of rabies vaccinations. (For example, many states require a rabies vaccination to obtain a dog license, and failure to get a dog license results in a fine.)

In sum, externalities can arise on the demand side of a market if the social costs and benefits of a consumption activity are not fully internalized by the participants directly involved in the exchange. If the consumption activity generates either external benefits or costs, the good or

5. The authors used a $1.66 million estimate of the willingness to pay for mortality reductions.

6. To continue our illustration, Manning et al. (1989) point out that the average cigarette tax of 37 cents per pack nearly pays for the 38 cents of external costs from smoking in the United States. Their estimate of the external costs of alcohol, 48 cents per ounce, is well above the current excise and sales tax average of 23 cents per ounce. They conclude that smokers compensate for their external costs, but drinkers do not.

FIGURE 9–2
External Benefits of Rabies Vaccines

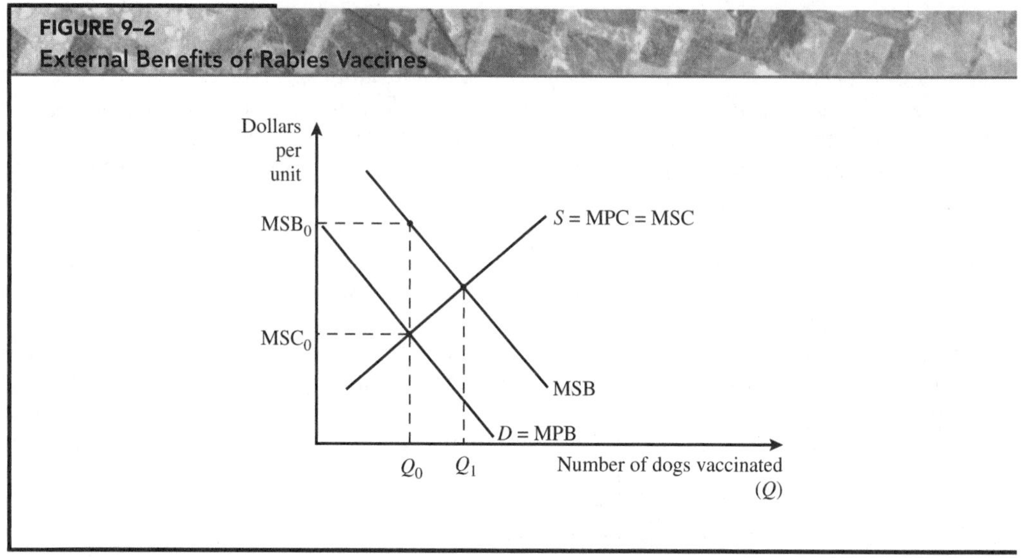

The graph captures the market for rabies vaccinations. In the process of consumers maximizing utility and producers maximizing profits, market equilibrium results in the outcome at Q_0 where marginal private benefit, MPB, equals marginal private cost, MPC. However, the market outcome is inefficient because at that point, marginal social benefit, MSB, exceeds marginal social cost, MSC, because of the external benefits caused by rabies vaccinations. An efficient allocation of resources occurs at Q_1 because MSB = MSC. Left alone, the market tends to underproduce goods that generate positive externalities in consumption.

service is likely to be under- or overproduced from a societal perspective. Consequently, government intervention may be necessary to correct the market's failure to allocate society's resources efficiently.

Supply-Side Externalities. As you now know, an externality creates an inefficient allocation of resources when the actions of one market participant affect another and no compensation is forthcoming. As in the case of a demand-side externality, the presence of an externality on the supply side usually distorts the allocation of resources in a market economy. A **negative supply-side externality** exists if a firm inflicts an uncompensated cost on another party in the process of production. In this case, a deviation arises between the marginal social cost and the marginal private cost of production. Because the firm bases its output decision on the private cost of production and not on the social cost, the good is usually overproduced. Figure 9–3 depicts this situation for a competitive market.

The demand curve, or marginal social benefit curve, is labeled D = MSB; the supply curve, or marginal private cost curve, is labeled S = MPC. The latter curve represents the amount it costs private industry to produce each additional unit of output. The MSC curve stands for the marginal social cost of production, and it lies above the MPC curve because it equals not only the marginal private cost of production but also the additional per-unit cost the firm inflicts on others. The distance between the two cost curves represents the per-unit dollar value of the cost imposed on society. The cost may reflect the greater health hazards from such factors as air pollution and toxic waste or higher time costs resulting from congested highways.

FIGURE 9–3
Negative Supply-Side Externality

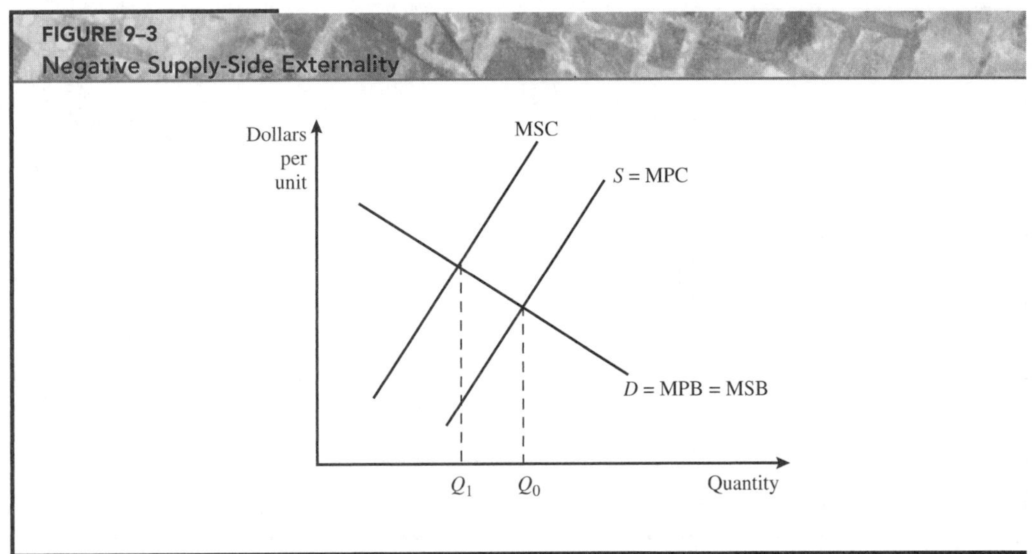

The graph captures a market where firms emit pollution as a by-product of production. Because of the external costs from pollution, marginal social cost, MSC, exceeds the marginal private cost, MPC, of production. In the process of consumers maximizing utility and producers maximizing profits, market equilibrium results in the outcome at Q_0 where marginal private benefit, MPB, equals marginal private cost, MPC. However, the market outcome is inefficient because at the point, marginal social cost, MSC, exceeds marginal social benefit, MSB, because of the external damages caused by the pollution. An efficient allocation of resources occurs at Q_1 because MSB = MSC. Left alone, the market tends to overproduce goods that generate negative externalities in production.

Profit maximization dictates that the good be produced up to point Q_0, where the marginal private cost equals the marginal social benefit, or the price. At Q_0, however, the marginal social cost of production exceeds the marginal social benefit of the product. From a societal perspective, resources are efficiently allocated if the Q_1 level of output is produced because the marginal social cost of production equals the marginal social benefit and the total social surplus is maximized. Because the market fails to assign the total social cost of production to the firm, the good is overproduced and resources are inefficiently allocated.

A classic example of a negative supply-side externality is acid rain. When fossil fuels are burned, they release sulfur and nitrogen oxides into the atmosphere; these substances combine with water to raise the acidic level of the water supply. Acid rain has caused extensive damage to marine and wildlife in certain regions of the country, such as New England. Because sulfur and nitrogen oxides can be carried hundreds of miles by wind currents, it is extremely difficult to assign costs to them. As a result, many of the producers of these emissions do not bear the full cost of production.

In the health care sector, the problem of hazardous waste disposal by hospitals can be analyzed in the context of a negative externality. This became a national issue in the summer of 1988, when vials of blood, used syringes, and other hospital waste washed up onshore at a public beach in New Jersey (Baker, 1988). When five of the vials of blood tested positive for AIDS antibodies, many people became concerned that hospitals were attempting to pass the high cost of waste disposal on to the public by not properly disposing of infectious waste. From the public's perspective, the cost of inappropriate disposal of medical waste was in terms of an increased risk of accidentally acquiring AIDS. Rutala et al. (1989) estimate that U.S. hospitals

FIGURE 9–4
Positive Supply-Side Externality

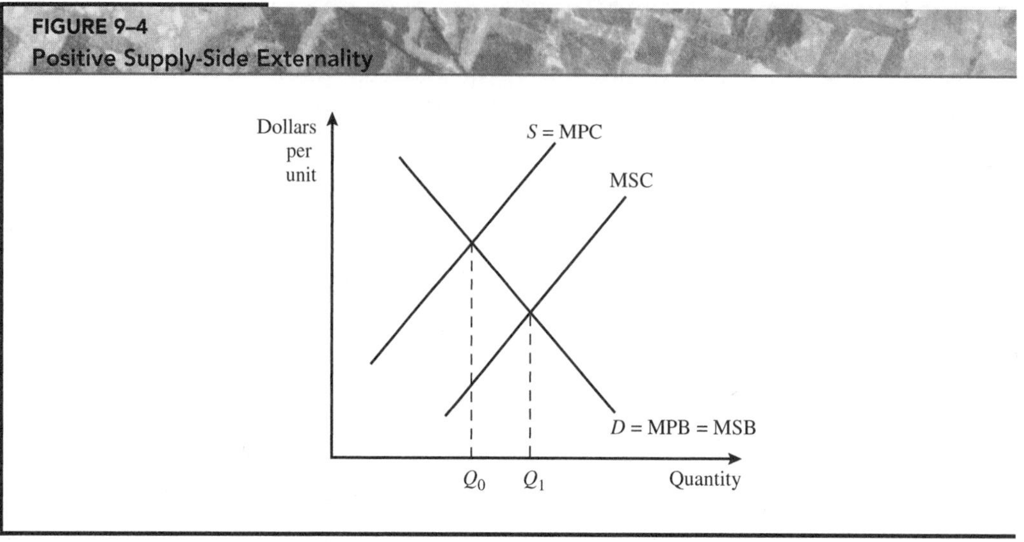

The graph captures a market where one firm generates external benefits for other firms in the market as a by-product of production. For example, suppose one firm discovers a more efficient production process and freely shares the idea with others. Because of the external benefits from the discovery, marginal social cost, MSC, is less than the marginal private cost, MPC, of production. In the process of consumers maximizing utility and producers maximizing profits, market equilibrium results in the outcome at Q_0 where marginal private benefits, MPB, equals marginal private cost, MPC (that is, the firm does not freely share the idea). However, the market outcome is inefficient because at that point, marginal social cost, MSC, is less than marginal social benefit, MSB, because of the external benefits that can potentially be generated by the firm. An efficient allocation of resources occurs at Q_1 because MSB = MSC. Left alone, the market tends to underproduce goods that generate positive externalities in production.

produce approximately 15 pounds of waste per patient per day and that infectious waste makes up 15 percent of that total. As a result, the Environmental Protection Agency (EPA), along with many states, regulates the hazardous waste disposal of hospitals in an attempt to properly assign costs.

A **positive supply-side externality** occurs if firms in one market (say, A) provide uncompensated benefits for firms in another market (say, B). In that case, the marginal social cost is less than the marginal private cost of production; that is, the MSC curve lies below the MPC curve in market A (see Figure 9–4). The distance between the two curves reflects the benefits received by the firms in market B. Since no compensation is paid to the firms in market A, they lack the incentive to produce the efficient amount of output. The profit-maximizing level of output equals Q_0, but at this amount the MSB exceeds the MSC. If total social surplus is to be maximized, output should expand to Q_1. Since the firms in market A are not financially rewarded for the benefits other firms receive, they do not produce up to the point where total social surplus is maximized.

The transfer of medical knowledge across international borders is a good illustration of a positive supply-side externality. For example, assume the research funded by one country leads to a major breakthrough in the treatment of cancer that significantly lowers medical costs. This advance in medical knowledge is likely to be written up in a medical journal and, in the absence of intellectual property rights, quickly adopted by other countries at little or no cost. The firm in the country that developed the treatment and incurred the cost of research is not compensated for the full benefit of the breakthrough. Consequently, private medical researchers in any one country may face an incentive to underproduce medical knowledge in the absence of government subsidies because they would fail to receive a suitable return on their research investment.

In conclusion, economic theory suggests that the presence of an externality on the supply side impedes the market's ability to allocate resources efficiently. This occurs because production decisions are based solely on the private cost of production incurred by the firm rather than on the social cost.

Taxes and Subsidies as Corrective Instruments. By using taxes and subsidies, government can alter economic incentives and correct the unconstrained tendency of the market to misallocate society's resources when externalities are present. Specifically, taxes and subsidies can be used to alter the price of a good and discourage either overconsumption or underconsumption. Market participants are forced to consider the true net social benefit of their actions. For example, government can encourage an efficient amount of cigarette consumption by imposing a per-unit tax, T, on cigarette manufacturers equal to the vertical distance between MPB and MSB at Q_1 in Figure 9–5. Because of the per-unit tax, the market price of cigarettes increases to P_1 and cigarette consumption falls to the socially efficient level (MSB = MSC). Cigarette producers receive P_2, the difference between the market price of P_1 and the per-unit tax (or vertical distance between the MPB and MSB) as after-tax revenues per unit.

Notice in this example that both sellers and consumers share the burden from the cigarette tax. The consumers pay the portion $P_1 - P_0$, and the sellers pay the portion $P_0 - P_2$. The sellers' portion of the tax burden typically results in a smaller profit margin or is shifted backward to input suppliers. In our example, the cigarette tax may force producers to pay lower wages to their

FIGURE 9–5
A Tax as a Corrective Instrument

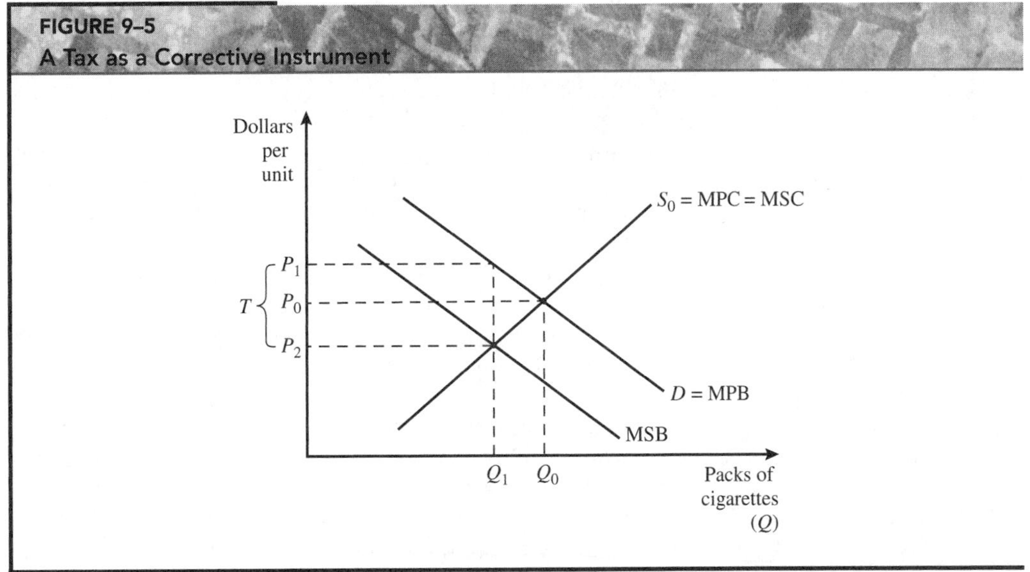

The graph captures the market for cigarettes. As before, an unfettered market results in the outcome where MPB = MPC at Q_0. Efficiency, however, exists at the point where MSB = MSC at Q_1. Government, in this case, can bring about a more efficient allocation of resources by setting a tax equal to the external damages caused by cigarette smoking at the efficient level. In this example, both consumers and producers share the tax burden. Consumers pay the portion $P_1 - P_0$ and producers pay $P_0 - P_2$. In general, the incidence of a tax depends on the relative demand and supply elasticities.

employees or lower the prices they pay to tobacco farmers. Whether consumers or producers pay a greater share of the cigarette tax depends on the relative magnitudes of the price elasticities of supply and demand. In general, when the price elasticity of demand (in absolute terms) exceeds the price elasticity of supply, the producer pays a greater fraction of the tax burden. The consumer incurs a relatively greater portion of the tax burden when the price elasticity of supply exceeds the price elasticity of demand.[7]

Governments face an incentive to tax goods for which demand is price inelastic. That is because the quantity demanded declines by a smaller percentage than the percentage increase in taxes when demand is price inelastic. Thus, the total tax revenue to government, the product of the per-unit tax and quantity, increases when demand is price inelastic. In fact, one reason "sin taxes" on cigarettes and alcohol products are so politically popular is that the demand for these two products is price inelastic, thus providing a fruitful source of revenues for government.

The point is that taxes or a threat of fines can be used to discourage socially harmful activities. In contrast, subsidies can be used to encourage socially beneficial activities that are otherwise undervalued in the marketplace. Recall that underproduction and underconsumption occur when marginal social benefit exceeds marginal private benefit. A subsidy that reduces price creates an incentive for more buyers to engage in a socially beneficial activity.

A Market Solution for Externalities? In the preceding section, we treated an externality as a situation where the market fails to allocate resources efficiently because a portion of the costs and benefits is not internalized by those participating in the exchange. Government is usually needed to tax a harmful activity or subsidize a beneficial one. In some situations, however, the market can automatically correct for any externalities because individuals—those who are harmed and those who benefit from the activity—bargain and come to agree on a mutually satisfying solution. As a result, the presence of an externality does not always require government intervention.

For this to happen, three conditions must hold (Coase, 1960). First, clearly specified property rights must be assigned to either the benefiting party or the harmed party. (Property rights are laws that describe what people can do with their property.) Second, the involved parties must have an equal amount of bargaining power; otherwise, one party in the ensuing negotiation may have an unfair advantage. Third, the transaction costs of negotiation, or bargaining costs, must be low to ensure that the bargaining actually takes place.

Figure 9–6 represents a situation where the bargaining between parties provides a solution to an externality problem. The horizontal axis measures the quantity of cigarettes, and the vertical axis reflects the associated dollar costs and benefits. The downward-sloping $NMPB_A$ curve shows the net marginal private benefit (MPB less the constant market price or, equivalently, the consumer surplus per cigarette) that person A receives from smoking cigarettes in a two-person dormitory room. MPC_B stands for the marginal private cost, or damages, that cigarette smoke imposes on person B. The curve is upward sloping to reflect the assumption that marginal private costs are likely to increase with a greater amount of cigarette smoking.

Suppose smoking is allowed in the dormitory rooms and person A is totally inconsiderate of person B's welfare. In this situation, person A is essentially granted property rights to the air in the room and faces a zero price for her actions (because the price per cigarette has been subtracted out from MPB). To maximize her utility, she smokes q_1 number of cigarettes, where

7. The answers to several questions at the end of the chapter provide the logic behind this statement. In general, it can be shown that the consumers' portion of the tax revenues equals ES/(ED+ES), where ES and ED stand for the price elasticities of supply and demand.

FIGURE 9–6
A Market Solution to an Externality

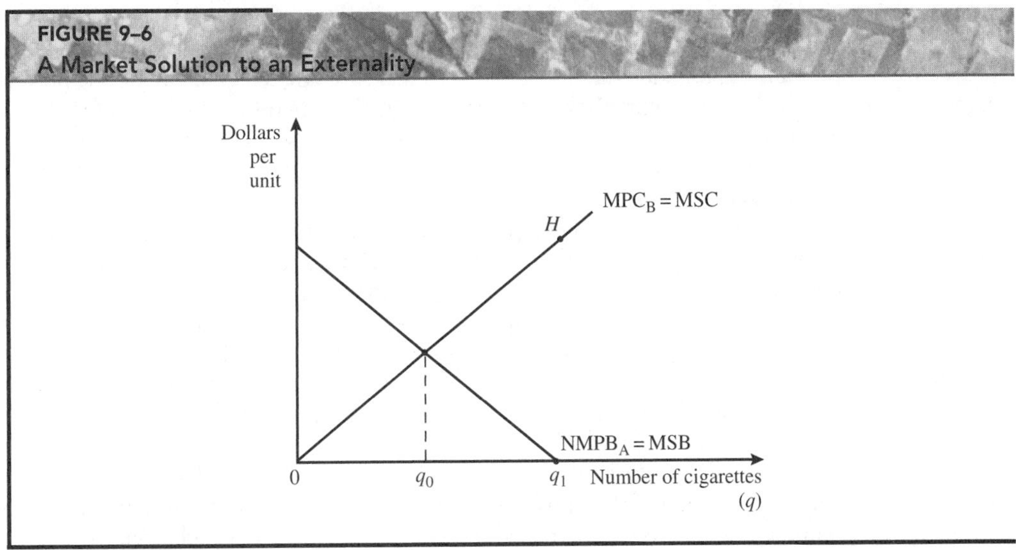

The graph shows the potential gains from two parties agreeing to some amount of cigarette smoking in a two-person dormitory room. The two curves represent the net marginal private benefit, NMPB, to one person and the marginal private cost, MPC, to another from different amount of cigarettes smoked. Person B, the harmed party, may bribe person A, the smoker, to refrain from smoking the amount of cigarettes represented by the horizontal distance $q_1 - q_0$ because the cost to person B outweighs the benefit to person A. Or, person A might pay person B to allow the amount of cigarette smoking represented by the horizontal distance represented by $q_0 - 0$ because the benefit to person A exceeds the cost to person B. The idea is that voluntary exchange can sometimes correct for an externality. The assignment of property rights to the air in the room determines who bears the externality costs.

NMPB equals zero. This amount of smoking, however, causes considerable harm to person B as indicated by point *H* on the MPC$_B$ curve.

Given this scenario, person B faces an incentive to bribe person A into smoking fewer cigarettes in the room, or at least smoking them when B is not around. As long as person A receives a sum of money (or some in-kind compensation of equal monetary value) greater than the NMPB for a given quantity of cigarettes, she is made better off by smoking less in the room and taking the bribe. According to Figure 9–6, person B is willing to pay a price, as indicated by the MPC, that is higher than the NMPB for all levels of cigarette smoking greater than q_0. For points to the left of q_0, NMPB exceeds MPC and person B is not willing to compensate person A enough for further reductions in smoking. As a result, bargaining ceases given the assignment of property rights. At q_0, the amount of smoking is optimal for both persons A and B.[8]

Now suppose college policy changes such that smoking is not allowed in the dormitory room unless all roommates consent. The nonsmoker, person B, is essentially assigned the property rights, and the origin in Figure 9–6 represents the initial position before bargaining takes place. At zero cigarettes, however, the marginal benefit to person A greatly exceeds the marginal cost to person B. Therefore, person A faces an incentive to bribe or compensate person B to accept some positive amount of smoking in the room. Person B might leave the room while person A smokes or install a smoke-eater mechanism in the room with some of the money received from person A. In any case, bargaining results in q_0 cigarettes, where NMPB$_A$ equals MPC$_B$. As Coase points

8. If MPC$_B$ exceeds NMPB$_A$ at all levels of cigarette consumption, no smoking takes place in the room.

out, the final outcome is invariant as to who is assigned the property rights. Both assignments lead to q_0 for an efficient outcome. The assignment determines who incurs the externality costs.

The "private market" reaches an efficient outcome in this case due to equal bargaining power. For example, if person A is physically larger than person B, the threat or actual use of violence might influence the relative bargaining power of the two parties. If so, physical violence rations the scarce air in the room, and the outcome is likely to be unsatisfactory to person B. Also, high transaction costs can prevent the exchange from taking place. If the group affected by the externality is large, free-rider effects will make cooperation on an efficient bribe difficult to achieve. For example, suppose three smokers and three nonsmokers share a suite of rooms in the dormitory. If the members of each group are heterogeneous, they may disagree on the appropriate payment, and the externality will remain uncorrected. Moreover, some individuals in the group may attempt to free-ride the bribes of others. In fact, some restaurants voluntarily designate smoking and nonsmoking areas due to the high transaction costs of negotiation among restaurant customers, among other reasons. Because the model does not apply to a large-group setting, the Coase theorem is limited in scope.

In any event, one lesson of the Coase theorem is that government is not *always* needed to correct for an externality. The assignment of property rights can produce an efficient outcome to an externality problem as long as bargaining costs are low. Government is needed only to assign and enforce property rights. Note that in the process of assigning property rights, government determines who "should" incur the externality costs.

Regulations

A government regulation that attempts to control either the price, quantity, or quality of a product or the entry of new firms into the marketplace represents another kind of government intervention. According to the public interest theory, the regulation is justified because a market imperfection exists that would otherwise cause a misallocation of society's resources. For example, insufficient consumer information often justifies government-imposed quality requirements. As another example, government might grant monopoly status to a firm and regulate its price because one large firm can produce output more cheaply than a large number of small firms (that is, a natural monopoly, such as an electric utility or a local telephone company). The effect of government regulations in medical markets is hard to predict. Whether government impedes or promotes efficiency and equity depends on a host of factors, such as the competitiveness of the market, the cost structure faced by the individual medical firm, objectives motivating medical decision makers, and whether the exclusion principle holds (that is, externalities, third-party payer, or public good considerations). In the next section, we examine the impact of a per-unit price ceiling within a supply and demand model assuming that consumers possess health insurance coverage—the most common situation in medical markets.

The Effects of a Per-Unit Price Ceiling. The price paid for a good or service is one item a third-party payer, such as the government, might regulate. Government might regulate the price by establishing a maximum price or reimbursement level. In that case, the government sets a **price ceiling** for a product, and producers are prohibited by law from charging a higher price to consumers covered under the ceiling. Figure 9–7 shows the effect of a price ceiling within a supply and demand model of a market for physician services.

As you know, the equilibrium price and quantity are determined at the intersection point of supply and demand in a typical nonmedical market. But because the model represents a medical market, we must also consider the impact of health insurance coverage. To simplify the

FIGURE 9–7
Effect of a Per-Unit Price Ceiling in a Supply and Demand Model

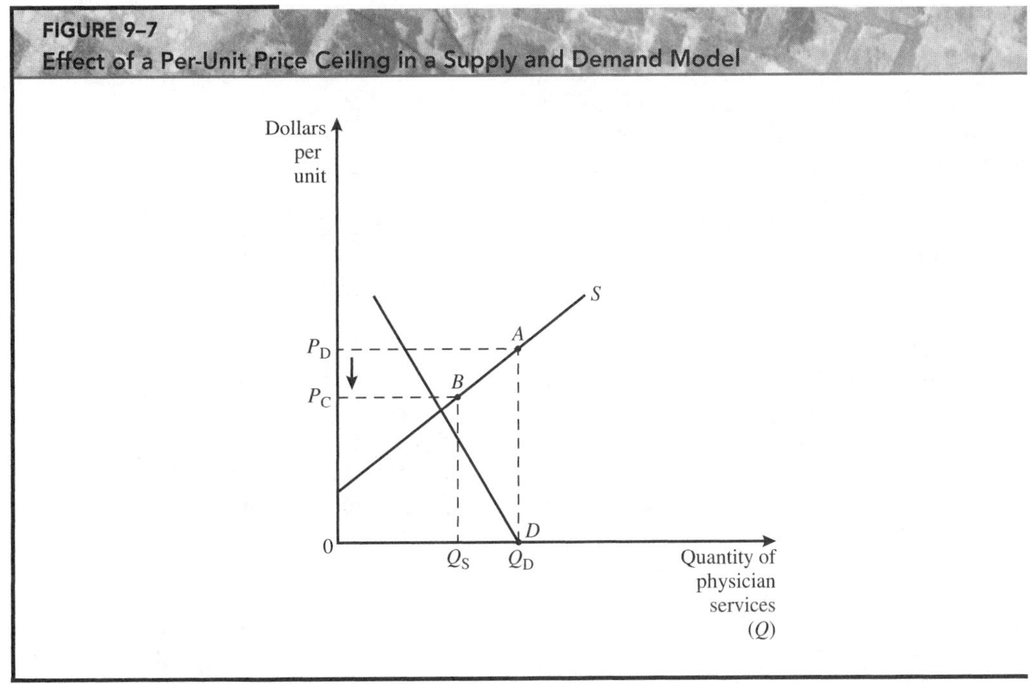

The graph represents the market for physician services. At a zero out-of-pocket price, consumers desire Q_D amount of physician services. If a third-party reimburses physicians at the price P_D, consumer demand is satisfied and no shortage occurs. If for cost containment reasons the government implements a price ceiling and lowers the price to P_C, physicians supply only Q_S amount of services and a shortage results in the market.

discussion, let's suppose consumers have complete rather than partial insurance coverage. Given the demand, consumers wish to purchase Q_D units of physician services (say, office visits) because they have full health insurance coverage and effectively pay a zero out-of-pocket price. Assuming a third party initially reimburses physicians a price of P_D, which is sufficient to elicit the amount of physician services demanded by consumers, expenditures on physician services amount to area P_DAQ_D0, the product of the reimbursement price of P_D and Q_D, the quantity demanded by consumers. In this case, no shortage of physician services exists because quantity supplied equals quantity demanded. Notice that expenditures on physician services exceed the level that results when consumers face the full market price for physician care at the intersection of supply and demand, as discussed earlier in the text.

Now suppose that for cost containment reasons the government sets a cap or reimbursement ceiling at P_C. Because of the positively sloped supply curve, the lower reimbursement rate creates an incentive for physicians to reduce the quantity supplied to Q_S and, as a result, expenditures on physician services fall to area P_CBQ_S0. Notice that because the reimbursement ceiling of P_C is set below P_D, quantity demanded exceeds quantity supplied and the price ceiling results in a shortage of physician services.

In a price ceiling situation where a shortage ensues and the price mechanism is not employed as a rationing device, some unintended outcomes may occur. For one, physicians may treat patients on a first-come, first-served basis even if some patients require more urgent attention than others. Physicians may also reduce the quality of visits in an attempt to lower costs. The quality reduction may mean a longer waiting time for a visit or shorter time spent with physicians during the actual visit. In addition, some unethical physicians may accept illegal side payments from wealthy people who want to jump to the front of the waiting line.

Political concerns may also dictate how a scarce medical service is rationed when a shortage exists. Perhaps politicians decide that medical services should be rationed on the basis of age, illness, or the amount of campaign contributions the individual donates. For example, in Great Britain, where price has virtually no rationing role, less rationing of medical care occurs for children than for adults. According to Aaron and Schwartz (1984), "Health expenditures per child in Britain are 119 percent of expenditures per prime age adult, whereas in the United States they are only 37 percent as much" (p. 97).

The point is that medical cost containment is typically not a free lunch. According to the preceding model, cost containment under plausible circumstances can result in shortages, longer waiting lines, nonprice rationing, and reductions in the quality of care. Society has to seriously consider the likely trade-offs before adopting cost containment strategies.

It should be mentioned that the exact behavioral response of the medical firm is more multidimensional than presented thus far and depends largely on the base to which the price ceiling is applied (Cromwell, 1976). Specifically, health care providers, in general, may react to a lower charge by adjusting the length of stay, number of patients, or quality of services. For example, if hospitals are paid according to a per diem price ceiling (that is, average revenue per patient-day), they may respond to a lower per diem charge by increasing the number of patient-days to obtain additional revenues and also by lowering quality. The number of patient-days can be increased by increasing the number of new admissions and/or increasing the average length of stay. By increasing the patient's length of stay, hospitals can use the profits received from the later days to subsidize the more costly, service-intensive earlier days and make greater profits.

As another example, hospitals (or nursing homes) that are reimbursed on a per-case or per-patient basis are likely to respond to a lower per-case charge by admitting more patients to obtain additional revenues and lowering quality and length of stay. In this regard, some observers have argued that harmfully low diagnosis related groups (DRG) payments, which are per-case reimbursements, have caused hospitals to release their Medicare patients "quicker and sicker."

In addition, some critics have argued that the DRG per-patient payment has created an incentive for patient dumping by hospitals. Although illegal in certain cases under the Federal Emergency Medical Treatment and Active Labor Act, **patient dumping** refers to the practice whereby private hospitals fail to admit severely sick patients and instead dump them on public hospitals. In practice, this may happen because the DRG payment is based on the historical cost of providing services to patients with an average level of sickness and does not necessarily cover the cost of providing hospital services to patients with severe illnesses.

In sum, the impact of a price ceiling on the performance of an industry is difficult to predict. Its precise impact depends on a host of factors including the extensiveness of third party involvement, the competitiveness of the market, and the base to which the price ceiling is applied. Experience in other markets, such as natural gas and housing, has taught economists that price controls often create unwanted shortages of goods and can cause other unintended effects such as reductions in quality, longer waiting lines, and discrimination against selected groups, for instance. Sometimes price controls are implemented as a means to contain costs. If so, policy makers should be aware that cost containment may come with a considerable trade-off. However, sometimes a price ceiling is adopted so more individuals can afford a particular good. The irony is that the price ceiling may lead to a shortage, such that the good or service becomes more affordable, perhaps, but less available. This situation should not be interpreted as suggesting that we should ignore individuals who are unable to pay for life's necessities. Instead, this situation suggests that more efficient ways of providing equity may exist. We consider some of these redistribution methods later in this chapter.

The Effects of Quality Regulations. Government may also attempt to regulate the quality of medical services when consumers are rationally ignorant. As mentioned earlier, quality differences show up in the structure, process, and outcomes of production. Because procedural and outcome guidelines are more difficult to set and enforce, quality regulations are typically directed at the structure of operation. For example, a public agency may require that medical workers be professionally licensed or may mandate a minimum staff-to-patient ratio. In both cases, the assumption is that a higher level of structural quality promotes increased quality at the process and outcome stages.

Regulations aimed at the quality of the employees typically mean higher costs of production and thereby reduce the supply of medical services in the medical marketplace. The reduction of supply occurs because the acquisition of a professional license requires a greater human capital investment by the medical employee and raises the cost of providing the medical service. Figure 9–8 shows the implications of a quality regulation, such as professional licensing. The original supply and demand curves for medical employees are S_0 and D_0 and the corresponding market wage and employment levels are W_0 and N_0, respectively. Professional licensing, which

FIGURE 9–8
Effect of Professional Licensure

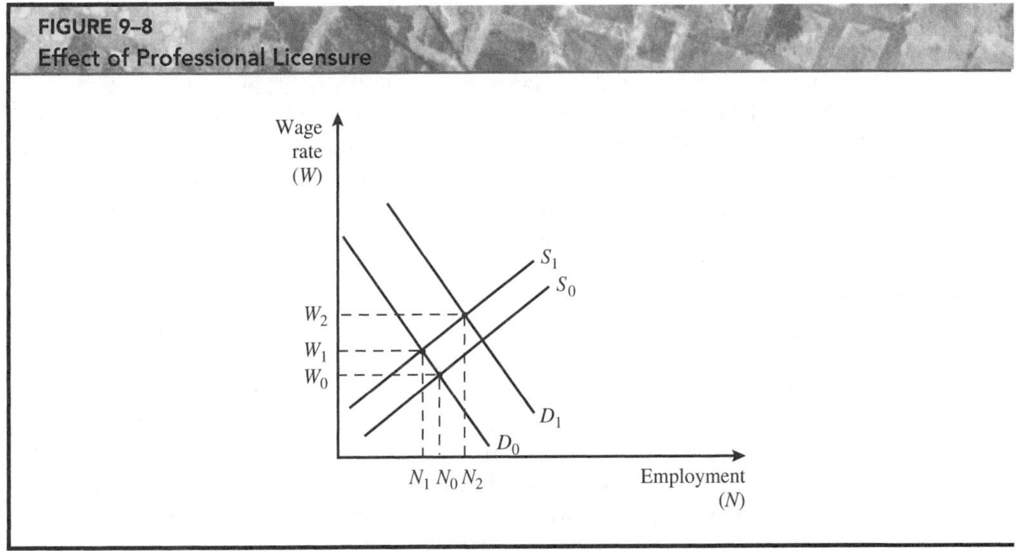

The graph represents a market for professional labor. Without occupational licensing, market equilibrium occurs at employment N_0 where D_0 intersects S_0. Occupational licensing potentially has two effects. First, the licensing requirement increases the human capital investment necessary to enter the occupation and thereby reduces supply from S_0 to S_1. Second, the higher wage of W_1 brought on by the supply reduction creates an incentive for professionals to improve their job performance. The quality assurance of occupational licensing, brought on by the improved job performance, leads to a greater demand for the output of the professional labor. As a result, demand increases from D_0 to D_1. If the demand shift exceeds the supply shift such that N_2 exceeds N_0, the occupational licensing reflects an efficient policy serving the public interest.

raises the cost of entering an occupation due to the increased human capital investment, reduces supply to S_1, and thereby raises the wage rate to W_1. The difference between W_1 and W_0 captures the **compensating wage differential** necessary to attract the marginal worker with the appropriate professional license to the labor market.

Two questions follow from the analysis. First, is professional licensing truly associated with increased procedural and outcomes quality? If not, the result may not justify the method of controlling quality. Second, was a professional group behind the implementation of the professional licensing requirement? This question follows because those inframarginal individuals in the labor group (particularly those who lack the required license but are grandfathered in) obviously gain from the higher wage rate.

Svorny (1987) provides an interesting way to analyze the second question by comparing a professional license to a trademark or brand name. All three of these devices may signal quality assurance to consumers. Specifically, Svorny argues that the higher wage resulting from the professional license creates a financial incentive for the typical medical worker to perform efficiently, satisfy patient wants, and provide a desirable amount and quality of output. This is because opportunistic behavior, when discovered, results in job termination and causes the medical worker to receive a low or negative return on the original human capital investment. The quality assurance generated by the higher wage, in turn, raises the marginal value of the employee's services to the consumer. The higher quality assurance can be represented by a shift to the right of the demand curve from D_0 to D_1 in Figure 9–8.

Due to the greater demand arising from the increased quality assurance, the wage rate increases further to W_2 and employment rises from N_1 to N_2. Svorny goes on to note that the model provides a useful test of whether professional licensure requirements (and other quality regulations) serve the public interest or some special interest group, such as the entrenched medical employees. If the quality regulation provides benefits (quality assurance) that exceed its cost (human capital investment), the shift of the demand curve to the right should be greater in magnitude than the shift of the supply curve to the left. Thus, employment should increase overall if society is made better off and the public interest is served by the quality regulation (that is, N_2 should exceed N_0). However, if the opposite occurs—the supply curve shifts to the left by more than the demand curve shifts to the right—the quality regulation favors special interests.

Svorny uses the analysis to test whether basic science certification and citizen requirements for medical licensure made any difference in the number of physicians per capita across the 48 contiguous states of the United States in 1965. She notes that both requirements potentially involve some degree of human capital investment that increases wages and establishes a future return to discourage opportunistic behavior. Using multiple regression analysis, Svorny finds an inverse relation between the presence of both requirements and the number of physicians. The theory suggests that an inverse relation is evidence for the special interest model of the regulatory process.

The implication is that these quality regulations result in lower rather than higher consumption of physician services. A lower consumption of physician services results because the licensure restrictions increased entry costs by more than they increased the consumer benefits from quality assurance. Overall, the study found evidence supporting the special interest group theory of the regulatory process.

Two interesting studies on the relationship between regulatory barriers and health care outcomes also deserve mentioning. Anderson et al. (2000) find empirically that physician income is higher in states with regulations restricting the practice of homeopathy, a type of alternative medicine. Kleiner and Kudrle (2000) find that tougher dental licensing does not improve dental health but does raise the price for consumers and the earnings of dental practitioners. Consequently, these studies also support the special interest theory of regulation.

Antitrust Laws

Government also intervenes in a market economy by enacting and enforcing antitrust laws. Antitrust laws are concerned primarily with promoting competition among the firms within an industry and prohibiting firms from engaging in certain types of market practices that may inhibit efficiency. The Sherman Antitrust Act, passed in 1890, is the cornerstone of all antitrust laws. Other antitrust laws, such as the Clayton Act of 1914, the Federal Trade Commission Act of 1914, and the Cellar-Kefauver Amendment of 1950, either clarify, reinforce, or extend the Sherman Act. The Sherman Act stipulates two important provisions:

> ***Section 1:*** Every contract, combination in the form of trust or otherwise, or conspiracy, in restraint of trade or commerce among the several states or with foreign nations, is hereby declared illegal.
>
> ***Section 2:*** Every person who shall monopolize, or conspire with any other person or persons to monopolize any part of the trade or commerce among the several states, or with foreign nations, shall be guilty of a misdemeanor.

Price Fixing, Boycotting, and Market Allocation. The Sherman Antitrust Act has been interpreted as prohibiting anticompetitive business practices, such as price fixing, boycotting, market allocations, and mergers, that promote inefficiencies and inequities in the marketplace. **Price fixing** occurs when business rivals in an industry abide to a collusive agreement, refrain from price competition, and fix the price of a good or service. Essentially, the firms collectively act as a monopolist, maximize joint profits, and, according to monopoly theory, create a higher price and a lower level of output. An agreement among a number of large hospitals to establish the price of various hospital services is an example of price fixing. Physicians who have been denied staff privileges frequently allege that the existing hospital physicians violated Section 1 of the Sherman Act by unlawfully conspiring to exclude them from the hospital (Jacobsen and Wiggins, 1992).[9]

A **boycott** is an agreement among competitors not to deal with a supplier or a customer. For example, suppose that in response to a Blue Shield ban on balance billing, the physicians in an area collectively agree not to offer services to Blue Shield patients.[10] While it is legal for any one physician to unilaterally refrain from dealing with Blue Shield, the combination is in violation of the Sherman Antitrust Act. In this case, the rival physicians are essentially trying to fix the price of medical services charged to Blue Shield subscribers.

Market allocation occurs when competitors agree not to compete with one another in specific market areas. This business practice can ultimately produce the same undesirable outcome that price fixing does, since each firm within the area is free to set a monopoly price and restrict output with no concern about competitive entry.

Price fixing, boycotting, and market allocations are *illegal per se;* that is, they are unreasonable by their very nature and therefore illegal. To be found in violation of the Sherman Act, the plaintiff must only prove that those practices took place.

An antitrust action against a number of health care providers in Alamogordo, New Mexico, provides a recent example of a price-fixing and boycotting agreement. In this case, the

---

9. See Felsenthal (1992) for an insightful discussion of how physicians and hospitals have attempted to fend off low-cost competitors, such as nurse-midwives, chiropractors, and optometrists.

10. A physician boycott of this kind occurred in *Kartell v. Blue Shield of Massachusetts,* 749 F.2d 922 (1984). See Frech (1988) for an economic assessment of this antitrust suit.

Federal Trade Commission (FTC) charged that a number of independent physicians and nurse anesthetists refused to deal individually with health plans and instead engaged in collective negotiations with them. Eighty-four percent of all physicians independently operating in the area and all nurse anesthetists participated in this arrangement. The collective price negotiations took place through a private agency that provided consulting and contracting services to a physician/hospital organization in the area. Through this private agency the health care providers orchestrated collective refusals to deal with payors that resisted their terms. The FTC argued that the joint negotiations did not enhance efficiency or consumer welfare. Those participating in the price-fixing and boycotting arrangement eventually settled by accepting the consent order of the FTC to discontinue their practice of collectively negotiating prices.[11]

Horizontal Mergers. The Sherman Act (in conjunction with Section 7 of the Clayton Act) has also been cited as a basis for preventing horizontal mergers among firms. A **horizontal merger** takes place when two or more firms in the same industry combine together. The economic concern is that a merger may harm consumers by making it easier for the remaining firms in the market to collude, expressly or tacitly (for example, by following the leader), and thereby force price above the competitive level.

Although a combination of two or more competitor firms can result in higher prices to the consumer, the merger may also benefit the consumer if economies exist with respect to large-scale production. Larger firms may not only produce with economies of scale and organizational economies but also have better access to technological innovations. Any cost or resource savings mean society can produce more output from a given amount of inputs. For example, according to hospital officials, a proposed merger of the 710-bed Iowa Methodist Medical Center and the 319-bed Iowa Lutheran Hospital in Des Moines "could save as much as $12 million annually during the first three years of the merger" (Burda, 1993, p. 24). Similarly, officials at St. Joseph Mercy and North Iowa Medical in Mason City claimed their proposed merger "would reduce their operating expenses by $2 million to $3 million per year." Thus, potential anticompetitive and procompetitive effects must be properly weighed when determining the social desirability of a merger. Assessing the net social benefits of a business practice such as a merger is referred to as the **rule of reason** doctrine.

The Williamson (1969) merger trade-off model in Figure 9–9 provides an insightful way to conceptualize the net social benefit of a horizontal merger. Suppose the market in some geographical area is competitive before the merger and the industry is characterized by constant costs. As a result, the market price and quantity of hospital services are P_0 and Q_0, respectively, where the demand curve intersects the original supply curve S_0. Now suppose a merger of two hospitals in the area makes it easier for the remaining firms to collude and reduce output to Q_1 and raise price to P_1. Relative to the original competitive equilibrium, a deadweight loss of area *bad* occurs. The deadweight loss reflects the social cost, C, associated with the merger.

Suppose that due to the horizontal merger and the associated greater production efficiency, the per-unit cost of producing hospital services declines from AC_0 to AC_1. Cost savings might accrue from economies of scale at the firm level, improved access to capital markets, purchasing discounts, or managerial economies. This reflects some important resource cost savings to society. Resources are saved and can be used for other purposes if a larger firm is more efficient in

11. See http://www.ftc.gov/opa/2004/09/whitesands.htm (accessed January 5, 2006).

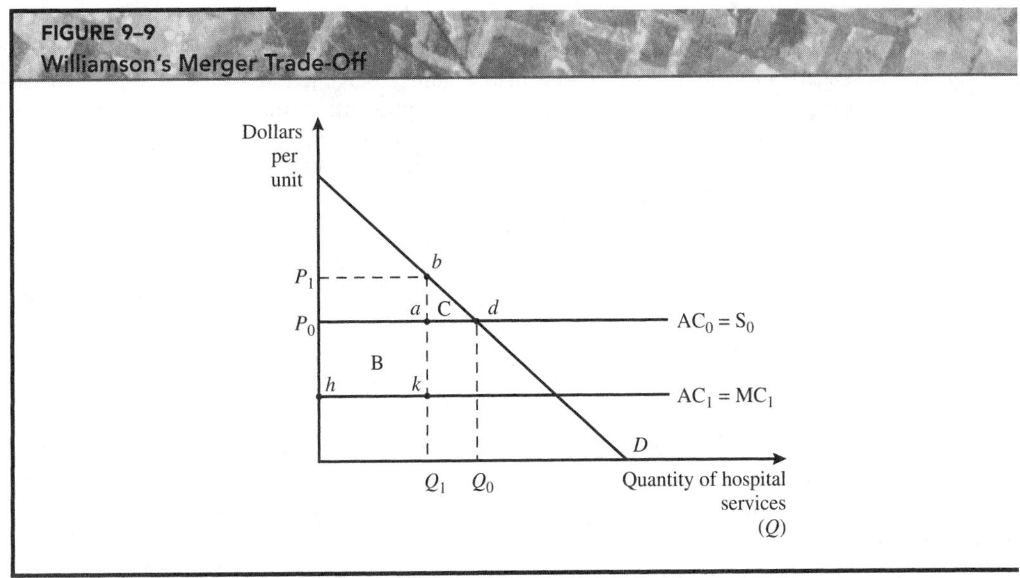

The graph represents the market for hospital services supposing a constant cost industry. Suppose the hospital market is initially in equilibrium at Q_0 where D intersects S_0. Now suppose two relatively large firms merge and the resulting collusion among the firms in the market causes output to fall to Q_1 and price to rise to P_1. The deadweight loss of bad represents the cost, C, of the merger. But suppose the merger also results in cost savings such that average costs falls to AC_1. The cost savings, represented by the area P_0akh, reflect the benefits of the merger. To determine whether if the merger provides net social benefits, the benefits of the merger must be compared to the costs of the merger.

production. Compared to the costs in a competitive market, the total resource cost savings is measured by area P_0akh. The area reflects the social benefit, B, that arises from the merger. The net benefit of the merger is found by subtracting the deadweight loss of area C from the resource cost savings of area B. As drawn, the merger provides positive net benefits to society. Of course, actual mergers may cause net benefits or losses depending on the relative magnitudes of the cost savings and deadweight losses. The bottom line is that a proposed horizontal merger should be given careful scrutiny using cost-benefit analysis.

Exclusive Dealing Contract. An *exclusive dealing contract* is another business practice that may impede efficiency and therefore violate antitrust laws. An exclusive dealing occurs, for example, when a manufacturer allows only one distributor to sell its product or products in a market area. Economists consider an exclusive dealing arrangement as one of several types of vertical restrictions that often take place between manufacturers and distributors. Vertical restrictions are viewed as an alternative to a vertical merger, where firms at different stages of production, such as a manufacturer and distributor, merge their operations. Other types of vertical restrictions include exclusive territories, resale price agreements, tying contracts (explained shortly), and franchise arrangements.

In general, vertical restrictions can have anticompetitive or procompetitive impacts and thereby potentially harm or benefit consumers. In terms of exclusive dealings, consumers may be harmed if rival manufacturers are foreclosed from offering their products through the distributor in a market area. The foreclosure limits competition and raises product prices.

However, exclusive dealing contracts can also reduce the free-rider problem that sometimes accompanies exchanges between manufacturers and distributors. For example, suppose that two manufacturers in the same industry, A and B, want to sell their reasonably similar products through a distributor in a market area. Further suppose that manufacturer A invests a considerable sum of money training the staff of the area distributor about the intricate details behind its product. Or, suppose that manufacturer A advertises the general availability of its product and provides a list of potential consumers to the distributor. Obviously, consumers gain from the advertising message and when they purchase quality products from an informed distributor. It also follows that manufacturer A may have to charge a higher price for its product to cover the training and advertising costs and the establishment and updating of the customer list.

However, the rival manufacturer, manufacturer B, may free-ride the investment of manufacturer A by selling its products to the same distributor at a lower price and receiving the benefits of a well-trained staff and the advertising at the distribution outlet. In fact, if no exclusive dealing contract existed such that each manufacturer faced an incentive to free-ride the first-mover investment of the other, much less training and advertising would take place and consumers would be potentially harmed. Exclusive dealings represent a solution to the underinvestment caused by this free-rider problem.

For example, in January 1999, the Department of Justice (DOJ) filed an antitrust lawsuit against Dentsply International, Inc., a dental supply company in York, Pennsylvania. The lawsuit alleged that Dentsply, which controlled more than 70 percent of the U.S. market for prefabricating artificial teeth over the previous ten-year period, illegally entered into exclusive dealing arrangements with its dealers. The DOJ claimed that the exclusive dealing contracts prevented independent dealers from selling other brands of false teeth, resulting in reduced competition and higher prices for false teeth. The DOJ cited that the Clayton Act of 1914 declares illegal various business practices that substantially lessen competition or tend to create a monopoly.

The courts have generally embraced a rule of reason approach to cases involving exclusive dealing arrangements. First, the manufacturer involved in the dealing must be shown to possess a critical degree of market power in the relevant market. Second, the exclusive arrangement must be shown to inhibit competition and harm consumers. The ultimate proof of inhibited competition is to show that consumers pay higher prices and receive fewer services because of the exclusive dealing contract. With that in mind, the DOJ (1999, p. 14) argued, "Dentsply's exclusion of its rivals has resulted in higher prices, loss of choice, less market information, and lower quality of artificial teeth."

The U.S. District Court for the District of Delaware ruled in 2003 that Dentsply International, Inc. did not violate federal antitrust laws. While the market power of Dentsply was recognized, the court ruled that the DOJ failed to prove that Dentsply's policy prevented competition in the market. The court pointed out that competing manufacturers could sell to their customers—the dental laboratories—directly or through new dealers. Moreover, Dentsply's dealers were free to leave Dentsply whenever they chose. Hence the court maintained that Dentsply had not used its market power in the artificial teeth market to create a market with artificially high prices and thus did not violate the Sherman Act under a rule of reason analysis.

Interestingly, the court was not convinced that Dentsply's exclusive dealing arrangement was necessary to protect its investment in the promotion of artificial teeth. Instead, the court found that Dentsply was motivated by anticompetitive intent when it adopted the policy in February 1993. But bad intent is not sufficient to find a firm in violation of antitrust laws when the conduct cannot harm competition, the court observed.

Tying Contract. Tying occurs when the seller of product A will sell A (the tying product) only if the buyer also purchases product B (the tied product). Similar to an exclusive dealing contract, both procompetitive and anticompetitive explanations can be offered for the use of a tying contract. Promoting high quality and reducing transaction costs are two of the several procompetitive explanations often offered for tying contracts. For instance, a vacuum cleaner may operate well only if a specific vacuum cleaner bag is used. Or, it may be logistically more costly for a seller to sell two products separately rather than together as a bundle. For example, a car typically comes with some type of radio already installed, and a computer typically comes with various programs already installed.

In terms of its potential anticompetitive effects, a tying contract theoretically can enable a seller to practice **price discrimination.** Price discrimination occurs when different customers are charged different prices for the same good. When practiced successfully, price discrimination allows a seller to transform some portion of what would have been consumer surplus with uniform pricing into additional profits. However, price discrimination works only when the firm possesses some degree of market power, can distinguish among buyers based on willingness to pay, and can prevent the product from being resold. In the case of a tying contract, the seller charges all consumers the same fixed price for the tying product (say, a vacuum cleaner) but then uses the tied product (vacuum cleaner bags) to reveal intensity of use and charges a higher per-unit price to buyers with greater intensity. In essence, the tying contract serves as a two-part tariff with a fixed charge for the tying product and a variable charge for the tied product.

Leveraging provides another anticompetitive explanation for tying contracts. Leverage theory suggests that a monopolist in one market may attempt to extend its market power into another market with the use of a tying contract. If buyers can purchase the tying product only if they buy the tied product, and if the tying product dominates its market, the logic is that the tied product will also dominate its market. The dominance results in greater profits for the company in the tied market and overall.

While potentially resulting in either procompetitive or anticompetitive effects, the courts have tended to apply a "modified" per se ruling, rather than a rule of reason, to cases involving tying contracts (Viscusi et al., 2000). Under a modified per se ruling, the plaintiff must show both that the seller possessed monopoly power and that the practice took place such that buyers were forced into a tying contract. Recall that for a per se violation, the plaintiff must show only that the practice took place (for example, price-fixing, boycotting, market-sharing arrangements) and that demonstration of monopoly power is unnecessary.

Jefferson Parish Hospital v. Hyde provides an example of an antitrust case involving a tying contract in a medical care setting (Lynk, 1994). In 1977, Dr. Hyde, a board-certified anesthesiologist, wanted to practice his services at East Jefferson Hospital and applied for privileges. The board of directors at the hospital, however, denied his application, citing that a contract had already been secured for all of the hospital's anesthesia requirements with Rioux & Associates. In response to the denial of admission, Dr. Hyde claimed that East Jefferson Hospital was in violation of the Sherman Antitrust Act. He argued that the hospital unnecessarily bundled operating and anesthesiology services as a type of tying contract and that the hospital had acquired monopoly power in the market for operating services in its market area. Therefore, consumers were forced into purchasing anesthesiology services through the hospital if they desired surgical services.

However, in 1984, a majority of justices on the Supreme Court ruled in favor of Eastern Jefferson Hospital, citing that the hospital had little market power. Therefore, the hospital had little to gain financially from any tying contract because, without market power, the hospital was unable to profitably practice price discrimination or use any leverage.[12] This case is interesting because a minority of justices expressed the opinion that no sound reason existed for treating operating and anesthesia services as separate services because patients are interested in purchasing anesthesia only when they receive surgical services. Therefore purposely tying the two together cannot result in greater profits because that's the way consumers desire the two services. Also the minority opinion expressed the view that it might be desirable in the future to replace the per se approach to tying contracts with a rule of reason.

Antitrust Enforcement. Although the Sherman Act was enacted in 1890, the health care field escaped its purview until the mid-1970s.[13] Up to that time, it was believed that members of the medical profession, like other professionals, such as lawyers and engineers, were exempted from antitrust laws. In the *Goldfarb v. Virginia State Bar* case of 1975, the Supreme Court unanimously rejected any claim to a professional exemption and stated,

> *The nature of an occupation, standing alone, does not provide sanctuary from the Sherman Act . . . nor is the public service aspect of professional practice controlling in determining whether section 1 includes professions.*

Some early signs appeared to indicate that the courts would aggressively enforce antitrust laws in health care markets. For example, in *Arizona v. Maricopa County Medical Society* in 1982, the Supreme Court condemned as price fixing the attempt by a professionally sponsored foundation to set a maximum price on the fees charged to member physicians for services underwritten by insurers that had agreed to abide by the foundation's fee schedule. Typically, when firms collude and pursue their joint interests, they agree to a price floor rather than a price ceiling. The foundation claimed that the maximum price was fixed for the benefit of the consumer. In this particular case, the Supreme Court invoked the per se illegality of price fixing, but opened the door to a possible rule of reason ruling in the future. The Court explained that the public service aspect and other features of the medical profession may require that a particular practice that could be properly viewed as a violation of the Sherman Act in another context be treated differently. The Court went on to explain that in *Maricopa,* the price-fixing arrangement was premised on neither public service nor ethical norms nor quality of care considerations.

Two merger cases prior to the mid-1990s, *Hospital Corporation of America v. FTC* (807 F.2d 1381 [7th Cir. 1986]) and *U.S. v. Rockford Memorial Corporation* (898 F.2d 1278 [7th Cir. 1990]) also demonstrated the Court's willingness to enforce antitrust laws aggressively and disallow horizontal mergers in the hospital services industry if they substantially lessen competition or tend to create a monopoly. In the *Rockford* case, for example, the U.S. government brought suit to prevent the horizontal merger of Rockford Memorial Corporation and Swedish American Corporation, both of which are not-for-profit institutions. Citing a high postmerger market share and, consequently, the potential for monopoly pricing, the Court ruled against the merger.[14]

However, not all health policy analysts believe that antitrust laws should be stringently enforced in the health services industries. Some argue that various institutions, such as third-party payments, not-for-profit organizations, and excessive government regulations, mean that antitrust laws are less applicable and necessary in health care markets than in other markets. With health

12. The hospital also couldn't gain financially because Rioux & Associates, the anesthesiology group, was reimbursed directly by payers.

13. See Havighurst (1983) and Kopit (1983) for a thorough discussion of the application of antitrust laws to the health care industry.

14. More discussion of merger policy in the hospital industry is provided in Chapter 13.

care costs continually increasing, many analysts claim that the enforcement of antitrust laws could actually worsen the situation as cost-minimizing joint ventures and mergers are discouraged. Indeed, legislation in Maine, Minnesota, Ohio, Wisconsin, and Washington allows hospitals to cooperate if the benefits of the proposed venture substantially outweigh the disadvantages of any reduction in competition (Felsenthal, 1993). In 1993, the Department of Justice and the Federal Trade Commission issued a joint statement of antitrust enforcement in health care markets, basically echoing the notion that the procompetitive and anticompetitive effects of various business activities, such as mergers, joint ventures, joint purchasing, and provider networks, will be weighed when making an antitrust determination.

Greaney (2002) argues that anti–managed care sentiment has reduced the enthusiasm for applying competitive principles in health care markets since the mid-1990s. With respect to the hospital industry, for example, Greaney points out that the Federal Trade Commission and Department of Justice won five of six cases challenging hospital mergers between 1984 and 1994. Many other mergers were settled or abandoned after government investigation spotlighted potential antitrust concerns. In contrast, federal and state antitrust enforcement agencies have lost all seven cases brought before the federal court since 1995. It remains to be seen how stringently and consistently antitrust laws are enforced in various health care markets once the backlash against managed care subsides.

Public Enterprise

Instead of indirectly influencing the structure, conduct, or performance of private industry, government may take a more direct role in health care provision by producing and distributing a specific health care service. For example, many local governments are responsible for providing county and city hospital services to local residents. In addition, some nursing homes and mental health facilities are operated by local or state government agencies. Moreover, the federal government runs and operates Veterans Administration and military hospitals. Despite the fact that the government may operate health care facilities, economic analysis is still useful for analyzing the many production decisions that take place. Valuable resources are used in production, and some type of economizing behavior occurs.

The primary difference between public enterprise and private, for-profit enterprise is the lack of a profit motive. Like not-for-profit entities, public health care providers may pursue goals other than profit maximization. The upshot is that public health care providers may not minimize the cost of producing a given quantity of medical care services or attempt to satisfy consumer wants. Of course, even public agencies are subject to least-cost constraints of various kinds. For example, bureaucrats and politicians are either directly or indirectly influenced by the consumer/voters' response to excessive taxation. The potential loss of job tenure may create a sufficient incentive for cost minimization even in public facilities.

Many analysts argue that public medical facilities are more likely to provide services to more severely ill patients. Unlike their for-profit (and even not-for-profit) counterparts, public medical facilities do not have to worry about the profit consequence of servicing high-cost patients. Therefore, public provision of medical services is often argued to be more equitable because all individuals, rich and poor, are provided with equal access to public facilities.

Lindsay (1976) develops a useful model of government enterprise that may explain why public hospitals tend to operate with lower per-unit costs of production than proprietary hospitals. The author assumes that politicians tie managerial compensation to the level of net social income that public organizations generate. Net social income, an analogue to profits in the private sector, is the difference between the social value of the output and the total cost of production. Higher managerial pay results from a higher level of net social income.

To estimate the value of the output provided by the public agency, politicians monitor the levels of various attributes associated with the product. Some attributes are observable and measurable; others are not. Bureau managers, in pursuit of higher pay, face an incentive to divert resources away from the production of attributes that are not easily measurable to those that are to increase the perceived social value of their output. Therefore, a financial incentive exists to make the output of public institutions contain too few "invisible" attributes, such as quality (as reflected in the number of staff visits to a hospital ward, words of encouragement, number of smiles, and so on), and too many visible attributes, such as quantity (for example, number of patients). In contrast, managers of private organizations are disciplined to a greater degree by the marketplace and forced by consumer demand to provide the desired level of quality. Price fails if private firms fail to satisfy the quality demands of customers, unlike in a public agency, where price is essentially fixed by politicians.

Lindsay's model of government enterprise predicts that the average cost of government enterprise—that is, total cost divided by visible output—will be lower than the comparable average cost of proprietary enterprise. The author offers some empirical evidence to support his view of government enterprise.

The Redistribution Function of Government

In addition to providing public goods, correcting for externalities, enforcing regulations and antitrust laws, and operating public enterprises, another function of government is to redistribute income more equitably because a pure market system cannot guarantee that everyone receives an adequate level of income. Some people own very little labor, capital, and land resources, and hence are often unable to generate a subsistence level of income in the marketplace. Redistribution involves taxing one group and using the resulting tax revenues to provide subsidies to another group. One may question why people in a free democratic society, such as that of the United States, support redistribution and rely on government to administer various programs. One justification for redistribution advanced by economists is the existence of interdependent utility functions such that donors get utility from increasing the welfare of recipients. More formally, when utility functions are interdependent, person A derives utility when person B is made better off. Person B might be made better off by receiving some income or benefits in kind, such as housing or food, from person A.

Consequently, redistribution takes place in a free society because it provides utility to both recipient and donor groups. Government must administer and require people by law to contribute to the redistribution scheme through taxation because some people in the donor group might otherwise attempt to free-ride the voluntary contributions of others. For example, person C may also derive utility if person B is made better off, but may attempt to free-ride by relying on the sole contributions of person A to finance the redistribution program. Person A, in turn, may decide not to voluntarily contribute to the redistribution scheme given that others, such as person C, will indirectly benefit but will not share in the overall costs. Given the likelihood of a free-rider problem on a large scale, redistribution tends to be underprovided in a free market. So, in effect, government acts as an intermediary or fiscal agent by legally stipulating and collecting the necessary taxes from the donor group and redistributing the income to the recipient group.

For a redistribution scheme to be considered equitable, the two principles of *vertical* and *horizontal equity* must be satisfied. **Vertical equity** means that "unequals are treated unequally." To determine whether this principle has been satisfied in practice, a standard of comparison must first be selected. In terms of financial equity, the usual standard of comparison is income. As a result, the principle of vertical equity is satisfied when people with higher incomes are treated differently from those with lower incomes. This principle by itself, however, does not establish whether the net taxes (that is, taxes less subsidies) of higher-income people should be higher or lower than those of people with lower incomes. Therefore, notions of fairness dictate that net taxes be based on "ability to pay"; that is, those with more ability to pay should incur a greater net tax liability.

Even this additional principle is ambiguous, because it is unclear how much more net taxes higher-income people should pay or whether taxes, when assessing burden, should be expressed in absolute terms or as a fraction of income. For example, suppose a household with $10,000 of income pays $2,000 in net taxes and another household with $100,000 pays $4,000 in net taxes. In absolute terms, the richer household pays more taxes. When taxes are expressed as a fraction of income, however, taxes comprise only 4 percent of the rich household's income compared to 20 percent of the poor household's income.

In practice, many consider that vertical equity is achieved when the net tax system is sufficiently progressive. A redistribution scheme is considered to be **progressive** if net taxes as a fraction of income increase with income. Ignoring the subsidy side of the redistribution issue, the federal income tax system comes closest to being a progressive tax scheme. The underlying belief is that higher-income individuals should pay more taxes in both absolute and relative terms.

In a **proportional** redistribution scheme, net taxes as a fraction of income remain constant with respect to income. The Medicare tax is a proportional tax because all payroll income is subject to a fixed percentage rate.

Finally, net taxes as a fraction of income fall with income if the redistribution scheme is **regressive.** A sales tax is generally considered to be a regressive tax because although everyone pays the same tax rate, consumption expenditures as a fraction of income tend to decrease with income.

Horizontal equity means that "equals should be treated equally." Using income as the standard of comparison, horizontal equity implies that individuals with the same income should pay the same amount of net taxes. If not, the resulting outcome is not fair according to the principle of horizontal equity.

With these principles of horizontal and vertical equity in mind, let's examine supply-side and demand-side subsidies as different ways to redistribute medical services.

Supply-Side Subsidies. A **supply-side subsidy** is essentially a grant of money from a third party that is aimed at reducing the internal costs of producing some consumer-oriented good or service. As an example, the subsidy may be awarded to an institution such as a public hospital or used to finance the education of an important labor input, such as a nurse or physician. A supply-side subsidy typically expands the production of a good in the marketplace by lowering the marginal private cost of production. Given a downward-sloping market demand curve, the price of the good to the consumer declines and quantity demanded increases.

In the absence of any positive externalities, economists generally argue that a supply-side subsidy leads to a misallocation of resources in a market economy. The subsidy distorts market prices and provides a false signal that production is cheaper than it really is. Output in the subsidized sector expands and resources are drawn from nonsubsidized sectors. Hence, too much output is produced in the subsidized sector and not enough resources are allocated to the nonsubsidized sectors. Some economists also argue that supply-side subsidies are an inequitable way of redistributing income. Because the subsidies are directed at the supply side of the market, individuals with different levels of income similarly benefit from the lower prices at the subsidized firms. Rich and poor alike end up paying the same price when redistribution takes place with a supply-side subsidy. Therefore, the principle of vertical equity is sometimes compromised with a supply-side subsidy.

Demand-Side Subsidies. Because a supply-side subsidy is often viewed as inefficient because it distorts resource allocation and as inequitable because it benefits all rather than only poor consumers, many economists favor **demand-side subsidies.** Often (but not always, as in the case of Medicare or the tax exemption on health care benefits) people must qualify for demand-side aid by passing a means test. A means test requires that a household of a certain size has a combined income below some stipulated level to be eligible for the aid. Tying eligibility to household income is one way to satisfy the principles of vertical and horizontal equity. In practice, however, the principle of horizontal equity is violated for Medicaid services because the 50 states specify different guidelines for income eligibility.

One type of demand-side aid is an **in-kind subsidy** that provides needy individuals with specific goods or vouchers for such items as food, housing, medical services, or transportation. The food stamp program, Medicare, and Medicaid are examples of in-kind subsidies. A second type of demand-side aid is a cash subsidy. People are granted a certain amount of income that they can use to purchase various goods and services of their own choice. Temporary Assistance for Needy Families (TANF) and the Supplemental Security Income (SSI) programs provide recipients with cash subsidies. The in-kind subsidy attempts to increase the quantity demanded of a specific good, whereas the cash subsidy is designed to increase the demand for various goods based on the recipient's preferences. Both programs are typically funded by taxes and do not directly affect the prices of the goods and services in the marketplace as long as the subsidized individuals are relatively few in number. A cash subsidy is preferred over in-kind aid if the goal of the donor group is to raise the utility of the recipients to the highest possible level for a given amount of transfer payments. The cash subsidy provides more utility per dollar because recipients are free to choose how they spend the money. If the donor group's goal is to ensure that the recipients consume at least a minimal amount of some specific goods, it can more easily target specific purchases with in-kind aid given the difficulty associated with enforcing spending restrictions on cash subsidies.

Welfare Loss of Taxation. So far we have been discussing the transfer side of the redistribution program. But we cannot overlook the fact that redistribution also involves taxation. That is, some group must be taxed to finance the transfer payments made to the recipient group. According to economic theory, a tax on a resource involved in production may cause a deadweight loss by creating a disincentive for individuals to commit those resources into production. In practice, the tax may fall on the income generated by a number of different resources including labor (such as personal income tax), business capital (corporate business tax), and land (property tax). In the following discussion we consider the impact of a tax on the employment of labor because the personal income tax generates most of the revenues received by both state and federal governments. The same analytical framework can be applied to taxes on other resources and revenue bases (such as sales) as well.

Figure 9–10 shows the supply of labor, S, in some hypothetical market. Notice that market supply is drawn as being upward sloping to suggest that laborers are willing to work more hours at a higher hourly wage rate. A higher hourly wage is necessary to induce more labor hours into production because workers are giving up leisure time. As leisure time diminishes and becomes scarcer with a movement up the labor supply curve, the increased work hours come at a higher opportunity cost. Hence increased wages are necessary to induce workers to commit more labor time into production.

We suppose that the hourly wage equals W before the tax is implemented such that laborers are willing to work L_0 hours. Total labor income equals the area formed by the rectangle WaL_00 and laborer (similar to producer) surplus equals the triangle formed by the area Wae. Laborer surplus equals the difference between labor income and the opportunity cost of leisure time, as measured by the area under the labor supply curve. Laborer surplus reflects the net benefit to the laborers from committing their time to production rather than leisure.

FIGURE 9–10
Impact of an Income Tax in a Labor Market

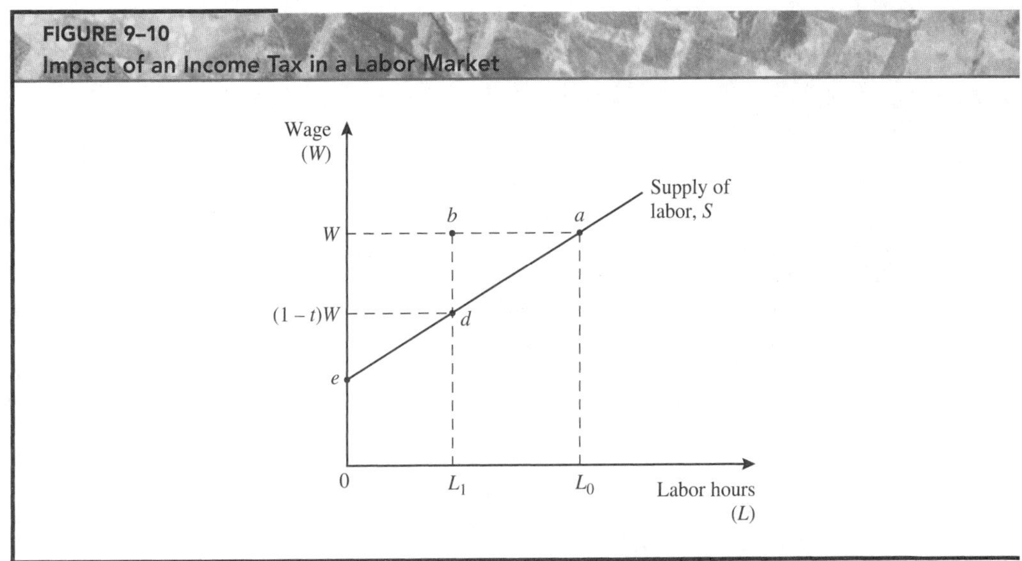

A tax on a productive resource such as labor tends to create an excess burden. Before the tax, laborers devote L_0 hours to production and receive labor surplus of *Wae* at an hourly wage of *W*. When the after tax wage falls to (1 – *t*)*W*, workers commit only L_1 hours to production. Labor surplus fall to the area [(1 – *t*)*W*]*de* and tax revenues equal the area *Wbd* [(1 – *t*)*W*]. Excess burden is measured by the area *bad* that is lost because of the tax.

Now suppose the government imposes a proportional tax on labor income of rate *t*. As a result, the after tax wage rate falls to $(1 - t)W$. For example, the tax rate may equal 20 percent such that workers keep 80 percent of the income they earn per hour. Given the supply of labor, at that lower after-tax wage rate, the hours supplied by workers falls to L_1 in the market. With the tax, notice that worker surplus now falls to the triangular area formed by $[(1 - t)W]de$. Also notice that the tax revenue to the government equals the area $Wbd[(1 - t)W]$. This income tax revenue might be used to finance the transfer payment programs we discussed earlier.

The negative aspect of the tax, however, is reflected in the area *bad,* the laborer surplus or net benefit that is lost because of the tax. This area is referred to as the *excess burden* of the tax. An excess burden results because worker choices between labor and leisure have been distorted such that less labor is committed to production and therefore fewer goods and services are produced in society. Alternatively, stated, if the labor supply curve captures the true marginal social cost of labor and *W* reflects the marginal social benefit of labor, then the amount of labor is not supplied at the point where MSC equals MSB. In short, an inefficient allocation of labor takes place because of the tax and this is reflected in excess burden.

The amount of excess burden created by the tax depends on the elasticity of the supply curve with respect to the wage rate. A more elastic (flatter) supply suggests that a tax imposes a larger excess burden. In fact, a perfectly inelastic supply indicates that a tax on labor income imposes no distortion on the choice between labor and leisure. However, empirical evidence typically lends little support for a perfectly inelastic supply of labor in various markets. The upshot is that taxes can create distortions in input markets and can cause inefficiencies. Thus decision makers must carefully weigh the benefits (equity) and costs (inefficiencies) associated with redistribution programs.[15]

15. A demand for labor is not specified because we are interested in showing only the excess burden of the tax and not the incidence of the tax.

SUMMARY

Government intervention is often necessary to correct situations where the market fails to allocate resources efficiently or distribute income fairly. In this context, government has been assigned the task of providing public goods, correcting externalities, redistributing income, and regulating the marketplace. We should keep in mind, however, that market failure is a necessary but not a sufficient condition for government intervention. Although markets may fail and impose costs on society, the costs of government intervention may be much greater. For example, it may cost the government $10 million in labor and capital costs to correct a problem in the marketplace that is imposing $8 million of damages on society. If so, it is efficient to leave the problem uncorrected. Also, both markets and governments fail in certain circumstances. One objective of economics is to determine which institution can provide which particular services in the most efficient and equitable manner.

CASE STUDIES

9-1 Managed Care Regulation

One of the most active areas of government regulation in recent years has been the regulation[16] of managed care organizations and health plans. Just as the last vestiges of classic utility regulation are giving way to reform—and in some cases complete deregulation—throughout the economy, state and federal legislators over the past decade have been increasingly viewing managed care regulation as the next best alternative to a national health system. For example, during a California Senate Insurance Committee hearing addressing health plan representatives, state senator Jackie Speier stated emphatically, "With more than 24 million people enrolled in managed care in California, you can't tell me that [health plans] should be treated any differently than any other public utility." In her comments, Senator Speier invoked the public interest rationale for economic regulation simply by emphasizing the number of California residents affected by managed care, which involves roughly 70 percent of the state population. State enactment of managed care regulations has diffused rapidly in the United States during the previous decade (Rogal and Stenger, 2001). Many states have enacted at least some form of legislation controlling various aspects of managed care business practices. Regulations typically address two concerns: the content of the benefit package offered by health plans (that is, coverage mandates, such as cancer screenings), and the operations of health plans (such as restrictions on the exclusion criteria for provider networks). As contracts between health plans and providers become more complex and widespread, state legislators are likely to view health plan operations increasingly as an entry point for regulations. Whereas the economic effects of regulation in general are well understood, the application of that body of knowledge to managed care regulation is considerably less developed.

16. "Utility Regulation" is used to distinguish between social regulations aimed exclusively at quality and safety and economic regulations aimed at controlling the economic aspects of markets and firms, including market structure, firm operations, and finances. The term "public-utility regulation," has its roots in its initial application in traditional utility industries such as electricity, water, and natural gas. The core features of utility regulation include an agency charged with overseeing a private industry, employing administrative controls on capacity, quality, costs, profits, or some combination of these. Economic regulation is often observed in industries where markets fail to operate freely and competitively or where the attributes of the markets, products, or services add layers of relatively high complexity to transacting and contracting among producers and consumers.

Questions for Discussion

1. *Why should managed care organizations be regulated?*
2. *The majority of managed care laws resemble those employed in other regulated industries. If some of the features of managed care regulations resemble economic regulation (that is, "public utility" regulation), to what extent might we expect some of the same classic problems associated with economic regulation, such as higher prices and inefficient input mixes?*

9-2 Waiting Lists

Several developed countries have centrally controlled "single payer" health systems. Examples include Canada and Great Britain. In these systems, access to health care services is limited mainly by the availability of physicians, hospital beds, equipment, and supplies. It is also limited by government decisions as to what kinds of care are necessary and appropriate. Few of these systems use financial incentives to control use (such as individual deductibles or coinsurance). The lack of price rationing and often limited availability of specialized personnel or equipment results in waiting lists for many types of services in many health systems, some of which are exceptionally long, at least by U.S. norms. For example, the mean waiting time for a magnetic resonance image (MRI) of the head in Canada in 1997 was 150 days, compared to 3 days in the United States (Bell et al., 1999). Blendon et al. (2002) report similar findings for hospitalizations for elective surgery in a number of countries. The percentage of survey respondents reporting waiting times of four months or more for elective surgery ranged from 23 percent (Australia) to 38 percent (United Kingdom), compared to only 5 percent in the United States (p. 188).

Mechanisms for managing waiting lists vary across health systems and by type of service. In some cases no explicit criteria are used to prioritize individual patients on waiting lists, while in others clinical criteria are used in an attempt to place those with a more immediate need for service closer to the front of the queue (Alter et al., 1999). The latter approach is often hampered by a lack of consensus among experts concerning specific clinical criteria for prioritization (Naylor et al., 1990). Moreover, an individual's placement on a waiting list is also influenced by nonclinical factors, such as nonclinical patient characteristics, characteristics of the referring physician or facility, and geographic location (Naylor et al., 1992; Naylor and Levinton, 1993; Naylor et al., 1993; Hughes and Griffiths, 1997; Arnesen et al., 2002). Although deaths attributable to delays in treatment are rare (Naylor et al., 1995), studies report high levels of anxiety among patients about perceived mortality risk during long delays (Llewellyn-Thomas et al., 1999). For many patients delays in treatment also delay the alleviation of symptoms, such as angina, osteoarthritis pain, or impaired vision. Bishai and Lang (2000) report willingness-to-pay estimates for a reduction in waiting time for cataract surgery to less than 1 month of $128 in Canada, $160 in Denmark, and $243 in Spain (all in 1992 U.S. dollars). In many of these countries, individuals with the means to do so can bypass queues by purchasing services from private providers (sometimes located in different countries).

Questions for Discussion

1. *Are waiting lists a good way to ration health care? Why or why not? What are the main benefits and drawbacks to waiting lists?*
2. *If some patients are willing to pay more for a better place on a waiting list, why not auction off waiting list spots? Should health care be treated differently from other auctioned services? Why or why not?*

9-3 Physician Organizations, Collective Action, and Antitrust

The Texas Surgeons Independent Practice Association (IPA) is a collection of several general surgery practice groups in the Austin area, comprising the majority of general surgeon private practitioners serving the Austin area. According to the Federal Trade Commission (FTC), from 1997 to 1999, Texas Surgeons IPA engaged in "actual or threatened concerted refusals to deal, and to negotiate collectively, in order to obtain higher prices from Blue Cross and Blue Shield of Texas and United Health Care of Texas." The FTC found that the actions of Texas Surgeons IPA had the effect of "depriving consumers of the benefits of competition" and ultimately increasing the costs of health care in the Austin area. A key element of the case was that Texas Surgeons IPA was not a risk-bearing entity (that is, it was paid for most of its work on a fee-for-service basis), and that the collective action among the groups was predominantly for the purpose of extracting higher prices from Blue Cross and United.

Questions for Discussion

1. *If Texas Surgeons IPA had been a risk-bearing entity, or if it had been collectively working on quality and administrative tasks, rather than price negotiations, the FTC probably would not have found fault with its actions. Why is it undesirable to have a group like Texas Surgeons IPA negotiate prices collectively?*
2. *Suppose Blue Cross and United were the only private third-party payers in the Austin area. Would Texas Surgeons IPA have been able to argue that its collective action was necessary to "level the playing field?" Why or why not?*

Review Questions and Problems

1. Discuss the two views of government intervention in a market-based health care system. What role does the politician play in both of these views?
2. Health officials have suggested that the spread of AIDS can be partly contained if more males use condoms while engaging in sexual intercourse. Use the concept of a demand-side externality to explain why the number of condoms sold in the United States is likely to be lower than the optimal number. Explain some ways the government might promote a more optimal use of condoms
3 The discussion on price ceilings supposed that the medical firm faces increasing marginal costs of production. Suppose a for-profit, monopolistic hospital is experiencing economies of scale (that is, downward-sloping average and marginal cost curves) in the relevant range. Show graphically and discuss in writing the problems associated with a price ceiling set where the demand curve intersects the marginal cost curve and a price ceiling set where the demand curve intersects the average cost curve. Think in terms of allocative efficiency and financial solvency.
4. Allied health professionals (for example, social workers) are required by law to possess a professional certificate in some states; in others, they are not. Assuming sufficient data exist, discuss how you might test empirically whether this law exists to protect the public interest or to provide benefits to special interests.
5. Minnesota and Tennessee, among other states, have recently begun to tax the sales of health care providers, such as hospitals and physicians. Analyze the incidence of this sales tax for three different scenarios: (a) The demand for medical services is completely inelastic, while the supply curve is positively sloped to the right; (b) the demand curve is downward sloping

and supply is completely inelastic (for this case, it is best to shift the demand curve downward by the amount of the per-unit tax); and (c) the demand curve is downward sloping and the supply curve is positively sloped. When does the consumer or the health care provider pay a larger portion of the tax? Why?

6. Do you think subsidies should be provided to lower the cost of a medical education? Why or why not? Use a graphical model in your explanation, if possible.
7. Answer the following questions regarding redistribution.
   A. Why must the government perform the redistribution function?
   B. What are horizontal and vertical equity?
   C. What are the differences among proportional, progressive, and regressive taxation?
   D. What are the three ways subsidies can be provided in practice?
   E. Comment on the relative efficiency and equity of these three methods.
8. Define *price fixing*, *boycotting*, *exclusive dealing contracts*, *tying contracts,* and *market allocations*. How have these business practices been viewed by the courts? Explain.
9. Discuss why the courts use a rule of reason when determining whether to allow a horizontal merger.
10. According to Lindsay (1976), why are the average costs of production likely to be lower for a public hospital than for an otherwise identical private hospital?
11. Suppose that the supply of labor is perfectly inelastic with respect to the wage rate in some labor market. Show graphically that no excess burden results from a tax on labor income. What does a perfectly inelastic supply of labor suggest about the opportunity cost of leisure time?
12. Suppose the laborers in a particular market are currently working 200 hours per week at a wage of $40 per hour. Further suppose that the government implements a 25 percent tax on labor income and that these same laborers are willing to work 180 hours at $30 per hour. Calculate the size of the excess burden resulting from this tax (you must know how to calculate the area of a triangle). Using this information, also calculate the elasticity of labor supply with respect to the wage rate. Average the two observations for hours worked and the wage rate when determining the base to calculate each percentage change. Now suppose that the laborers are willing to work 100 hours at $30 per hour. Recalculate the excess burden from a 25 percent tax on labor income and the wage elasticity of labor supply. What does this exercise suggest about the relation between excess burden and the supply of labor?

CEBS Questions

■ *CEBS Sample Question on Subject Matter from CEBS Course 9 Study Manual*

1. Using the special interest group theory, identify the likely winners and losers from a favorable tax treatment policy for long-term care premiums. (pages 230–232)

■ *CEBS Sample Exam Questions*

1. In a supply and demand model, what is the effect of a fee-for-service third-party price ceiling on physician services? (Assume consumers have full health insurance.)
   A. The quantity demanded will exceed the quantity supplied and a shortage of physician services will be created.
   B. The price of physician services will increase.
   C. Supply and demand will not apply after the price ceiling is imposed.

D. The demand curve for physician services will become kinked.
E. Prices for physician services will become more volatile.

2. The Sherman Antitrust Act has been interpreted as prohibiting anticompetitive business practices in health care that include which of the following?
   I. Boycotting
   II. Profit maximization
   III. Price fixing
      A. I only
      B. III only
      C. I and II only
      D. I and III only
      E. I, II, and III
3. All the following are reasons for government intervention in a market-based health care system EXCEPT:
   A. Provision of public goods.
   B. Correction for externalities.
   C. Enforcement of regulations and antitrust laws.
   D. Redistribution of income.
   E. Improvement in managerial quality.

■ *Answer to Sample Question from Study Manual*

Owners of nursing homes, providers of services to such facilities, individuals suffering from debilitating diseases such as Alzheimer's and strokes and their family members would be the winners. The loss of revenues resulting from such a policy would produce losers in the section of the population that relies heavily on public welfare programs and public funding.

■ *Answers to Sample Exam Questions*

1. A is the answer. The lower price creates an incentive for physicians to reduce the quantity supplied and for expenditures on physician services to decline. See pages 242–243 of the text.
2. D is the answer. Statements I and III are correct. Statement II is false; the act doesn't prohibit businesses from maximizing profits. See page 247 of the text.
3. E is the answer. The government doesn't exercise its instruments of taxation and subsidies in the market to alter the performance of managers. See page 232 of the text.

Online Resources

To access Internet links related to the topics in this chapter, please visit our web site at **www.thomsonedu.com/economics/santerre**.

References

Aaron, Henry J., and William B. Schwartz. *The Painful Prescription: Rationing Hospital Care*. Washington, D.C.: The Brookings Institution, 1984.

Alter, D. A., A. Basinkski, E. Cohen, and C. D. Naylor. "Fairness in the Coronary Angiography Queue." Canadian Medical Association Journal 161, no. 7 (1999), pp. 813–17.

Anderson, Gary M., Dennis Halcoussis, Linda Johnston, and Anton D. Lowenberg. "Regulatory Barriers to Entry in the Healthcare Industry; the Case of

Alternative Medicine." *Quarterly Review of Economics and Business* 40 (2000), pp. 485–502.

Arnesen, K. E., J. Erikssen, and K. Stavem. "Gender and Socioeconomic Status as Determinants of Waiting Time for Inpatient Surgery in a System with Implicit Queue Management." *Health Policy* 62, no. 3 (2002), pp. 329–41.

Baker, James N. "Blood in the Water." *Newsweek*, July 18, 1988, p. 35.

Becker, Gary S. "A Theory of Competition among Pressure Groups for Political Influence." *Quarterly Journal of Economics* 93 (August 1983), pp. 371–400.

Bell, C. M., M. Crystal, A. S. Detsky, and D. A. Redelmeier. "Shopping Around for Hospital Services: A Comparison of the United States and Canada." *Journal of the American Medical Association* 279, no. 13 (1999), pp. 1015–17.

Bishai, D. D., and H. C. Lang. "The Willingness to Pay for Wait Reduction: The Disutility of Queues for Cataract Surgery in Canada, Denmark, and Spain." *Journal of Health Economics* 19, no. 2 (2000), pp. 219–30.

Blendon, R. J., C. Schoen, C. M. DesRoches, R. Osborn, K. M. Scoles, and K. Zapert. "Inequities in Health Care: A Five-Country Survey." *Health Affairs* 21, no. 3 (2002), pp. 182–91.

Burda, David. "Flurry of Merger Plans Has Eyes Focused on Iowa." *Modern Healthcare*, April 12, 1993.

Coase, Ronald. "The Problem of Social Cost." *Journal of Law and Economics* 3 (October 1960), pp. 1–44.

Cromwell, Jerry. "Hospital Productivity Trends in Short-Term General Nonteaching Hospitals." *Inquiry* 11, no. 2 (1976), pp. 181–87.

Department of Justice. "United States of America vs. Dentsply International." Civil Action No. 99-005, 1999, http://www.usdoj.gov/atr/cases/f2100/2164.htm (accessed June 18, 2002).

Felsenthal, Edward. "Antitrust Suits Are on the Rise in Health Field." *The Wall Street Journal*, October 29, 1992, p. B1.

———. "New Rules Let Hospitals Start Joint Ventures." *The Wall Street Journal*, May 14, 1993, p. B1.

Frech, H. E. "Monopoly in Health Insurance: The Economics of *Kartell v. Blue Shield of Massachusetts*." In *Health Care in America*, ed. H. E. Frech. San Francisco: Pacific Research Institute for Public Policy, 1988, pp. 293–322.

Greaney, Thomas L. "Whither Antitrust? The Uncertain Future of Competition Law in Health Care." *Health Affairs* 21 (March/April 2002), pp. 185–96.

Havighurst, Clark C. "The Contributions of Antitrust Law to a Procompetitive Health Policy." In *Market Reforms in Health Care*, ed. Jack A. Meyer. Washington, D.C.: American Enterprise Institute, 1983, pp. 295–322.

Hughes, D., and L. Griffiths. "'Ruling In' and 'Ruling Out': Two Approaches to the Micro-Rationing of Health Care." *Social Science and Medicine* 44, no. 5 (1997), pp. 589–99.

Jacobsen, Raymond A., Jr., and Robert B. Wiggins. "Denials of Staff Privileges Face Increased Antitrust Scrutiny." *Health Care Management Review* 17 (fall 1992), pp. 7–15.

Kleiner, Morris M., and Robert T. Kudrle. "Does Regulation Affect Economic Outcomes? The Case of Dentistry." *Journal of Law and Economics* 43 (October 2000), pp. 547–82.

Kopit, William G. "Health and Antitrust: The Case for Legislative Relief." In *Market Reforms in Health Care*, ed. Jack A. Meyer. Washington, D.C.: American Enterprise Institute, 1983, pp. 323–31.

Lindsay, Cotton M. "A Theory of Government Enterprise." *Journal of Political Economy* 84 (October 1976), pp. 1061–77.

Llewellyn-Thomas, H., E. Theil, M. Paterson, and C. D. Naylor. "In the Queue for Coronary Artery Bypass Grafting: Patients' Perceptions of Risk and 'Maximal Acceptable Waiting Time.'" *Journal of Health Services, Research, and Policy* 4, no. 2 (1999), pp. 65–72.

Lynk, William J. "Tying and Exclusive Dealing: *Jefferson Parish Hospital v. Hyde*." In *The Antitrust Revolution*, 2nd ed, eds. J. E. Kwoka, Jr., and L. J. White. New York: HarperCollins, 1994.

Manning, Willard G., et al. "The Taxes of Sin: Do Smokers and Drinkers Pay Their Way?" *Journal of the American Medical Association* (March 17, 1989), pp. 1604–9.

Musgrave, Richard A., and Peggy B. Musgrave. *Public Finance in Theory and Practice.* New York: McGraw-Hill, 1989.

Naylor, C. D., A. Basinski, R. Baigrie, B. Goldman, and J. Lomas. "Placing Patients in a Queue for Coronary Revascularization: Evidence for Practice Variations form an Expert Panel Process." *American Journal of Public Health* 80, no. 10 (1990), pp. 1246–52.

Naylor, C. D., and C. M. Levinton. "Sex-Related Differences in Coronary Revascularization Practices: The Perspective from a Canadian Queue Management Project." *Canadian Medical Association Journal* 149, no. 7 (1993), pp. 965–73.

Naylor, C. D., C. M. Levinton, R. Baigrie, and B. Goldman. "Placing Patients in the Queue for Coronary Surgery: Do Age and Work Status Alter Canadian Specialists' Decisions?" *Journal of General Internal Medicine* 7, no. 5 (1992), pp. 492–8.

Naylor, C. D., C. M. Levinton, S. Wheeler, and L. Hunter. "Queueing for Coronary Surgery During Severe Supply-Demand Mismatch in a Canadian Referral Centre: A Case Study of Implicit Rationing." *Social Science and Medicine* 37, no. 1 (1993), pp. 61–67.

Naylor, C. D., K. Sykora, S. Jaglai, and S. Jefferson. "Waiting for Coronary Artery Bypass Surgery: Population-Based Study of 8517 Consecutive Patients in Ontario, Canada." *Lancet* 346, no. 8990 (1995), pp. 1605–9.

Ohsfeldt, Robert L., and Stephan F. Gohmann. "The Economics of AIDS-Related Health Insurance Regulations: Interest Group Influence and Ideology." *Public Choice* 74 (July 1992), pp. 105–26.

Peltzman, Sam. "Toward a More General Theory of Regulation." *Journal of Law and Economics* 19 (August 1976), pp. 211–40.

Rogal, D., and R. Stenger. "The Challenge of Managed Care Regulation: Making Markets Work?" Washington, D. C.: Academy for Health Services Research and Health Policy, 2001.

Rosen, Harvey S. *Public Finance.* Homewood, Ill.: Richard D. Irwin, Inc., 1995.

Rutala, William A., Robert L. Odette, and Gregory P. Samsa. "Management of Infectious Waste by U.S. Hospitals." *Journal of the American Medical Association* 262 (September 22–29, 1989), pp. 1635–40.

Stigler, George J. "The Theory of Economic Regulation." *Bell Journal of Economics and Management Sciences* 2 (1971), pp. 137–46.

Svorny, Shirley V. "Physician Licensure: A New Approach to Examining the Role of Professional Interests." *Economic Inquiry* 25 (July 1987), pp. 497–509.

Viscusi, E. Kip, John M. Vernon, and Joseph E. Harrington. *Economics of Regulation and Antitrust,* 3rd ed. Cambridge, Mass.: MIT Press, 2000.

Williamson, Oliver E. "Economies as an Antitrust Defense: Reply." *American Economic Review* 59 (December 1969), pp. 954–59.

GOVERNMENT AS HEALTH INSURER

"No longer will older Americans be denied the healing miracle of modern medicine. No longer will illness crush and destroy the savings they have so carefully put away over a lifetime so they might enjoy dignity in their later years. No longer will young families see their own income, and their own hopes eaten away simply because they are carrying out their deep moral obligations to their parents, and to their uncles, and to their aunts. . . . No longer will this Nation refuse the hand of justice to those who have given a lifetime of service and wisdom and labor to the progress of this progressive country." (Speech by President Lyndon Johnson on July 30, 1965, at the Truman Library in Independence, Missouri, upon signing into law the Medicare and Medicaid programs, as quoted in DeParle [2000])

And thus began the Medicare and Medicaid programs, the most important domestic legislation of the post–World War II era. The legislation was the political brainchild of Congressman Wilbur Mills and was referred to as a "three-layer cake." The first layer was the Johnson administration's proposed Medicare plan, a mandatory program to cover the hospital costs of the elderly and referred to as Part A. The second layer, called Medicare Part B, which was initially proposed by the AMA and Republicans who were opposed to the mandatory program, was designed to provide voluntary coverage to the elderly for physician costs; the third layer, Medicaid, expanded federal assistance to states for public insurance coverage of the poor elderly and disabled, and parents and their dependent children (DeParle, 2002).

These two public health insurance programs have continued to evolve and change over the years. The total costs of the Medicare and Medicaid programs, when combined, totaled more than $550 billion in 2003, or approximately one-third of all national health expenditures. All indications are that these figures are going to increase in the future. Recent estimates have the total price tag for the Medicaid and Medicare programs increasing to $1.4 trillion by 2014 (Heffler et al., 2005). This represents an increase of more than 148 percent in a little more than a decade! Needless to say, elected officials are going to have their hands full over the next few years as they try to balance the desire to provide high-quality health care against competing needs and the want to hold the line on any major tax increases.

Given the importance of the Medicaid and Medicare programs, this chapter:

- describes the structure and operation of the Medicaid and Medicare programs
- discusses recent reforms that have taken place in the Medicaid and Medicare programs

The information presented should be useful to you in your role as a concerned citizen, health care policy maker, or future recipient of Medicare services.

WHY DOES THE GOVERNMENT PRODUCE HEALTH INSURANCE?

In the case of the Medicare and Medicaid programs, which are the focus of this chapter, government acts as a *producer* of health insurance for certain segments of U.S. society (elderly people, some disadvantaged groups, and people with certain disabilities). As a producer, government collects the tax and/or premium revenues, bears some residual risk, and establishes the reimbursement paid to health care providers.[1] Economists normally argue that government should intervene when a market fails to allocate resources efficiently or distribute income equitably. As we saw in earlier chapters, an inefficient allocation of resources occurs when a small number of powerful sellers dominate the industry, barriers to entry are substantial, consumers lack perfect information, or the exclusion principle does not hold (as for externality or public good considerations). An inequitable distribution of income results when some people lack the production characteristics needed to generate a sufficient level of income in the private marketplace.

Usually, when markets fail, government intervenes by either subsidizing the prices of goods and services when inequities are present (for example, through food stamps and housing allowances) or regulating the production of goods and services when inefficiencies otherwise exist in an unregulated environment (such as electric utilities). That is, government typically subsidizes or regulates private production instead of directly producing the good or service. Consequently, the current system of public production of health insurance for certain population segments raises the following two related questions:

1. What is the source of market failure in the private health insurance industry that necessitates government intervention?
2. Why does the government act as a producer of health insurance for certain population segments?

Since individual buyers tend to internalize the benefit (that is, financial security or access value, see Chapter 6) that health insurance provides, it appears that externality or public goods considerations can be ruled out. Also, as Chapter 11 confirms, the private health insurance industry appears to be reasonably competitive because of the large number of competitive fringe insurers and because self-insurance represents an alternative for large employers. In addition, barriers to entry are low, so a monopoly market structure cannot substantiate government intervention. Ruling out the exclusion principle and monopoly structure leaves imperfect information as the primary economic rationale for government intervention in the health insurance industry.

In particular, consider that public health insurance presently coexists with private for-profit and private not-for-profit health insurance in the United States. As we saw in Chapter 4, different forms of ownership may coexist in markets where imperfect information exists and demands for services are heterogeneous. The imperfect information exists because some consumers lack the information they need to understand the technical terms and conditions contained in health insurance policies. Think about it. The description and explanation of health insurance nomenclature, such as deductibles, copayments, benefit coverage, and maximum liability can be mind-boggling for even the most educated individuals (Garnick et al., 1993).

Individual consumers who are uninformed may feel vulnerable to noncompetitive behavior on the part of for-profit insurers and therefore may prefer to deal with not-for-profit insurance providers that they perceive as being less likely to profit from consumer ignorance. However, not

1. The government often pays private health insurance companies to "administer" public health insurance. Private health insurers process the claims and pay the stipulated amounts to health care providers.

all people are uninformed. Some people are fairly knowledgeable or belong to group policies represented by informed individuals. Informed consumers may be willing to deal with for-profit health insurance providers, especially when offered quality coverage at a low price.

As a result, it is likely that government acts as a producer of health insurance in the United States as a result of informational problems and an associated demand for government-produced health insurance by certain population segments. It should be noted that the Medicare and Medicaid programs were originally structured to provide health insurance to the "medically needy"—elderly, disabled, and poor individuals—a unique group in society. As a producer, the government not only subsidizes the health insurance to promote equity but also helps to avoid the inefficiencies normally associated with information imperfections in the private health insurance market.[2]

The Medicaid Program

The Medicaid program is designed to provide medical coverage to certain individuals with low incomes. Federal and state governments jointly share the cost of the program, but states administer the program and have wide latitude in determining eligibility and the medical benefits provided. As a result, it is difficult to describe the program except in the broadest of terms.

Eligibility under the Medicaid program is determined at the state level and varies extensively across states. At a minimum, states must provide medical coverage to most individuals covered under other federal income maintenance programs, such as the Temporary Assistance for Needy Families and Supplemental Security Income programs, to receive matching federal funds. Among other additional requirements, states must provide coverage to children under age 6 and to pregnant women whose family incomes are below 133 percent of the federal poverty level, and to all children born after September 1983 who are under age 19 and are in families with incomes at or below the federal poverty level. The federal government also requires that certain basic medical benefits be provided, such as (but not limited to) inpatient and outpatient hospital services, physician services, prenatal care, and vaccines for children.

As you can see from Table 10–1, the total number of Medicaid recipients hovered between 21 and 23 million throughout most of the 1970s and 1980s. At the close of the 1980s, however, things changed dramatically as economic growth stagnated throughout the country and changes in the Medicaid program expanded eligibility. From 1990 to 2002, the number of Medicaid recipients nearly doubled to almost 50 million individuals. A breakdown of recipients in 2002 shows that the single largest group was dependent children under age 21, accounting for 47.7 percent of the recipients. The next largest group, with 25.7 percent of the recipients, was adults in families with dependent children. Individuals with permanent and total disabilities (15.6 percent) and individuals age 65 and older (9.2 percent) constituted the next two largest groups of Medicaid recipients.

A look at total vendor payments by group tells a slightly different story. The lion's share of vendor payments went to individuals with permanent and total disabilities (43.0 percent). The next largest group was elderly people, with 24.2 percent of total payments, followed by dependent children with 14.6 percent. Finally, adults in families with dependent children accounted for 10.9 percent of the Medicaid payments. The change in order between the two groupings based on total recipients and total costs reflects the high cost of caring for elderly and disabled individuals. For

2. Due to imperfect information, adverse selection problems are also associated with the private provision of health insurance. See Chapter 11.

TABLE 10–1
Total Number of Medicaid Recipients and Total Vendor Payments for Medicaid, Selected Years 1972–2002

Year	Total Number of Recipients (millions)	Total Vendor Payments (millions)
1972	17.6	$ 6,300
1975	22.0	12,242
1980	21.6	23,311
1985	21.8	37,508
1990	25.3	64,859
1995	36.3	120,141
1998	40.6	142,318
2002	49.7	213,491

SOURCE: U.S. Department of Health and Human Services, Social Security Administration. *Annual Statistical Supplement*, 2004, Table 8.E.

example, in 2002 the average Medicaid payment for elderly and disabled people was $10,870 and $11,407, respectively. For dependent children the average payment was only $1,271; for adults it was $1,771. Much of the difference is explained by the high cost of nursing home care for elderly and disabled Medicaid recipients.

The Financing and Cost of Medicaid

Medicaid is financed jointly by the federal and state governments, with the federal portion varying between a low of 50 percent and a potential high of 83 percent. States with the lowest per capita income receive the largest federal subsidy. In 2005, eleven states were reimbursed at the minimum level. Mississippi received the largest subsidy (77.08 percent), followed by West Virginia (75.27 percent). The average share subsidized by the federal government in 2001 was 57 percent.

The cost of the Medicaid program has increased substantially over time. As Table 10–1 indicates, the Medicaid program cost a little more than $6 billion in 1972 and that figure ballooned to more than $213 billion by 2002. A number of reasons account for this large increase in cost. First and foremost was a significant rise in the number of enrollees, especially between 1990 and 2002, when the number of enrollees nearly doubled. The increase was primarily due to a number of changes in the Medicaid program that extended coverage to children and pregnant women. For example, federal mandates dictated that by 1990 Medicaid coverage was to be extended to children under age 6 and pregnant women in families with incomes below 133 percent of the federal poverty line.

Another reason for the increase in cost was a significant increase in medical prices, which forced states to increase reimbursement rates to medical care providers. High rates of medical price inflation and technological advances largely account for the increase in medical prices. Another factor was the increase in the number of elderly and disabled individuals in need of long-term care.

Efforts on the part of states to increase federal funding of Medicaid also contributed to rising Medicaid costs. As you can imagine, these efforts were met with some resistance from the federal government, which has had its own budgetary difficulties. Some of these efforts have been dubbed "Medicaid maximization" and involve shifting state-run health programs into the Medicaid program so that they will qualify for matching federal funds. Mental health and mental retardation services were the most common services shifted into state Medicaid programs (Coughlin et al., 1994).

Finally, **disproportionate share hospital payments** contributed to the rise in Medicaid expenditures. This was a way for states to acquire federal funds and help defer the expenses of hospitals that cared for a disproportionately high number of low-income individuals. Coughlin et al. describe these programs as follows:

> *Providers, usually hospitals, donated funds or paid a tax to the state. The states would then use the donations or tax revenue to make Medicaid payments and, in the transaction, receive federal matching dollars. Generally the programs operated so that providers were held harmless; that is, providers were refunded their full donations or tax contribution. Most often they received a bonus. (p. 485)*

Do Differences in the Medicaid Program Make a Difference?

To receive federal funds to support the Medicaid program, the federal government mandates that certain populations receive medical coverage and that certain basic medical services be included in the coverage. After these minimum requirements are met, states are free to change the program to meet their individual needs. As a result, Medicaid programs vary widely across the country in terms of eligibility requirements, medical services covered, and payments to providers. In addition, the program has gone through a number of changes at the federal level that have involved relaxing eligibility requirements to provide health care coverage to needy populations, specifically children and pregnant mothers. The basic question arises as to whether differences in the program over time and across states have any impact on the health of Medicaid-eligible populations. For the sake of consistency, we focus on studies looking at poor children and their mothers.

In two related studies, Currie and Thomas (1995) and Cutler and Gruber (1996) found that expanded Medicaid eligibility for low-income children improved access to health care. Specifically, Currie and Thomas found that Medicaid coverage decreased the probability that a child failed to have a routine checkup within the past year by 15 percent. Looking at the Medicaid programs of thirteen states, Long and Coughlin (2001/2002) found that significant differences existed across states in terms of access to and use of health care by children with Medicaid coverage even after controlling for demographic, socioeconomic, and health factors. Completing the circle, Kronebusch (2001) examined the impact of policy changes across states from 1979 to 1998. He found that recent federal policy changes have increased Medicaid enrollment of children nationwide and at the same time have decreased state-level variations in enrollment patterns over time. However, significant state-level policy differences still existed.

The evidence also indicates that Medicaid fees vary widely across the country and are generally lower than comparable private or Medicare rates. If the rates are set too low by state authorities, access problems are created for individuals covered under Medicaid. If rates are too low, profit-maximizing health care providers may find it in their best interest not to participate in the Medicaid program at all. That's because their time may be better spent servicing the medical needs of more lucrative private-pay or Medicare patients. Low Medicaid fees may also impact the quality of the care provided to Medicaid patients. Take the case of the physician who finds the Medicaid fee for a well-child office visit to be below some acceptable level. To make up the difference, the physician may spend less time with the child than otherwise would be the case and at the same time minimize the level of beneficial services provided.[3] In either case, the overall quality of care provided to children on Medicaid is adversely impacted because the physician is being compensated at a level below the comparable private-pay or Medicare rate.

Curious about the precise extent to which Medicaid fees vary across states, Zuckerman et al. (2004) report on changes in Medicaid physician fees from 1998 through 2003. The authors find that the average Medicaid fee varied widely across the country. Developing an index that equaled 1.00 for the national average, they find that fees ranged from a low of 0.56 for New Jersey to a high of 2.28 for Alaska. Ten states had Medicaid fees that were at least 25 percent greater than the national weighted average; three states had fees that were at least 25 percent lower than the national weighted average. The survey also uncovered that Medicaid fees lag behind comparable Medicare fees, as the average Medicaid-to-Medicare ratio for the entire country equaled 0.69 in 2003. Despite these rather dismal figures, the authors note that Medicaid fees did increase by 27.4 percent from 1998 through 2003.

The evidence appears to suggest that Medicaid fees have a direct impact on the level of medical care provided to Medicaid recipients. Utilizing a data set on physician practices from the late 1980s and early 1990s, Baker and Royalty (2000) found that a 10 percent increase in Medicaid fees resulted in a 2.4 percent increase in office-based physician visits for poor patients. Taking the discussion one step further, Currie et al. (1995) and Gray (2001) establish a connection between Medicaid fees and health care outcomes. The first study finds that a 10 percent increase in the Medicaid-to-private-fee ratio for obstetricians/gynecologists lowered the infant mortality rate by between 0.5 and 0.9 percent. In the second study, Gray (2001) finds a relationship between Medicaid physician fees and birth outcomes. According to his estimates, a 10 percent increase in the average relative Medicaid fee decreased the risk of low birthweight for a newborn by 0.074 percent and the risk of a very low birthweight by 0.035 percent.[4]

Finally, with the expanded eligibility of vulnerable populations in the Medicaid program beginning in the mid-1980s, there has been some concern as to whether the Medicaid expansion has "crowded out" private insurance. For example, in the 1980s Medicaid coverage was expanded to a number of low-income pregnant women and children. Might it be that those who became eligible for Medicaid would have otherwise opted for private insurance? Blumberg et al. (2000) point out that crowding out can occur if some people elect to drop private insurance coverage and become eligible for Medicaid, or if others who are uninsured opt for Medicaid as opposed to private insurance.

A study by Cutler and Gruber (1996) finds significant levels of crowding out. In particular, the authors discover that about 50 percent of the Medicaid enrollment from 1987 to 1992 resulted in a decrease in private insurance coverage. More recent studies have estimated more modest levels of crowding out. For example, Dubay and Kenney (1997) find that 14 percent of the increase in Medicaid coverage for pregnant women caused crowding out, while Yazici and Kaestner (2000) estimate that almost 19 percent of the increase in Medicaid enrollment resulted in crowding-out of private insurance. Finally, Blumberg et al. (2000) estimate the displacement impact to be a very modest 4 percent. Collectively, these studies suggest that while there appears to be a certain amount of crowding out, the bulk of the increase in Medicaid enrollment in recent years came from the ranks of the uninsured.

---

3. The economics of price differentials resulting from the Medicaid program are discussed in more detail in Chapter 15. The interested reader is urged to jump to the section on the dual market model and apply the model to the current pricing problem.

4. A low birthweight is less than 2.5 kg., a very low birthweight is less than 1.5 kg.

This body of literature is extremely helpful to policy analysts because it suggests that any meaningful policy initiative aimed at improving health outcomes among needy populations by expanding Medicaid coverage must involve not only a careful look at eligibility requirements but also Medicaid fees. Naturally, this information is not likely to be greeted kindly by politicians and taxpayers because it implies an increase in both the number of enrollees in the Medicaid program and the cost per enrollee.

The State Children's Health Insurance Program

In 1996 approximately 42 million people in the United States were without health insurance coverage and almost a quarter of that group were children under age 18. Feeling the political pressure to address what some felt was a national disgrace, Congress enacted the State Children's Health Insurance Program (SCHIP) as part of the Balanced Budget Act of 1997. The ultimate objective of SCHIP is to decrease the number of uninsured children by providing federal funds to states that initiate plans to expand insurance coverage to low-income, uninsured children. The federal government has committed approximately $40 billion to the program over a ten-year period from 1998 through 2007. As of 2001, state allotments were based on the number of low-income and low-income uninsured children in the state, adjusted by a geographic cost factor. SCHIP is designed to give states considerable latitude when addressing the problem of uninsured children. Each state that elects to participate in the program must submit a plan for approval that articulates how it intends to utilize the funds. States have the option of expanding insurance coverage through their existing Medicaid programs, developing separate child health insurance programs, or using a combination of the two.

Now that SCHIP has been in existence for nearly a decade, researchers have begun to assess the impact of the program. Kenney and Chang (2004) argue that despite its young age, SCHIP has had a positive impact on the health and well-being of the young. In just a few years every state and a number of territories have managed to adopt SCHIP in some form. According to the Centers for Medicare & Medicaid Services, as of 2006, 56 states and territories have approved plans that are evenly divided among the three options. In addition, many states have implemented plans to improve enrollment and enhance retention. For example, some states have developed media campaigns to increase awareness of the program, while others have streamlined the application process. Still others have relaxed admission standards. Clearly, much research needs to be done to determine which strategies work best at expanding enrollments in SCHIP.

A study by Kronebusch and Elbel (2004) can serve as a valuable guide to future researchers concerning the factors that impact enrollment in SCHIP. Using survey data from the *Current Population Survey* in 2001, they find that SCHIP plans administered as part of the Medicaid program enroll more children than stand-alone or combination programs. Why that is the case is not fully understood. The authors also find that removing the asset test and allowing applicants to self-report income positively impacts enrollment. Understandably, lengthy waiting periods and higher premiums negatively impact enrollments. Surprisingly, streamlining the application process by allowing mail-in and telephone applications has no impact on enrollments.

Kenney and Chang (2004) also note that SCHIP currently provides insurance coverage to millions of children. Enrollment in the program increased sharply when the program first began and has continued to increase in recent years, albeit at a lower rate. More than 4.4 million children were enrolled in SCHIP during some part of the first quarter of 2005. With expanded insurance coverage has come greater access to health care. Based on a survey of new enrollees in three states (Florida, Kansas, and New York), Dick et al. (2004) find that new enrollees have greater access to medical care along with enhanced satisfaction.

Despite these achievements, Kenney and Chang (2004) point out that SCHIP suffers from a few shortcomings. For one thing, millions of children still remain without health insurance. According to the Bureau of the Census, 8.4 million children were without health insurance in 2002. While not all of these children are eligible for insurance coverage under SCHIP, much more can be done to improve enrollments. Lo Sasso and Buchmueller (2004) estimate that only 9 percent of children that are income eligible gained insurance through SCHIP from 1996 through 2000. Evidence also indicates that the expansion of SCHIP enrollees substituted public health insurance coverage for private coverage. While it is difficult to determine the extent to which this substitution takes place, Lo Sasso and Buchmueller (2004) find that nearly half of the increase in SCHIP enrollments resulted in a crowding out of private insurance. Other shortcomings with SCHIP include uncertainty in funding sources (remember that the program is funded at the federal level only through 2007) and the fact that few states have the resources to estimate the full impact of SCHIP on the eligible population.

The Medicare Program

The primary objective of the Medicare program is to improve access to medical care for elderly people by underwriting a portion of their medical expenditures. Anyone age 65 or older is eligible for the program.[5] The program is made up of four distinct components: Part A, the Hospital Insurance program, which is compulsory; Part B, the Supplementary Medical Insurance program, which is voluntary; Part C, the Medicare Advantage Program, which gives individuals the opportunity to participate in private health insurance plans; and Part D, which provides a drug benefit plan.

The Hospital Insurance portion of the program primarily covers (1) inpatient hospital services, (2) some types of posthospital care, and (3) hospice care. The number of people age 65 and older covered under Part A has increased rapidly over the years and reflects the growing elderly population. In 1966, when the program first began, slightly more than 19 million elderly individuals were enrolled, and by 2004 the number of Medicare enrollees had grown to almost 35 million.

The Supplementary Medical Insurance program provides benefits for (1) physician services, (2) outpatient medical services, (3) emergency room services, and (4) a variety of other medical services. Although Part B of Medicare is voluntary and requires a monthly premium to participate, a large number of elderly people have elected to purchase the insurance. During the initial year of the program, slightly more than 17 million elderly people participated and by 2004 the number had increased to slightly more than 33 million, almost matching the number of enrollees in the compulsory portion of Medicare. This trend reflects the fact that the federal government heavily subsidizes the cost of the supplementary insurance program.

The Medicare Advantage program, formally known as the Medicare + Choice program, provides Medicare beneficiaries the choice to join private insurance plans in an attempt to improve the efficiency and quality of health care services. Finally, Part D is voluntary for most individuals (for dually eligible Medicaid/Medicare individuals it is mandatory) and offers Medicare beneficiaries prescription drug benefits for a heavily subsidized monthly premium.

5. In addition, the Medicare program covers some individuals younger than age 65 who are severely disabled or have kidney disease.

The Financing and Cost of Medicare

Since its inception, total expenditures on the Medicare program have increased at a brisk pace. In 1966 the federal government spent $7.7 billion on the Medicare program; by 1980 this figure had increased almost fivefold to $37.8 billion. As of 2003, total expenditures exceeded $274 billion, with an average rate of increase of 8.4 percent from 2000 through 2003. The rise in Medicare expenses through the years is explained by an increase in both the number of enrollees and reimbursement per enrollee, with the latter accounting for the majority of the increase.

Figure 10–1 displays the major funding sources for the Hospital Insurance program. The main source of funding has been a payroll tax of 2.9 percent, which employees and employers share equally. The payroll tax accounted for approximately 85 percent of total revenues in 2003. The second-largest revenue source has been interest income emanating from the Federal Hospital Insurance Trust Fund, which was established at the inception of the program and which has built up over the years. Interest income topped $15.8 billion in 2003 and accounted for 9 percent of total receipts. Income from the taxation of benefits accounted for another 5 percent of total receipts. The remaining receipts, "Other" in Figure 10–1, made up 1 percent of total receipts and included transfers from the railroad retirement account, reimbursements from general revenues for uninsured people and military wage credits, and premiums of voluntary enrollees.

Medicare beneficiaries face a number of financial incentives similar to those of the privately insured to curb expenses. As we learned in Chapter 5, the out-of-pocket price, as captured by the size of the deductible and coinsurance, inversely affects the quantity demanded of medical care.

FIGURE 10–1
Receipts for the Hospital Insurance Program, 2003

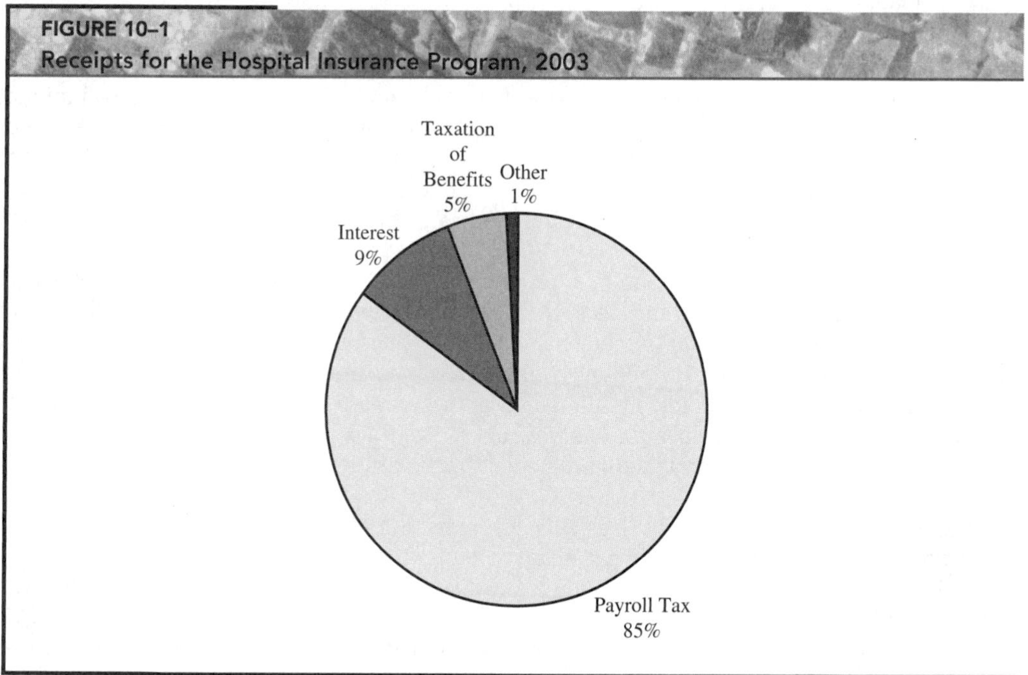

SOURCE: U.S. Department of Health and Human Services, Social Security Administration. *Annual Statistical Supplement, 2004.*

TABLE 10–2
The Cost Sharing for Medicare, Selected Years 1966–2006

	Hospital Insurance			Supplementary Medical Insurance		
	Deductible	Daily Coinsurance		Payment		
	1–60 days	61–90 days	After 90 days	Annual Deductible	Coinsurance Rate	Monthly Premium
1966	$ 40	$ 10	—	$ 50	20%	$ 3.00
1970	52	13	26	50	20%	5.30
1980	180	45	90	60	20%	9.60
1990	592	148	296	75	20%	28.60
2001	792	198	396	100	20%	50.00
2006	952	238	476	124	20%	88.60

SOURCE: U.S. Department of Health and Human Services, Social Security Administration. *Annual Statistical Supplement, 2001;* and Centers for Medicare & Medicaid Services web site (http://www.cms.hhs.gov).

The first three columns in Table 10–2 supply deductible and coinsurance information for Part A of Medicare. In 1966 the deductible was $40. It increased steadily through the years and by 2006 it equaled $952. Once the deductible is met, Medicare covers all inpatient hospital expenses for the first 60 days. For days 61–90, the enrollee is required to pay a daily coinsurance payment equal to 25 percent of the inpatient hospital deductible, or $238. After day 90, Medicare no longer covers hospital inpatient expenses. However, each enrollee is provided with an additional 60-day lifetime reserve. The reserve can be used only once and has a daily coinsurance rate of 50 percent for inpatient hospital deductible, which equaled $476 a day in 2006. Notice that once the deductible is met, the coinsurance rate is initially zero and then increases with the number of hospital inpatient days. Clearly, the intent of Medicare Part A is to provide insurance coverage for short-term hospital stays.

The supplementary Medical Insurance program, or Part B of Medicare, is financed partly through premium payments for enrollees. In 2003, total revenues exceeded $89.9 billion, with premium payments contributing 24 percent of the total. According to Figure 10–2, the largest source of revenues has been contributions by the government and represents the extent to which the federal government subsidies premiums. Over the years, the government has consistently provided approximately 74 percent of total revenues. The final source has been interest income from a trust fund, which has provided only a small fraction of revenues over the years (2 percent in 2003).

Despite the rapid growth in enrollees over the years, Supplementary Medical Insurance premiums had to increase to provide the necessary revenues. As noted earlier, this is largely because expenditures per enrollees grew at a much faster pace than the number of new enrollees. According to Table 10–2, the monthly premium was $88.60 in 2006, up from $3 a month in 1966. In addition, the enrollee is obligated to pay an annual deductible equal to $124 and a coinsurance rate equal to 20 percent on most charges.

Given that the monthly premium is set below the expected benefits to be paid because of the rather generous government subsidy, Medicare-eligible recipients have a strong incentive to

FIGURE 10–2
Receipts for the Supplementary Medical Insurance Program, 2003

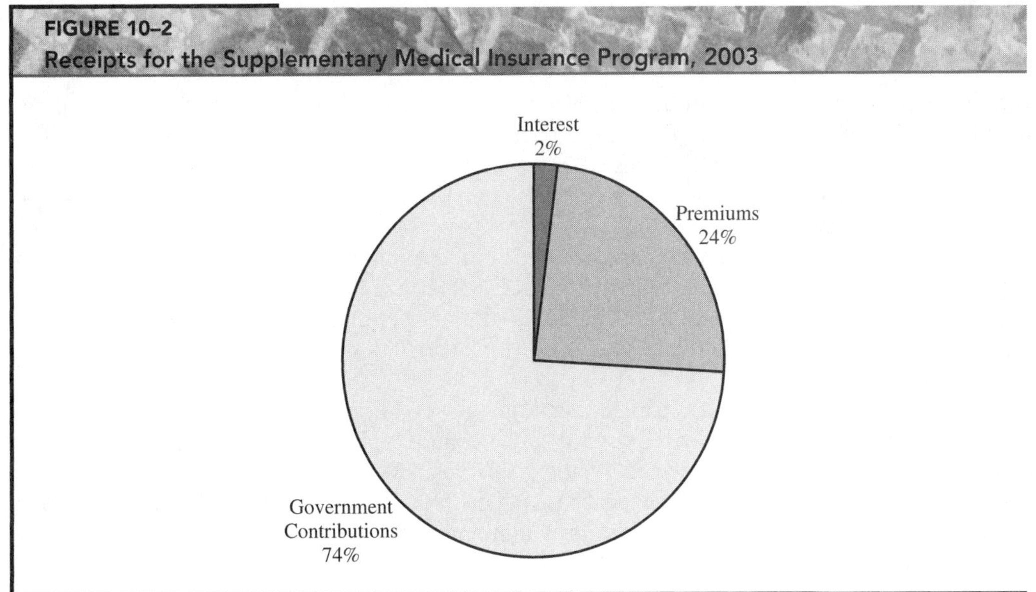

SOURCE: U.S. Department of Health and Human Services, Social Security Administration. *Annual Statistical Supplement, 2004*.

enroll in the Supplementary Medical Insurance program. The heavily subsidized premium, coupled with a modest annual deductible and a 20% coinsurance rate, explains why the national enrollment figures for Part B of Medicare, which is voluntary, nearly match those of Part A, which is compulsory.

The new Medicare Part D drug benefit, which began January 1, 2006, provides Medicare beneficiaries the opportunity to purchase private insurance plans that provide coverage for prescription drugs. Part D is set up such that the federal government funds approximately 75 percent of the basic prescription drug coverage, while the remaining 25 percent is funded from premiums collected from enrollees. According to the Congressional Budget Office (http://www.cbo.gov), the prescription drug program is estimated to cost the federal government in the neighborhood of $400 billion from 2006 through 2013. Monthly premium rates for the basic drug coverage are estimated to run around $37 for 2006 (MedPAC, 2005).

Medicare Program Reforms

Facing a growing federal deficit and an elderly population frustrated by ever-rising deductibles, copayments, and premiums, Congress was forced to alter the Medicare program over the years. The objective has always been to contain costs while at the same time improving access to medical care for elderly people. Instead of going through the tedious process of examining each policy change, we focus on three of the most significant reforms to the Medicare program. The first major reform took place in 1983, when a new payment system for hospitals was implemented based on diagnosis-related groups (DRGs). The second was the passage of the Omnibus Budget Reconciliation Act of 1989, which significantly altered the method of payment to physicians.

Finally, the Balanced Budget Act of 1997 radically expanded plans available to beneficiaries and the rate of managed care.

Diagnosis-Related Groups. In just five years (1975 to 1980), Medicare expenditures on inpatient hospital services grew by more than 120 percent from $8.8 billion to $19.5 billion (U.S. Department of Health and Human Services, 1993). In reaction to the expenditure increase. Congress instituted a prospective payment system (PPS) to compensate hospitals for medical services provided to Medicare patients.

Under the PPS, Medicare patients are classified based on their principal diagnosis into one of approximately 560 or so diagnosis-related groups (DRGs) on entering a hospital. The prospective payment received by the hospital is a fixed dollar amount per discharge and largely depends on the DRG classification with adjustments made for factors that contribute to cost differences across hospitals.

In particular, Medicare sets a separate operating and capital payment rate for every discharge. These rates "are intended to cover the operating and capital costs that efficient facilities would be expected to incur in furnishing covered inpatient services" (MedPAC, 2002, p. 12). In most cases, the payment is established by multiplying a base payment by the relative weight for each DRG. The payment rate is then modified to account for variations in input prices across the country and a number of hospital and case-specific attributes.

Each DRG weight reflects the average cost of medical care for that particular medical problem relative to the average Medicare case. The DRG weight is an index number, based on the total medical charges, that reflects the relative costs across all hospitals of providing care to the average patient in a particular DRG. The higher the DRG weight, the greater the prospective payment. In 2006, the relative weight ranged from a low of 0.0987 for DRG 448 (an allergic reaction for someone under age 18) to a high of 19.8 for DRG 541 (extracorporeal membrane oxygenerator or tracheostomy with mechanical vent). The five most common DRGs, accounting for 19 percent of all short-term hospital discharges in 2004, are shown in Table 10–3.

TABLE 10–3
Five Most Common DRGs for 2004

DRG #	Description	Total Discharges
127	Heart failure and shock	699,142
089	Simple pneumonia and pleurisy, with age greater than 17 and with complications and/or comorbidities	554,672
209 210	Major joint and limb reattachment procedures of lower extremities	464,512
088	Chronic obstructive pulmonary diseases	415,743
182	Esophagistic, Gastroenteritis, and miscellaneous digestive disorders	293,770
Total Top 5 DRGs		2,427,839
Total DRGs		12,216,080

SOURCE: http://www.cms.hhs.gov.

Prior to 1983, hospitals were paid on a retrospective basis for the actual medical services provided. As discussed in Chapter 4, under a retrospective payment system, health care providers bill for actual costs incurred. Economists have long argued that a retrospective payment system has the potential to drive up medical costs for two reasons. First, a retrospective system provides little incentive for cost efficiency, because hospitals are not penalized for any excess costs of production; higher costs can simply be passed on to the third-party payer. Second, when payment is based on the type and quantity of medical services actually provided, an incentive likely exists for hospitals to provide unnecessary medical services. For example, a patient may stay an additional day in the hospital to recuperate from surgery even if it is not medically necessary. The hospital earns additional profits due to the longer stay.

With a prospective system, fees are set in advance on a per-case basis. Hospitals essentially become price takers and face a perfectly elastic demand curve for Medicare patients. Inefficient behavior is no longer tolerated because hospitals are unable to pass higher costs on to the third payer, which in this case is the government. Under the PPS, hospitals that provide medical care at a cost below the preset fee retain the difference, whereas hospitals that incur costs in excess of the preset fee must sustain the loss. Naturally, inefficient hospitals have a difficult time operating in such an environment.

Finally, because compensation is now on a per-case basis, rather than a per-item basis, hospitals have the incentive to provide only necessary medical services. Any hospital that elects to provide additional medical services, such as allowing the patient to stay an additional day to recuperate after surgery, receives no additional compensation and thus has no economic incentive to provide those services (see the discussion surrounding Figure 4–2).

Medicare's PPS appears to have successfully diminished the overall rate of growth in hospital expenditures. Over the eight years prior to the inception of the PPS (1977 to 1984), expenditures for the hospital insurance program grew at an average annual rate of more than 15 percent. The rate dropped to 8.75 percent over the eight years immediately after the program was put in place (1985 to 1992). However, most of the decrease in the rate of growth took place when the program was first introduced. In particular, the average annual rate of growth in expenditures was only 5.1 percent from 1985 through 1988. The relative increase in Medicare hospital spending after 1988 may indicate that the ability of the PPS to control the costs may have waned over time as hospitals began to learn how to work the system. One way hospitals have learned to work the system is to place their patients into higher-weighted DRGs and raise their case-mix index to increase reimbursement. Artificial increases in the case-mix under the PPS are referred to as DRG creep.

Much has been written concerning the impact of the DRG program on the market for hospital services.[6] Foremost on the minds of many researchers is whether the Medicare prospective payment system has had a deleterious effect on the health status of Medicare patients. They fear that hospitals may react to the Medicare price controls by providing a lower quality of medical care. After reviewing the literature on the subject, however, Feinglass and Holloway (1991) conclude that there "is little direct, generalizable evidence that PPS has reduced the quality of care of Medicare patients" (p. 107).

Closely related to the issue of quality is the impact of the DRG system on admissions and length of stay. Economic theory suggests that hospitals may react to the fixed PPS price by attempting to increase admissions as a way to raise revenues. (See the discussion in Chapter 9.) In fact, just the opposite occurred after the PPS was implemented. The number of admissions under

6. For a review of the literature, consult Coulan and Gaumer (1991), Feinglass and Holloway (1991), or Chapter 13 in this text.

Medicare actually dropped by 11 percent during the first eight years of the PPS, and a large portion of the decrease took place within the first two years (Hodgkin and McGuire, 1994). The reason for the drop in admissions is difficult to explain. Feinglass and Holloway (1991) attribute the decline to the implementation of utilization review programs that screen the use of inpatient medical services and to the switch to outpatient facilities as a result of the PPS. The switch to outpatient treatment is substantiated by the fact that hospital outpatient surgery for Medicare patients doubled between 1983 and 1985 (Feinglass and Holloway, 1991). The new payment system also shortened the average length of stay for inpatient hospital visits. Estimates indicate that the average length of stay fell by 14.6 percent from 1982 to 1985 (Feinglass and Holloway, 1991).

The decline in admissions, coupled with the decrease in average length of stay, caused the overall number of inpatient days for Medicare clients to decrease by 20.7 percent from 1982 to 1988 (Schwartz and Mendelson, 1991). The decline in inpatient days during the mid-1980s largely explains the decrease in the overall rate of growth in Medicare hospital expenditures discussed earlier. The more recent increases in the overall rate of growth in Medicare expenditures may also indicate that the cost savings resulting from fewer inpatient days have largely been exhausted. The unsustained reduction of Medicare expenditures led Muller (1993) to report that the "effectiveness of the reforms began to diminish by 1986" (p. 298).

In the early years, the prospective payment system has also had a significant negative impact on the overall financial condition of hospitals. Financial impacts are to be expected, since hospitals are no longer able to bill Medicare for medical services on essentially a cost-plus basis. Fisher (1992) examines the financial performance of more than 4,600 hospitals that were continuously involved with the PPS from 1985 through 1990. Overall, the proportion of hospitals that reported profits dropped marginally from 77.2 percent in 1985 to 72.4 percent in 1990. However, the proportion of hospitals that reported Medicare profits dropped more dramatically over the same period, from 84.5 percent in 1985 to 40.7 percent in 1990. Fisher also finds a positive correlation between overall profitability and Medicare PPS inpatient net profits.

The Omnibus Budget Reconciliation Act of 1989. As the cost of Part B escalated over the years, Congress responded with various changes, including freezes on physician payments and annual limits on increases in fees. Despite these cost containment measures, Medicare expenditures for physician services continued to rise, placing an even greater financial burden on both the federal government and the elderly population. Forced into action, Congress passed the Omnibus Budget Reconciliation Act of 1989, or OBRA 1989, which was directed at restructuring the physician payment system. The act contained four major provisions:

1. A new payment system was established that bases compensation primarily on resources utilized.
2. A procedure was established for Congress to monitor the rate of growth in physician fees over time.
3. Limits were put on charges physicians may assess patients that are beyond the amount paid by Medicare.
4. The Agency for Health Policy Research was established to develop outcomes research and provide guidelines.

Each of these changes is discussed in turn next.

Resource-Based Relative Value Scale System. At the core of OBRA 1989 was a new fee schedule introduced in 1992. Prior to OBRA 1989, physicians were compensated based on the usual, customary, or reasonable (UCR) or the customary, prevailing, and reasonable (CPR) method.

Under this method, physicians were paid the lowest of the bill submitted, the customary charge of the physician, or the prevailing rate in the area for services provided. The general consensus was that the UCR-CPR method of payment contributed to the increase in physician expenditures over the years. According to Yett et al. (1985), the UCR-CPR method of payment creates an incentive for physicians to increase their fees over time to raise what constitutes the reasonable rate in the future. The inflationary bias is especially acute when the overall rate of inflation is high.

In addition, the UCR-CPR method was criticized for creating distortions in relative prices of various types of physician services. Fees for technical procedures were overvalued, whereas fees for evaluations and management services were undervalued. As a result, primary care physicians, who generally provide more evaluation-type services such as physical exams, were being compensated less than specialists, who provide more technical services such as surgery. The price differential tended to distort physicians' income and potentially had an impact on the composition of physician services provided (Oliver, 1993).

The **resource-based relative value scale (RBRVS)** system of fees considers the time and effort of physician work, or physician resources, necessary to produce physician services. The relative work values are based on the research of William Hsiao and colleagues at Harvard University (Hsiao et al., 1988) and make up approximately half of the total value of physician services under the new fee schedule. The other half is accounted for by practice and malpractice expenses. A conversion factor that translates the scale into a fee schedule has also been developed. Yearly adjustments are made in the conversion factor to account for inflation and any other changes that take place.

Since the RBRVS fees are now based on relative work effort, the new fee schedule no longer provides a historical momentum for future fee increases. That is because past fee increases no longer provide the basis for future increases by inflating the "reasonable" rate. Also, a resource-based fee schedule no longer provides physicians with an incentive to supply more technical medical procedures, such as surgery, than evaluation and management services, such as office visits with established patients, which are more time consuming. As a result, physicians who provide primary care should see Medicare revenues increase, whereas those who provide more specialty types of care should see revenues decrease. This view is substantiated by the fact that in 1992, family practitioners saw fees increase by 10 percent while specialty surgeons endured an 8 percent decrease (Physician Payment Review Commission, 1993). Such changes are likely to have a major impact on the types and volume of physician services provided at the margin and the relative incomes of physicians in various specialties.

The RBRVS fee schedule is not without its critics, however. According to Hadley (1991), the entire approach is inconsistent with the theory of cost. A resource-based method determines the value of a service primarily by physician work effort and fails to consider input prices. Thus, contrary to the theory of costs presented earlier, input prices play no role in determining the marginal and average costs of production or the supply and prices of physician services. An example similar to the one developed by Hadley proves this point. In 1993, slightly more than 38,000 general surgeons were practicing in the United States. What would have happened had this number doubled by 1994, *ceteris paribus*? Supply and demand theory suggests that the average fee for surgical services would have dropped as the supply of general surgeons increased, or the supply curve would have shifted to the right. With a resource-based payment scheme, however, lower surgical fees do not result from a greater supply of surgeons because fees are based on work effort. Input prices play no role in determining market price.

Also, one might criticize the resource-based fee schedule on the grounds that it constitutes a price control. If relative fee schedules are set incorrectly, shortages or surpluses of different physician services may result. For example, more generous relative fees for primary care services may encourage an oversupply of those services and an undersupply of specialist services in the future. Consequently, considerable care must be taken when establishing the appropriate fees for the different services.

Medicare Volume Performance Standards. In an attempt to gain more control over the growth of Medicare expenditures, Congress adopted a Medicare volume performance standards (VPS) system that establishes expenditure limits. Each year Congress establishes a target rate of growth for physician expenditures under Medicare, or a VPS. The target considers such items as inflation, the number and ages of enrollees, barriers to access, the level of inappropriate care given, changes in technology, and any legislated changes in the program. Whether the target was met in a given year is used as a basis for determining the extent to which fees are updated the following year through the conversion factor. In other words, if the actual rate of growth in physician expenditures exceeds the VPS in a given year, the increase in physician fees for the following year may be set lower than planned through updates in the conversion factor. If, on the other hand, the actual rate of increase is below the target, the increase in fees may move upward (Physician Payment Review Commission, 1993).

The benefits from a VPS system are twofold. First, the VPS gives Congress a mechanism with which to control the rate of growth of physician expenditures. Second, the VPS gives physicians, as a group, the incentive to provide appropriate care. If excessive amounts of inappropriate care are provided, overall expenditures are driven upward, and this dampens the extent to which fees are increased in the future. Critics, however, point out that the system provides inappropriate incentives to physicians because it fails to take physician practice style into account. Given the wide variation in practice styles, a uniform payment system provides inequitable payments for medical services. In addition, a free-rider problem may exist because such a large number of physicians participate in the system. No one physician has the incentive to eliminate inappropriate care because there is no direct relationship between individual physician behavior and future fee increases (Holahan and Zuckerman, 1993; Miller and Welch, 1993). Ginsburg (1993) responds to the latter criticism by pointing out that the intent was to directly influence the behavior of physician organizations rather than that of individual physicians. The general idea is that the VPS will put pressure on physician organizations to monitor and control individual physician behavior.

Limits on Balance Billing and the Assignment Issue. Faced with the prospect that the new RBRVS fee schedule, along with the expenditure caps, could inhibit access to medical care by forcing up out-of-pocket payments for Medicare recipients, Congress put specific limits on the amount physicians can charge patients above the Medicare rate. When Part B was initially implemented, physicians were allowed to balance-bill patients for charges in excess of the established Medicare fee on a case-by-case basis. When this occurred, the physician was responsible for collecting the entire fee from the patient, and the patient received directly from Medicare a reimbursement check equal to the allowable fee less the 20 percent copayment. Under those circumstances, the physician bore the total risk of nonpayment.

To minimize the level of balance billing and therefore improve access to medical care, Medicare gave physicians the option to accept the assignment of benefits. Physicians who accept **assignment** give up the right to balance-bill, but in return receive a payment directly from Medicare equal to the preset fee minus any deductibles or copayments. The remainder of the bill had to be collected directly from the patient. The decision to accept assignment presents physicians with a classic risk-return trade-off. Physician who opt to balance-bill and not accept assignment receive higher fees but take on the added risk of nonpayment by patients.

The assignment rate, as measured by the percentage of total claims submitted that were assigned, hovered around 60 percent during the earlier years of the Medicare program. However, the rate fell thereafter and bottomed out at around 50 percent in the late 1970s. In response to the lower assignment rate, Congress passed the Medicare Participating Physicians program in 1984, which altered the method of assignment. Now physicians had to elect to either participate or not participate. Physicians who elected to participate had to accept assignment for all patients covered under Part B. Those who opted not to participate were still free to accept assignment on a case-by-case basis. To encourage participation, Congress provided a variety of incentives. For example, nonparticipating physicians had their fee schedule frozen under Medicare, while participating physicians saw a modest increase. These changes brought about the desired outcome, as the assignment rate increased from 53.9 percent in 1983 to 59 percent in 1984 and 68 percent in 1985. Later Congress made further changes in favor of participation. For example, the Omnibus Budget Reconciliation Act of 1986 placed maximum limits on the amount nonparticipating physicians could charge Medicare patients. As a result, the assignment rate reached 81 percent in 1990.

Fearing that the new fee schedule, along with voluntary performance standards, would cause the assignment rate to fall as physicians felt the pinch of more stringent price controls, OBRA 1989 placed even further constraints on the ability of physicians to practice balance billing. By 1991, physicians could not bill patients in excess of 125 percent of the Medicare rate. This rate fell to 120 percent in 1992 and to 115 percent in 1993 for most services. It should be noted that in 1993, the actual balance-billing rate was only 109.25 percent because nonparticipating physicians received only 95 percent of the Medicare fee for participating physicians (115 percent times 95 percent).

As of 2003, the assignment rate reached 99 percent for all physician charges covered by Medicare. In return for accepting assignment, physicians currently receive three major benefits. First, they can directly bill Medicare for services rather than collect their fees directly from Medicare beneficiaries. Second, participating physicians receive a 5 percent increase in payment on allowed charges; finally, they can have their practice information posted on the Medicare web site (MedPAC, 2005).

Health Outcomes Research. Finally, OBRA 1989 calls for the government to take a more active role in outcomes research for the purpose of developing practice guidelines. The long-run objective is to contain the growth of physician and hospital expenditures in the future by minimizing the uncertainty surrounding alternative medical treatments. Outcomes research "involves not only the investigations of the link between medical care and outcomes, but also activities aimed at establishing which providers or systems of health care deliver a better quality of care than others" (Guadagnoli and McNeil, 1994, p. 14).

Payers are pressing for outcomes research so that medical guidelines can be developed to contain costs by eliminating ineffective medical care. Whether this will happen is open to question. For one thing, there is some debate concerning the level of inappropriate care. Some recent studies suggest that it is much lower than previously thought. For another, Guadagnoli and McNeil (1994) contend that outcomes research may force up costs because it may uncover some costly medical procedures that currently are underutilized. Physicians desire medical guidelines because they will aid them in treatment decisions and potentially diminish the possibility of malpractice suits. Another issue is whether guidelines can be effectively developed and implemented given the complexity of developing appropriate data sets and the difficulty in transferring this information into specific recommendations (Guadagnoli and McNeil, 1994). Many illnesses are patient specific, and consequently appropriate treatment cannot be standardized.

Balanced Budget Act of 1997. Despite the many changes in the Medicare program, many felt that rising Medicare costs throughout the 1990s could have jeopardized the financial viability of the program. One estimate indicated that if nothing were done, the trust fund for Part A of Medicare would be exhausted by 2001 (Physician Payment Review Commission, 1997). A glance at Table 10–4 indicates that the growth in expenditures had been rather uneven during the years preceding the Act. For example, while expenditures for inpatient and physician services grew at annual rates of 9.2 and 6.0 percent from 1991 through 1995, expenditures for skilled nursing facilities, home health care, and hospice grew at annual rates in excess of 30 percent. Realizing that something needed to be done, Congress enacted the Balanced Budget Act of 1997 (BBA). The centerpiece of the legislation was the **Medicare + Choice (M+C)** program, which significantly increased the types of insurance plans available to participants and altered the way in which Medicare pays for those plans. The M+C program changed Medicare in four important ways (Christensen, 1998):

- The number of capitation plans available to beneficiaries was greatly expanded.
- The conditions that participating plans must fulfill were relaxed.
- The method of calculated payment rates to plans was adjusted.
- The enrollment process for beneficiaries was changed.

To extend the range of options available to beneficiaries, the BBA allowed a number of alternative types of health insurance plans to participate in the program. Previous to this, only health maintenance organizations were allowed to offer risk-based insurance plans to Medicare participants. Now PPOs, PSOs, FFS plans, and MSAs will be allowed to participate, greatly expanding the range

TABLE 10–4
Average Annual Growth Rates in Medicare Expenditures, 1991–1995

Medical Service	Average Annual Rate of Growth, from 1991–1995
Part A	
Inpatient services	9.2%
Skilled nursing facility	37.7
Home health care	30.6
Hospice	37.4
Part B	
Physician services	6.0
Outpatient services	12.0
Home health care	29.4
Laboratory services	5.8

SOURCE: Physician Payment Review Commission. *Annual Report to Congress*, 1997, Table 1–1.

of options available to consumers.[7] To participate, plans must be licensed under state law and at a minimum cover the same medical services currently covered under the traditional Medicare fee-for-service plan. In an attempt to make it easier for plans to participate, the BBA made two changes. First, it dropped the fifty-fifty rule that required that at least half of the plan's enrollment come from the private sector. Second, it lowered the minimum enrollment requirements for PPOs to participate in the program (Christensen, 1998).

The BBA also significantly changes the method for calculating the monthly capitation payment received by private health plans that enter into contracts with Medicare. HMOs that contracted with Medicare prior to 1998 received a monthly capitation payment equal to 95 percent of the average expected costs of similar beneficiaries who were enrolled in the traditional Medicare plan (calculated at the county level).[8] In addition, capitated payments were further adjusted based on a number of factors, including age, gender, and Medicaid enrollment status prior to 1998.

However, analysts realized that this earlier M+C compensation scheme posed a number of methodological problems. First and foremost was the fact that the capitation payments did not consider the health status of the enrollees. To rectify this problem the BBA required that Medicare capitation payments be risk-adjusted beginning in the year 2000. In addition, the old method for setting the capitation payment had the problem of establishing payment rates that were highly variable from year to year within any given county. That variability tended to discourage companies from participating in the program because it was simply too difficult to project enrollment and profitability. To decrease the level of uncertainty and, therefore, encourage more plans to participate, the BBA mandated a new payment method that is based on the beneficiary's relative expected health care costs plus county of residence. In determining relative expected medical costs, Medicare considers seven characteristics: age, sex, whether the beneficiary has end-stage renal disease, whether the beneficiary is on Medicaid, whether the beneficiary is institutionalized, whether the beneficiary is covered by an employer-sponsored plan, and a health risk factor based on diagnoses made during any Medicare-covered hospital stays in the past year. The county-level payment is calculated as the highest of a blend of the local and national rate, a minimum payment amount (or floor) or a minimum increase from the previous year's county rates (MedPAC, 2002).

Success with the price controls on inpatient hospital and physician services also prompted Congress to call for prospective payment schedules for skilled nursing facilities, hospital outpatient facilities, home health agencies, and rehabilitation facilities in the BBA legislation. These payment schedules were to be developed and put in place with the last implemented in October 2000 for rehabilitation facilities.

The BBA also addressed some issues with regard to Part B of the Medicare program. As we discussed previously, OBRA 1989 mandated a resource-based relative value scale system of payment for physician services. Practice and malpractice expenses were still based on historical charges. The BBA required that a resource-based method of payment be extended to practice expenses starting in 1999 and malpractice expenses in 2000.

In addition, the BBA replaces the volume performance standard with a new system that ties conversion factor updates to a sustainable growth target. This target is tied to the rate of medical inflation, changes in fee-for-service enrollment, growth in the overall economy, and any changes in spending resulting from any modifications in government policy. The old way of basing

7. PPO stands for *preferred provider organization:* PSO stands for *provider-sponsored organization.* FFS stands for *fee-for-service,* and MSA stands for *medical savings account.*

8. The logic is that health maintenance organizations have a cost advantage over traditional fee-for-service organizations. Since they should be able to provide medical services at a reduced cost, Medicare reduces the payment by 5 percent.

updates in the conversion factor on the volume performance standard system had come under criticism in recent years for a number of reasons. First, under the volume performance standard system, separate conversion factors were used for primary services, surgical services, and non-surgical services, thus distorting relative payments across physician services over time. To remedy this problem a single conversion factor has been established (MedPAC, 1998).

Most important, however, was the fact that the volume performance standards were generating spending targets that were much too low. Previously, the target was based on the growth in the volume and intensity of physician services minus any legislated deduction to slow the rate of growth in spending. In recent years the growth in volume and intensity slowed down while at the same time the legislated deduction was increased. "As a result, performance standards, which originally were well above the gross domestic product growth are now projected to drop well below" (Physician Payment Review Commission 1997, p. 252). Beginning in 1999 the updates in the conversion factor will be determined by a sustainable growth rate system that will be tied more closely to the overall economy. The idea is to link spending for physician services under Medicare more closely to what the economy can afford to finance over time while changes have been made in the conversion factor in recent years, the method of determining physician fees remains essentially intact.

Realizing that the drastic changes called for by the BBA may cause undue hardship on health care providers, Congress passed the Balanced Budget Refinement Act, or BBRA, in 1999. Among other things, the BBRA increased Medicare spending by approximately $16 billion from 2000 through 2004 and delayed the implementation of several of the prospective payment systems called for by the BBA. In additions, the legislation decreased the reductions for managed care, disproportionate share payments, and indirect education payments. The overall objective of the legislation was to provide health care providers more time to transition into many of the changes called for in the BBA of 1997.

Medicare Prescription Drug Improvement and Modernization Act of 2003

The Medicare Prescription Drug Improvement and Modernization Act of 2003 (MMA) was a momentous piece of legislation because it calls for major structural changes to expand the role of private insurance plans in Medicare (Davis et al., 2005). The general consensus is that the original M+C choice program did not meet expectations in expanding the rule of private insurance in Medicare. First and foremost, the program experienced a significant drop in participating plans. The number of contracts fell from a maximum of 348 in 1998 to 148 early in 2002. This drop in contracts was matched by a significant fall in M+C enrollees. Over the same four-year period, between 300,000 and one million individuals lost coverage through the M+C program annually (MedPAC, 2002). In addition, many of the plans that elected to stay with the M+C program were forced to either curtail benefits or increase premiums because increases in Medicare payments did not keep up with the rising cost of health care. Needless to say, this created an additional incentive for enrollees to switch back to the traditional Medicare program. The program has also failed to generate any cost savings for Medicare. According to MedPAC (March 2002), the average spending per enrollee in the M+C program was about 4 percent higher than in the traditional Medicare plan in 2001 after controlling for the demographic attributes of the beneficiaries. While the estimates did not control for health status of recipients, they provide some preliminary evidence of a lack of cost savings.

In reaction to these problems, the MMA made significant changes in the types of private insurance plans that can participate in the Medicare program and the method of payment, along with renaming the M+C program the Medicare Advantage (MA) program. The most significant change in plan participation is the addition of regional PPOs. As of 2006, 26 PPO regions have been established in the United States. To encourage the creation of regional PPOs, a number of financial incentives have been created, including a certain degree of risk sharing for two years and a stabilization fund. The goal is to increase participation in private plans by offering Medicare enrollees more choice, especially those located in rural areas where local MA plans may be unavailable. It is also hoped that the PPO option will attract additional enrollees by offering them the ability to choose medical care providers that are inside or outside the medical network. If you recall, HMOs have been criticized for restricting choice to in-network medical care providers.

The MMA also instituted a new method for calculating payment rates in an attempt to stabilize the number of private firms taking part in the Medicare program. The objective is to set the rate high enough to attract private firms and low enough to contain costs.[9] Under the new system beginning in 2006, the Centers for Medicare & Medicaid Services establish a benchmark against which private plans bid. The benchmark for each plan is based primarily on the average spending for beneficiaries enrolled in the traditional Medicare program at the county level. If the plan covers enrollees from multiple counties, then the benchmark is a weighted average of Medicare expenditures per enrollees across counties. If the submitted bid is above the benchmark, the benchmark becomes the level of payment. Finally, if the submitted bid is below the benchmark, then Medicare shares 75 percent of the difference with the private plan, provided that the funds are used by the private insurance company to enhance benefits, reduce cost sharing, or cut premiums. The remaining 25 percent of the difference is retained by the government (MedPAC, 2005).

The MMA of 2003 also establishes Part D of Medicare, which provides prescription drug coverage to Medicare enrollees beginning January 1, 2006. This piece of legislation is significant for two reasons. First, it calls for the largest onetime increase in benefits in the history of the Medicare program. As stated earlier in the chapter, the Congressional Budget Office estimated the cumulative cost of the program to the federal government to be around $400 billion from 2006 through 2013. Second, the legislation calls for significant structural changes in the Medicare program. Specifically, it is the first time in the history of the program that a major benefit is offered that is not available through the traditional Medicare program (Davis et al., 2005).

Under part D, Medicare beneficiaries have two options to obtain prescription drug coverage. They can remain in the traditional Medicare program under Part A and purchase a private stand-alone prescription drug plan, or they can join a Medicare Advantage (MA) plan that offers medical and prescription drug coverage. Under the standard benefit package, the beneficiary pays a monthly premium to a private insurer, estimated to be around $37 for 2006. The premium payment is intended to cover approximately 25 percent of the total cost of the drug benefit across beneficiaries. The remaining 75 percent of the cost is subsidized by the federal government.

The standard benefit package for 2006 includes an annual deductible of $250 and a 25 percent copayment for the next $2,000 in prescription drug expenses. Thus if a beneficiary has drug expenses of $2,250 for the year, the insurance plan covers $1,500 and the beneficiary has an out-of-pocket expense of $750 (the deductible of $250 plus 25 percent of $2,000). For drug expenses between $2,250 and $5,100 per year, the coinsurance rate is 100 percent and the beneficiary is responsible for any additional amount up to $2,850. This gap in coverage has been referred to in the popular press as the **doughnut hole** because it represents a gap in insurance

9. MedPAC (2005) couches the issue in terms of the quest of financial neutrality, which occurs when the Medicare program pays the same amount per enrollee regardless of plan choice.

coverage. For all drug expenses beyond $5,100 per year, the beneficiary receives catastrophic insurance coverage and the coinsurance rate drops from 100 to 5 percent. In other words, the catastrophic benefit comes into play only after the beneficiary pays a total out-of-pocket drug expense of $3,600 for the year.

Figure 10–3 provides an illustration of the doughnut hole in which drug expenditures are measured on the horizontal axis and the coinsurance rate is measured on the vertical axis. The shaded area represents the percentage of each dollar spent on drugs that is the responsibility of the beneficiary. Notice that the out-of-pocket price is 100 percent for the first $250 in drug expenditures. Once the deductible has been fulfilled, the coinsurance rate drops to 25 percent and remains there up to the point where the total drug costs reach $2,250. After that point, the beneficiary is in the "doughnut hole" and the coinsurance rate increases to 100 percent. Catastrophic coverage takes hold for any drug expenses beyond $5,100 and the coinsurance rate drops to 5 percent.

Three points of clarification need to be discussed before we move on. First, premium and cost-sharing subsidies are provided by the federal government to beneficiaries with limited incomes. Second, the premium payments and coverage may vary across plans to reflect geographical differences in the cost of drugs and more generous benefit packages. Third, premiums, deductibles, and other out-of-pocket thresholds are projected to increase in the future to reflect increases in per capita drug spending over time.

FIGURE 10–3
Coinsurance Rate for the Standard Benefit Package Under Part D of Medicare for 2006

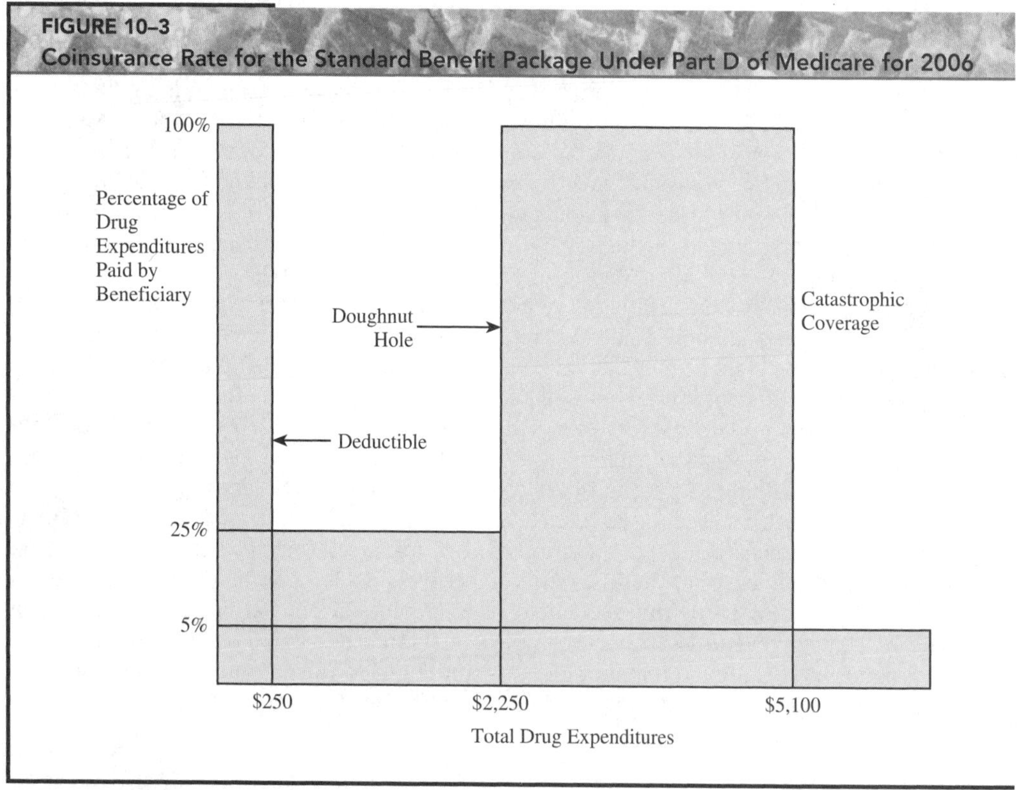

SOURCE: Rexford E. Santerre and Stephen P. Neun.

While it is difficult to discuss the implications of the new Medicare drug benefit with few hard facts at this early date, a study commissioned by the Henry J. Kaiser Family Foundation (2004) lends some preliminary insights. According to the study's findings, of the 29 million beneficiaries estimated to participate in Part D in 2006, 10 percent will have zero drug expenditures, while an additional 36 percent will not meet the deductible of $250. Of the remaining 54 percent, 30 percent will have drug expenses between $250 and $2,250, 14 percent will be the doughnut hole and have drug expenses between $2,250 and $5,100, and 10 percent will have drug expenses in excess of $5,100.

The study also estimates that 30 percent of the enrollees, or 8.7 million elderly, will qualify for some type of low-income subsidy. For the remaining 20-million-plus enrollees, on average their out-of-pocket expenditure on drugs is projected to drop from $1,495 to $1,081 in 2006 as a result of MMA. While preliminary, these findings suggest that the majority of those who participate in Part D of Medicare will spend less out-of-pocket on drugs in 2006 than would otherwise be the case.

SUMMARY

This chapter focuses on Medicaid and Medicare, two public health insurance programs that account for a high and rising share of total health care costs in the United States. The Medicaid program has seen tremendous change in recent years and these changes have placed a number of states in rather precarious positions. States all across the country have been forced to control costs and at the same time meet federal mandates that call for the relaxation of eligibility requirements for certain segments of the poor. Most have turned to managed care as a way to contain Medicaid expenditures. Whether managed care offers the solution to Medicaid cost containment will most likely be a lively source of debate in the near future.

The Medicare program has also experienced significant change in the recent past. First and foremost the Medicare program over the last few decades has moved away from a fee-for-service method of payment as its major method of payment to a prospective payment system in an attempt to contain costs. This movement started with the implementation of the diagnosis-related group payment program in the 1980s and was followed by the resource-based payment program for physician services in the 1990s. More recently, prospective payment systems have been adopted for many other types of medical services covered by Medicare. The Medicare program has also turned to managed care with mixed results in the hopes of containing costs. Most recently, the passage of the MMA of 2003 calls for expanding the role of private insurance in Medicare and the extension of prescription drug coverage to the elderly.

CASE STUDIES

10-1 Advertising of MCOs—Information or Persuasion?

While everyone agrees that advertising is a fact of life in today's business environment, economists have long debated whether advertising enhances or diminishes society's overall well-being. As we learned in Chapter 8, proponents argue that advertising provides consumers with additional information that can be used to make an informed decision, the result being a more efficient allocation of resources brought about through enhanced competition. Critics contend that advertising results in anticompetitive outcomes by creating artificial wants, habit buying, and barriers to entry. A recent study by Neuman et al. (1998) may rekindle that debate. Neuman et al. analyze newspaper and television ads placed by HMOs. They also review the presentations at marketing seminars to gain an understanding of the marketing strategies employed by HMOs to attract Medicare-eligible customers. According to their findings, HMOs convey the message that they can provide more benefits at a lower cost than traditional Medicare plans. More important, the authors conclude that HMOs have developed and implemented marketing strategies based on attracting healthy seniors. To support their conclusion they cite the fact that "nearly half of all television ads include images of physically active seniors, in the midst of strenuous activities such as mountain biking, swimming and jogging up stairs" (p. 135). In addition, "none of the newspaper and television ad images includes beneficiaries in hospital beds or wheelchairs or with walkers, canes, or obvious handicaps or illnesses" (p. 135). They also report that in almost all cases the font size used in the fine print that appeared in TV and newspaper ads was smaller than the smallest print recommended for individuals age 65 and older. What is even more astonishing is that one out of three seminars to prospective enrollees were held in facilities that were not wheelchair accessible. Overall, the evidence supports the proposition that HMOs face strong incentives to enroll healthy seniors and to avoid those with greater potential medical needs.

Questions for Discussion

1. *The research by Neuman et al. suggests that insurers face strong financial incentives to enroll healthier patients. But can plans realistically be expected to maintain a healthier risk pool?*
2. *Suppose health plan X is successful in a campaign to enroll a disproportionate share of healthy seniors. After one year, what will happen when high-risk enrollees of health plan Y observe that health plan X's premiums grew more slowly (which they would have to in order to keep the low-risk enrollees)?*

10-2 Medicare Advantage[10]

In 2005, many of the nation's largest health insurance companies greatly improved their insurance policies for those receiving Medicare. In an attempt to gain more customers, insurance companies are adding extras such as vision benefits and gym memberships and offering lower or no premiums at all. This insurance activity was part of the federal government's renewed effort to transfer Medicare recipients into privately run managed care plans known as Medicare Advantage. As of November 2005, only 13 percent of those using Medicare received their benefits through an Advantage plan. The risks to the new Advantage plans lie in the possibility for later cutbacks in funding, which could lead insurers to cut back on coverage. However, at this time, the government is spending hundreds of dollars more for each person using a Medicare Advantage plan than for those in traditional Medicare. In rural areas where Medicare Advantage plans are scarce, there are usually three to four plans for people to choose from thanks to preferred provider organizations (PPOs). PPOs provide benefits for services outside a person's network of "preferred" doctors, but those services usually come at a higher cost. Some insurers are also beginning to market "special needs" plans that are designed for those with severe chronic disease or for those who fall under federal or state Medicaid programs as well. Seniors who use Medicare Advantage over traditional Medicare can potentially save up to $100 a month.

---

10. Source: Vanessa Fuhrmans and Sarah Lueck, "Insurers Sweeten Health Plans for Seniors," *The Wall Street Journal*, November 8, 2005.

Questions for Discussion

1. *Compared to traditional Medicare, what are the main advantages to seniors enrolled in Medicare Advantage?*
2. *Why are private health plans interested in enrolling Medicare recipients?*
3. *What are the policy advantages of enrolling Medicare seniors in private plans? Can there still be benefits even if the per-enrollee costs are higher in the Medicare Advantage plan?*
4. *Discuss the relationship between benefit packages (including the amenities offered by some Medicare Advantage plans) and selection bias. Do gym memberships and prescription drug benefits attract the same kind of enrollee?*

Review Questions and Problems

1. Using economic theory, justify the need for the Medicaid and Medicare programs.
2. Discuss the methods states use to contain Medicaid costs.
3. Discuss the importance of Medicaid fees in determining the success of the Medicaid program in improving health outcomes of the poor.
4. What is the Medicaid crowding-out problem and why is it important?
5. In 1983, Congress adopted the prospective payment system (PPS) to compensate hospitals for medical services. Prior to that point, hospitals were paid on a retrospective basis. Provide the economic justification for such a move.
6. Explain some of the advantages and disadvantages of the resource-based method of payment for physician services under Medicare.
7. The muffler on your car suddenly needs repair, and there are only two automobile repair shops in town. You drive to the first shop, and the mechanic tells you to leave the car and he will repair it. Payment will be due when you pick it up. A mechanic at the second shop looks at your car and guarantees that she will charge you only $99.95 to repair the muffler, as advertised. Which repair shop is likely to provide costly needless repairs to your car, and why? Which one may underprovide quality? In your answers, discuss the concepts of prospective and retrospective payment for services.
8. What is the assignment problem? How have recent changes in the Medicare program addressed the problem?
9. Discuss how health outcomes research is supposed to contain rising medical costs.
10. Explain how the Medicare + Choice program alters the role of private insurance in the Medicare program.
11. What factors explain the disappointing results from the Medicare + Choice program?
12. How does the Medicare Advantage program differ from the Medicare + Choice program?
13. What is the doughnut hole?
14. Why is Medicare Part D considered such a major change to the Medicare program?

CEBS Questions

■ *CEBS Sample Question on Subject Matter from CEBS Course 9 Study Manual*

1. What are ways in which Congress over the years has encouraged physician participation in the Medicare program? (pages 280–281)

■ *CEBS Sample Exam Questions*

1. Not counting the 60-day lifetime reserve, Medicare covers hospital inpatient expenses for a maximum of:
   A. 30 days
   B. 60 days
   C. 90 days
   D. 120 days
   E. 360 days

2. The Balanced Budget Act of 1997 contained which of the following major changes in the Medicare program?
   I. The Act limited reimbursement of Medicare expenditures to two-thirds the cost of comparable services in 1995, the base year of cost measurement.
   II. The Act expanded the number of alternative types of risk-based health insurance plans eligible to participate in the plan.
   III. The Act changed the method of calculating the monthly capitation payment received by private health insurance plans that enter into risk contracts with Medicare.
   A. II only
   B. III only
   C. I and II only
   D. II and III only
   E. I, II, and III

3. All the following statements regarding Medicaid financing, costs, and fees are correct EXCEPT:
   A. The cost is financed jointly by the federal and state governments.
   B. Scant evidence exists that Medicaid fees have an impact on health care outcomes.
   C. Federal mandates, such as required coverage of children and pregnant women, have increased Medicaid expenditures.
   D. Medicaid fees vary widely across the country and are generally lower than comparable private or Medicare rates.
   E. Disproportionate share hospital payments have contributed to the rise in Medicaid expenditures.

Answer to Sample Question from Study Manual

The ways in which Congress has encouraged physician participation has been by guaranteeing reimbursement minus any deductibles or copayments directly from Medicare, by placing limits on the amount nonparticipating physicians could charge Medicare patients, and by placing constraints on balance billing. Also, as of 2003, participating physicians receive a 5 percent increased in payment on allowed charges and they can have their practice information posted on the Medicare website.

Answers to Sample Exam Questions

1. C is the answer. Except for the 60-day lifetime reserve, after the 90th day Medicare stops paying hospital inpatient expenses. See page 274 of the text.
2. D is the answer. The first statement is false but the other two are true. The Medicare + Choice program introduced by the act increased the types of insurance available to the Medicare participants and required that Medicare capitation payments be made on a

risk-adjusted basis beginning in the year 2000. Modifications were made to the Medicare + Choice program by the Medicare Prescription Drug Improvement and Modernization Act of 2003 (MMA). The modifications were changes in the types of insurance plans that can participate in the Medicare program and the method of payment. The MMA also renamed the program Medicare Advantage (MA). See pages 282–285 of the text.

3. B is the answer. Studies seem to suggest that Medicaid fees have a direct impact on the level of medical care provided to Medicaid recipients. See pages 268–271 of the text.

ONLINE RESOURCES

To access Internet links related to the topics in this chapter, please visit our web site at **www.thomsonedu.com/economics/santerre**.

REFERENCES

Baker, Laurence, and Anne Beeson Royalty. "Medicaid Policy, Physician Behavior, and Health Care for the Low-Income Populations." *Journal of Human Resources* 35 (summer 2000), pp. 480–502.

Blumberg, Linda J., Lisa Dubay, and Stephen A. Norton. "Did the Medicaid Expansions for Children Displace Private Insurance? An Analysis Using the SIPP." *Journal of Health Economics* 19 (January 2000), pp. 33–66.

Christensen, Sandra. "Medicare + Choice Provisions in the Balanced Budget Act of 1997." *Health Affairs* 17 (July/August 1998), pp. 224–31.

Coughlin, Teresa A., et al. "State Responses to the Medicaid Spending Crisis: 1988 to 1992." *Journal of Health Politics, Policy and Law* 19 (winter 1994), pp. 837–64.

Coulan, R. F., and G. L. Gaumer. "Medicare's Prospective Payment System: A Critical Appraisal." *Health Care Financing Review* (annual supplement, 1991), pp. 45–77.

Currie, Janet, and Duncan Thomas. "Medical Care for Children: Public Insurance, Private Insurance and Racial Differences in Utilization." *Journal of Human Resources* 30 (1995), pp. 135–62.

Currie, Janet, Jonathan Gruber, and Michael Fischer. "Physician Payments and Infant Mortality: Evidence from Medicaid Fee Policy." *American Economic Review* 85 (1995), pp. 106–11.

Cutler, David M., and Jonathan Gruber. "Does Public Insurance Crowd Out Private Insurance?" *Quarterly Journal of Economics* 111 (May 1996), pp. 391–430.

Davis, Karen, Marilyn Moon, Barbara Cooper, and Cathy Schoen. "Medicare Extra: A Comprehensive Benefit Option for Medicare Beneficiaries." *Health Affairs* Web Exclusive, (October 4, 2005).

DeParle, Nancy Min. "Celebrating 35 Years of Medicare and Medicaid." *Health Care Financing Review* 22 (fall 2000), pp. 1–7.

Dick, Andrew W., et al. "SCHIP's Impact in Three States: How Do the Most Vulnerable Children Fare?" *Health Affairs* 23 (September/October 2004), pp. 63–75.

Dubay, Lisa, and Genevieve Kenney. "Did Medicaid Expansion for Pregnant Women Crowd Out Private Insurance?" *Health Affairs* 16 (January/February 1997), pp. 185–93.

Feinglass, Joe, and James J. Holloway. "The Initial Impact of the Medicare Prospective Payment System on U.S. Health Care: A Review of the Literature." *Medical Care Review* 48 (spring 1991), pp. 91–115.

Fisher, Charles R. "Hospital and Medicare Financial Performance under PPS, 1985–1990." *Health Care Financing Review* 14 (fall 1992), pp. 171–83.

Garnick, Deborah W., et al. "How Well Do Americans Understand Their Health Coverage?" *Health Affairs* 12 (fall 1993), pp. 204–12.

Ginsburg, Paul B. "Refining Medicare Volume Performance Standards: Commentary." *Inquiry* 30 (fall 1993), pp. 260–64.

Gray, Bradley. "Do Medicaid Physician Fees for Prenatal Services Affect Birth Outcomes?" *Journal of Health Economics* 20 (July 2001), pp. 571–90.

Guadagnoli, Edward, and Barbara J. McNeil. "Outcomes Research: Hope for the Future the Latest Rage?" *Inquiry* 31 (spring 1994), pp. 14–24.

Hadley, Jack. "Theoretical and Empirical Foundations of the Resource-Based Relative Value Scale." In *Regulating Doctors' Fees: Competition, Benefits and Control under Medicare*, ed. H. E. Frech III. Washington, D.C.: AEI Press, 1991.

Heffler, Stephen, Sheila Smith, Sean Keehan, Christopher Borger, M. Kent Clemens, and Christopher Truffer. "U.S. Health Spending Projections for 2004–2014." *Health Affairs*, Web Exclusive, February 23, 2005.

Henry J. Kaiser Family Foundation. "Estimates of Medicare Beneficiaries' Out-of-Pocket Drug Spending in 2006." November 2004.

Hodgkin, Dominic, and Thomas G. McGuire. "Payment Levels and Hospital Response to Prospective Payment." *Journal of Health Economics* 13 (1994), pp. 1–29.

Holahan, John, and Stephen Zuckerman. "The Future of Medicare Volume Performance Standards." *Inquiry* 30 (fall 1993), pp. 235–48.

Hsiao, William C., et al. "Results and Policy Implications of the Resource-Based Relative-Value Scale." *New England Journal of Medicine* 319 (September 29, 1988), pp. 881–88.

Kenney, Genevieve, and Debbie I. Chang. "The State Children's Health Insurance Program: Successes, Shortcomings, and Challenges." *Health Affairs* 23 (September/October 2004), pp. 51–62.

Kronebusch, Karl. "Children's Medicaid Enrollment: The Impact of Mandates, Welfare Reform, and Policy Delinking." *Journal of Health Politics, Policy and Law* 26 (December 2001), pp. 1217–22.

Kronebusch, Karl, and Brian Elbel. "Enrolling Children in Public Insurance: SCHIP, Medicaid and State Implementation." *Journal of Health, Politics, Policy and Law* 29 (June 2004), pp. 451–49.

Lo Sasso, Anthony T., and Thomas C. Buchmueller. "The Effect of State Children's Health Insurance Program on Health Insurance Coverage." *Journal of Health Economics* 23 (2004), pp. 1059–82.

Long, Sharon, K., and Teresa A. Coughlin. "Access and Use by Children on Medicaid: Does State Matter?" *Inquiry* 38 (winter 2001/2002), pp. 409–22.

Medicare Payment Advisory Commission (MedPAC). *Report to the Congress: Medicare Payment Policy*. Vols. I and II. Washington, D.C., March 1998.

———. *Medicare Payment Policy Report to Congress*. Washington D.C., March 2002.

———. *Medicare Payment Policy Report to Congress*. Washington, D.C., March 2005.

———. *Medicare Payment Policy Report to Congress*. Washington, D.C., June 2005.

Miller, Mark E., and W. Pete Welch. "Growth in Medicare Inpatient Physician Charges per Admission, 1986–1989." *Inquiry* 30 (fall 1993), pp. 249–59.

Muller, Andreas. "Medicare Prospective Payment Reforms and Hospital Utilization." *Medical Care* 31 (1993), pp. 296–308.

Oliver, Thomas R. "Analysis, Advice, and Congressional Leadership: The Physician Payment Review Commission and the Politics of Medicare." *Journal of Health Politics, Policy and Law* 18 (spring 1993), pp. 113–74.

Physician Payment Review Commission. *Annual Report to Congress*. Washington, D.C.: PPRC, 1993.

———. *Annual Report to Congress*. Washington, D.C: PPRC, 1997.

Schwartz, William B., and Daniel N. Mendelson. "Hospital Cost Containment in the 1980's." *New England Journal of Medicine* 324 (April 11, 1991), pp. 1037–42.

U.S. Department of Health and Human Services, Social Security Administration. *Annual Statistical Supplement, 1993*. Washington, D.C., 1993.

———. *Annual Statistical Supplement, 2001*. Washington, D.C., 2001.

———. *Annual Statistical Supplement, 2004*. Washington, D.C., 2004.

Yazici, Esel Y., and Robert Kaestner. "Medicaid Expansions and the Crowding Out of Private Health Insurance among Children." *Inquiry* 37 (spring 2000), pp. 23–32.

Yett, Donald E., William Der, Richard L. Ernst, and Joel W. Hay. "Fee-for-Service Reimbursement and Physician Inflation." *Journal of Human Resources* 20 (spring 1985), pp. 278–91.

Zuckerman, Stephen, Joshua McFeeters, Peter Cunningham, and Len Nichols. "Changes in Medicaid Physician Fees, 1998–2003: Implications for Physician Participation." *Health Affairs*, Web Exclusive, June 23, 2004.

PART 3

INDUSTRY STUDIES

CHAPTER 11

THE PRIVATE HEALTH INSURANCE INDUSTRY

Our pal Joe was sort of lucky. Sure he suffered a heart attack. That in itself can be a medically frightening and painful experience. But as a federal employee, Joe and his family were covered by a sound and generous health insurance policy, so at least they did not have to bear the sharp psychological sting of the financial insecurity that can result from an unexpected medical occurrence.

However, Leo, Joe's brother, was not so fortunate. You see, Leo worked as a machinist in a specialty parts fabrication shop that employs five workers. Given the competitive nature of the market for specialty machined goods, Leo's employer was financially unable to sponsor any health insurance for the workers. But Leo and his wife, Sarah, really didn't care about the lack of health insurance anyway. They were both in their early fifties, which is relatively young by today's standards, and seemed to be in great health. They had built up a small nest egg of $100,000 and planned on using the money to support an early semi-retirement in which Leo would quit his job and open a machine shop in his garage. At age 65 both Leo and Sarah would be eligible for Medicare and then they were all set—or so they thought.

Then all hell broke loose. Sarah found a lump in her breast! A visit to a local doctor confirmed her most feared suspicion. She was diagnosed with a cancerous tumor. Since Sarah had not received annual mammograms due to what she considered an unnecessary out-of-pocket expense, the cancer was at an advanced stage. It was too late for a simple lumpectomy or chemotherapy; a radical mastectomy was deemed the necessary treatment. Not only were Leo and Sarah distraught over Sarah's physical and mental well-being, but also saddened that their hard-earned life savings would be completely wiped out.

This story raises a number of important questions:

1. Who exactly are the uninsured? That is, are specific groups or individuals, such as employees of small businesses, at a greater risk of being uninsured than others?
2. Suppose that Leo had participated in a group health insurance policy with his employer but decided to change jobs. Would he and Sarah be immediately eligible for health insurance with the new employer, especially with Sarah's condition already diagnosed?
3. If Leo did not have a group health insurance policy with his employer, would he face higher health insurance premiums or would Sarah be excluded from the policy?

This chapter deals with these questions, among others, and raises a host of other problems and issues pertaining to the private health insurance industry. The examination is couched in terms of the structure, conduct, and performance paradigm discussed in Chapter 8. Specifically, this chapter:

- provides a brief history of the private health insurance industry
- analyzes the structure of the private health insurance industry in terms of the number and types of sellers, buyer characteristics, barriers to entry, and other factors

- describes the conduct of firms in the private health insurance industry with respect to pricing methods, managed care effects, and risk selection
- assesses the performance of the private health insurance industry with regard to the number of insured and uninsured, pricing, and moral hazard

A Brief History of the Private Health Insurance Industry

The modern private health insurance industry started around 1929 when Baylor University in Dallas began accepting insurance premiums from local schoolteachers to cover any medical services provided at the university hospital (Temin, 1988).[1] The idea quickly spread during the Great Depression of the 1930s as a number of hospitals adopted similar financing methods. Shortly thereafter, the American Hospital Association created and organized several insurance plans, named Blue Cross, which allowed subscribers free choice among the hospitals within a given city. Corresponding to the alleged public service nature of Blue Cross plans, premiums were determined by community rating. The Blue Cross plans enjoyed a virtual monopoly position in the hospital insurance market throughout the 1930s.

The hospital insurance market expanded and the level of competition intensified during World War II, when the federal government imposed wage and price controls. Because wage increases were restricted, the only way employers could attract additional laborers was to offer fringe benefits, such as private health insurance. Initially, employers did not report the value of the fringe benefits to the Internal Revenue Service, but eventually regulations were passed requiring employers to include the value of medical care as part of reported wage income. By that time, however, workers had become accustomed to the tax-exempt status of medical insurance and expressed considerable alarm. Congress responded, and health insurance has remained tax exempt ever since (Friedman, 1992).

Commercial insurance companies were slow to branch off into the health insurance market because they were uncertain about its profitability (Sapolsky, 1991) and doubted whether medical care was an insurable risk due to the difficulty in predicting losses accurately (Iglehart, 1992). The Blue Cross experience demonstrated the viability of health insurance to commercial insurers. By the time the commercials entered the industry in the late 1940s, Blue Cross plans were viewed as pro-union, having established a strong union allegiance. As employers looked to alternative sources for private health insurance, commercial plans searched for clients. The commercial insurance segment later grew as the rate of union membership declined among workers and experience rating became more common among employer groups. According to Temin (1988), "Blue Cross accounted for only two-thirds of hospital insurance by the war's close, and it had less than half of the market in the 1950s and 1960s" (p. 89).

Today the private health insurance industry is the source of funds for 36 percent of all health care expenditures, providing coverage to roughly 70 percent of the population. The modern health insurance industry is very pluralistic, composed of many different types of health plan providers that include health maintenance organizations, preferred provider organizations, self-insurers, third-party administrators, and traditional insurers with and without utilization review. Some of these insurers are not-for-profit entities, whereas others are for-profit organizations. Moreover, many of them rely on different methods of reimbursing health care providers for

1. According to Sapolsky (1991), a few paternalistic employers, including General Motors and Procter & Gamble, established welfare programs with medical benefits for their employees prior to 1926.

medical services rendered to their subscribers. The rest of this chapter examines the structure, conduct, and performance of the private health insurance industry.

The Structure of the Private Health Insurance Industry

As noted in Chapter 8, structure is an important feature of an industry because it influences the conduct and performance of the member firms. In the following discussion, we take a closer look at some of the structural characteristics associated with the private health insurance industry.

Number, Types, and Size Distribution of Health Insurers

Private health insurance in the United States involves many different health insurers, including commercial carriers, Blue Cross/Blue Shield (BCBS) plans, HMOs, and other types of managed care plans. Several practices of private health insurers are worth noting. First, a private health insurer, such as a commercial company or BCBS, normally offers its subscribers a choice among traditional plans and various types of managed-care plans. Second, insurers may specialize in either group or individual health insurance, or may choose to offer both. Lastly, private health insurers often are licensed to underwrite and sell health insurance in more than one state.

At the national level, data suggest that a relatively large number of insurers offer private health insurance in the United States. Specifically, Chollet et al. (2003) estimate that 2,151 insurers participated in the group health insurance industry and 643 insurers operated in the individual health insurance market in 2001. Also, these researchers report that independent HMOs, with a 42 percent market share of earned premiums, dominated the group health insurance market, whereas BCBS plans, with more than half of all earned premiums, dominated the individual health insurance market in 2001. Commercial insurers, although more numerous in both markets, held national market shares of only 19 and 23 percent in the group and individual segments of the health insurance industry, respectively. At the end of 2004 the ten largest health insurers in terms of enrollment (with approximate national market shares shown in parentheses)[2] were WellPoint, Inc. (13.3%), UnitedHealth Group, Inc. (9.9%), Aetna, Inc. (5.9%), Health Care Services Corp. (5.2%), CIGNA HealthCare, Inc. (4.5%), Kaiser Permanente (4.3%), Humana, Inc. (2.7%), WellChoice, Inc. (2.5%), BCBS of Michigan (2.4%), and Health Net, Inc. (1.9%).

While many sellers of health insurance exist at the national level, Robinson (2004) and others point out that the health insurance industry is characterized by a few large sellers at the state level. For example, out of 47 states and Washington, D.C., the three largest health insurance companies accounted for at least 50 percent of enrollment in 43 states in 2003. In 39 states, the top three insurers accounted for 60 percent or more of enrollment, and in only 1 state did the top three insurers account for less than 40 percent. Robinson also finds that the HHI exceeded 1,000 in all but 3 states and exceeded 1,800 in all but 14 states. Recall from Chapter 8 that economists often consider four-firm concentration ratios in excess of 40 percent and HHIs in excess of 1,000 as reflecting mild oligopoly.

Chollet et al. (2003) further show that high market concentration characterizes both the group and individual segments of the health insurance industry. In fact, the individual health insurance industry appears to be even more highly concentrated than the group segment. Chollet et al. also note that a large number of sellers with tiny market shares operate in both segments of the health insurance industry. That is, the smallest 50 percent of all group health insurers collectively held

2. http://www.aishealth.com/MarketData/MCEnrollment/MCEnrol_mc01.html (accessed October 24, 2005).

less than 3 percent of the market in 2001. Likewise, the smallest 50 percent of all individual health insurers accounted for only 8 percent of earned premiums. Economists refer to the large number of firms with tiny market shares that coexist with one or a few dominant firms as the **competitive fringe** of an industry.

The GAO (2005) finds similar evidence concerning the concentrated nature of the small-group health insurance market at the state level in 2004. Small-group health insurance is defined differently by the states but the definition typically allows for less than 50 employees in a plan. The study found that the median number of licensed carriers in the small-group market was 28 per state. When combined, the five largest insurers represented more than 75 percent of the market in 26 of the 34 states providing information. In all but 2 states, the five top insurers covered 60 percent or more of those receiving health insurance in the small-group insurance segment. Similar to the study by Chollet et al., another implication of the GAO study is the existence of a large competitive fringe of health insurers in the small-group segment of the industry.

Thus far, available data suggest that the private health insurance industry is highly concentrated when the state is treated as the relevant geographical market. However, Kopit (2004, p. 29) explains that "health insurance markets are local, because they are derivative of the provider networks used by the plan. In a state the size of Rhode Island, the geographic market could be the entire state, but in larger states such as Pennsylvania, the sale of health insurance products in Pittsburgh does nothing for local employers in Philadelphia or even Harrisburg." For this reason, the relevant geographical market for the health insurance industry is typically defined more narrowly for antitrust purposes as the metropolitan statistical area (MSA).

At the MSA level, the American Medical Association (AMA) offers one of the more comprehensive studies on the structural competitiveness of the private health insurance industry.[3] In 2004, the AMA study analyzed 92 of the roughly 320 MSAs in the United States and treated the relevant product market as being both broad (combined HMO/PPO products) and narrow (separate HMO and PPO products). Based on a broad product market definition, the AMA established that the HHI exceeded 1,800 in 86 of the 92 MSAs analyzed. Recall that an HHI in excess of 1,800 indicates a highly concentrated industry. Moreover, the AMA found that the HHI exceeded 1,800 in 88 of the 92 MSAs based on the narrow HMO product definition and in all of the MSAs for the narrow PPO product definition. Therefore, similar to the findings of the more aggregated statewide studies, the AMA finds that high concentration characterizes the health insurance industry in most major MSAs of the United States.

Consequently, the contemporary private health insurance industry appears relatively concentrated in most market areas of the United States. However, for some large employers, self-insurance offers an alternative to purchased health insurance. Large employers with self-insured plans assume the financial risk associated with paying medical claims, although third-party administrators may administer the plan for a fee. Alternatively, large employers may self-fund their plans but purchase stop-loss insurance to cover the risk of large losses or severe adverse claims experiences. About 54 percent of all workers were covered by fully or partially self-funded plans in 2005, rising from 44 percent as recently as 1999.[4] Self-insured plans expanded over time because they are exempt from paying premium taxes, which can run as high as 2 percent. Self-funded plans also expanded because they are subject to the Employee Retirement Income Security Act (ERISA) of 1974, which exempts self-insured plans from providing state-mandated benefits.

3. See the executive summary at http://www.ama-assn.org/ama/pub/category/9573.html (accessed January 6, 2006).

4. Employer Health Benefits 2005 Annual Survey, http://www.kff.org/insurance/7315/sections/ehbs05-10-1.cfm (accessed October 25, 2005).

A **health insurance mandate** is a requirement that an insurance company or a health plan covers specific benefits, health care providers, or patient populations. For example, mandates may include providers such as chiropractors, podiatrists, social workers, and massage therapists; benefits such as mammograms, well-child care, alcohol abuse treatment, acupuncture, and hair prostheses (wigs); and populations such as adopted and noncustodial children.

The Council for Affordable Health Insurance has identified more than 1,800 mandated benefits and providers as of 2005. Mandated benefits may apply only to certain types of coverage and typically vary from state to state. For example, a mandated benefit may exempt individual or small-group coverage or may apply to only insurance companies that are domiciled within a state. The most common mandated benefits are those for mammograms (50 states), maternity stays (50 states), breast reconstruction (48 states), diabetic supplies (47 states), emergency services (46 states), alcohol treatment (45 states), and mental health parity (42 states).[5]

The welfare implications of state health insurance mandates can be debated on both efficiency and equity grounds. In particular, inefficiencies may result if the costs of these state mandates are not justified by their benefits. That is, while these state mandates make health insurance coverage more comprehensive, they can also lead to higher premiums and, consequently, a reduction in the number of people covered by insurance if consumers perceive that the benefits of the additional coverage do not exceed the additional premium costs. In addition, horizontal and vertical inequities may be created because ERISA exempts self-funded plans but not purchased plans from state mandates. For example, workers in large firms, which are more likely to be covered by self-funded plans, may pay lower premiums than otherwise similar workers in small firms because of the ERISA exemption from state mandates. Given these efficiency and equity concerns, the desirability of state mandates continues to be debated by analysts and policy makers.

Barriers to Entry

Although the data portray the private health insurance industry as being relatively concentrated, theory tells us that health insurers may face an incentive to behave efficiently if they face a threat from potential competitors. Potential competition makes it more difficult for existing firms to collude and raise price because they encounter the likelihood that new entrants may break into the market by offering a better deal to their customers. The likelihood of potential competition depends on the height of any barriers to entry. When high enough, barriers deter the entry of new firms.

In the private health insurance industry, scale economies in administering health insurance may serve as a barrier to entry. Scale economies enable existing firms with large volumes of output to underprice new, low-volume competitors and discourage their entry. As discussed in Chapter 8, pricing to deter entry is referred to as limit pricing. Blair et al. (1975) examine the existence of economies of scale by using multiple regression analysis to investigate the relationship between administration expenses and the size of insurance output for a sample of 307 insurance companies in 1968. If per-unit administrative costs decline with output, that would be evidence that scale economies exist in the administration of health insurance.

As a measure of average administrative costs, the authors use total operating costs divided by health insurance premiums. As a measure of the size of health insurance output, they selected the dollar value of premiums written. While premiums written captures both insurance output and price differences across firms, the use of premiums is legitimate if output is homogeneous and competitive pressure forces firms to charge the same price. Blair et al. find that per-unit

5. Council for Affordable Health Insurance, http://www.cahi.org/index.asp (accessed October 25, 2005).

administrative costs were inversely related to output, as measured by premiums, suggesting that long-run economies of scale exist in the administration of health insurance. The policy implication of the empirical findings is that the administration of health insurance should be centralized among a few insurance companies if the goal is to minimize administrative costs. If this finding can be generalized, another implication is that incumbent firms face an advantage over new entrants because of scale economies.

However, in a follow-up study, Blair and Vogel (1978) use survivor analysis (Stigler, 1958) to examine the existence of economies of scale in the provision of health insurance. **Survivor theory** supposes that firm-size classes with expanding populations are more efficient than those with shrinking populations over time. Firms in expanding size classes have obviously met and survived the market test. The survivor test, unlike the econometric test discussed earlier, reflects overall economies in the provision of health insurance, not just scale economies associated with the administrative function. To conduct the survivor test, Blair and Vogel construct seven firm-size classes for commercial health insurers based on real premium volume. They then analyze the percentage of commercial health insurers falling into the various size classes over the period 1958 to 1973.

The authors found that the percentage of firms and total premium volume fell in the smallest firm-size category over time. The other six firm-size classes either grew or remained relatively constant as a percentage of either total premium volume or total firms. Thus, the results of their survivor test suggest that the optimal size extends over quite a large range of output, except for the smallest size category, providing support for constant returns to scale over a relatively vast range of output. According to Blair and Vogel (p. 528), the econometric and survivor tests, taken together, indicate that the administrative scale economies "must have been swamped by diseconomies elsewhere" in some other function(s), such as risk bearing, marketing, and so on. Hence, this study suggests that scale economies do not provide incumbent firms with a relative advantage over new entrants.

Wholey et al. (1996) examine whether HMOs experience scale economies by using a national sample of HMOs over the period 1988 to 1991. They recognized the multiproduct nature of HMO insurance by allowing for both non-Medicare and Medicare coverage. Like Blair and Vogel (1978), Wholey et al. find that small HMOs face scale economies associated with both non-Medicare and Medicare beneficiaries but the scale economies are exhausted relatively quickly. Thus, incumbent insurers do not benefit from scale economies.

In general, entry barriers do not seem to seriously impede entry into the health insurance industry. About 40 health insurance companies operate within the typical state, although most of these insurers make up the competitive fringe (Chollet et al., 2003). Also, the sunk costs of entering the health insurance industry appear to be relatively low because health provider networks can sometimes be rented from incumbent sellers and many lines of the insurance business are fairly fungible. This latter point refers to the idea that it may not be that costly for existing insurance companies to switch among alternative lines of insurance business such as life, health, and disability, for example, in reaction to changes in expected profits. The threat of competitors switching among product lines may inhibit companies in any one line from setting price far above the marginal costs of production.

While inter-industry entry barriers are not particularly limiting, intra-industry entry barriers may exist. Intra-industry barriers prevent or slow sellers from moving from the competitive fringe into the concentrated core of an industry. In the case of health insurance, a few major players such as Aetna, CIGNA, and WellPoint tend to dominate the industry, and the market shares of these dominant sellers tend to be fairly stable over time. It may be that some intra-industry mobility barriers are preventing small health insurers from gaining additional market share. Brand names and advertising are sometimes credited with creating intra-industry mobility barriers. We consider this possibility when we discuss the dominant firm pricing model.

Consumer Information

One of the likely noncompetitive features of the private health insurance industry concerns consumer knowledge. Recall that when individuals possess imperfect information they may pay higher prices and/or receive lower quality when compared to a situation with perfect information. For people belonging to a group plan, this problem may not be as severe since specialists, such as human resource managers or union representatives, often provide individuals with the information to make more educated choices. However, people purchasing individual plans may lack the technical information needed to accurately assess the true value of a health insurance policy. For instance, an individual may be confronted with numerous plans, each offering slightly different benefits, exclusions, and out-of-pocket payments.

Prior to the Omnibus Budget Reconciliation Act (OBRA) of 1990, the market for medigap insurance provided a good example of the importance of consumer information when purchasing insurance. Medigap policies are purchased by individuals to cover any medical payments not reimbursed by Medicare, such as the monthly premium under Part B. Prior to the act, insurers were allowed to offer any number of medigap policies. Reinhardt (1992) pointed out that these policies have been so difficult to comprehend that "many of the elderly have been induced to buy multiple, duplicate policies—probably an intended byproduct of an intended confusion" (p. A5). Reinhardt goes on to note the low payout rate (percent of premiums paid out as benefits) and therefore higher price among commercial insurers for medigap policies (66 percent on average compared to 93.4 percent for traditional Blue Cross/Blue Shield policies) and on small business insurance plans (as low as 77 percent for firms with fewer than 20 employees).

Included as part of the Omnibus Budget Reconciliation Act of 1990 was a provision to reform the medigap market. The legislation attempted to provide more informed consumer choice and thereby promote competition in the medigap market. The law stipulated that after July 1992 only ten standard insurance policies, based on increasing levels of comprehensiveness, could be sold as Medicare supplements to individuals. The basic belief was that ten policies represented sufficient choice and that standardization would facilitate comparisons and promote informed buying of medigap policies.

According to McCormack et al. (1996), the legislation had the intended impact. After the law when into effect, consumer complaints declined considerably in various states because shopping for a policy became easier and more straightforward. Many of those interviewed believed that consumer confusion declined as a result of standardization and because consumers were able to make more informed decisions. In addition, the researchers found that the price of medigap insurance declined, as theory suggests when consumers make more informed decisions. Specifically, the price of an individual medigap policy fell from an average of $1.29 per benefit dollar during the period 1990–1992 to an average of $1.27 for the period 1993–1994.

However, other individual health insurance policies are not as standardized as medigap policies are now. Those not covered by Medicare and who purchase individual plans often face a choice among a multitude of plans with varying benefits, clauses, and exclusions. Although diversity of choices often provides utility, diversity can also be costly when it leads to confused choice. Consequently, informational imperfections may result in some noncompetitive behavior in the individual policy segment of the private health insurance industry.

THE CONDUCT OF THE PRIVATE HEALTH INSURANCE INDUSTRY

From a structural perspective, the private health insurance industry appears to resemble an oligopoly with a relatively large competitive fringe. Although 40 health insurers sell group policies in the typical state, only a few insurers account for a relatively large proportion of earned premiums. Entry barriers do not seem to seriously impede entry into the industry, which probably accounts for the relatively large competitive fringe. The low entry barriers and large competitive fringe most likely help maintain a significant amount of price competition within the industry. Now we examine how a reasonably competitive market structure affects the conduct of private health insurers as the structure, conduct, and performance paradigm suggests it should. Among the behavioral aspects discussed are pricing, managed care effects, rate setting, cherry-picking behavior, and adverse selection.

The Dominant Insurer Pricing Model

According to the data on the number and size distribution of health insurers in the United States, the health insurance industry in most market areas resembles a tight oligopoly with a relatively large competitive fringe. For various reasons, some health insurers have become quite dominant over time while others have remained fairly small in terms of market share. Business organizations typically become dominant in their market for various reasons including sheer luck, technical and pecuniary economies, superior performance, or mergers with other organizations. Let us elaborate.

Like individuals, some organizations are just luckier than others. Mere chance may mean several successive years of tremendous growth such that a relatively small organization can be quickly transformed into a much larger one. Once the firm is relatively large, it becomes difficult for smaller competitors to catch up.

Organizations may also become dominant as they strive for survival in the marketplace by attempting to exploit any economies from larger size. Technical economies refer to any economies of scale or scope that may be conferred to a larger organization. Pecuniary economies occur when large organizations purchase inputs and supplies at a lower price than similar but smaller organizations. If a very large size is necessary to fully exploit technical and pecuniary economies in a particular industry, firms in that industry will seek a large size over time to survive in a competitive market. Thus, a few dominant firms may evolve and be observed in industries characterized by vast technical and pecuniary economies.

Some analysts refer to the existence of a few dominant firms that result from seeking the gains from large size as the Rule of Three. The Rule of Three states, "In competitive, mature markets, there is room for only three major players along with several (in some markets, many) niche players" (Sheth and Sisodia, 1998, p. A22). The large dominant firms are volume-driven generalists who compete across a wide range of differentiated, name-brand products and services while the smaller organizations either are niche players or produce standardized versions of the name-brand products. According to Sheth and Sisodia, the Rule of Three can be observed in the beer, cereals, tires, insurance, aluminum, oil, chemicals, and airline industries, among others. Note the inclusion of the insurance industry among those affected by the Rule of Three.

Superior performance may also provide a business with a dominant market share. Superiority may result from an excellent product or a low-cost production process. Microsoft represents a good example of dominance resulting from a superior product. In fact, many analysts argue that a superior product tends to provide the best explanation for dominance, although various business tactics and strategies such as limit pricing or persuasive advertising must be employed to prevent dominant market shares from eventually receding (recall the example of Johnson & Johnson in Chapter 8).

Finally, organizations may become dominant in a particular market through horizontal or vertical integration. Recall that horizontal integration takes place when firms producing similar products merge together. As discussed in the context of the Williamson model in Chapter 9, horizontal mergers benefit consumers if cost savings and lower prices result from the larger size. However, monopoly pricing may occur if the larger size confers market power onto the firm. Vertical integration involves the combination of firms that produce at successive stages of production, or stated differently, among buyers and sellers. A merger between a hospital and a group physician practice or a hospital and a nursing home represent examples of vertical integration. Chapters 13 and 14 discuss vertical integrations in the context of the hospital and pharmaceutical industries, respectively. Let us just note here that vertical integration may also have procompetitive and anticompetitive impacts on consumers.

Now that we have some idea about how one or a few firms may grow to dominate an industry, an interesting question emerges concerning how a dominant firm may influence the price of a good or service in a market when a competitive fringe of sellers also exists. When a dominant firm operates in a market with a competitive fringe, economists often use the dominant firm pricing model to analyze how market price and quantity are determined. The dominant firm pricing model involves the following assumptions.

The first assumption is that only one dominant firm exists in the industry. While few markets, even health insurance markets, are characterized by a single dominant firm, this model still holds if the few dominant firms act in a concerted fashion by either overtly or tacitly coordinating their prices. Two, the dominant firm is assumed to be a low-cost producer relative to the rest of the firms in the competitive fringe. In fact, the dominant firm gains its dominance in this model because of its favorable position as a low-cost producer. Third, the model assumes that a fixed number of firms constitute the competitive fringe and that each firm can be treated as being a price taker. Fourth, the dominant firm is assumed to know industry demand and how much the competitive fringe firms will collectively supply at various prices. Finally, all firms, including the dominant firm and those in the competitive fringe, are assumed to produce a homogeneous product, which sells at an identical price.

Figure 11–1 provides a graphical depiction of the dominant firm pricing model in the context of a market for health insurance. The quantity of health insurance (perhaps the number of policies written) is shown on the horizontal axis, and dollar values are shown on the vertical axis. Market demand is represented by the downward-sloping demand curve labeled D and the supply of the fringe firms is captured by the upward-sloping curve S_F. To maximize profits, the dominant firm must determine how much health insurance to sell and what price to charge given the market demand for health insurance and the competitive fringe supply.

Let's suppose that ACME Insurance Company represents the dominant health insurer in some market area. To maximize profits, ACME must first determine its residual demand. Residual demand equals the amount of health insurance left over for ACME in the market after deducting the amount of health insurance offered for sale by the competitive fringe insurers. Mathematically, ACME's residual demand is found by subtracting the quantity supplied of the competitive fringe insurers from market demand at each and every price. Figure 11–1 reflects the graphical derivation of the residual demand curve facing ACME. At a price represented by point A, ACME's residual demand equals zero because the fringe supply insurers completely satisfy market demand at that price. Oppositely, at a price indicated by point B, market demand equals ACME's residual demand because at that price, the competitive fringe insurers do not produce and sell any health insurance. In fact, at any price below point B, market demand also represents ACME's residual demand.

FIGURE 11–1
Dominant Insurer Pricing Model

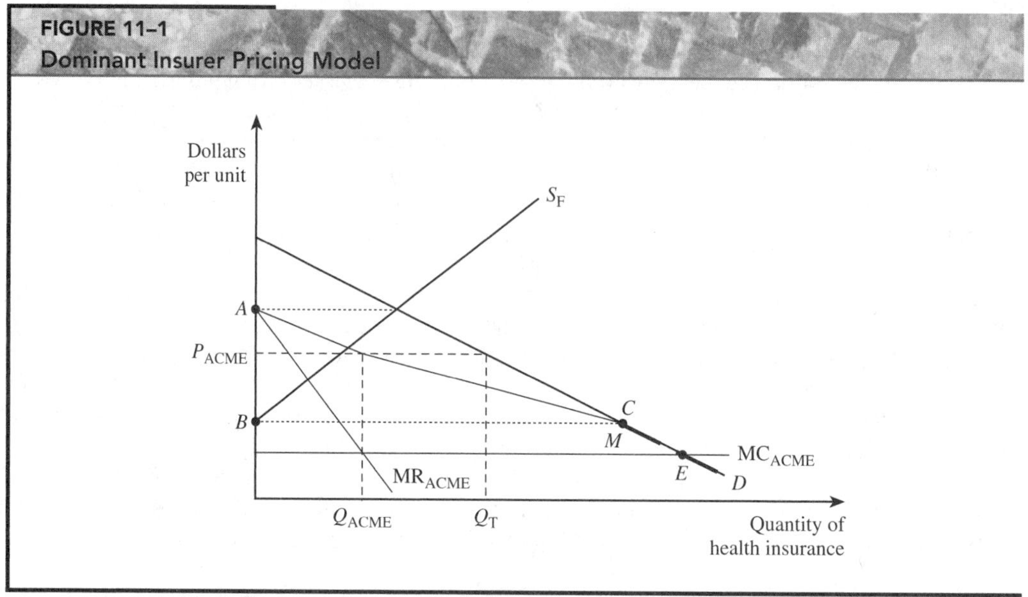

D represents the market demand curve for health insurance and the supply of the competitive fringe firms is labeled as S_F. ACME Insurance, the dominant firm in the market, derives its residual demand by subtracting the fringe supply from market demand at each and every price. At the price represented by point *A*, ACME offers no insurance on the market whereas ACME completely fills market orders for health insurance at a price indicated by point *B*. ACME's residual demand is thus found by the curve labeled as *A-C-M-E*. Following the usual procedure for a linear demand curve, ACME's marginal revenue curve, MR_{ACME}, is derived from its demand curve. ACME is assumed to be a lower-cost producer than the competitive fringe and assumed to produce with constant marginal costs so the marginal cost curve is drawn as MC_{ACME}. To maximize profits where MR = MC, ACME sells Q_{ACME} amount of health insurance and charges P_{ACME}. The fringe firms take the price set by ACME and produce the rest of the market output indicated by the horizontal distance between Q_{ACME} and Q_T.

ACME's residual demand curve can be derived by drawing a line from point *A* to point *C*, opposite *B* on the market demand curve, and connecting it to the segment of the market demand curve labeled as *ME*. Thus, *A-C-M-E* represents ACME's kinked residual demand curve. Let's assume that section *AC* of ACME's demand curve represents the relevant range for price, so the kink in its demand curve plays no role in the analysis. Given this assumption, ACME's marginal revenue curve can be derived from its demand curve. Recall from Chapter 8 that the marginal revenue curve shares the same intercept as a linear demand curve but has twice its slope (in absolute terms). Following this procedure, ACME's marginal revenue curve is graphically depicted and labeled as MR_{ACME}.

One of the assumptions behind this model is that the dominant firm is a low-cost producer. As a result, ACME's marginal cost curve is drawn below the fringe supply. Following the empirical studies previously discussed, it is further assumed that ACME produces health insurance with constant marginal costs, so a horizontal marginal cost curve is drawn.

To maximize profits, ACME sells the amount of health insurance indicated by Q_{ACME} because marginal revenue equals marginal costs at that point. ACME charges a price of P_{ACME} for its health insurance. As price takers, the competitive fringe accepts the price set by ACME and produces the rest of the market demand as indicated by the horizontal distance between Q_{ACME} and

Q_T. Conceptually that horizontal distance is the same as the one between the origin and the quantity read off the fringe supply curve at a price of P_{ACME}.

Several implications can be drawn from the dominant firm pricing model. First, market price is lower because of the dominant firm. In our example, market price would be determined by the intersection of market demand and fringe supply at point *A* in Figure 11–1 if ACME, with its lower costs, did not exist. However, if ACME acted competitively and charged a price corresponding to its marginal costs of production, market price would be even lower. In fact, if ACME set a price corresponding to its marginal costs, the competitive fringe would be driven from the market according to the graphical model in Figure 11–1.

Second, the model implies that a larger competitive fringe causes the price set by the dominant firm to fall. In Figure 11–1, a larger competitive fringe can be treated as a fringe supply located further to the right. If so, the residual demand facing ACME shifts downward to the left and thus market price falls. Third, a more elastic fringe supply also puts downward pressure on the market price set by the dominant firm according to the model. For example, if the fringe supply in Figure 11–1 becomes flatter (more elastic) but pivots off of the same vertical point, ACME's residual demand shifts downward to the left and price declines.

In sum, the dominant firm pricing model is a useful conceptual device when considering the pricing behavior of a market characterized by a single dominant firm or a few dominant firms and containing a competitive fringe. The model suggests that even a dominant firm must consider the reaction of the smaller firms when setting prices. Moreover, the model predicts that the dominant firm faces more pressure to set a low price when the competitive fringe market share is greater and when the fringe supply is more responsive to price.

Other Issues Relating to the Pricing of Health Insurance

The dominant firm pricing model is useful for analyzing the market forces that help determine the price or health insurance premium paid by consumers. However, for the sake of manageability, the model ignores some of the complexities actually involved in the setting of premiums.

In practice, a private health insurance company sets the premium equal to the expected benefits to be paid out (E[BEN]), plus any marketing and administrative expenses (ADMIN), federal, state, and local taxes (TAX), and profits (PROFIT), or

(11–1) $$\text{Premium} = \text{E[BEN]} + \text{ADMIN} + \text{TAX} + \text{PROFIT}.$$

The dollar benefits the insurance company expects to pay out are equal to the actual benefits, BEN, plus some forecast error, *e*; that is,

(11–2) $$\text{E[BEN]} = \text{BEN} + e.$$

Since people can expect to receive some of their premiums back in the form of reimbursed medical expenditures, health economists sometimes measure the price of insurance, or loading fee, using the ratio of premiums to actual benefits paid out, or Premium/BEN. The ratio can be obtained by substituting Equation 11–2 into Equation 11–1 and dividing by the actual dollar benefits paid out, or

(11–3) $$\text{Price} = 1 + \frac{\text{ADMIN} + \text{TAX} + \text{PROFIT} + e}{\text{BEN}}.$$

The price of health insurance reveals the average amount that must be spent in premiums to receive one dollar in benefits. For example, a price of \$1.25 means the representative individual pays \$1.25 to receive \$1 in benefits, on average. The remaining 25 cents is the loading fee. The magnitude of the loading fee depends on a host of factors, including the administrative technology, tax laws, any forecast errors, and the competitive nature of the market for private health insurance (Sindelar, 1988).

In a competitive market, the loading fee is driven to a normal level, that is, a level that is sufficient to pay for necessary administrative and marketing costs, taxes, and a normal profit rate (if a for-profit insurer). Given that the health insurance industry seems reasonably competitive, at least in the group health insurance market, incentives most likely exist for some degree of price competition among health insurers.

However, many health insurers now compete not only on the basis of price (loading fee) but also on the ability to control health care costs—the actual health benefits paid out. Prior to the 1980s, the not-for-profit Blue Cross plans dominated many markets and were controlled by hospital interests. Lacking incentives, Blue Cross plans pursued a policy of encouraging complete health insurance coverage. The policy led to high hospital prices and medical costs and elevated health insurance premiums (Hay and Leahy, 1987). Now most insurers are forced by the cost consciousness of their payers, such as employers, to control health benefits paid out by adopting managed care practices. Thus, competition has created an incentive for health insurers to hold down both the loading fee and actual medical benefits paid out.

In trying to contain both the loading fee and benefits paid, health insurers now face an interesting trade-off. Managed care contains health care costs (or benefits paid out) most effectively through various administrative functions such as utilization review. However, more spending on administrative functions leads to a higher loading fee (see Equation 11–3). Economic principles suggest that an insurer chooses the optimal amount of an input by equating its marginal benefit and marginal cost. Certainly a profit-maximizing insurer would never knowingly implement a policy or function for which its program costs exceed its benefits in terms of additional revenues or cost savings. For example, when the backlash mounted against the restrictive cost-control practices of MCOs in the 1990s, companies began to abolish "preauthorization," the practice of making doctors get permission for certain tests or treatments. Most companies realized that they were spending millions of dollars each year assessing the practice decisions of physicians, yet ultimately denied only 2% of their requests.

Hence any further push for cost containment means that managed care activities will continue to increase in scope and, consequently, larger loading fees are likely to result. The magnitude of the premium level, the sum of benefits paid out, and the loading fee reflects the overall success or failure of managed care activities. With that idea in mind, the following section discusses the role and effects of managed care organizations.

Managed Care Organizations and Insurance Premiums

Managed care organizations (MCOs), which include HMOs and PPOs, integrate the delivery of health care with the insurance function. Advocates have claimed that MCOs are capable of reducing the level and growth of health insurance premiums. The reduction of health insurance premiums comes about in two ways. First, MCOs of various kinds, by design, are expected to moderate the scope of the moral hazard problem by adopting various financial incentives and management strategies aimed at both consumers and health care providers, as discussed in Chapter 6. Examples include utilization controls and negotiated price discounts from health care providers. Competition among MCOs pressures each managed care insurer to set premiums closer to the actual costs of servicing its own subscribers. Second, the competition from MCOs motivates traditional insurers to make similar improvements in utilization and costs and to reduce their premiums or face the prospect of losing business.

As will be discussed in Chapter 13, a host of studies (for example, Manning et al., 1984; Rapoport, 1992; Miller and Luft, 1994) have found that MCOs, especially HMOs, attain medical cost savings of about 15 to 20 percent through a reduced hospital-intensive practice style.[6] The question is whether the reduced medical costs brought about by managed care translate into lower premiums systemwide. According to Morrisey (2001), the answer to this question depends on the degree to which employers change plans in response to lower premiums, the extent to which competition among managed care plans leads to lower managed care premiums, and how lower managed care premiums influence the premiums of traditional insurers. As discussed in Chapter 6, the few studies examining choice of plans from the perspective of the employer found relatively high premium elasticities ranging as high as −8 when multiple plans are offered and employees must pay more for expensive plans. Consequently, available studies, for the most part, suggest that employers do respond to lower premiums.

In terms of whether managed care premiums decline, some economists point out that the greater administrative costs (loading fee) associated with MCOs may swamp any medical cost savings (benefits paid out) as previously pointed out. McLaughlin (1988) argues that the health insurance market initially responded to managed care insurance with cost-increasing rivalry, not price competition, as both traditional and managed care insurers have chosen to compete on service offering rather than on price.

Feldman et al. (1993) note that "many companies accuse HMOs of 'shadow-pricing,' that is, setting their premiums just below that of commercial carriers. HMOs can profit from shadow pricing if they tend to enroll a disproportionate share of young, healthy workers in the firm" (p. 781). The authors compared the weighted average HMO and fee-for-service (FFS) premiums in firms that offer both HMOs and FFS plans to the premium of FFS-only firms. They found that offering a HMO plan raises rather than lowers the average premium of an insurance policy for family and single coverage. Insurance premiums rise if HMOs skim the healthiest patients and thereby drive up FFS costs and premiums (Baker and Corts, 1995).

Studies using more recent data, however, support the notion that competition among managed care companies has led to lower managed care premiums. Wholey et al. (1995) use multiple regression analysis to examine the impact of HMO competition and penetration on the level of HMO premiums in various metropolitan areas of the United States for the years 1988 to 1991. The authors find that a greater number of HMOs in the market area resulted in lower HMO premiums. Higher penetration of HMOs was also found to be associated with reduced HMO premiums.

As a complementary study, Pauly et al. (2002) analyze the impact of competition among HMOs on their profitability using a sample of 262 U.S. metropolitan areas in 1994. Competition is measured by the number of HMOs and also by the relative size distribution of the various HMOs in each metropolitan area. The authors find that greater competition among HMOs tends to be associated with lower profit rates, as measured by metropolitan areawide HMO profits divided by the comparable premium revenues. For example, their simulation showed that profits decline by about 12 to 30 percent if one new HMO enters the market with a 10 percent share. The authors also found that high profitability did not persist over the period 1994 to 1997, suggesting that entry and expansion forced HMOs to actively compete.

Empirical studies have also examined whether lower managed care premiums influence the premiums of traditional insurers and systemwide premiums levels. Wickizer and Feldstein (1995) used multiple regression analysis to isolate and examine the impact of the HMO market

6. See the various health care industry studies in the following chapters for detailed information about the relation between managed care and medical cost savings.

penetration rate on the growth of indemnity premiums for 95 insured groups over the period 1985 to 1992. They found empirically that the HMO penetration rate had an inverse impact on the growth of indemnity premiums. As an illustration, they estimate that the real rate of growth in premiums would be approximately 5.9 instead of 7 percent for the average group located in a market where the HMO penetration rate increased by 25 percent. The authors concluded by noting that their results "indicate that competitive strategies, relying on managed care, have significant potential to reduce health insurance premium growth rates, thereby resulting in substantial cost savings over time" (p. 250).

Baker et al. (2000) investigate the impact of HMO market penetration on the costs of employer-sponsored health insurance. Using data for more than 20,000 private employers in both 1993 and 1997, the authors find that costs for employer health plans were about 8 to 10 percent lower in metropolitan areas with an HMO market penetration rate above 45 percent than ones with HMO market penetration rates below 25 percent. The result reflects both lower HMO premiums and lower premiums for non-HMO plans in markets where the HMO penetration rate exceeds 25 percent. This latter result refutes the notion that HMOs achieve savings by only selecting the healthiest and least expensive patients because, if so, non-HMO premiums would increase with greater HMO penetration.

In sum, MCOs, particularly HMOs, have achieved sizeable medical cost savings from various utilization and cost-control techniques. Recent studies have tended to find that these cost savings have translated into lower premiums provided that a sufficient degree of competition exists among HMOs. In addition, recent evidence suggests that systemwide premiums savings result from increased penetration and competition of HMOs.

Do HMOs Possess Monopsony Power?

One way that MCOs might reduce medical costs is by forcing health care provider reimbursement rates below the competitive level. Theoretically, an outcome like that can occur when one or a few MCOs enjoy a sizeable amount of buying power within a market. The lower reimbursement rates, in turn, may discourage providers from offering services on the market. This reduction of medical services may seriously compromise the quantity and quality of care received by the people in an area.

When payers possess enough buying power to drive price below the competitive level, market power is said to exist on the demand side of the market. The extreme case is that of a monopsony when only one buyer of a good or service exists in a market. Oligopsony is a situation involving a few dominant buyers of a product. When a monopsony exists in an otherwise competitive marketplace, economic theory suggests that both the price and quantity of the product are lower than the competitive model predicts. Figure 11–2 clarifies the economic logic behind this point by examining the impact of a hypothetical monopsonist in the market for hospital services. The price and quantity of inpatient days are shown on the vertical and horizontal axes, respectively. Market demand and supply are labeled *D* and *S*, respectively (ignore the MFC curve for now).

In a competitive market consisting of a large number of buyers and sellers, each individual buyer and seller acts as a price taker. For example, suppose we view the market for hospital services as containing a relatively large number of hospitals supplying services and a large number of health insurance companies negotiating hospital prices on behalf of subscribers. If each health insurer and each hospital represents only a tiny fraction of the total market, all market participants can be treated as price takers. In effect, each health insurer faces a horizontal individual supply curve (rather than market supply) of hospital services and, given its inconsequential

FIGURE 11–2
Monopsony Model of the Market for Hospital Services

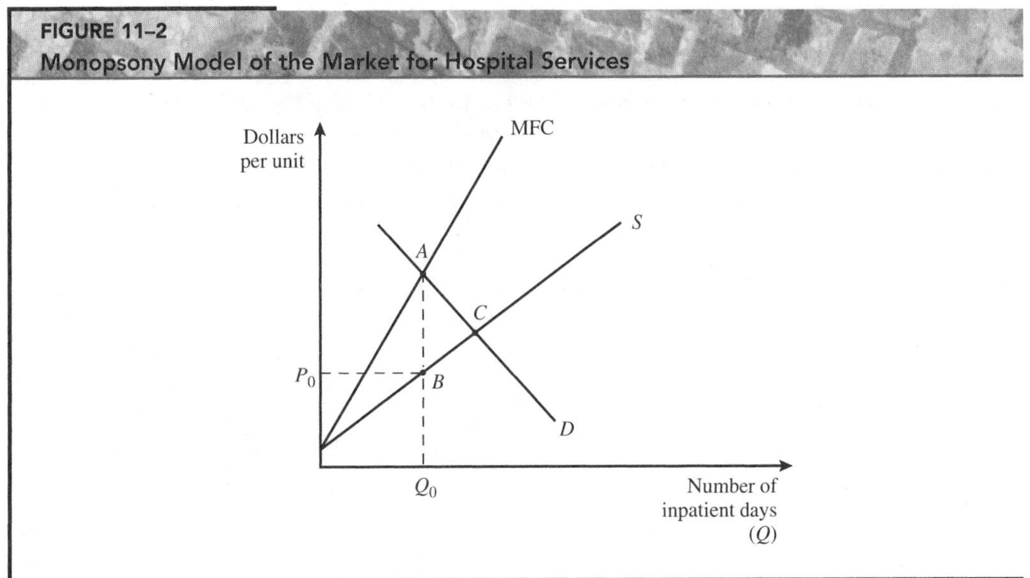

Point *C* in the graph indicates the competitive outcome when all market participants are price takers. The MFC curve represents the incremental cost of purchasing an additional patient day when the insurer has monopsony power. In this case, the monopsonist purchases hospital inpatient days up to the point where the demand curve crosses the marginal factor cost curve, Q_0, and pays P_0. Notice that when the buyer has monopsony power both price and quantity are lower than the competitive level.

market share, can purchase hospital services without influencing its market price. Each hospital, also as a price taker, faces a horizontal or perfectly elastic demand for its product and cannot influence the market price of hospital services. As all of the hospitals and health insurers each act as price takers, competitive equilibrium occurs at point *C* in Figure 11–2, as supply and demand theory suggests.

Now, instead of a large number of health insurers with tiny individual market shares, suppose only one health insurer, as a monopsonist, covers all of the people and represents the only purchaser of hospital services in an area. However, continue to suppose the existence of a large number of hospitals with relatively small market shares such that each hospital can be treated as a price taker. As a monopsonist, the health insurer faces the market supply curve for hospital services, which is positively sloped reflecting the higher costs for hospitals when supplying additional inpatient days. The positively sloped supply curve means that the monoponist must pay a higher price to negotiate a greater number of inpatient days at the beginning of the contract period. Assuming that a uniform price is set for each and every day, a monopsonistic health insurer must pay a higher price not only for any higher cost additional patient days but also for the other lower-cost patient days. Since the monopsonist must pay a higher price for each and every day when purchasing an additional inpatient day, the total incremental cost to the insurer of purchasing an additional day exceeds the average cost per inpatient day as revealed by the supply curve. As a result, the marginal factor cost (MFC) associated with an additional patient day lies above market supply, as depicted by the MFC curve in Figure 11–2. The MFC reflects the additional costs of both the marginal and "inframarginal" days from the perspective of the monopsonist insurer. Inframarginal in this case, refers to the "previous" days.

To determine the profit-maximizing amount of inpatient days to purchase from the hospitals, the monopsonistic health insurer equates demand to marginal factor cost. In the figure, the profit-maximizing number of inpatient days occurs at Q_0. The price necessary to attract this number of inpatient days from the various hospitals in this area can be read off the supply curve as P_0. Thus monopsony theory suggests that a single buyer pays a lower price and purchases a lower quantity than the competitive level typically indicates. A deadweight loss equal to the triangular area *ACB* results from the monopsonistic distortion, reflecting an inefficient allocation of resources. Monopsony, like monopoly, is clearly undesirable from a societal point of view.

Feldman and Wholey (2001) investigate whether HMOs have monopsony power in the markets for ambulatory and inpatient hospital services. They use a data set containing all of the HMOs in the United States from 1985 through 1997. The authors use multiple regression analysis to investigate the importance of an HMO as a buyer on both the price paid and utilization. Feldman and Wholey rightfully argue that monopsony theory predicts that *both* price and quantity should decline with the importance of an HMO as a buyer. Finding that price declines is not enough to indicate monopsony power because HMOs, through their buying power, may simply "beat back" or countervail the monopoly power of medical suppliers rather than drive price below the competitive level.

In their study, HMO buying power for hospital services is measured by the percentage of community hospital days in the market area that is purchased by each HMO. HMO buying power for ambulatory services is measured by the number of ambulatory visits purchased by the HMO per 1,000 active physicians in the market area. The dependent variables in the various regression equations are the prices paid by individual HMOs for ambulatory care and inpatient hospital days and, as utilization measures, the annual number of ambulatory visits and hospital days per member. Feldman and Wholey also control for a host of other supply and demand factors in the regression equation that influence price and utilization. Their empirical results show that HMO buying power over hospitals has a negative and significant effect on hospital price per day but no impact on the price of ambulatory visits. They also find that HMO buying power led to increased hospital use but had no statistically significant effect on ambulatory visits. Feldman and Wholey note that their results support the "monopoly busting" and not the monopsony view of HMO buying power. They also suggest that HMO buying power has improved the efficiency of markets for hospital services. Consequently, their study finds that the typical HMO does not possess monopsony power.

Rating of Premiums, Adverse Selection, and Risk Selection

As shown in Equation 11–1, health insurers consider the expected medical benefits to be paid out when establishing health insurance premiums. How closely the premiums paid by a particular person mirrors her expected medical benefits depends on whether the insurance company uses community or experience rating or some combination of the two rating methods when setting premiums. When an insurance company practices community rating, expected medical benefits are based on the risk characteristics of the entire plan membership and not the health history or risk status of a particular person. However, even pure community-rated premiums may differ across individuals because of geographical location due to cost-of-living considerations, type of contract (individual or family), and benefit design (level of copayments, coinsurance, deductibles, and benefits covered).

In contrast, when premiums are determined by experience rating, insurers place individuals, or a group of individuals, into different risk categories based on various identifiable personal characteristics, such as age, gender, occupation, and prior illnesses. Premiums are then based on geographical location, type of contract, and benefit design but also on the relation between risk category and expected health care costs as determined by using historical data. Under experience rating, individuals or groups of individuals pay a price closer to their expected medical benefits.

Analysts and policy makers continue to debate the relative merits of community and experience rating of premiums in terms of their efficiency and equity considerations. For example, some analysts point out that experience rating of premiums is more efficient because it creates an incentive for people to adopt favorable lifestyles. That is, if people are required to pay more for health insurance because they smoke cigarettes or drink excessively, for example, they will be more inclined to practice good health behaviors. Advocates of experience rating also note that high-risk people might be more wealthy than low-risk people, and thus community-rated premiums can end up redistributing income from the poor to the rich. For example, young low-income individuals may cross-subsidize wealthy elderly individuals when premiums are community rated.

Advocates also point out that experience rating can reduce the practice of adverse selection to some degree. **Adverse selection** occurs when high-risk consumers, who know more about their own health status than insurers do, subscribe to an insured group composed of lower-risk individuals. To secure low premiums, the high-risk consumers withhold information concerning their true health status. Once these consumers are insured, the insurer has no alternative but to increase premiums for all plan subscribers in the next period due to the higher utilization rates of high-risk consumers. As low-risk subscribers leave the higher-priced policies, "musical insurance plans" may develop as high-risk individuals follow low-risk individuals in pursuit of lower premiums. In addition, some insurers may find it difficult to earn a normal profit. Alternatively, some low-risk individuals may eventually find it cheaper to self-insure. If so, high-risk individuals end up in homogeneous pools paying high premiums or being excluded from health insurance coverage (Rothschild and Stiglitz, 1976). Insurers can prevent adverse selection to some degree by limiting people's ability to change plans or through prior screening and experience rating.

Figure 11–3 shows how community rating of premiums can lead to cross-subsiding of insurance costs and inefficiencies at least temporarily. In the figure, varying premium levels are shown on the vertical axis and the amount of insurance coverage is measured along the horizontal axis. We begin by assuming that two equally sized low-risk, D_L, and high-risk, D_H, groups are demanding insurance coverage but both groups belong to the same plan, at least initially. Notice that both demands are downward sloping to indicate that more coverage is purchased at a lower premium regardless of risk category. Also note that the high-risk group possesses a greater demand for insurance coverage at each premium level. The greater demand of the high-risk group reflects the greater expected medical benefits to be paid out on their behalf by the insurer at each level of coverage relative to the low-risk group.

Further suppose that the administrator (for example, the employer), by considering the welfare of the average person in the plan and the trade-off between premiums and wage income, chooses the level of coverage indicated by Q_0. Given that points C (= \$1,000) and E (= \$3,000) reflect the likely benefits paid out to the two groups at Q_0 amount of coverage, the insurance company charges a uniform community rated premium of P_0 (= \$2,000) per enrollee that averages the risk status and medical costs of the two groups.

Notice at the premium of P_0 that the low-risk group prefers less insurance coverage as indicated by point A in Figure 11–3. Stated differently, low-risk individuals are required to purchase more insurance than they find optimal at a price of P_0. In addition, the figure shows that low-risk individuals cross-subsidize the costs of high-risk individuals. The size of the cross-subsidy paid by the low-risk group is measured by the vertical distance between their willingness to pay for Q_0 amount of coverage at point C (= \$1,000) and point F (= \$2,000), the actual premium they are required to pay.

FIGURE 11–3
Community Rating of Premiums and Cross-Subsidization

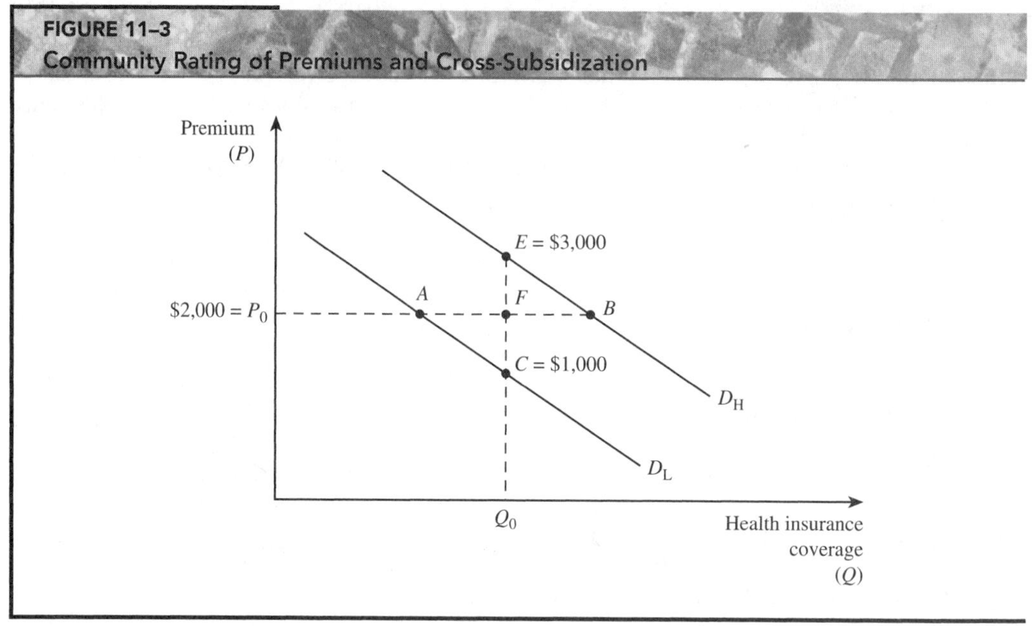

Suppose the employer offers Q_0 amount of coverage at a premium of $2,000 to all of its employees. If so, low-risk employees, as reflected in the demand curve, D_L, cross-subsidize high-risk employees, D_H. If low-risk employees have other choices, they opt out of the plan and the premium eventually rises to $3,000.

Also note that high-risk individuals prefer more insurance coverage at a premium of P_0 as indicated by point *B*. Thus the model suggests that both groups could be made better off in separate plans at the existing price of P_0. But the model suggests that high-risk individuals would end up paying a higher premium in the absence of the cross-subsidy from the low-risk individuals. The unsubsidized premium, in turn, prices some of the high-risk individuals out of the insurance market.

In the longer run, the community-rated premium situation in Figure 11–3 may not represent a stable equilibrium, particularly when individuals are free to choose among alternatives. For example, low-risk individuals may seek out other insurance plans in which a lower premium conforms more closely to their expected medical benefits paid out. Or if low-risk individuals are not free to select among policies, they may choose to self-insure if that is an option. Consequently, if health insurance is not mandatory, theory suggests that low-risk individuals will try to leave community-rated health plans such that high-risk individuals will find themselves in more homogenous pools and paying a higher premium for their coverage or excluded from coverage.

However, advocates of community rating of premiums view the situation differently and argue that experience rating of premiums is both inequitable and inefficient. Experience rating is deemed inequitable because some people are charged a higher price for health insurance simply because of their poor health status. The inequity of experience rating is particularly acute when poor health status is uncontrollable rather than a function of a chosen adverse lifestyle.

Advocates of community rating further claim that experience rating of premiums encourages insurers to engage in risk selection or cherry-picking behavior. It has been pointed out that if insurers practiced community rating of premiums and accepted all applicants for coverage, they would be more interested in creating systemwide medical cost savings rather than choosing among individual low-risk subscribers. More specifically, many health care experts believe that competition among insurers, in conjunction with experience rating, provides an incentive for insurers, as a group, to offer health insurance to healthy individuals but deny coverage to people with poor health. The best cherries (the healthy) are picked off the tree, while the worst are left dangling. The reasoning behind the cherry-picking behavior is rather straightforward. Facing increased market competition, insurers are forced to lower premiums. One way to lower premiums is to insure only low-risk individuals. The result is that health insurance companies tend to compete for low-risk individuals, that is, healthy people. Those in poor health are either denied access to health insurance or charged prohibitively high prices.

Individuals who belong to large, employment-based group policies, which are the predominant form of private health insurance in the United States, are relatively insulated from this problem. While premiums for experience-rated group policies are adjusted annually based on the actual claims experience of the group and changes in medical care prices, the total cost is distributed equally among all group members, thus minimizing the burden for any one individual.

In contrast, people who lack access to large-group coverage have difficulty obtaining health insurance at comparable premiums. People who apply for insurance, either individually, as a family, or through small businesses, are usually subject to stringent insurance underwriting procedures because providing insurance to these individuals is much riskier. A health status questionnaire or physical exam is normally required. Depending on the resulting risk status of the individual(s), insurance companies usually offer health insurance at an increased premium and/or exclude coverage for any preexisting conditions for a period of one year or more. Preexisting conditions are serious illnesses that were diagnosed before the policy took effect and might include cancer, heart disease, AIDS, or care for low-birthweight babies. Conditions that trigger higher rates vary widely across insurance companies but routinely include such common conditions as hypertension, allergies, arthritis, and asthma. Thus, for individual purchasers of health insurance, especially those with chronic health problems or high-risk conditions, high premiums may be an obstacle to obtaining coverage.

Health insurers may practice cherry-picking (or equivalently, cream-skimming) behavior in a number of subtler ways depending on what information they possess (Van De Ven and Ellis, 2000). If unable to identify the health risks of individuals in the market and what the precise health risks are, insurers may structure their health insurance coverage so high-risk individuals reveal themselves. For example, the benefits package may not cover prescription drugs or may contain high out-of-pocket expenses. If insurers know the precise health risks for conditions such as AIDS but not the risk characteristics of specific individuals, they may not contract with physicians known to treat patients with high-cost illnesses. Finally, if insurers can predict unprofitable individuals, marketing strategies might be focused away from high-risk individuals and towards low-risk individuals.

While this view of cherry-picking behavior and access denial is generally accepted at face value, empirical studies on this topic have been relatively lacking. One of the few studies to date, by Beauregard (1991), used data from the 1987 National Medical Expenditure Survey to estimate the number of uninsured people who were denied private health insurance or could purchase only limited coverage because of poor health. Beauregard's study found that benefit denial is not as widespread as typically believed. In particular, only a very small proportion of the uninsured population, less than 1 percent, was found to have ever been denied private health insurance due to poor health. However, the author cautions that the figure does not include currently insured individuals whose policies exclude coverage for preexisting conditions.

Pollitz et al. (2001) provide a very compelling study concerning access to coverage for those in less-than-perfect health in the individual health insurance market. The study involves seven "hypothetical" health insurance applicants, aged 12 to 62, of both genders, and with different preexisting conditions such as hay fever, depression, prior knee injury, and "HIV-positive status". Although the specific conditions are not representative of the general population, they are similar to those experienced by a large number of people. Sixty applications for each hypothetical person were submitted to nineteen insurance companies in eight market areas around the country, including six Blue Cross/Blue Shield plans, six HMOs, and seven national or regional commercial carriers.

Each insurer was asked to underwrite the applications. Underwriting involves determining whether to cover someone and on what terms. The participating insurers responded to these hypothetical applications by accepting the applicant for standard coverage at a standard rate for a healthy person, rejecting the applicant, offering coverage with special restrictions on covered benefits, or offering coverage at a higher-than-standard premium. Carriers were asked for information about their most frequently sold policies in each individual market with a $500 annual deductible and a $20 office visit copayment. Carriers were also asked to provide the standard premium rate for policies with these features corresponding to the age and gender of the seven hypothetical applicants for the healthiest applicants.

The results from the experiment were insightful. Of the 420, only 43 (10 percent) applications resulted in standard coverage at the standard rate. The applications were rejected 154 times, with the HIV applicant accounting for 60 of the rejections. Of the accepted applications (63 percent), most imposed benefit restrictions (118 applications), premium surcharges (56), or both (49). The researchers found that the results varied somewhat across states, with different state rules explaining some of the difference.

The results of their study imply that consumers who are in less-than-perfect health clearly face significant barriers to obtaining health insurance coverage in the individual health insurance market. Insurance companies often decline to cover people who have preexisting conditions, and when they offer coverage, they frequently impose limitations and or raise premiums. Higher premiums can often price people with preexisting conditions out of the individual market.

Guaranteed Renewability in the Individual Health Insurance Market

Individual health insurance offers two advantages over group health insurance. First, unlike employer-sponsored plans, the consumer has considerable choice over the specifics of the health insurance policy. Second, an individual health insurance plan offers more portability in the sense that coverage can be retained even if a person changes jobs. However, we learned in the preceding discussion that individual health insurance also has various disadvantages associated with it such as adverse selection, experience rating, and risk selection (that is, cream skimming). But Patel and Pauly (2002) explain that individual health insurance contracts can be written with a guaranteed renewability clause such that adverse selection, experience rating, and cream skimming present less of a problem for individuals and insurance companies.

Guaranteed renewability is a contractual feature in an insurance policy that requires the insurer to (1) sell another policy on the anniversary date of the current period, and (2) charge a premium for that policy that is not affected by any individual loss experience or change in the insured person's circumstances during the current period. This feature means that the insurer cannot re-underwrite an insurance contract on renewal. However, the insurer has the right to increase premium rates for the underwriting class in which a policy is initially placed (for example, based on age and gender).

It stands to reason that higher premiums are charged when an insurance contract offers the guaranteed renewability (GR) feature. In essence, the consumer is purchasing two policies for a single premium. The first policy pays for the claims experienced during the current term and the second policy covers the claims of individuals in the rating class who become above-average risks at some point.

Patel and Pauly explain that the GR feature helps solve some of the problems associated with the individual market when risk varies among individuals. Because of GR, people are individually protected against unexpected jumps in premiums relating to the onset of a chronic condition. That is, once a person becomes chronically ill, the GR provision means that he has locked into a premium that is independent of his individual health status, and therefore experience rating cannot be practiced on renewal. This feature does not protect people against age adjustments, which are predictable. Also, GR does not protect against rising health care costs because marketwide risks cannot be reduced through pooling.

The GR feature reduces the likelihood of adverse selection because people who start off expecting average risks and then learn of higher risk in the next period cannot capitalize on that information by purchasing more coverage at the GR rate. Also, people who remain a low risk are not priced out of the market because the initial premium includes the expected higher risks in future periods that they have already agreed to pay. In effect, premiums in the next period are unaffected by individuals who become chronically ill and remain in the plan, because premiums have been established with that likely transition in mind.

Cream skimming also becomes less likely because of the GR feature. Individuals with higher risks have a legal right to stick with the policy; insurers cannot legally deny them coverage. In addition, those who remain average risks face a premium they should be willing to pay because it reflects the likelihood that they themselves may become chronically ill at some point.

Patel and Pauly point out some problems potentially associated with the GR feature. First, if buyers possess inside information about their health conditions when purchasing the initial policy, the GR feature will not stop adverse selection from taking place. Hence, people should be encouraged to purchase individual health insurance early in their lives. In fact, the lock-in feature of GR provides an incentive for people to purchase health insurance coverage while still in good health rather than waiting to be diagnosed with a chronic condition.

Second, if consumers become high risk before seeking insurance, they will be charged high premiums. In this case, social transfers may be necessary for low-income, chronically ill individuals. This is another reason why people should be encouraged to seek out health insurance with the GR feature early in their lives. Third, insurers may not abide by the terms of the contract or may lower quality or service to discourage high risks from renewing. In addition, insurers may raise premiums for an insured class of individuals more than experience dictates, and then offer lower rates to lower risks once they threaten to leave the plan. Practices like those, however, are illegal and can tarnish the image of insurers and thereby lower the market value of their companies. In any case, some regulations and monitoring of health insurers may be necessary.

Patel and Pauly point out that the Health Insurance Portability and Accountability Act (HIPAA) of 1996 requires guaranteed renewability but is silent about limiting the rates charged at renewal. Specifically, HIPAA does not require that premiums be the same for all insured people in a rating class. However, based on their survey, Patel and Pauly find that almost all states require GR and that premiums are the same for all people within the same rating class. Furthermore, they find that re-underwriting would be challenged by most state governments.

Individual health insurance offers the benefits of more choice and increased portability. However, individual health insurance is characterized by the problems of adverse selection, risk selection, and experience rating. Guaranteed renewability is a contractual feature in individual health insurance plans that can deal with these three problems to some degree.

The Performance of the Private Health Insurance Industry

The structural characteristics of the private health insurance industry imply that individual insurers may be pressured to behave in a reasonably competitive manner. While a few large health insurers typically dominate the industry in most market areas, low barriers to entry and a large competitive fringe likely create incentives for price competition. Health insurers in the group health insurance segment of the industry face additional pressure to behave competitively because large employers may self-insure.

According to some of the topics covered in the conduct section, unfettered competition in the private health insurance industry may not be completely desirable. One reason is that unchecked price competition may encourage health insurers to practice cherry-picking behavior and deny coverage to individuals with preexisting conditions. Such behavior limits the ability of the private health insurance industry to provide universal health insurance coverage, which is a primary goal of many health policy makers. In addition, some critics have claimed that the private health insurance industry has failed to contain health care costs.

In this section, we examine evidence on the performance of the private health insurance industry more thoroughly. We consider measures and issues relating to the price and quantity of health insurance and the profitability of health insurers.

The Price of Private Health Insurance in the United States

One indicator of the performance of an industry is the price of the product being sold. At a point in time, economic theory suggests that consumer surplus is maximized when prices are set equal to the marginal costs of production. In contrast, when prices are set above marginal cost, consumer welfare is reduced. Economic theory also implies that prices adjust over time in response to any changes in demand or the costs of production. In fact, these price variations serve an important purpose by allocating resources to their best uses, coordinating demand and supply, and rationing goods to the highest bidder.

We mentioned in Chapter 6, and previously in this chapter, that the price of health insurance is sometimes measured by the loading fee, the portion of the premium payment above expected medical benefits. However, once MCOs began to dominate the industry, health insurers were expected to compete among themselves not only on the basis of the loading fee but also by controlling moral hazard as represented by the size of the medical benefits paid out.

As discussed earlier, moral hazard refers to a situation in which individuals, once they are covered by health insurance, change their behavior because they are no longer financially responsible for the full cost of their actions (Pauly, 1968). In particular, people may choose to pursue activities that increase the probability and/or magnitude of the loss covered by health insurance. To the individual consumer, the current health insurance premium represents a sunk cost and is unaffected by her spending on medical care services. In addition, any one individual is likely to believe that her own medical spending in isolation does not affect the future premiums of the insured group. However, if a sufficient number of people act in a similar fashion and increase their spending on medical services due to the moral hazard situation, future insurance premiums increase to reflect the greater benefits paid out.

Seidman (1982) likens the moral hazard problem to restaurant bill splitting. If two people have lunch together and decide to split the bill, each person may realize that he is paying only half of the cost of every additional dollar spent on the meal. Therefore, each individual might purchase the higher-priced imported beer rather than the lower-priced domestic beer or order the restaurant specialty rather than the less expensive special of the day. Of course, if both people behave similarly and overspend, the restaurant bill is higher than it would be if they paid separately for their own meals. Also, each person's share of the bill falls as the size of the sharing group increases (say, from two to six). As a result, the incentive to overspend increases with the size of the group, *ceteris paribus,* when the bill is split.

In terms of the market for medical services, moral hazard results from five types of actions. First, at any point in time when an insured event takes place, the quantity demanded of medical services may exceed the amount the consumer would buy if she had to pay the full cost. Quantity demanded may be greater because the insured consumer faces a price that lies below the marginal cost of the medical service. We discussed this type of moral hazard in Chapter 6 when we compared the conventional and Nyman models of the demand for health insurance. The extent to which quantity demanded increases depends on the price elasticity of demand. A more elastic demand results in greater quantity demanded as a result of the reduced out-of-pocket price, *ceteris paribus.*

Second, the moral hazard problem may show up over time as consumers have less incentive to guard against an insured event. Reductions in preventive activities such as exercise or dieting may raise the probability of an illness occurring. Moral hazard may arise from a third type of behavior that deals with technological advances in medical care. Third-party payments may encourage the development and adoption of new technologies offering low-benefit, high-cost care (Weisbrod, 1991). The adoption and diffusion of these high-priced technologies, in turn, causes the demand for health insurance and the range of services covered by health insurance to increase. A vicious cycle encompassing health insurance, technology, and rising medical costs is set in motion.

Moral hazard results in a fourth behavioral change as insurance lowers the consumer's incentive to monitor the behavior of health care providers. Less monitoring gives the health care provider the ability to prescribe unnecessary tests or surgery when a financial incentive exists to engage in opportunistic behavior or supply inducement of this sort. Since the consumer's out-of-pocket costs are largely unaffected by the unnecessary services, the consumer has little incentive to seek a second opinion. Finally, a moral hazard effect occurs when insurance lowers the consumer's incentive to shop around and find the lowest price for medical services.

To effectively control claim costs, the managed care insurer must adopt and implement various consumer and health care provider financial incentives and management strategies to prevent these five types of moral hazard behavior. But recall from our discussion of the Nyman model in Chapter 6 that not all moral hazard may be inefficient. Therefore, health insurers want to discourage only those types of behavior that result in the marginal cost of medical care exceeding marginal benefit. Also recall that financial incentives and management strategies result in either higher administrative costs or lower premium rates because the health insurance product effectively offers less insurance coverage to consumers. The successful MCO competes by appropriately balancing the trade-off between premium revenues, the administrative expense load, and medical benefits paid out. Hence, the premium rate provides a better indication of the price of health insurance than the loading fee because it reflects both the size of the medical benefits paid out and the expense load, which must be properly balanced by the successful MCO. It is interesting to note that the premium captures the price of health insurance in the Nyman model because it reflects how much income (and all other goods) a person in good health must willingly give up to claim an income transfer if he becomes ill.

Figure 11–4 provides annual estimates of the average real premium and the average real premium as a percentage of real income per capita for the period from 1960 to 2003. The data in the figure suggest that the price of health insurance increased dramatically over the 43-year period both in real terms and as a fraction of income. Indeed, as a fraction of income, health insurance

FIGURE 11–4
Average Premium Payment per Privately Insured Individual and as a Percentage of Income, 1960–2003

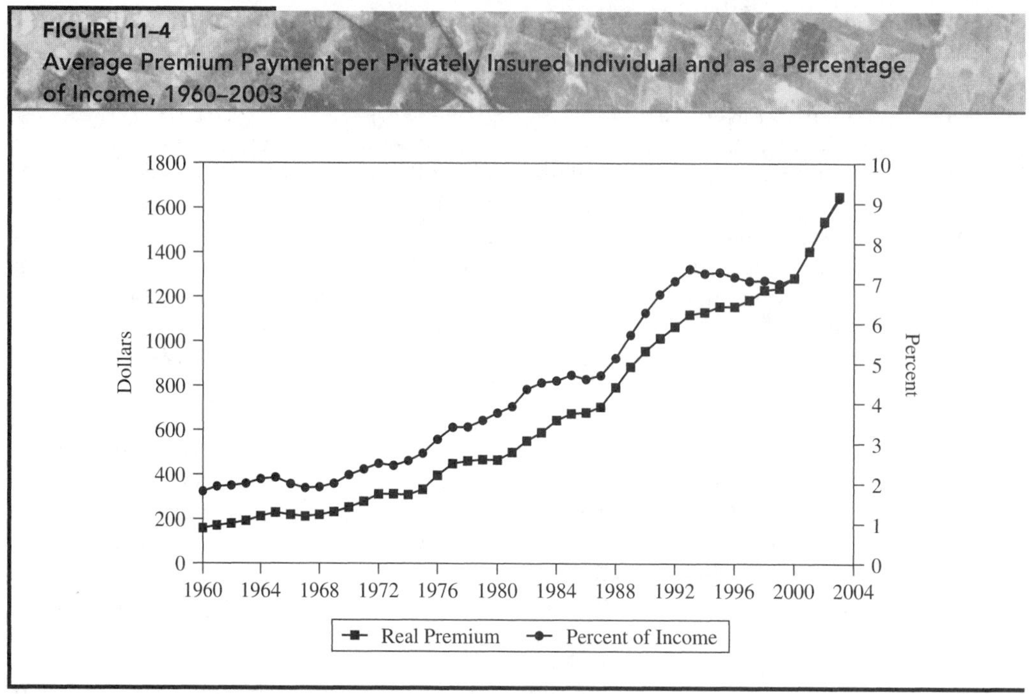

SOURCE: Authors' estimates based on data from the Research and Statistics section of the website at the Centers for Medicare and Medicaid Services, Health Care Industry Update: Managed Care Washington, D.C.: CMS, March 24, 2003. http://www.cms.gov.

premiums increased from slightly less than 2 percent in 1960 to about 9 percent in 2004. However, some periods experienced much faster growth in the price of health insurance than others. The period from 1987 to 1993 stands out in the figure because real premiums grew at a significantly faster rate than during the previous periods both in real terms and as a fraction of income. During this period enrollment in managed care plans expanded, with the percentage of workers in traditional plans declining from 73 to 46 percent.[7] Reflecting the shift to managed care plans, this period was characterized by intense innovation in new strategies to control moral hazard (Danzon, 1992). That is, MCOs adopted various financial incentives and management strategies, such as utilization review, case management, and selective contracting, with the intent of reining in medical claim costs. The costs of implementing these strategies appear as claims administration costs and can raise the premium payment, as discussed earlier, if not offset by commensurate reductions in medical benefits paid out. Apparently these earlier initiatives to control moral hazard were not very effective on an industry-wide basis, given that real premium increased rapidly during this period.

The next six years tell a different story concerning the effectiveness of MCOs at controlling medical claims costs. During the period from 1993 to 1999, real premium growth slowed both in real terms and as a fraction of income. In fact, the percentage of income devoted to health insurance premiums actually declined slightly during this period. The mid- to late 1990s is considered to represent the "heyday" of managed care because a relatively large percentage of insured individuals

7. Kaiser Family Foundation, http://www.kff.org/insurance/7315/sections/upload/7375.pdf (accessed November 1, 2005).

were enrolled in restrictive managed care plans, which relied heavily on supply-side strategies such as utilization controls. In fact, 52 percent of all workers were enrolled in HMOs or POS plans in 1999. While these restrictive plans cost more to administer, the medical cost savings more than compensated for the rise in administration costs such that the health insurance premium rate tended to grow much less quickly during this period than in previous periods.

However, beginning in 1999, medical care consumers and providers felt adversely impacted by the restrictive supply-side policies adopted by MCOs. For instance, both consumer and provider groups complained that MCOs should not be allowed to preauthorize medical services, set the number of days that a patient can stay within a hospital, or determine which drugs to reimburse. This backlash resulted in a significant exodus of consumers from more restrictive to less restrictive managed care plans. For example, from 1999 to 2005, the percentage of insured workers in PPO plans increased sharply from 39 to 61 percent. As people voted with their feet and wallets, managed care organizations of all types, including HMOs, subsequently began changing their financial and management strategies away from tight supply-side controls (such as preauthorization and narrow networks of providers) and toward looser demand-side strategies such as higher copays or coinsurance rates. This change in strategy by MCOs resulted in more choice for consumers and, not surprisingly, led to higher health insurance premiums. In particular, note in Figure 11–4 that health insurance premiums exploded after 2000 both in real terms and as a percentage of income.

All in all, it appears that MCOs accomplished what they initially were expected to do. By design, MCOs are supposed to control moral hazard costs, something the indemnity plans prior to the 1980s were not designed to accomplish. However, the necessary supply-side controls were viewed by medical care consumers and providers as being unduly restrictive and the emphasis eventually changed toward demand-side controls. The data in Figure 11–4 suggest that the demand-side controls have been relatively ineffective at controlling the growth of premiums thus far. Perhaps the learning curve is fairly flat and more time must pass before the effects of demand-side controls can be observed. After all, it did take some time for the effects of supply-side controls to show up in slower premium growth.

Before leaving this topic, it should be mentioned that rising health insurance premiums do not necessarily reflect inefficiencies in the private health insurance industry. Prices naturally rise in a competitive market when willingness to pay increases, as revealed by demand, and costs increase, as reflected in supply. For example, people have become insured for many more types of medical care and to a greater degree in terms of lower out-of-pocket costs over the years. In addition, new medical technologies have been very successful at saving, enhancing, and extending lives (Cutler and McClellan, 2001). Hence the demand for health insurance coverage may be rising over time because people wish to gain access to these expensive life-saving medical technologies (Nyman, 2003; Santerre, 2006). As such, a rising price of health insurance may signify success in both the medical and insurance markets and does not necessarily indicate failure. Moreover, any attempts at regulating the price of health insurance might mean less access to new medical innovations and, subsequently, a reduction in the quantity and quality of lives compared to what could have been otherwise.

The Underwriting Cycle of Health Insurance. Complicating the interpretation of any short-term changes in health insurance premiums is a phenomenon called the underwriting or profitability cycle. Private health insurers have generally experienced three consecutive years of underwriting gains, followed by three consecutive years of underwriting losses, in the group health insurance market. The underwriting cycle holds for both commercial insurers and not-for-profit Blue Cross and Blue Shield plans.

Health insurance premium increases are shown to follow the underwriting cycle with a lag of about two years (Gabel et al., 1991). Rather than consistently and moderately rising, premiums appear to cycle over a six-year period with three consecutive years of rapid premium growth during the so-called hard market phase followed by three successive years of slowing premium growth during the soft market phase. Seeking to explain the root cause of the underwriting cycle, Gabel et al. point to three broad causes: supply and demand forces, industry pricing actions, and external factors. According to these authors, supply and demand forces can affect the profitability of health insurers in two ways.

First, because of relatively free entry into health insurance markets, firms enter the market in times of excess profits. As a result, price falls and some firms experience losses and exit the market. Exit reduces supply, price increases, and profits return. The cycle begins once again. Second, Samuelson's (1939) "cobweb" model may explain the cycle. When the price of health insurance is relatively high in the present period, insurers act on the information by deciding to sell more insurance policies in the next period. The greater supply, in turn, leads to lower prices in the next period, especially because the demand for group health insurance is relatively price inelastic and modest supply changes lead to dramatic price changes. Hence, current prices affect future supply decisions, and this linkage results in a continual cycling of prices and profits.

Industry pricing actions consider that insurers may reduce prices to increase market share and raise them later to compensate for past losses. In addition, actuarial pricing techniques often extrapolate the recent past to the future from recent claims experience. If decision makers form "adaptive expectations" of this kind, they systematically overestimate true premiums in periods of falling claims and underestimate true premiums in periods of rising claims. According to Gabel et al., this type of pricing behavior, although irrational, has been shown to result in a cyclical profitability pattern.

Another industry pricing explanation supposes that all insurers tacitly collude at first and follow the pricing pattern of the leader firm(s). At some point, however, individual firms are tempted to reduce prices to gain greater market share, and the informal cartel breaks down. Eventually, the pattern repeats itself. Finally, external factors, including underlying claims events and general economic conditions, may cause the profitability cycle. That is, medical care costs and general factors ranging from the budget deficit, national unemployment, and interest rates may follow a business cycle pattern and generate the insurance profitability cycle.

As you can see, economists have offered a number of alternative theories for the underwriting cycle in the health insurance industry. Very few studies, however, have tried to empirically determine which of these competing theories provide a better explanation for the cycle. Born and Santerre (2005) use national data for the United States over the period from 1960 to 2002 to compare the predictive power of some of these theories. Among their empirical results, they find that fluctuations in medical claims costs primarily determine the cycling of insurance premiums.

Grossman and Ginsburg (2004) point out that, beginning in the 1990s, the traditional underwriting cycle seemed to break, with longer and more uneven periods of gains and losses and less extreme fluctuations in profitability. They argue that the traditional underwriting cycle broke down because of structural changes in the health insurance industry and because of a closer relationship between cost trends and premium adjustments. More specifically, they argue that consolidations among insurance companies have reduced the amount of price competition in the industry. They also point out that more experience with managed care products and electronic processing of provider claims have enabled insurance companies to better predict medical claims costs. Grossman and Ginsburg anticipate that health insurance premiums may be higher but less volatile if insurance companies continue to consolidate in the future. They also anticipate that the underwriting cycle will not disappear and will be characterized by more muted swings in the future.

An important lesson from this discussion is that premium increases must be properly interpreted in the context of the underwriting cycle. To say that premium increases are low this year does not mean that some trend of low premium increases has set in. Rather, the low premium increases of today may mean that tomorrow's premium increases will be larger if the profitability cycle continues to hold.

Output of Private Health Insurance in the United States

Private Health Insurance Coverage. Another measure of the performance of an industry is the amount of output provided. Incentives should exist so suppliers produce the optimal amount of a product—neither too much nor too little. In the case of the private health insurance industry, optimal provision implies that the right number of people is covered by private health insurance. Theoretically, the efficient number of insured individuals occurs at the level where the marginal social benefit and marginal social cost of health insurance coverage are equal. Those pushing strongly for universal health insurance coverage in the United States apparently believe that marginal social benefit exceeds costs at all levels of the population.

Table 11–1 offers some data on the percentage of people with private health insurance coverage in the United States for selected years from 1940 to 2004. Private insurance plans are defined as all supplemental, comprehensive, and catastrophic insurance policies, including those individually purchased, both by the non-elderly and elderly (for example, medigap) and group policies sponsored by employers or trade associations. A number of observations can be drawn from the data. For one, notice that the number of privately insured individuals increased overall from 9 percent to roughly 69 percent of the population from 1940 to 2004. The tremendous jump in private insurance coverage during the 1940s reflects the point made at the beginning of this chapter that employers offered health insurance as a tax-exempt fringe benefit during the wage and price control period of World War II.

The 1950s and 1960s witnessed further huge increases in private insurance enrollments. Enrollments in private insurance expanded, in part, because of the declining health insurance prices during that time as a result of experience-rated premiums. According to Morrisey (2001), "commercial insurers identified employer groups that had lower than average claims experience and offered them premiums lower than those charged by the then dominant carrier, Blue Cross" (p. 209).

Also, notice that the percentage of people covered by private health insurance reached a peak of more than 76 percent in the mid-1970s but declined thereafter. In fact, because of the decline, the percentage of the population covered by private health insurance increased by a mere 1.3 percentage points over the entire 44-year period from 1960 to 2004. Several factors account for the decline in the percentage of privately insured individuals after the mid-1970s.

One simple reason for the relative decline in private health insurance coverage is the growing percentage of the population aged 65 years and older in the United States. Recall that Medicare took effect in the late 1960s and that people become automatically eligible for Medicare on reaching age 65. Medicare recipients made up 13.7 percent of the population in 2004 but only around 10 percent in 1975, for instance. It should be noted, however, that many people covered by Medicare also purchase medigap coverage from private insurance carriers. Those who purchase medigap coverage are included in the figures reported in Table 11–1 as also possessing private health insurance coverage, and most elderly people have some medigap coverage. Thus, Medicare coverage cannot explain much of the decline in the percentage of the population covered by private health insurance since 1975.

TABLE 11–1
People with Private Health Insurance Coverage, Selected Years, 1940–2004

Year	Number (millions)	Percentage of Population
1940	12.0	9.1%
1945	32.0	22.9
1950	76.6	50.3
1960	122.5	67.8
1970	154.3	75.3
1975	164.8	76.3
1980	169.7	74.7
1985	176.3	74.1
1990	182.1	73.2
1995	185.9	70.3
2000	201.1	71.9
2004	291.2	69.1

SOURCE: Health Insurance Association of America (HIAA). *Source Book of Health Insurance Data 1999/2000.* Washington, D.C.: HIAA Insurance Association of America, 2001, Table 2–10; and U.S. Census Bureau, "Health Insurance Coverage 2004," http://www.census.gov/hhes/www/hlthins/hlthins.html.

Rising health insurance premiums provide the second and probably most significant reason for the decline in private health insurance coverage. As we saw previously, health insurance premiums rose rapidly from the mid-1980s to early 1993. This caused many employers, mostly small businesses, to either raise employee contributions or drop health insurance coverage altogether. Health insurance premiums also increased sharply after 2000 in response to the backlash against restrictive managed care plans, as shown in Table 11–1. This spike in health insurance premiums may account for part of the fall in the percentage of the population covered by private health insurance after 2000. Notice that enrollment in private health insurance increased as a percentage of population over the period from 1995 to 2000, when real premiums as a percentage of real income per capita marginally decreased.

A third explanation for declining private coverage deals with occupational shifts from traditionally higher-coverage manufacturing sector jobs to lower-coverage service sector jobs. However, Long and Rodgers (1995) find that employment shifts explain about only 15 percent of the decline in employer-provided private health insurance coverage. The final reason for declining coverage is the growing fraction of people covered by Medicaid. For example, less than 8 percent of the population was covered by Medicaid in 1980. Several expansions took place in the Medicaid program, and this percentage figure blossomed to almost 13 percent by 2004 (DeNavas-Walt et al., 2005). While many people became eligible for Medicaid coverage because they lost private health insurance coverage for the reasons previously mentioned, several studies find that Medicaid program expansions created a financial incentive for some families to drop their private health insurance coverage in favor of Medicaid. As discussed further in Chapter 10, public coverage tends to crowd out private coverage and may have caused some of the decline in health insurance coverage since the mid-1970s.

Who Are the Uninsured? The U.S. Census Bureau began collecting data on insurance coverage on a systematic basis beginning in 1987. Those interviewed by census officials are asked a series of questions regarding whether they were covered in the previous year by insurance and by what type of insurance. People are considered insured if they were covered by any type of health insurance for part or all of the previous year, and everyone else is considered uninsured for the entire year. Research shows that health insurance coverage is underreported for a variety of reasons by the Census Bureau. Some people, for example, report their insurance coverage status at the time of their interview rather than their coverage status during the previous calendar year.

With this caveat in mind, data reported by the Census Bureau over the last ten years suggest that between 14 and 16 percent of the U.S. population tends to be uninsured for the entire year (DeNavas-Walt et al., 2005). Being uninsured is not without significant personal and social costs. The uninsured sometime face the sharp psychological sting from the financial insecurity that can result from an unanticipated medical occurrence. In addition, uninsured individuals are more likely to find themselves in the emergency room of a hospital, sometimes after it is too late for proper medical treatment, with their resulting poorer health and shorter lives causing sizeable social costs. As an illustration, Miller et al. (2004) estimate a lower-bound dollar value of the health forgone because of uninsurance in the United States at $65 to $130 billion per year. Thus, reducing the uninsured population seems a legitimate social goal, and identifying why some people are without private health insurance coverage becomes a valuable endeavor for public policy purposes. Policy makers generally wish to know which groups and individuals are more at risk so that policies might be properly designed to reduce the number of people who are uninsured.

Logic suggests that people are without private health insurance for a variety of reasons. We learned in Chapter 6 that people alter their purchasing of health insurance in response to changing economic circumstances such as the price of insurance or their income just as they change their demands for other goods and services. That is, some people choose to be without private health insurance coverage or choose only minimal coverage. For example, an individual may decide to self-insure because she expects to gain little from market-provided health insurance as a result of its high price relative to expected medical benefits. Behavior of this kind may account, at least partly, for the 31.4 percent of the population between ages 18 and 24 that do not have health insurance coverage. Some in this age group normally expect to receive very little in terms of medical benefits reimbursed and may have to cross-subsidize the higher premium costs of more elderly individuals.

Others may be without private health insurance coverage for reasons other than its voluntary nature. By borrowing from the different classifications for unemployment offered by labor economists, three categories of uninsurance can be specified, although admittedly these classifications are not mutually exclusive in the context of uninsurance. First, some people may lack private health insurance coverage during a particular time period because they become frictionally uninsured. **Frictional uninsurance** occurs when a person terminates one job that offered health insurance and is searching for another job or waiting to become eligible for insurance at a new job. Seventy-three percent of employees covered by health insurance work for companies that require a waiting period averaging three months before extending medical insurance benefits to a new employee (Steinmetz, 1993).

In fact, the Consolidated Omnibus Budget Reconciliation Act of 1985 (COBRA) was developed expressly with frictional uninsurance in mind by requiring employers with more than 20 workers to allow former employees and their dependents the option to retain their health insurance coverage for up to eighteen months after terminating employment. However, given that this act requires the frictionally uninsured to pay the full premiums and an administrative fee of 2 percent, only about 20 percent of those eligible extend their health insurance under COBRA while between jobs (Madrian, 1998).

Frictional uninsurance also occurs when people are temporarily without private health insurance because of a mismatch of information. Because of imperfect information, consumers take time to shop around for the right insurers while health insurers search for the right customers. It stands to reason that insurance agents and brokers can impact the number of individuals frictionally uninsured and the duration of frictional uninsurance by providing timely and reliable information (Conwell, 2002). Within the context of frictional uninsurance, Swartz et al. (1993) find that monthly family income, educational attainment, and industry of employment in the month prior to losing health insurance are the characteristics with the greatest impact on the duration of a spell without health insurance.

Second, structurally uninsured individuals constitute another category of those without private health insurance. Included in the **structurally uninsured** category are individuals who are without private health insurance on a long-run basis because of chronic illnesses, preexisting conditions, employment that does not offer health insurance coverage, and/or insufficient income. For example, noncoverage rates tend to fall as household income rises. Slightly more than 24 percent of households with annual incomes of $25,000 or less lacked health insurance coverage of any kind in 2004. The comparable figure for households with annual incomes of $75,000 or more was only 8.4 percent. In addition, 19.7 percent of all blacks and 32.7 percent of all Hispanics were uninsured in 2004 compared to a rate of only 11.3 percent for non-Hispanic whites. Blacks, and particularly Hispanics, are more likely to accept casual employment in small firms that are less likely to offer health insurance coverage to their employees.

Swartz (1994) stresses that the duration of the spell without health insurance coverage is another important consideration. She estimates that the median spell without health insurance coverage is about six months. A median uninsured spell of six months means that 50 percent of all spells without insurance are rather short and end before six months. However, another 50 percent of spells last longer than six months. At least 28 percent of uninsured spells last more than one year, and 15 to 18 percent last more than two years. Those with long uninsured spells are clearly among the structurally uninsured.

Finally, individuals who are cyclically uninsured make up the last category of those without private insurance. **Cyclical uninsurance** pertains to individuals (and their families) who change insurance status as they drift in and out of jobs offering group health insurance benefits as the macroeconomy normally expands and contracts in the short term. Cyclically uninsured individuals tend to possess few skills and may fluctuate between working in small and large firms over the course of the business cycle. For example, part-time workers and those without a job are more likely to be uninsured compared to those who work full-time. Specifically, about 25 percent of part-time workers and 26 percent of the unemployed lack health insurance coverage compared to a figure of 18 percent for full-time workers in 2004.

Job Lock. While employer-sponsored group health insurance offers several advantages over individual health insurance, such as lower premiums and informed purchasing, group insurance also offers some disadvantages. First, workers are typically unable to choose among a variety of health insurance products. Instead, they must choose among a few products already narrowed down by their employer.

The second disadvantage is that workers cannot take their employer-sponsored insurance policy to their next place of employment. This nonportability of employer-sponsored health insurance could mean that the next employer does not offer any insurance at all. Or the employer at the next job may not offer the same plan, particularly a plan with the same out-of-pocket payments or network of health care providers. In addition, long waiting periods, preexisting conditions, and the potential for less extensive health coverage at the new job all increase the financial risk associated with extensive unanticipated medical events, making the move to a new job a costly endeavor. Thus, some workers may become locked into their current jobs because of variations in the insurance products sponsored by different employers. The resulting job lock disrupts the proper functioning of a macroeconomy because workers are discouraged from switching to jobs where they are more efficient producers. This immobility of labor resources can lead to a lower level of labor productivity and national income. Whether job lock severely inhibits job mobility is of interest to many health care policy makers.

As one might imagine, it is not easy to determine empirically whether, and how frequently, job lock occurs in practice. Researchers must carefully control for all other factors affecting job turnover decisions other than health insurance, such as initial wages and expected wage offers at new employment, job security, other fringe benefits, experience, education, and workers' and dependents' health status. In addition, employer-provided health insurance may be correlated with other unobservable job attributes also affecting job choice (such as workplace conditions and collegiality), which makes it difficult empirically to distinguish between association and causation.

Gruber and Madrian (2002) review eighteen empirical papers on the topic that differ with respect to sample coverage, explanatory variables, methodology, and identification strategy (that is, distinguishing between association and causation). Overall they claim that the empirical literature on the relationship between health insurance and job choice is certainly not unanimous. About an equal percentage of studies finds evidence supporting and not supporting the hypothesis that health insurance reduces job mobility. Of the papers uncovering a statistically significant relationship, Gruber and Madrian note a consistent finding that health insurance reduces job mobility by 25 to 50 percent. While these authors believe that job lock exists as a result of their extensive review (and their own research in this area), they stress that it is unclear whether these effects result in large welfare or efficiency losses.

Health Insurance Portability and Accountability Act of 1996. Concern over the nonportability of health insurance, lengthy waiting periods for preexisting conditions, and insurance benefit denial led to the passage of the Health Insurance Portability and Accountability Act (HIPAA) in 1996. The basic idea behind HIPAA was to make it more difficult for health insurers to segment insurance risk pools and deny or revoke access to specific individuals or groups on the basis of health status. Considered by many as the most significant federal health care reform legislation since the passage of the Medicare and Medicaid programs in 1965, HIPAA created the first national standards for the availability and portability of group and individual health insurance coverage.

Prior to HIPAA (or the Kassebaum-Kennedy Act), uniform standards were lacking in the health insurance industry for two reasons. First, states had been granted authority over health insurers within their jurisdictions by the McCarran-Ferguson Act of 1945 (Nichols and Blumberg, 1998). Some states chose to aggressively regulate and set standards in the health insurance industry; others did not. Second, the federal government has full responsibility for self-insured plans under the Employee Retirement Income Security Act (ERISA) of 1974. States are therefore unable to regulate the health insurance of a large percentage of U.S. workers. Furthermore, no federal regulations existed regarding the availability and portability of health insurance for self-insured plans.

HIPAA has wide-sweeping implications, as the law generally applies to all health plans, including large- and small-group plans, state-regulated plans, self-funded ERISA plans, indemnity and HMO plans, and individual plans. The major provisions as they relate to the health insurance industry are as follows:

Guaranteed Access and Renewability

1. With certain exceptions, insurers participating in the small-group market (2 through 50 employees) cannot exclude a small employer or any of the employer's eligible employees from coverage on the basis of health status.
2. Eligibility or continued eligibility of any individual to enroll in a group plan, regardless of size, cannot be conditioned on the following health-related factors: health status, medical condition (physical or mental), claims experience, receipt of health care, medical history, genetic information, or evidence of insurability or disability.
3. Individuals within a group plan cannot be charged a higher premium based on their health status. This requirement does not restrict the amount an employer may be charged for coverage under a group plan.
4. Except for certain specific exceptions (such as fraud, nonpayment, and discontinuance of market coverage), all group coverage in both the small- and large-group markets and individual coverage must be renewed.
5. Generally, individual insurers must provide coverage to individuals coming off group insurance if the individual had previous coverage for eighteen months, was not eligible for other group coverage, was not terminated from the previous plan due to nonpayment, and was not eligible or had exhausted COBRA-type coverage.
6. Individual insurers must guarantee to provide at least two policies. These two policies may be the insurer's most popular plans, based on premium volume, or a package of lower-level and higher-level coverage plans based on actuarial averages. The latter plans must be covered under a risk-spreading mechanism. States may elect to institute an approved alternate mechanism to provide the transition from group to individual coverage.

Portability

1. Employees moving from one employer to another (and individuals coming off group coverage to individual coverage) are protected against a newly imposed preexisting condition limitation. In general, a plan may not impose a new preexisting condition if no more than 63 days have passed between covered jobs, not including any applicable employer waiting period for new hires. The plan must also give credit for the portion of the preexisting condition satisfied under a prior plan, which can include individual coverage, dependent coverage, and so on.
2. The maximum exclusion period for preexisting conditions is no more than twelve months, or eighteen months for a late enrollee. The look-back period to determine a preexisting condition is no more than six months prior to the person's enrollment date.
3. Preexisting condition exclusions may not apply in the case of pregnancies, or for newborns and adopted children who are covered by insurance 30 days from the date of birth or adoption.

By setting national standards, proponents hope that HIPAA encourages health insurers to compete more on the basis of efficiency and quality than on risk selection. Moreover, by setting national standards for availability and portability, it is hoped that there are greater opportunities for risk pooling. Opponents fear that the reforms will raise the price of health insurance to individuals and thereby reduce the number of insured individuals. It should be pointed out that

HIPAA does not change how health care is delivered or how it is financed. Moreover, HIPAA does not increase access to health insurance for the uninsured or regulate the rates that health plans can charge (Atchinson and Fox, 1997). While HIPAA represents a major step, advocates of health care reform believe that much more work remains to be done in health insurance markets.

Profitability in the Private Health Insurance Industry

As mentioned throughout this text, resources are scarce at a point in time so any economic system must seriously address how these scarce resources should be allocated to different purposes. In a market system, resources are allocated to alternative uses based on supply and demand forces. In long-run equilibrium, if the market is perfectly competitive, price reflects the marginal benefit associated with consuming, and also the marginal cost of producing, the last unit of output. In the absence of any externalities, the market outcome represents efficiency because price or marginal social benefit equals marginal social costs. Also, if the market is perfectly competitive, and therefore entry barriers are nonexistent, the representative firm earns no more than a normal economic profit because competition among firms drives price down to equal average total costs.

It follows that the efficiency of an industry can be judged, to some degree, by the excessiveness of its economic profits. That is, if actual economic profits are greater than the normal level, it may indicate that firms in the industry exploit their market power by restricting output and raising price above the marginal costs of production. If so, consumer welfare is harmed and resources are misallocated from a societal point of view.

Lerner (1934) provides an alternative but related way of thinking about market power. In the context of a monopoly, Lerner argues that market power can be measured by how high price, P, can be elevated above the marginal costs, MC, of production. He shows mathematically that the ability to elevate price above costs depends on the price elasticity of market demand, E_M, facing the monopolist. Specifically, the Lerner index of monopoly power, L, can be written as

(11–4)
$$L = \frac{(P - MC)}{P} = \frac{1}{|E_M|}.$$

The Lerner index implies that the markup of price above marginal cost as a percentage of price is inversely proportional to the price elasticity of market demand (in absolute terms). That is, the ability to elevate price above marginal cost is limited by the responsiveness of consumers to a price increase. For example, supposing that price elasticity of market demand equals −2.0, the Lerner index suggests that the markup of price above cost equals 50 percent of the price. If, instead, the price elasticity of market demand was more elastic and equaled −10.0, the index indicates that the markup falls to only 10 percent of price. It stands to reason that firms, facing many substitute producers or products, are unable to elevate price very high above the marginal costs given a more elastic demand for their products. In fact, the Lerner index for a perfectly competitive firm equals zero because it faces a perfectly elastic demand. Thus, the Lerner index is often treated as a measure of market power.

If we assume that marginal costs equal average total costs (that is, a horizontal per unit cost curve), the Lerner index can be rewritten as

(11–5)
$$L = \frac{(P - ATC)}{P}.$$

Multiplying both the numerator and the denominator of the right-hand term by Q/Q, the following expression can be obtained:

(11–6)
$$L = \frac{Q(P - ATC)}{QP} = \frac{(TR - TC)}{TR} = \frac{\pi}{TR}.$$

Equation 11–6 indicates that the Lerner index can be approximated by the ratio of economic profits to total revenues or sales. A higher value for the ratio of economic profits to sales indicates that the firm or industry possesses greater market power.

Given the strong theoretical underpinnings, it should not be surprising that economists often use profit rates to draw inferences about the market power of real-world firms and industries. In practice, other measures of profitability, such as profits as a fraction of stockholder equity or total assets, are examined in addition to the profit return on sales when the necessary data are available. Using several bases to measure profit rates represents a sound practice because profits sometimes differ across firms and industries simply because of variations in production methods (labor versus capital intensive) or reliance on debt versus equity financing, for example.

To gain some insight into the market power of private health insurers and to show the limitations associated with using profits as a measure of market power, Table 11–2 provides figures representing the profitability of selected major publicly traded health insurance companies during the 2000 to 2002 period. Averages for the industry and consolidated Blue Cross/Blue Shield results are also reported in the table. The top of the table shows profit margins (profits/sales); the bottom depicts the returns on stockholder equity. Both of these profitability figures are commonly reported by industry analysts as measures of performance.

Notice that, except for the consolidated Blue Cross/Blue Shield results, health insurers typically earned positive profit rates during that period of time. For example, the figures suggest that 6.2 percent of WellPoint's sales resulted in profits and also that WellPoint earned 22 cents of profits on each $1 of stockholder equity, on average, over the three-year period from 2000 to 2002. The other major health insurers did slightly better or worse than WellPoint in terms of their return on sales or equity. Aetna's relatively dismal performance at the time reflects how it "crashed and almost burned as a result of excessive acquisition growth" (Robinson, 2004, p. 19). The negative return on sales for the consolidated Blue Cross/Blue Shield companies may reflect that some of the plans organized on a not-for-profit basis are driven by their charitable mission, or absence of a profit motive, to contain costs.

At first blush, one might conclude from the figures reported in Table 11–2 that most health insurers possess significant market power because their profit rates, especially the returns to equity, are greater than zero. However, several factors must be considered before drawing this inference. First, the reported rates represent accounting and not economic profits. Recall from Chapter 7 that economic profits consider the opportunity cost of all resources and not just resources that are purchased by companies. Alternatively stated, accounting profits do not reflect the opportunity cost of resources that are owned by businesses such as buildings, land, and equipment. Hence accounting profits generally overstate economic profits and sometimes complicate comparisons across companies. For example, CIGNA appears to have earned a lower profit margin than WellPoint over the three-year period. However, CIGNA may rent many of its buildings whereas WellPoint owns more of its buildings. As a result, the rental payments for the buildings reduce CIGNA's accounting profits but not WellPoint's. Once the opportunity costs of the buildings owned by WellPoint are considered, economic profit margins are more comparable.

Second, we must also consider that even perfectly competitive firms earn a normal economic profit rate. Profit-maximizing firms must receive at least a normal return on their capital or they will exit the industry to earn a higher return elsewhere. Thus, we must allow for some economy-wide,

TABLE 11–2
Accounting Profit Margin and Accounting Return on Equity of Major Health Insurers, 2000–2002

	WellPoint	Anthem	United Health Group	Aetna	CIGNA	Average of 18 Health Insurers	Blue Cross/ Blue Shield Average
Profit Margin Three-Year Average, 2000–2002	6.2%	6.7%	7.0%	1.6%	5.8%	3.6%	−0.8%
	WellPoint	**Anthem**	**United Health Group**	**Aetna**	**CIGNA**	**All Publicly Traded Health Insurers**	
Return on Equity Three-Year Average, 2000–2002	22.4%	14.9%	25.2%	0.9%	20.4%	19.9%	

SOURCE: James C. Robinson. "Consolidation and the Transformation of Competition in Health Insurance." *Health Affairs* 23 (November/December 2004), pp. 1–24; and Centers for Medicare and Medicaid Services. *Health Care Industry Update: Managed Care*. Washington, D.C.: CMS, March 24, 2003.

competitive rate of return. For example, industries in the general economy may normally earn a 6 percent return on their capital. Any economic profits received after allowing for a 6 percent return on capital might then be considered as being excessive or above the normal amount.

Third, investments in some industries are riskier than in others. Economic theory suggests that risk-averse investors require a risk premium to invest in more risky industries, *ceteris paribus*. Thus, observed differences in profit rates across industries may reflect differences in risk. This means that the economic profits rate must be adjusted for risk before inferences about relative profitability can be made. For example, an industry rate of return on capital of 8 percent may reflect a 6 percent normal return and a 2 percent risk premium.

Finally, economic theory suggests that a perfectly competitive industry earns a normal rate of return in the long run. However, favorable and unfavorable industry or economy-wide shocks may cause actual (and risk-adjusted) economic profits to deviate from the long-run normal rate in the short run. Also, short-run profits and losses should not persist in the long run because firms eventually enter and exit markets if barriers are low. Returning to the figures in Table 11–2, the period from 2000 to 2002 represented an upswing in the underwriting cycle faced by health insurers. So the relatively high profit rates observed for this period are normally balanced out by relatively low profit rates during the downswing of the underwriting cycle. Hence, we must be careful not to draw any strong conclusions about profitability from a simple snapshot of industry performance. That is, we must determine whether excessive economic profitability persists over time before drawing any conclusions about market power.

In sum, economic theory indicates that economic profits should be greater than zero when firms possess and exploit their market power. As a result, profit rates, such as those reported in Table 11–2, are sometimes used to draw inferences about the market power and efficiency of firms and industries. However, from an economic perspective, it is important to assess the long-run risk-adjusted industry economic rate of return to the long-run risk-adjusted economy-wide competitive rate of return before the presence of market power can be properly detected.

SUMMARY

Recent data suggest that the private health insurance industry is highly concentrated but with a large competitive fringe in most market areas. However, health insurance is fairly homogeneous, at least within a particular product line, such as traditional or managed care health insurance. While state regulations and administrative economies exist, barriers to entry do not appear to be particularly binding on the entry of new health insurance companies, perhaps because existing insurance companies can easily switch among alternative insurance product lines (health, casualty, life, and so on). Group plans also face the prospect that large employers may self-insure.

Individual buyers may possess imperfect information regarding the quality of health insurance. However, the information problem is much less severe in the group insurance submarket. Thus, overall the market for private health insurance appears to be reasonably competitive. While the market demand for health insurance is found to be inelastic, an individual insurer is likely to face a highly elastic demand curve given the relative ease of entry and available substitutes.

Competitive insurance markets in conjunction with experience rating can give rise to cherry-picking behavior, in which only healthy individuals are offered adequate health insurance coverage. Less-healthy people are denied access to health insurance, are not covered for preexisting conditions, or are charged prohibitively high prices. While this problem is much more pronounced in the individual health insurance market, guaranteed renewability may offer a solution.

In terms of performance, the relative price of private health insurance has tended to rise over the long run. This rise in health insurance premiums may reflect the access value generated by health insurance and the notion that the demand for health insurance is derived from the demand for good health, which tends to be highly valued by consumers. During the short term, the period between 1993 and 1999 witnessed an abrupt slowdown in premium growth because of the successful cost containment efforts of MCOs. However, the backlash against MCOs after 2000 led to less restrictive supply-side policies and consequently a return to rapidly rising health insurance premiums once again.

Some output problems continue to prevail in the market for private health insurance. A significant percentage of Americans lack health insurance coverage. Others are locked into their jobs because of variations in health insurance coverage offered by different employers. People are uninsured for a variety of reason, so no one single type of policy action can be expected to reduce the uninsurance rate to zero in a voluntary health insurance system.

Finally, the profitability of the private health insurance industry was discussed. We learned that profit rates are often used as an indicator of the market power or efficiency of industries. In fact, the Lerner index provides the theoretical underpinnings for using profit rates as a measure of market power. Before drawing any conclusions about the relative efficiency of an industry from profits, however, we must make sure that the opportunity cost of all resources, risk, normal rates of return, and the proper time frame are all considered.

CASE STUDIES

11-1 Ride a Skateboard? We Have a Health Plan for You[8]

Health insurance companies have started to take a new look at the 45 million uninsured people in the United States. These "potentially insurable people" represent a large untapped market, consisting of college students, part-time workers, and middle-income workers. The industry has recently realized that many of the uninsured are the same healthy Americans that were once covered in employer health plans. Applying marketing techniques from consumer products, insurers are segmenting the uninsured into specialized markets. For example, in 2004, Blue Cross of California launched Tonik, a line of health insurance with plans such as "Thrill-Seeker," "Calculated Risk-Taker," and "Part-Time Daredevil" that targeted uninsured young adults. Although many of the plans cover catastrophic illnesses and a set number of doctor visits or preventive services, they often have high deductibles and more restrictions. Some critics consider plans such as Blue Cross's Tonik undesirable because they take advantage of young, healthier people, in turn making it harder and more expensive for the sick, uninsured population to get insurance. On the other hand, many feel that having even a limited health insurance plan is better than having no health insurance at all.

Questions for Discussion

1. *Critics of youth-oriented plans argue that they "skim off" healthy people from other plans, leaving the other plans with an older and sicker mix of patients. Explain how such a process might work, and explain why it is pervasive in the health insurance industry. Do you agree with the critics of youth-oriented plans? Why or why not?*
2. *The article tells the story of a young person who stopped snowboarding and motorcycle riding because he had no health insurance. The same young person, after purchasing one of the Tonik plans, said that he could now begin snowboarding again. Identify and describe the common problem in health care business and economics that is illustrated by this person's decision to resume snowboarding.*
3. *Critical to insurers' ability to market to different segments of the population is flexibility in what is included in the benefit package. What are some impediments to what can and cannot be included in benefit packages?*

11-2 Health Plans and Consumer Satisfaction[9]

In an annual survey conducted online in the United States during April 2005, The Harris Poll asked adults whether a list of different industries were generally doing "a good job or bad job of serving their consumers." Most Americans were pleased with the service provided by supermarkets, but they were dissatisfied with the oil industry. Interestingly, of the industries that scored

8. Source: Vanessa Fuhrmans, "Health Insurers' New Target," *The Wall Street Journal*, May 31, 2005.
9. Source: The Harris Poll, "Americans Rank Supermarkets Highest for Serving Consumers," *The Wall Street Journal*, April 27, 2005.

lowest in terms of serving their customers, three were health care related (pharmaceuticals, managed care, and health insurance); the other two were tobacco and oil. Managed care companies and health insurance companies each posted six consecutive declines in customer ratings over the 2000–2005 interval. Overall, most industries improved their scores from 2004 but the oil industry scored worse than the previous year, presumably reflecting the public's dismay with higher gasoline prices. Telephone companies showed the most improvement since 2004, most likely due to the decline in telemarketing following the Do Not Call Registry. Pharmaceuticals recovered 17 points in 2005, but were still 47 points lower than they were in 2004.

Questions for Discussion

1. *Identify some of the important changes in the health care industry over the past ten years that may, to some extent, explain the poor customer satisfaction ratings of managed care organizations and health insurance companies.*
2. *Some studies have shown that people dislike managed care but like their own health plan. Indeed, some credit the demise of the Clinton health plan to an aversion of many people to part with their current health insurance arrangements. What might explain this seemingly counterintuitive finding?*
3. *Explain the likely relationship between adverse selection, the ability of managed care organizations to control costs, and consumer dissatisfaction with managed care.*

11-3 Illness-Specific Coverage[10]

In recent years insurers have introduced new critical care insurance policies that pay a lump sum that can be used to cover many costs related to illness if the policy holder is diagnosed with a health condition the policy covers, such as cancer, a heart attack, or a stroke. The plans are typically used for expenses that include copayments, travel, experimental treatments, or wages of family members. Payouts for the policies average around $25,000, which can cost from $300 to $500 a year, but some policies pay out as much as $100,000. The policies have been popular in Canada, England, and South Africa and are now just coming to the United States. Critics fear that insurers' aggressive marketing for the plans might scare people into purchasing the policies when they do not really need them, forcing people to spend money that could be better put toward savings, investments, or fitness programs that may help reduce a person's risk of getting sick. Critics also feel that comprehensive health and disability insurance might be just as effective for most people. The new insurance polices have several limitations, including not allowing the policies to be issued to people after ages 59 or 65, and if the policies are issued after this time, the payout is cut in half while the premiums stay the same. On the flip side, some insurers offer a "return of premium" option with the policies, which means that if a person who purchases the policy dies from a condition or accident that the policy does not cover, the company will refund the premiums.

Questions for Discussion

1. *Who is likely to purchase a critical care policy? Do such policies fill a gap in existing coverage, or do they offer different kinds of benefits?*
2. *Discuss the role, if any, of adverse selection in the marketing and sales of critical care policies.*
3. *Why are these policies popular in countries like Canada and England?*

10. Source: Rachel Emma Silverman, "Critical Care, the Insurance Industry's Latest Push," *The Wall Street Journal,* July 14, 2005.

Review Questions and Problems

1. Many economists point to moral hazard as the primary reason underlying rising health care costs in the United States.
   A. Explain the general argument behind moral hazard.
   B. Explain the five ways in which moral hazard takes place (explain with a graph when possible).
   C. How does price elasticity of demand influence the moral hazard problem?
   D. Explain how an insurer could reduce the scope of the moral hazard problem by introducing a consumer copayment.
   E. What two considerations determine the optimal copayment rate?
2. Many economists argue that the group health insurance industry is reasonably competitive. Based on various determinants of industry structure, explain the reasoning underlying this view.
3. Explain how health insurance mandates may result in inefficiencies and inequities.
4. Fully explain the two reasons the individual health insurance market may be less competitive than the group health insurance market.
5. Blair et al. (1975) find that substantial economies of scale exist in the administration of health insurance, yet survivor analysis finds no scale economies in the provision of health insurance. How can this inconsistency be explained?
6. Verbally and graphically explain how a profit-maximizing dominant health insurer determines the premium to charge for its policies.
7. Explain how the competitive fringe influences the premiums charged by a dominant health insurer.
8. Explain why someone may make the following seemingly contradictory statement: "High administrative costs are good because they sometimes lead to lower costs of providing health insurance."
9. Private insurers tend to experience three consecutive years of profits followed by three consecutive years of losses. What are the various explanations offered for this profit cycle?
10. Managed care plans tend to lower health care costs, yet the level and growth of managed care premiums are similar to those of traditional fee-for-service insurance plans. How can that be explained?
11. What does *cherry-picking behavior* mean? What does the evidence suggest about this type of behavior? Why is it less troublesome in the group health insurance market?
12. What does *adverse selection* mean? How does this type of behavior impose costs on society?
13. Explain why experience rating may be more efficient and equitable than community rating. Explain why community rating may be more efficient and equitable than experience rating.
14. Explain how the contractual feature of guaranteed renewability may lessen some of the problem that results when risk varies among the insured.
15. How is the price of health insurance measured? Why? What happened to the price of health insurance in the United States from 1993 to 1999? What happened to the price of health insurance after 1999? Why?
16. Explain how a monopsonist determines the price paid for and the quantity purchased of a good or service. According to Feldman and Wholey (2001), do HMOs have monopsony power? Why or why not?
17. Describe the typical uninsured person.
18. Explain the difference between voluntary and involuntary uninsurance and between frictional, structural, and cyclical uninsurance.
19. What were the main reasons behind the Health Insurance Portability and Accountability Act? What are the main features of the act?

20. Explain why accounting profit rates cannot be used to draw inferences about the market power of real-world firms and industries.
21. Suppose the accounting profit margins reported in Table 11–2 for the major health insurers are correct from an economic perspective. Use the Lerner index to back out the implied price elasticity of demand facing each health insurer.

CEBS Questions

■ *CEBS Sample Question on Subject Matter from CEBS Course 9 Study Manual*

1. Describe how the Omnibus Budget Reconciliation Act (OBRA) of 1990 addressed the problem of Medicare consumers lacking the necessary technical information to purchase medigap insurance policies. (page 301)

■ *CEBS Sample Exam Questions*

1. Which of the following statements on health insurance rating methods is correct?
   A. According to its supporters, experience rating can reduce the practice of adverse selection.
   B. Pure community rated premiums do not consider geographical location to differentiate across individuals.
   C. Experience rating can lead to inefficiencies in the short term.
   D. Advocates of community rating believe that experience rated premiums can result in the distribution of income from the poor to the rich.
   E. Supporters and opponents of experience rating agree that the method deals more equitably with issues arising from variations in health status.
2. Which of the following is (are) correct statements regarding barriers to entry to the health insurance industry?
   I. Scale economies in administering health insurance may serve as a barrier to entry.
   II. Lack of managerial expertise has been shown to be a significant barrier to entry.
   III. Entry barriers do not seem to seriously impede entry into the health insurance industry.
      A. I only
      B. III only
      C. I and II only
      D. I and III only
      E. I, II, and III
3. The Health Insurance Portability and Accountability Act of 1996 contains all the following features EXCEPT:
   A. Health insurers that meet specified quality and quantity standards qualify for partial reimbursement of increased costs created by the legislation.
   B. Insurers in the small group market cannot exclude any of the employer's eligible employees from coverage on the basis of health status.
   C. Individuals with a group plan cannot be charged a higher premium based on their health.
   D. With some exceptions, all group coverage must be renewable.
   E. There is a maximum exclusion period for preexisting conditions.

■ *Answer to Sample Question from Study Manual*

Prior to OBRA of 1990, Medicare beneficiaries who wanted to purchase medigap insurance found it difficult to differentiate among the provisions and limitations of a myriad of policies being sold. It was not unusual for individuals to purchase policies that duplicated other policies or, worse, that failed to provide supplemental Medicare coverage. OBRA of 1990 reformed the medigap market. It mandated that only ten standard policies based on increasing levels of coverage could be sold. The standardization enabled the consumer to assess the value and incremental cost of each of the ten policies.

■ *Answers to Sample Exam Questions*

1. A is the answer. Insurers can prevent adverse selection to some degree by limiting individuals' ability to change plans or through prior screening and experience rating. See pages 310–314 of the text.
2. D is the answer. Statements I and III are correct. Scale economies enable existing insurers to underprice new, low-volume competitors and discourage new entrants. However, despite the scale economies barrier, there appears to be no overly restrictive barriers that deter new entrants. See pages 299–301 of the text.
3. A is the answer. All statements are true except A. The act makes no provisions for subsidizing high-performing insurers. See pages 325–327 of the text.

ONLINE RESOURCES

To access Internet links related to the topics in this chapter, please visit our web site at **www.thomsonedu.com/economics/santerre**.

REFERENCES

Atchinson, Brian K., and Daniel M. Fox. "From the Field: The Politics of the Health Insurance Portability and Accountability Act." *Health Affairs* 16 (May/June 1997), pp. 146–50.

Baker, Laurence C., Joel C. Cantor, Stephen H. Long, and M. Susan Marquis. "HMO Market Penetration and Costs of Employer-Sponsored Health Plans." *Health Affairs* 19 (September/October 2000), pp. 121–28.

Baker, Laurence C., and Kenneth S. Corts. "The Effects of HMOs on Conventional Insurance Premiums: Theory and Evidence." National Bureau of Economic Research, Working Paper no. 5356, November 1995, pp. 1–33.

Beauregard, Karen M. *Persons Denied Private Health Insurance Due to Poor Health.* AHCPR Pub. No. 92–0016, 1991.

Blair, Roger D., and Ronald J. Vogel. "A Survivor Analysis of Commercial Health Insurers." *Journal of Business* 51 (July 1978), pp. 521–29.

Blair, Roger D., Jerry R. Jackson, and Ronald J. Vogel. "Economies of Scale in the Administration of Health Insurance." *Review of Economics and Statistics* 57 (May 1975), pp. 185–89.

Born, Patricia, and Rexford E. Santerre. "Unraveling the Health Insurance Underwriting Cycle." Mimeo, University of Connecticut, September 22, 2005.

Centers for Medicare and Medicaid Services. *Health Care Industry Update: Managed Care.* Washington, D.C.: CMS, March 24, 2003.

Chollet, Deborah J., Fabrice Smieliauskas, and Madeleine Konig. "Mapping State Health Insurance Markets, 2001: Structure and Change." Washington,

D.C.: Academy for Health Services Research and Health Policy, September 2003.

Conwell, L. J. "The Role of Health Insurance Brokers." Issue Brief #57. Washington, D.C.: Center for Studying Health System Change, October 2002.

Cutler, David M., and Mark McClellan. "Is Technological Change in Medicine Worth It?" *Health Affairs* (September/October 2001), pp. 11–29.

Danzon, Patricia M. "Hidden Overhead Costs: Is Canada's System Really Less Expensive?" *Health Affairs* 11 (spring 1992), pp. 21–43.

DeNavas-Walt, C., B. D. Proctor, and C. H. Lee. "Income, Poverty, and Health Insurance Coverage in the United States: 2004." U.S. Census Bureau, *Current Population Reports*, P60-229. Washington, D.C.: U.S. Government Printing Office, 2005.

Feldman, Roger, Bryan Dowd, and Gregory Gifford. "The Effect of HMOs on Premiums in Employment-Based Health Plans." *Health Services Research* 27 (February 1993), pp. 779–811.

Feldman, Roger, and Douglas Wholey. "Do HMOs Have Monopsony Power?" *International Journal of Health Care Finance and Economics* 1 (2001), pp. 7–22.

Friedman, Milton. "The Folly of Buying Health Care at the Company Store." *The Wall Street Journal*, February 3, 1992, p. A14.

Gabel, Jon, Roger Formisano, Barbara Lohr, and Steven Di Carlo. "Tracing the Cycle of Health Insurance." *Health Affairs* (winter 1991), pp. 49–61.

General Accounting Office. "Private Health Insurance: Number and Market Share of Carriers in the Small Group Health Insurance Market in 2004." 6A0-06-155R. Washington, D.C.: GAO, October 13, 2005.

Grossman, Joy M., and Paul B. Ginsburg. "As the Health Insurance Underwriting Cycle Turns: What Next?" *Health Affairs* 23, no. 6 (2004), pp. 91–102.

Gruber, Jonathan, and Brigette C. Madrian. "Health Insurance, Labor Supply, and Job Mobility: A Critical Review of the Literature." Working Paper no. 8817. Cambridge, Mass.: National Bureau of Economic Research, March 2002.

Hay, Joel W., and Michael J. Leahy. "Competition among Health Plans: Some Preliminary Evidence." *Southern Economic Journal* 50 (January 1987), pp. 831–46.

Health Insurance Association of America (HIAA). *Source Book of Health Insurance Data 1999/2000*. Washington, D.C.: HIAA, 2001.

Iglehart, John K. "The American Health Care System—Private Insurance." *New England Journal of Medicine* 326 (June 18, 1992), pp. 1715–20.

Kopit, William G. "Is There Evidence That Recent Consolidation in the Health Insurance Industry Has Adversely Affected Premiums?" *Health Affairs* 23 (November/December 2004), pp. 29–31.

Lerner, Abba P. "The Concept of Monopoly and the Measurement of Monopoly Power." *Review of Economic Studies* 1 (1934), pp. 157–75.

Long, Stephen H., and Jack Rodgers. "Do Shifts toward Service Industries, Part-Time Work, and Self-Employment Explain the Rising Uninsured Rate?" *Inquiry* 32 (spring 1995), pp. 111–6.

Madrian, B. C. "Health Insurance Portability: The Consequences of COBRA." *Regulation* (Winter 1998), pp. 27–33.

Manning, Willard, et al. "A Controlled Trial of the Effect of a Prepaid Group Practice on Use of Services." *New England Journal of Medicine* 310 (June 7, 1984), pp. 1505–10.

McCormack, Lauren A., Peter D. Fox, Thomas Rice, and Marcia L. Graham. "Medigap Reform Legislation of 1990: Have the Objectives Been Met?" *Health Care Financing Review* 18 (fall 1996), pp. 157–74.

McLaughlin, Catherine G. "Market Responses to HMOs. Price Competition or Rivalry?" *Inquiry* (summer 1988), pp. 207–18.

Miller, Robert H., and Harold S. Luft. "Managed Care Plan Performance since 1980." *Journal of the American Medical Association* 271 (May 18, 1994), pp. 1512–19.

Miller, W., E. R. Vigdor, and W. G. Manning. "Covering the Uninsured: What Is It Worth?" *Health Affairs*, Web Exclusive (March 31, 2004), pp. w4-157–w4-167.

Morrisey, Michael A. "Competition in Hospital and Health Insurance Markets: A Review and Research Agenda." *Health Services Research* 36 (April 2001), pp. 191–222.

Nichols, Len M., and Linda Blumberg. "A Different Kind of 'New Federalism'? The Health Insurance

Portability and Accountability Act of 1996." *Health Affairs* 17 (May/June 1998), pp. 25–42.

Nyman, J. A. *The Theory of Demand for Health Insurance.* Stanford, Calif.: Stanford University Press, 2003.

Patel, Vip, and Mark V. Pauly. "Guaranteed Renewability and the Problem of Risk Variation in Individual Health Insurance Markets." *Health Affairs*, Web Exclusive (August 28, 2002), pp. w280–w289.

Pollitz, Karen, Richard Sorian, and Kathy Thomas. *How Accessible Is Individual Health Insurance for Consumers in Less-Than-Perfect Health?* Report prepared for the Kaiser Family Foundation, Georgetown University Institute for Health Care Research and Policy, June 2001.

Pauly, Mark V. "The Economics of Moral Hazard: Comment?" *American Economic Review* 58 (June 1968), pp. 531–37.

Pauly, Mark V., Alan L. Hillman, Myoung S. Kim, and Darryl R. Brown. "Competitive Behavior in the HMO Marketplace." *Health Affairs* 21 (January/February 2002), pp. 194–202.

Rapoport, John, et al. "Resource Utilization among Intensive Care Patients." *Archives of Internal Medicine* 152 (November 1992), pp. 2207–12.

Reinhardt, Uwe. "The Market Won't Make Health Insurers Efficient." *Norwich Bulletin*, April 12, 1992, p. A5.

Robinson, James C. "Consolidation and the Transformation of Competition in Health Insurance." *Health Affairs* 23 (November/December 2004), pp. 11–24.

Rothschild, Michael, and Joseph Stiglitz. "Equilibrium in Competitive Insurance Markets: An Essay on the Economics of Imperfect Information." *Quarterly Journal of Economics* 90 (November 1976), pp. 630–49.

Samuelson, Paul A. "Interactions between the Multiplier Analysis and the Principle of Acceleration." *Review of Economics and Statistics* 21, no. 2 (1939), pp. 75–78.

Santerre, Rexford E. "Examining the Marginal Access Value of Private Health Insurance." *Risk Management and Insurance Review* 9(2006), pp. 53–62.

Sapolsky, Harvey M. "Empire and the Business of Health Insurance." *Journal of Health Politics, Policy and Law* 16 (winter 1991), pp. 747–60.

Seidman, Laurence S. "Health Care: Getting the Right Amount at the Right Price." *Business Review*, March–April 1982.

Sheth, Jagdish, and Rajendra Sisodia. "Only the Big Three Will Thrive." *The Wall Street Journal*, May 11, 1998, p. A22.

Sindelar, Jody L. "The Declining Price of Health Insurance." In *Health Care in America*, ed. H. E. Frech III. San Francisco: Pacific Institute for Public Policy, 1988, pp. 259–91.

Steinmetz, Greg. "Number of Uninsured Stirs Much Confusion in Health-Care Debate." *The Wall Street Journal*, June 9, 1993, p. A1.

Stigler, George J. "The Economies of Scale." *Journal of Law and Economics* 1 (October 1958), pp. 54–71.

Swartz, Katherine. "Dynamics of People without Health Insurance." *Journal of the American Medical Association* 271 (January 5, 1994), pp. 64–66.

Swartz, Katherine, John Marcotte, and Timothy D. McBride. "Personal Characteristics and Spells without Health Insurance." *Inquiry* 30 (spring 1993), pp. 64–76.

Temin, Peter. "An Economic History of American Hospitals." In *Health Care in America*, ed. H. E. Frech III. San Francisco: Pacific Research Institute for Public Policy, 1988, pp. 75–102.

Van De Ven, Wynand P. M. M., and Randall P. Ellis. "Risk Adjustment in Competitive Health Plan Markets." In *Handbook of Health Economics, Volume 1*, eds. A. J. Culyer and J. P. Newhouse. Amsterdam: Elsevier Science, 2000.

Weisbrod, Burton A. "The Health Care Quadrilemma: An Essay on Technological Change, Insurance, Quality of Care, and Cost Containment." *Journal of Economic Literature* 29 (June 1991), pp. 523–52.

Wholey, Douglas, Roger Feldman, and Jon B. Christianson. "The Effect of Market Structure on HMO Premiums." *Journal of Health Economics* 14 (1995), pp. 81–105.

Wholey, Douglas, Roger Feldman, Jon B. Christianson, and John Engberg. "Scale and Scope Economies among Health Maintenance Organizations." *Journal of Health Economics* 15 (1996), pp. 657–84.

Wickizer, Thomas M., and Paul J. Feldstein. "The Impact of HMO Competition on Private Health Insurance Premiums." *Inquiry* 32 (fall 1995), pp. 241–51.

CHAPTER 12
THE PHYSICIAN SERVICES INDUSTRY

Throughout the 19th century, the physician services industry was largely unregulated. Many physicians were practicing without proper medical training, primarily because the country was dotted with numerous medical schools of questionable quality. In reaction to this state of affairs, the American Medical Association (AMA) was founded in 1847. At its inception, the organization adopted the improvement of medical education in the United States as its major goal. Although improvements were made over the years, significant changes did not take place until the turn of the 20th century. The impetus for change was the Flexner Report published in 1910 by the Carnegie Foundation.

Concerned that not enough was being done to improve medical education, the Carnegie Foundation, with the blessing of the AMA, asked Abraham Flexner to conduct a study of the medical schools in Canada and the United States. The final report, commonly referred to as the Flexner Report, was highly critical of the medical training provided by an overwhelming majority of the schools in North America. The report was so controversial that Flexner received threats on his life. As a result of the report, many low-quality medical schools were forced to improve or close their doors. In addition, states began to take the role of licensing physicians more seriously (Raffel and Raffel, 1989). Thus, the formation of the AMA, coupled with the Flexner Report, ushered in the modern regulated physician services industry, which requires an individual to fulfill strict educational and licensing requirements before being allowed to practice medicine.

Over the past quarter century, the scope and complexity of physician services have increased dramatically, and this has had a profound impact on the structure and performance of the industry. Increases in demand for medical services and the introduction of many new, costly technologies have increased expenditures on physician services fiftyfold since 1960. Nearly gone are the days when an appointment with the doctor meant a visit to a self-employed male physician who owned a solo fee-for-service practice. Today, almost one out of four physicians is female and only about one-quarter of all physicians are self-employed and operating a solo practice. Multiphysician practices are the norm, and physicians who wish to survive are now forced to negotiate with MCOs for additional patients, adjust to many new and different fee schedules, and subject themselves to utilization reviews.

In keeping with the methodology laid out in the previous chapter, this chapter employs the structure-conduct-performance paradigm to analyze the ever-changing physician services industry. The first part of the chapter describes the current structure of the industry. In particular, it looks at the number and specialty distribution of physicians, examines the mode of practice, analyzes methods of payment, reviews the reimbursement practices of managed care buyers, and concludes with a discussion of the production and cost of physician services. The conduct section of the chapter discusses the impact of compensation schemes on physician behavior and examines geographic variations in the use of physician services. In addition, it looks at the supplier-induced demand hypothesis, reviews the physician practice hypothesis, and explores the implication of a quantity-setting model on physician behavior. The conduct section finishes with an analysis of the impact of managed care on physician behavior. The performance section traces expenditures on physician services over time, reviews the utilization of physician services, and discusses the growth of physician income over time.

The Structure of the Physician Services Industry

Because the conduct of buyers and sellers depends directly on the structure of the market, we begin with an analysis of the structure of the physician services market. Among the structural elements, we look at the number and specialty distribution of physicians, along with the organization arrangements adopted by physicians to produce medical services. Next we review the sources of physician revenues and examine the impact of managed care on the physician services market. Finally, we analyze barriers to entry and the production of physician services.

The Number of Physicians in the United States

It seems only logical to begin our analysis of the market for physician services with a look at the supply of physician labor, the primary input in the production of physician services.[1] According to Figure 12–1, the United States experienced a substantial increase in the number of physicians from 1975 to 2003. In 1975, a total of 353,742 physicians were in the United States; by 2003 that number had increased by more than 120 percent to 871,535.

To get a clearer picture of the impact of this increase in physician labor on the delivery of patient care, we need to look at a breakdown of physicians by major professional activities. According to Figure 12–1, almost 80 percent of all physicians, 691,873, were involved in direct patient care in 2003. That percentage has remained remarkably stable over time. The remaining 20 percent of the physicians were engaged in other activities such as medical teaching, administration, or research.

Although the absolute supply of physicians in the United States increased in recent years, it is impossible to make inferences regarding the relative supply of physicians without comparing the increase in physician labor to the overall increase in population. One crude measure of the relative supply of physician labor is the physician-to-population ratio. Data supplied by the AMA[2] indicate that the number of total nonfederal patient care physicians per 100,000 civilians increased substantially from 134 in 1970 to 238 in 2003, an increase of almost 80 percent. Put in other terms, in 1970 there was one patient care physician for every 747 people in the civilian population in the United States and by 2003 that number had dropped to 430 individuals.

It is apparent that the United States experienced a significant increase in physician labor over the last three decades. The increase outpaced the overall increase in the population and has led to a greater relative supply of labor, as measured by an increase in the physician-to-population ratio. Despite this increase in physician supply, however, the problem of a geographic maldistribution of physicians in the United States still persists, albeit to a lesser degree than previously was the case. According to a GAO study (2003c), the growth in physician supply was felt in metropolitan as well as nonmetropolitan areas across the country. Throughout the 1990s, all

1. As we will see later in the chapter, physician services are produced with a combination of various inputs, including physician labor, nurse labor, clerical staff, physician assistants, and lab technicians.

2. American Medical Association, *Physician Characteristics and Distribution in the U.S., 2005* (Chicago: AMA, 2005), Table 5–16.

FIGURE 12–1
Number of Physicians in the United States, 1975–2003

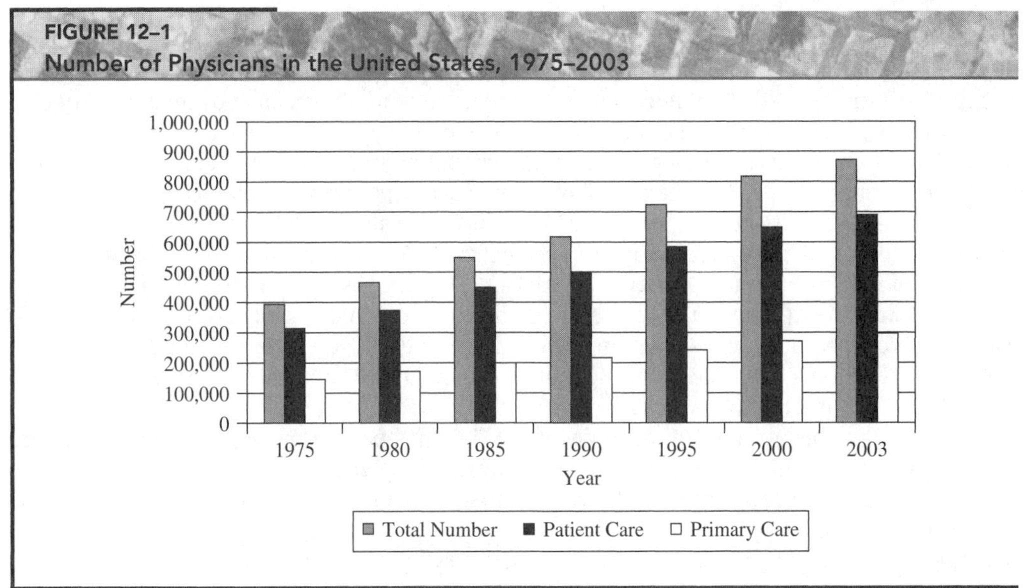

SOURCE: American Medical Association, *Physician Characteristics and Distribution in the U.S., 2005* (Chicago: AMA, 2005).

nonmetropolitan areas and 301 out of 318 metropolitan areas saw increases in the number of physicians per 100,000 people. Of the 17 metropolitan areas that experienced decreases in the relative supply of physicians, only 2 had an absolute decrease in the number of physicians. These results are largely confirmed by Rosenthal et al. (2005), who compare the location patterns of physicians in 1999 and 1979. For example, they find that "even in the most remote categories of counties, with an urban population of less than 2,500 and not adjacent to a metropolitan area, the mean distance to the nearest physician of any type was less than 5 miles" in 1999 (p. 1943).

Together, these findings indicate that geographic access to physician services has improved over time in the United States. Despite this good news, the GAO finds that disparities in physician supply between metropolitan and nonmetropolitan areas still exist.[3] Interestingly, nonmetropolitan counties with a large town experienced a greater percentage increase in physicians per 100,000 people than metropolitan and nonmetropolitan (including rural) counties without a large town during the 1990s. Overall, these findings are consistent with a study by Carpenter and Neun (1999) that examines the factors that influence the location decision of young primary care physicians. It appears that young physicians have a preference for small to medium-sized cities as opposed to either sparsely populated communities or major metropolitan areas. Young physicians also favor counties where the crime and poverty rates are low and taxes are not excessive. Finally, they prefer to locate in counties where there is a strong academic presence and the cost of living is moderate.

3. We need to keep in mind that these findings do not take into account any local geographic disparities in physician supply that may exist within counties.

Distribution of Primary Care and Specialty Care Physicians in the United States

Figure 12–1 provides additional information on the number of physicians providing primary care in the United States as defined by the AMA to include family practice, general practice, internal medicine, obstetrics and gynecology, and pediatrics, but excluding subspecialties within each of these general specialties. While the overall number of active primary care physicians in the United States increased from 144,861 in 1975 to 293,701 in 2003, the proportion of active primary care physicians decreased from approximately 40 percent in 1975 to 34 percent in 2005. The implication is that the number of specialty physicians in the United States over the last three decades increased at a faster pace than the number of primary care physicians. AMA data on the distribution of physicians by major specialties (not shown) indicate that the single largest category is internal medicine with 147,646 physicians in 2003. Other specialties of note include general surgery, 37,844; psychiatry, 40,334; and anesthesiology, 38,478.

Many analysts believe the United States has too many specialists and too few primary care physicians and that the problem has worsened over time. According to Schroeder (1992), the growth in the number of specialists relative to primary care physicians is one reason health costs are so high in the United States. Specialists are more prone to overutilize costly new, high-technology medical procedures that drive up medical costs. Higher surgery rates and a greater availability of medical technology in the United States relative to other industrialized nations are used as evidence to support this hypothesis. To prove his point, Schroeder (1984, 1992) compares the proportion of specialists in the United States to that of various Western European countries in 1980. He finds the proportion of specialists in Belgium, Germany, the Netherlands, and the United Kingdom to lie between 25 and 50 percent. In the United States, the proportion of specialists was slightly more than 60 percent, substantially higher than in most other developed nations.

Another study (GAO, 1994) finds basically the same thing for 1990. For example, the report found that 58 percent of the doctors in the United Kingdom are in primary care. It is interesting to note that one developed nation has a lower percentage of primary care physicians than the United States. According to the GAO report, only 18 percent of the physicians in Sweden are considered primary care doctors.

Whether the United States has more or less than the efficient level of primary care physicians is difficult to determine objectively. One way researchers have attempted to answer this question is by first establishing the medical need for primary care physicians—that is, how many primary care physicians are needed to deliver adequate care to the population. However, from an economic perspective, demand rather than need is really at issue. Next, the most cost-effective way to deliver physician services must be determined. Only after this has been established can one determine the total number of primary and nonprimary care physicians clinically needed to provide medical services to the entire population. These estimates must then be compared to the actual number of primary and nonprimary care physicians practicing in the United States to determine whether a surplus or a shortage of specialists exists. Obviously, the process of calculating the optimal number of many specialists is complicated and laced with value judgments.

Weiner (2004) takes on this challenge when he attempts to determine whether the supply of physician labor in the United States is adequate to meet the needs of the population. To establish need, he examines the physician staffing patterns adopted by eight large prepaid group practices (PGPs), at Kaiser Permanente and two other health maintenance organizations that were serving more than eight million enrollees in 2002. Weiner assumes in his analysis that PGPs provide an adequate amount of physician care in the most cost-efficient manner due to the financial incentives they face. In other words, he assumes that large PGPs provide the appropriate amount and type of physician care at least cost.

The goal is to assess the adequacy of the physician workforce in the United States by comparing the physician/population ratios for a select group of PGPs to the overall national average. Before making the comparison, however, Weiner adjusts the PGP physician/population ratios to reflect demographic differences between the PGPs in the sample and the U.S. population as a whole and to accommodate the use of outside referrals by PGPs. After making these adjustments, he finds that the PGPs in the sample have physician-to-population ratios that are between 22 and 37 percent lower than the overall U.S. ratio. In addition, he finds that the difference in the physician-to-population ratios between the PGPs in the study and the national average for primary care physicians is much less than for specialty care physicians. The major inference from these findings is that PGPs may be able to provide medical care to the general population with far fewer physicians than is currently the case.

While these results are interesting, Salsberg and Forte (2004) caution that we not overextend Weiner's findings and conclude that the United States has too many physicians. Significant differences exist between the ways physician activities are organized in PGPs and in the country as a whole that limit comparisons between physician workforce patterns in PGPs and that of the entire U.S. physician workforce. For one thing, PGPs tend to serve a distinct subset of the U.S. population, which was not adequately accounted for in Weiner's study. For example, enrollees in PGPs are more likely to be employed and therefore have fewer chronic illnesses than the general population. As a result, they require fewer physician services. More important, however, is the fact that the work responsibilities of physicians differ widely across the medical community and are not fully reflected in the staffing patterns of PGPs. As Salsberg and Forte point out, a significant number of physicians conduct clinical research, teach medical students, or provide medical care to individuals with very high needs. These are generally not the duties of PGP physicians. Given these considerations, it is inappropriate to apply the PGP physician staffing ratios to the nation as a whole because they fail to capture the overall scope of physician activities. The challenge, according to the authors, is to determine "which elements of the PGP system contribute to greater efficiencies and effectiveness" (p. 74) in the delivery and financing of medical services and selectively apply them to other delivery systems.

Politzer et al. (1996) look to the future to estimate whether the United States will have an adequate supply of physicians in the year 2020. To establish need, the authors conducted a statistical technique called meta-analysis on five alternative projection methods already developed in the literature. Meta-analysis allows them to establish bands of physician requirements for primary and specialty care physicians. Physician supply projections were based on a number of factors, including the number of first-year residency positions likely to exist in the future. The authors conclude that the "future physician supply does not appear well-matched with requirements" (p. 181). For example, assuming a 30/70 ratio of generalists to specialists and an increase in U.S. medical graduates equal to 110 percent of their 1998 levels, the authors project a shortage of approximately 33,000 primary care physicians by the year 2020. The same set of assumptions also generates a surplus of specialists.

Another study with many of the same authors (Gamliel et al., 1995) reaches the same conclusion. According to the results from this study, in all likelihood there will be an overall surplus of physicians of between 56,000 and 71,000 doctors by the year 2020, which will be due primarily to an oversupply of specialists. The problem of an oversupply of physicians is further complicated by the fact that the authors forecast a shortage of primary care physicians in the future.

Cooper et al. (2002) and Cooper (2004) take a very different approach to projecting the adequacy of physician supply and develop a macroeconomic forecast based on four trends that greatly impact the supply of and use of physician services. First and foremost, they consider the strong relationship between the growth of physician supply and economic growth over time. Next, they factor in the impact of population trends, physician work efforts, and the capacity of nonphysician health care professions to provide medical care. Their results are thought-provoking because they contradict conventional wisdom that the United States has too many physicians. According to their results, a substantial shortfall of approximately 200,000 physicians is likely to exist in the United States by the year 2020.

Clearly, these results point to a need for a better understanding of factors that are likely to impact the demand for and supply of physician services in the coming years. The strong likelihood of a mismatch between physician supply and demand also raises some interesting policy questions. For example, what role should the government play in correcting any imbalances that may exist in our health workforce given the fact that it has traditionally subsidized the education of many health care professionals, including physicians? Also, what role should the market play in correcting any labor market imbalances?

Mode of Practice

Economists view the provision of physician services as a production process that involves a multitude of inputs aside from physician labor. It includes other labor inputs, such as nurses, nurse practitioners, physician assistants, medical technicians, and receptionists, along with various nonlabor inputs, such as office space, medical supplies, and diagnostic equipment. In light of this view, it is extremely important to distinguish between physician labor as a strategic input in the production of medical services and the firm, or production arrangement, adopted by physicians to produce medical care. Self-employed profit-maximizing physicians act as entrepreneurs when they combine various inputs, including their own labor, to produce medical care for their patients.

Data from the AMA (1998, 2003) provide a glimpse of the modes of practice utilized by physicians from 1989 to 2001. The figures indicate that the majority of physicians are self-employed. In 1989 slightly more than 70 percent of all physicians were self-employed, and by 2001 this number had dropped to just under 60 percent. This drop appears to have resulted primarily from a decrease in the proportion of physicians operating solo practices. By 2001, fewer than 33 percent of all physicians, excluding those practicing in institutional settings, were engaged in a solo practice. There was also a decrease in the percentage of self-employed physicians involved in practices with two or three physicians. A greater percentage of self-employed physicians are now involved in larger practices with four or more physicians.

Based on this information there appears to be a trend away from smaller practices toward larger, multidoctor modes of production. This trend might reflect the economies of scope offered by large multidoctor, multispecialty practices or economies of scale in the production of physician services. We review some empirical evidence concerning economies of scale later in the chapter.

By far the greatest change in recent years has been an increase in the proportion of physicians who are not self-employed but are paid on a salary basis. By 2001, 35.1 percent of all physicians were paid on a salary basis, an increase of approximately 12 percentage points from 1989.

Buyers of Physician Services and Methods of Remuneration

A review of the methods of remuneration provides insight into the number and types of buyers of physician services and the extent to which any one buyer, or group of buyers, may exhibit some degree of market power. In 2003, 33.3 percent of all expenditures on physician and clinical services emanated from the government sector, with Medicare making up 60 percent of that total. This is in sharp contrast to the market for hospital services, in which the government sector accounted for nearly 60 percent of total revenues (see Chapter 13). This suggests that although the government sector is clearly a major player in the physician services market, its ability to exercise market power may not be as great as in the market for hospital services.

Rising health care costs have forced politicians to reevaluate the Medicare and Medicaid programs. For example, after much debate Congress passed the Omnibus Budget Reconciliation Act (OBRA) in 1989, which, among other things, called for major changes in Part B of the Medicare payment system, which provides compensation to physicians for medical services rendered to elderly patients. As of 1992, physicians are now compensated based on resources utilized rather than on the "usual, customary, or reasonable" rate. This Medicare reimbursement scheme for physician services, referred to as the *resource-based relative value scale system,* is reviewed in Chapter 10. OBRA 1989 was followed by the Balanced Budget Act of 1997, which extended the resource-based method of payment to include practice and malpractice expenses.

The private sector accounted for about 66.8 percent of physician revenues in 2003, with almost 50 percent coming from private insurance companies. Of the remaining 17 percent, a little more than 10 percent represents out-of-pocket payments and about 7 percent comes from other private sources. This is somewhat different from the hospital services market, in which out-of-pocket payments account for 3.2 percent of total revenues. The relatively higher out-of-pocket expenses for physician services are not too surprising, because insurance theory suggests that insurance coverage is lower for more predictable and lower-magnitude losses.

Overall, the private sector accounts for a much greater share of revenues in the physician services market than it does in the hospital services market. This is largely because out-of-pocket payments are a more important source of funds for physicians than for hospitals. This is not to say, however, that the government plays only a minor role in the physician services market. On the contrary, the recent Medicare reforms indicate that the federal government intends to play a more active role in this market for years to come.

Reimbursement Practices of Managed Care Buyers of Physician Services

Managed care, which embodies a broad set of policies designed by third-party payers to control the utilization and cost of medical care, has had a profound impact on the physician services market. Through the use of alternative compensation schemes, utilization reviews, quality controls, and the like, MCOs hope to modify the behavior of physicians to contain costs. These control mechanisms diminish the autonomy physicians traditionally enjoyed in practicing medicine, and, as a result, many physicians have resisted the movement toward managed care. Despite these reservations, managed care presently has a major impact on the allocation of resources in the physician services market.

The strong presence of managed care in the physician services market is reflected in the fact that 88 percent of all physicians practicing medicine in 2001 had at least one managed care contract. A more detailed look at the data confirms the significant role of managed care in the physician services market. The proportion of physicians with a minimum of one managed care contract varied little across regions of the country, practice size, or specialty in 2001. For example, the rate of contract involvement for physicians ranged from a high of 92 percent in New England to a low of 82 percent in the East South Central region. In relation to practice arrangement, there appears to be a weak but positive connection between practice size and managed care involvement. Finally, for almost all specialties the percentage of physicians with one or more managed care contract topped 90 percent; the lowest was psychiatry, with slightly more than 62 percent having signed at least one contract (American Medical Association, 2003).

Managed care also appears to account for a significant proportion of revenues generated by physicians. In 2001, 41 cents out of every dollar generated by practicing physicians was the result of some type of contractual arrangement with an MCO.

Barriers to Entry

It is generally accepted that substantial barriers to entry in the market for physician services impede competition primarily by legally limiting the supply of physicians. Before being allowed to practice medicine, a person must meet a minimum educational requirement (usually a degree from an accredited medical school), participate in an internship or a residency program at a recognized institution, and pass a medical exam. These various requirements entail substantial time and money costs and raise the opportunity cost of becoming a medical doctor. Advocates for these legal restrictions base their argument on the public interest theory. Market failure brought about by an asymmetry of information between patient and physician concerning the appropriateness and quality of medical care justifies the need for government intervention. Because consumers generally have imperfect information concerning the medical care received given its technical sophistication, they are sometimes unsure about the appropriateness and quality of physician services. As a result, the market cannot be relied on to weed out incompetent doctors or those who would take advantage of their position and prescribe needless and costly medical care.

The necessity of government intervention has also been justified based on the possibility that a negative supply-side externality will occur if incompetent physicians are allowed to practice medicine. For example, if an incompetent physician misdiagnoses a patient infected with the AIDS virus due to a faulty test, others may contract the virus. As a result, government intervention is necessary to ensure that consumers will not become innocent victims of medical malfeasance.

Over the years, proponents of the special interest theory, including Kessel (1958), Moore (1961), Friedman (1962, 1980), and Leffler (1978), have argued that barriers exist primarily to protect the economic interests of physicians. By restricting supply through the creation of educational and training barriers to entry, physicians have succeeded in generating economic profits. As evidence, these analysts point to high physician salaries. Control of medical licensure is the primary mechanism physicians use to restrict their numbers. In the United States, the licensure of physicians is under the control of the states, and most states have medical boards composed of physicians who establish, review, and maintain the criteria for obtaining a license to practice medicine. The fact that these requirements control the process of becoming a physician rather than encourage the maintenance of medical knowledge has been used as evidence to support the special interest interpretation of these restrictions.[4]

Control over medical licensure is not the only method physicians use to maintain their market power. Physicians as a group play a critical role in the accreditation of medical schools. For example, the Liaison Committee on Medical Education, the main accrediting body of medical schools, is composed of seventeen people, six of whom are representatives of the American Medical Association (Wilson and Neuhauser, 1985). By maintaining control over the number of medical schools, physicians are in a position to indirectly restrain the supply of their services.

4. The same argument can be made for lawyers and certified public accountants, who are required to pass the bar exam and CPA exam, respectively.

The establishment of limits on the use of physician extenders is yet another method physicians employ to protect their economic interests. Physician extenders, such as physician assistants and nurse practitioners, have the medical training necessary to perform a number of medical tasks traditionally carried out by the physician.[5] Production theory indicates that when more than one variable input is utilized in the production of physician services, a cost-conscious firm combines these inputs to produce in the most cost-efficient manner. For example, let's suppose a staff-model HMO faces an increase in wages for physicians. To counteract this increase, the HMO may attempt to substitute physician extenders for physicians in the production of certain medical services.[6] To limit the possibility of this occurrence, physicians may flex their political muscle to legally limit the duties of physician extenders. The goal would be to legally constrain the marginal rate of technical substitution between physicians and physician extenders to near zero.

Given many of the recent changes in medical care, Svorny (1992) questions the need for medical licensure in the physician market. She believes market incentives can now be relied on to ensure an efficient level of quality. In particular, Svorny points to changes in medical liability, the rapid growth in for-profit medical care providers, the increased use of brand names, and the growth in employed rather than self-employed physicians as lessening the need for the licensure of physicians.

For example, recent legal decisions have shifted some of the liability for medical malpractice away from physicians and toward institutions, such as hospitals and HMOs. As a result, hospitals and HMOs now have a greater incentive to monitor the behavior of physicians who practice medicine on their premises by assessing the quality of care provided. Institutional liability decreases the need for licensing because it is now in the self-interests of hospitals to weed out incompetent physicians.

The growth in for-profit medical care providers may have the same effect. Because at least one owner has a financial stake in a for-profit medical institution, there may be a greater incentive to oversee the performance of physicians than in a not-for-profit institution, which is run by a board of directors who have no financial commitment to the institution. The expanded use of brand names by hospitals, group practices, and HMOs also increases the incentive for these institutions to more closely monitor the performance of physicians. An incompetent physician can financially hurt the institution by damaging its reputation and tarnishing its image, which took a substantial amount of time and money to establish. Much goodwill is at stake, and hence there is an increased incentive to dismiss incompetent physicians.

The growing use of employed as opposed to self-employed physicians also provides medical institutions with an increased incentive to monitor the activities of physicians. Naturally, it is in the interests of these institutions to eliminate physicians providing low-quality or unnecessary medical care. In addition, because the physician is a salaried employee, the incentive to provide unnecessary care has been diminished. According to Svorny, all these changes have lessened the need for the licensure of physicians because market forces can now be relied on to force doctors to provide quality medical care at least cost.

---

5. A physician assistant must study for two years in an accredited physician assistant program and pass a certification exam before being allowed to practice. A nurse practitioner is a licensed registered nurse who has received an additional one or two years' training and passed a certification exam. In terms of duties, the difference between the two labor inputs is one of emphasis. Physician assistants concern themselves primarily with the direct application of medical care, whereas nurse practitioners deal mostly in education and wellness.

6. This is one reason why the physician-to-population ratios for managed care organizations tend to be lower than the national averages, as we saw earlier.

These institutional and structural changes imply a weakening of barriers to entry into the physician services market. If this is indeed the case, the level of competition should have intensified over time. To test for this phenomenon, Noether (1986) developed a system of stock and income equations to depict behavior in the physician services market. According to her results, competition in the physician services markets has increased since 1965, and this increase has caused the supply of physician labor to increase by 6 to 20 percent and physician incomes to fall by 19 to 45 percent. All this indicates that the degree of market power in the hands of physicians has waned in recent years.

Production, Costs, and Economies of Scale

Thus far, we have focused primarily on the supply of physicians. In this section, the perspective changes from the physician as an input in the production of medical services to the physician as an entrepreneur: one who makes allocation decisions concerning the most cost-effective way to produce medical services. Unfortunately, the literature on the production and cost of physician services is rather thin compared to the multitude of studies on the hospital services market.

The most comprehensive studies on the production of physician services were carried out by Reinhardt (1972, 1973, 1975). In these studies, the author estimates a production function for physician services using data from a survey of doctors in 1965 and 1967. Given the controversy surrounding the most appropriate means to measure output in the physician services market, the author employed three measures of physician output: total weekly patient visits at the office, home, or hospital; weekly office visits; and annual gross billings to patients. Inputs included physician labor, as measured by total practice hours per week; number of auxiliary personnel; medical supplies; and capital equipment. In addition, a host of control variables were included in the estimated equations.

The regression results with total patient visits as a measure of output are particularly interesting. To no one's surprise, Reinhardt finds physician labor to be highly correlated with output, with an elasticity of output to physician time equal to 0.70.[7] Capital inputs appeared to have a far smaller impact on output. The capital elasticity of output was estimated at 0.05. The effect of auxiliary personnel appeared to be somewhat greater than that of capital, with an elasticity of approximately 0.32. Finally, Reinhardt finds that physicians in group practices were about 5 percent more productive in terms of patient visits than physicians in a solo practice.

In a more contemporary study, Brown (1988) also examines the factors that influence physician output. He finds, among other things, that group practice physicians were 22 percent more productive than their counterparts in solo practices. These estimates are substantially greater than Reinhardt's and justify the organizational movement in the physician services market away from solo practices that we discussed earlier in the chapter. Solo practices face some difficulty in competing with group practices with such a significant productivity disadvantage.[8]

Brown's study also uncovers some interesting results concerning the efficient use of auxiliary personnel. According to Brown, the estimated marginal products for various labor inputs clearly show that physicians, registered nurses, and practical nurses are the most productive inputs, whereas secretaries, technicians, and physician assistants are the least productive inputs in the production of physician services. To determine whether physicians are utilizing inputs

7. This output elasticity means that the output of physician services increased by 7 percent for each 10 percent increase in physician hours, assuming all other factors remain constant.

8. The cost differential may reflect the value, or utility, that a proprietor/physician places on working independently and being her own boss. Otherwise, why would the proprietor/physician remain in the less profitable solo practice?

efficiently, we must compare the marginal product per dollar spent on each input. Recall from Chapter 7 that the firm is optimally utilizing all inputs if the marginal product of the last dollar spent on each input is equal across all inputs. Brown shows that the marginal product per dollar spent for physicians' time equals 0.114 and is higher than the marginal product to price ratio for all other inputs except licensed practical nurses. Thus we can conclude that physicians overutilize auxiliary personnel. For licensed practical nurses, the evidence suggests that they are underutilized, with a marginal product per dollar spent of 0.129.

Estimating a more general production function than Reinhardt, Thurston and Libby (2002) find that the marginal product of an additional hour of physician labor equals 0.55 office visits per week. Like Brown, Thurston and Libby also find the marginal productivity to be highest for nurses among nonphysician personnel such as administrative and clerical workers and technicians and aides. In particular, they find that the employment of one additional nurse increases physician office visits by between seven and eight visits per week. They also find the marginal productivity of capital, as measured in thousands of dollars, to equal 0.19, suggesting that the average physician practice would have to invest approximately $5,000 in capital equipment to generate an additional office visit per week.

The literature also suggests that moderate economies of scale exist in the production of physician services. A study by Pope and Burge (1996), which estimates the gross revenue production function for self-employed physicians, finds the lowest-cost practice size to be 5.2 physicians. The lowest-cost practice size is somewhat higher than the average practice size of 2.4 physicians in their sample. The authors also find that group physicians have the ability to handle 17 percent more office visits than physicians in a solo practice. Escarce and Pauly (1998) also find the presence of economies of scale in the production of physician services. In particular, they find that a 10 percent increase in physician services causes total costs, as measured by the sum of nonphysician input costs and the opportunity cost of physician labor, to increase by 6 percent. Contradicting these results, Defelice and Bradford (1997) find no statistical difference in efficiency between solo practice and group practice physicians.

The literature on survivor analysis also indicates the existence of economies of scale in the production of physician services. As it pertains to the market for physician services, survivor analysis examines the distribution of practice sizes over time to determine which practice size produces medical services most efficiently. Studies by Frech and Ginsburg (1974) and Marder and Zuckerman (1985) indicate that solo and two-physician practices are inefficient at the margin relative to group practices. Relying on more recent data, Marder and Zuckerman also find medium-sized groups to be less efficient than large practices (100 or more physicians). They go one step further and suggest that economies of scale may exist for practices as large as 100 physicians. Referring to our earlier discussion on the mode of practice, these results explain why the proportion of solo and two- and three-person practices decreased from 1989 to 1997 relative to physician practices with four-to-eight and more than eight people.

Before closing, we need to complete our discussion by noting the work of Rosenman and Friesner (2004). Using data envelopment analysis (DEA), they look at the efficiency of physician services across specialty and multispecialty physician practice groups. The authors find that single-specialty physician practices tend to be more efficient than multispecialty practices and these findings hold regardless of whether the specialty practice provides primary or specialty care.

Taken together, this body of research suggests that multiphysician practices have a cost advantage over solo practices and that economies of scale exist in the production of physician services at least up to the three-to-seven physician practice size. However, the ability of physicians to organize across specialties may be limited by scope diseconomies. Thus while the average practice size of physicians within specialties may rise in the future, there is a question as to whether the trend will continue across specialties.

Summary of the Structure of the Market for Physician Services

Whether the physician services market is measured based on real expenditures or the number of physicians practicing medicine, it has increased dramatically in size over the past three decades. Since 1970, the number of physicians and real expenditures on physician services in the United States have more than doubled. The increase has outpaced the overall growth in the economy and the general population, as illustrated by the significant increase in the physician-to-population ratio from 148 in 1970 to 238 in 2003 per 100,000 total population.

The increase in physician labor in the United States has not been without controversy. Some people believe the United States has too many specialists and too few generalists. This issue is likely to play an integral role in the health care reform debate over the coming years. There is also considerable debate as to whether there will be a shortage of physicians in the future.

The mode of practice in the physician services market has also changed significantly in recent years. There appears to be a movement away from single- and two-physician practices and toward multiphysician practices with four or more physicians. In addition, significant growth appears to be occurring in the number of salaried physicians. In all probability, this trend reflects changing economic conditions in the health care field. For example, productivity studies and survivor analysis studies indicate the existence of economies of scale that confer a distinct cost advantage on large multiphysician practices.

MCOs also appear to play a key role in the physician services market. Almost 90 percent of all physicians have at least one contract with an MCO. The growing presence of MCOs in the physician services market may also partly explain the growth of multiphysician practices relative to smaller ones. Since larger practices have a cost advantage over smaller practices, they are in a better position to negotiate price discounts with MCOs.

Despite the presence of barriers to entry, such as medical licensure, the physician services market has become even more competitive over time as large, institutional buyers challenge the authority of independent physicians. This has caused some policy makers to call for the elimination of these barriers. As the market for physician services becomes more competitive, perhaps market forces can be relied on more heavily to dispose of incompetent or unprofessional doctors.

THE CONDUCT OF THE PHYSICIAN SERVICES INDUSTRY

Now that we have established the market determinants of behavior, or the structure of the physician services industry, we are in a position to discuss the conduct of that market. As you know, market structure interacts with economic objectives to establish conduct. We will look at the supplier-induced demand hypothesis, McGuire's quantity-setting model, the effects of various compensation schemes on physician behavior, geographical variations in the utilization of physician services, and the impact of managed care practices.

The Supplier-Induced Demand Hypothesis

Without a doubt, one of the most talked-about issues in health economics over the years has been whether the **supplier-induced demand (SID) hypothesis** can be used to explain physician behavior. The basic premise of the SID hypothesis is that physicians abuse their role as medical advisors to advance their own economic self-interests. This involves prescribing medical care beyond what is clinically necessary and can include such items as additional follow-up visits, an excessive number of medical tests, or even unnecessary surgery. According to the model, consumers are relatively ill-informed concerning the proper amount of medical care to consume because an asymmetry of information exists regarding the various health care options available. The asymmetry forces consumers to rely heavily on the advice of their physicians for guidance. This implies that physicians are not only suppliers of physician services but also play a major part in determining the level of demand for those services. For example, physicians advise patients about how frequently they should have office visits, medical tests, and appropriate treatments. This situation places physicians in a potentially exploitative position. Physicians may be able to manipulate the demand curves of patients to advance their own economic interests.

For example, assume the market for physician services is initially in equilibrium in Figure 12–2, where equilibrium occurs at point (Q_0, P_0) and Q represents the quantity of physician services. Now assume for some reason an increase occurs in the number of practicing physicians. This increase in the number of physicians causes the supply curve to shift to the right from S_0 to S_1, which in turn forces the average price of physician services to fall from P_0 to P_1. Faced with an increase in competition along with a loss in income, physicians may exercise their ability to influence patients' behavior by inducing them to demand more services. The increased demand may involve more office visits, additional tests, or even unnecessary surgery. As a result, the demand for physician services increases from D_0 to D_1. In the end, the price of physician services could actually increase, as shown in Figure 12–2, where the new equilibrium price and quantity equal P_2 and Q_2, respectively.

FIGURE 12–2
The Supplier-Induced Demand Model

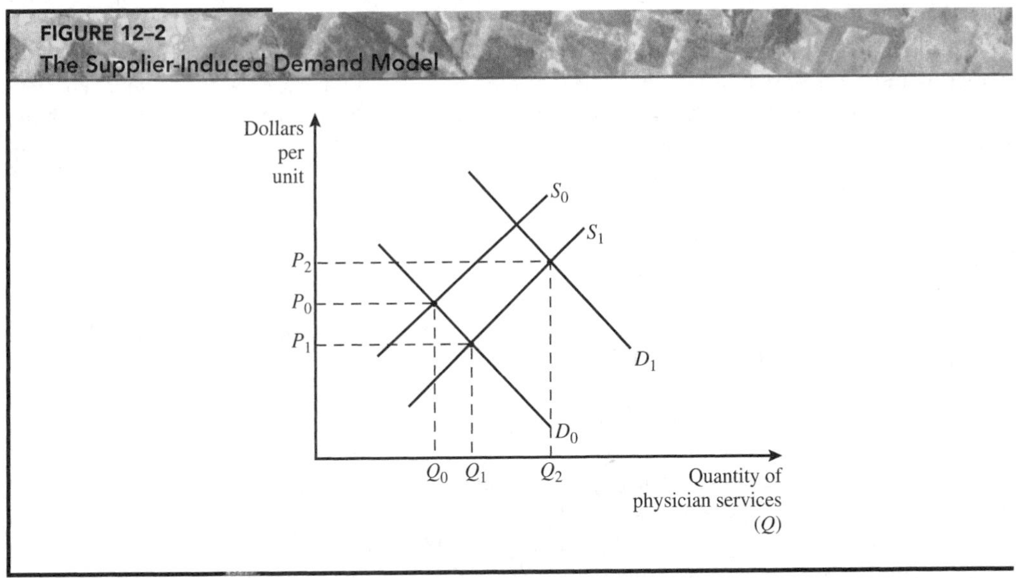

Assume initially that the market for physician services is in equilibrium at point (Q_0,P_0) off the D_0 demand curve and the S_0 supply curve. Now assume that there is an increase in the number of physicians practicing medicine and the supply curve for physician services shifts outward from S_0 to S_1. Under ordinary circumstances, the equilibrium price for physician services would fall to P_1 while the equilibrium quantity would increase to Q_1. In reaction to the decrease in the price of medical services, however, physicians induce the demand for their services and cause the demand curve to shift outward to D_1. The result is that the equilibrium price and quantity for physician services increases to (P_2, Q_2).

The SID model can also be described in the context of the principal–agent theory. The principal–agent theory is traditionally used to explain the interaction between the managers of a major corporation, who are the agents, and its stockholders, who are the principals. The fiduciary responsibility of the agent is to manage the firm in the best interest of the principal, and that means maximizing profits. Due to an asymmetry of information between the principal and the agent, the manager is likely to have more information than the stockholders concerning the true operation and performance of the firm. In this situation, the manager has the opportunity to shirk his responsibilities to the stockholders by not seeking to maximize profits. Instead, the manager may use company funds to advance his self-interests. Advancing self-interests may involve such things as higher pay, a large support staff, or a more luxurious office.[9]

Concerning the doctor–patient relation, the physician is hired to address the health concerns of the patient, the principal. Specifically, the physician, as agent, is given the responsibility of demanding medical services on behalf of the patient, who possesses much less information concerning the appropriateness of medical care. Given that patients are typically covered by health insurance and the physician's personal financial interests are at stake, the physician has the opportunity to exploit the situation by persuading the patient to consume more medical care than is clinically necessary. The increased medical services most likely do no harm, but they do mean increased income for the physician-agent.

The task of reviewing the empirical evidence on the SID hypothesis is daunting given the extensive work on the subject. In one of the earlier studies, Fuchs (1978) uncovers substantial support for the supplier-induced demand hypothesis. In particular, he estimates that a 10 percent increase in the supply of surgeons, as measured by the surgeon-to-population ratio, leads to a 3 percent increase in the per capita surgery rate. Cromwell and Mitchell (1986) also find evidence that surgeons induce demand. However, their estimates are substantially smaller than Fuchs's. They estimate that a 10 percent increase in surgeon density leads to only a 0.9 percent increase in surgeries and a 1.3 percent increase in elective surgeries per capita. Rossiter and Wilensky (1984) and McCarthy (1985) also uncover evidence that substantiates the inducement hypothesis, although the magnitude of the inducement is estimated to be marginal. Looking at the issue of physician ownership of ancillary services, Mitchell and Sass (1995) also find evidence of induced demand. According to their findings, physical therapy clinics in Florida owned by physicians required 50 percent more visits from patients than those clinics that received no referrals from owners, with no discernible difference in the quality of care across ownership structures. A partial list of additional studies that corroborate the inducement hypothesis includes Grytten and Holst (1990), Hemenway and Fallon (1985), Tussing (1983), and Tussing and Wojtowycz (1986).

A number of the more recent studies do not support the supplier-induced demand hypothesis. For example, Escarce (1992) employs Medicare enrollment and physician claims data to test the inducement hypothesis. The results indicate that increases in the supply of surgeons are associated with increases in the demand for initial contacts with surgeons but have no impact on the demand for services among surgery patients in terms of intensity of use. Thus, the author attributes the greater demand for surgeries to improvements in access, lower time costs, and better quality. These conclusions do not support the inducement hypothesis. Recent studies by Carlsen and Grytten (1998) and Grytten and Sorensen (2001) also do not support the SID hypothesis. Using data collected in 1998 from Norway, Grytten and Sorensen test how two different groups of physicians in Norway have reacted to increased competition. The first group

9. In the case of corporate managers, incentive contracts (such as bonus pay) might be designed to align the manager's personal interests with the actions desired by stockholders.

comprised contract physicians who were compensated on a fee-for-service basis. Presumably, they had an incentive to induce the demand for medical services when faced with increased competition. The second group included salaried physicians who had little incentive to induce demand. According to their empirical results there is no evidence that either group of physicians induced the demand for medical services when faced with increased competition. They conclude from their results that there is little evidence to support the SID hypothesis in the delivery of medical services by primary care physicians in Norway.

There are three reasons why empirical support for the SID hypothesis has been waning in recent years. First, older studies tended to rely on aggregate data that made it difficult to discern the extent to which variations in the consumption of physician services can be attributed to induced demand. For example, increased consumption in physician services attributed to induced demand may have resulted from decreased waiting times or travel costs. More recent studies generally employ physician-based practice data. Second, more recent studies rely on more sophisticated models and estimating techniques that allow researchers to more accurately control for other market conditions such as time costs and price effects. Finally, more recent studies utilize contemporary data sets and all agree that the ability of physicians to manipulate demand has diminished in recent years with the growth of managed care.

It is obvious from this brief overview of the literature that the issue of whether physicians possess the ability to induce demand is unlikely to be resolved in the near future. Overall, the evidence suggests that although physicians may possess the ability to induce demand, the extent to which they can do so is much less now then initially thought.

McGuire's Quantity-Setting Model

McGuire (2000) develops an interesting model of physician decision making that is based on monopolistic competition. Recall that many sellers exist in a monopolistically competitive industry, but each seller faces a downward-sloping demand curve because of imperfect substitutability among the products offered by the various sellers. In the case of physicians, imperfect substitutability may simply result from location if consumers value convenience. McGuire's model treats physicians as being quantity setters and shows that physicians respond to a lower administered price by increasing quantity supplied. Interestingly, the inverse relation between price and quantity supplied is obtained in McGuire's model without resorting to supplier inducement of demand.

Figure 12–3 provides a graphical illustration of McGuire's quantity-setting model. The horizontal axis represents the quantity of physician services and the vertical axis measures the dollar value of cost and benefits. To make the model easier to explain, let's pretend that the analysis represents how Dr. Maxwell determines price and quantity. The downward-sloping curve, MB, identifies the marginal benefit of the physician services provided by Dr. Maxwell to a typical patient. The horizontal curve, MC, represents Dr. Maxwell's constant marginal cost of producing physician services.

To make this basic model even easier, suppose for now that the patient has no insurance and pays the full price for the physician care. According to McGuire's model, Dr. Maxwell retains a patient by providing at least the amount of net benefits that the patient would receive from an alternative physician. Suppose NB_0, the shaded area, represents the net benefit that the patient would receive from an alternative physician. Dr. Maxwell has to select the price and quantity that maximizes her profits and also provides the patient with at least NB_0 amount of net benefits. In graphical terms, Dr. Maxwell attempts to raise price up vertically above MC and slide quantity over horizontally as much as possible to maximize profits yet provide at least NB_0 amount of net benefits.

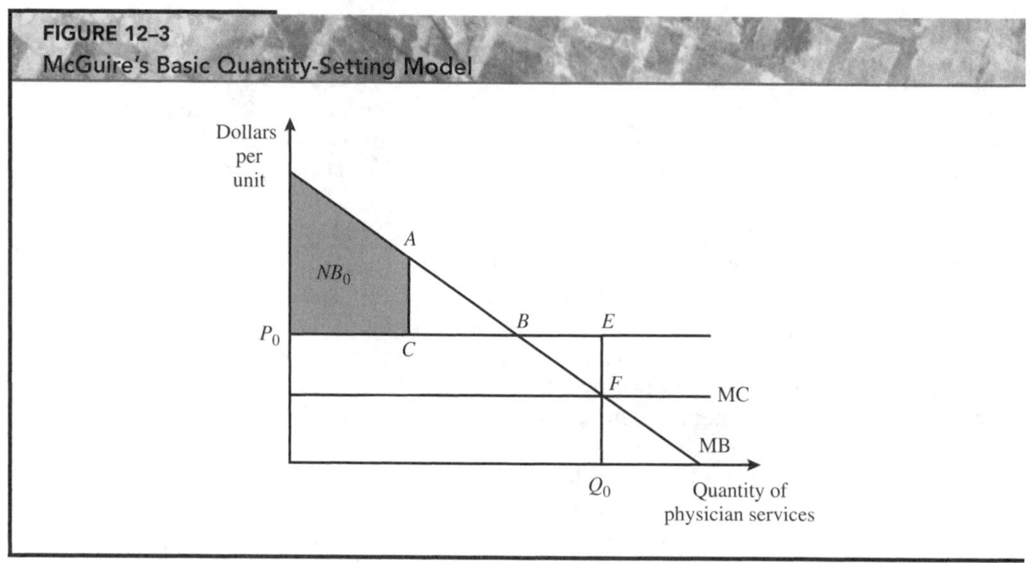

The MB curve represents the marginal benefits the consumer receives from consuming each additional unit of medical care and the MC curve equals the marginal cost of producing physician services. NB_0 represents the net benefit the consumer receives if she visits an alternative physician. Dr. Maxwell chooses P and Q such that profits are maximized and the consumer receives at least NB_0 amount of net benefits. Thus, Dr. Maxwell will require the average consumer to consume no more than Q_0 amount of medical care at price P_0. At this combination of price and quantity the patient is indifferent between having all or none of the care provided by Dr. Maxwell.

Following this logic, Dr. Maxwell chooses a price no greater than P_0 and a quantity not to exceed Q_0. Notice that at this combination of price and quantity the consumer is indifferent between having all or none of the care provided by Dr. Maxwell. That is, the patient's net benefits lost by having Dr. Maxwell provide Q_0 amount of care, area *BEF*, is exactly equal to the net benefits not received by the patient if Dr. Maxwell does not provide any care at all, area *ABC*. Any further increase in quantity causes the patient to visit an alternative physician where net benefits are greater.

The model predicts that greater competition causes profits to decline. Notice that Dr. Maxwell's profits equal the rectangular area formed by the difference between price and marginal cost over the range of quantity provided or Q_0. Both price and quantity are influenced by the level of competition in the industry as indicated by NB_0. If the market for physician services becomes more competitive, NB_0 increases. If NB_0 increases, price, quantity, and profits all decline; otherwise Dr. Maxwell loses the patient to a competitor. In a perfectly competitive situation, NB_0 equals the area below MB but above MC and Dr. Maxwell is forced by competition to price and produce the quantity of services at the point where MB equals MC. At the opposite extreme, If NB_0 equals zero, Dr. Maxwell faces no competition and can act like a monopolist and extract all of the patient's net benefits.

An interesting aspect of the McGuire quantity-setting model concerns how Dr. Maxwell responds to a regulator or third-party administrator with the power to lower price. In McGuire's model, Dr. Maxwell reacts to a lower administered price by increasing quantity supplied because the doctor need only provide a fixed level of net benefits to the patient. Hence, the model predicts that quantity increases in response to a lower regulated price. It is interesting to note that

FIGURE 12–4
McGuire's Quantity-Setting Model with Administered Pricing and Insurance

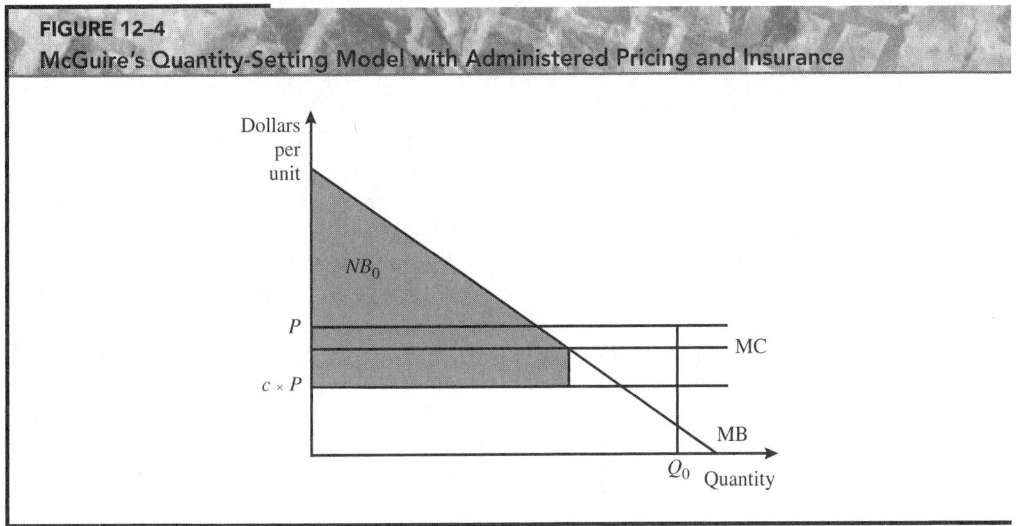

The MB and MC curves represent the marginal benefit and marginal cost curves, respectively. The price ceiling, *P*, which is established by a third party, lies above the MC curve to ensure physician participation in the plan. The $c \times P$ line represents the out-of-pocket price for physician services. Dr. Maxwell chooses the quantity of services, Q_0, such that the patient is indifferent between receiving all or no care from the doctor and profits are maximized.

an inverse relationship exists between price and quantity supplied in McGuire's basic model, much as the supplier-induced demand theory also predicts. In this case, however, the inverse relationship occurs without requiring demand inducement.

McGuire extends this basic model to include a third-party administered price and insurance coverage. A graphical illustration of the extended model is provided in Figure 12–4. We suppose that the consumer pays coinsurance equal to $c \times P$, where c represents the coinsurance rate and P equals the fixed price set by the third party. Notice that the third-party payer sets price above marginal cost to encourage Dr. Maxwell to participate in the health plan. The shaded area NB_0 once again represents the net benefit provided to the patient from an alternative physician. Dr. Maxwell no longer chooses price because it is set by the third-party payer, but she does select the quantity of services that maximizes her profits and provides at least NB_0 amount of net benefits to the patient.

The amount Q_0 gives Dr. Maxwell the best choice of quantity. At that quantity of services the patient is indifferent between all or no care provided by Dr. Maxwell and Dr. Maxwell's profits are maximized. Like the basic model, the extended analysis predicts that Dr. Maxwell responds to a lower administered price by increasing quantity supplied as long as price remains above marginal cost.

The Impact of Alternative Compensation Schemes on Physician Behavior

Concern for growing health care costs has caused third-party payers, both private and public, to seek new ways to reimburse physicians. The traditional fee-for-service method of payment has fallen out of favor because it creates an incentive for overutilization of medical care as the SID and McGuire models suggest. The problem becomes particularly acute when the fee-for-service method of reimbursement is combined with a nominal, or zero, consumer copayment, because under these circumstances consumers have little incentive to monitor the behavior of their physicians. To rectify this problem, many managed care providers and private insurance companies have adopted alternative physician reimbursement schemes.

Based on a survey of more than 100 managed care plans in 1994, Gold et al. (1995) uncover some interesting information concerning the methods presently used to recruit and compensate physicians. More than 70 percent of the managed care plans in the sample said they utilized a careful selection process when recruiting new physicians. More than 60 percent of all plans considered qualitative information, such as professional reputation or patterns of care, during the selection process. However, only 37 percent of the plans reviewed any quantitative data from indemnity claims and/or hospital discharge data when selecting a new doctor.

As we might expect, staff-model HMOs rely more heavily on a salary-based method of payment, whereas IPA HMOs tend to rely on other methods of payment. According to the study, 28 percent of staff-model HMOs used a salary-based method, while only 2 percent of the IPA HMOs used this method of compensation. Fee-for-service was the main form of compensation for PPOs, with 90 percent of the PPOs in the sample stating that it was the predominant form of payment for physician services.

Sixty percent of all plans in the survey used some type of risk-sharing mechanism when compensating physicians, which included some form of capitation payment, or withholdings or bonuses. Withholdings generally involve more sophisticated reimbursement schemes in an attempt to control costs. According to Hillman (1987), MCOs may direct premiums into a series of special-purpose funds after deducting administrative costs. These funds pay for such items as physician services, hospital services, and outpatient laboratory tests. Sometimes, a specific portion of the payment directed to physicians is withheld until the end of the fiscal year, when it can be established whether there is a surplus or a deficit in the remaining funds. If a surplus exists, the MCO generally returns the withheld portion to the physicians. If a deficit exists, the MCO applies all or part of the withheld funds against the loss. By establishing such a compensation system, the MCO creates a direct financial relationship between its own economic viability and the clinical behavior of its physicians. Those physicians who overutilize medical resources and drive up costs receive less compensation.

With a system of bonuses, the MCO gives a portion of any surplus remaining at the end of the year to physicians to elicit cost-effective behavior. Hellinger (1996) states that some MCOs also set up special-purpose referral accounts to pay for the cost of specialists. Primary care physicians may receive some portion of any unused funds in these accounts at the end of the accounting period. The objective is to control the high cost of specialty care by providing primary care physicians with a financial incentive to limit referrals.

A recent study by Rosenthal et al. (2002) provides additional information concerning the many compensation schemes currently in use. Based on a survey of physician organizations in California that included medical groups, independent practice associations, and other types of physician organizations, the authors find that fee-for-service contracts play only a minor role in revenue generation. The overwhelming majority of the revenue (84 percent) generated by physician organizations resulted from capitation contracts. They also find that bonuses and withholds were a common form of compensation. About one out of six physician organizations used bonuses and withholds based on the cost of care, while one-quarter of the physician organizations based bonuses and withholds on the quality of care provided. In addition, about half of the physician organizations used some form of profit sharing, while 13 percent employed productivity bonuses. Similarly, Stoddard et al. (2002) find that 32 percent of physicians involved in practices with two or more physicians faced performance-based incentives such as profiling and patient satisfaction in 1999, while 72 percent were subject to productivity incentives. Overall, they find that physicians are more likely to face incentives that may encourage the use of their services, such as patient satisfaction measures, rather than financial incentives aimed at restricting care.

A study by Grumbach et al. (1998) also points to the importance of financial incentives in physician compensation. According to a survey of primary care physicians involved in managed care, almost 40 percent of the doctors received at least some income based on incentives. Among the incentive factors considered were use of referrals, use of hospital services, quality of care provided, patient satisfaction, and productivity. The study also reported that more than half of the physicians felt some pressure from managed care organizations to limit referrals, while three-quarters felt pressure to increase the number of patient visits.

Hillman et al. (1989) use samples of more than three hundred MCOs to examine the impact of alternative physician compensation schemes on the utilization of medical services and firm profitability. The authors regress a host of explanatory variables on three measures of MCO performance: the rate of hospitalization, visits per enrollee, and the break-even status of the MCO. The first two variables gauge the utilization of medical resources, and the last measures profitability. The independent variables fall into three categories: physician compensation variables, MCO descriptors, and market characteristics. A total of eleven variables control for the various types of compensation schemes used.

Overall, the results indicate that financial incentives affect the medical decisions of physicians and therefore the utilization of medical resources. In terms of utilization of medical services, hospitalization rates are found to be inversely related to whether physicians are paid on a salary or capitation basis. MCOs that used a salary-based method of compensation had 13.1 percent fewer hospitalization days per 1,000 enrollees per year than those using the more traditional fee-for-service methods. Likewise, the capitation method of payment is associated with 7.5 percent fewer hospitalization days. Visits per enrollee are also found to be inversely related to the use of financial penalties. For example, MCOs that established a referral fund whereby the individual physicians were at risk for any deficits had 10.5 percent fewer visits per enrollee, on average. The relationship between type of compensation scheme and profitability, as measured by the break-even status of the HMO, was far from clear. Hillman et al. (1989) attribute these findings to the fact that profitability depends on many factors other than the utilization of medical resources. Be that as it may, this work is important because it establishes that clinical decisions are based at least in part on the financial incentives physicians face. This is not to suggest that physicians necessarily jeopardize the welfare of their patients; rather, in some circumstances, physicians consider their own self-interests when making marginal clinical decisions.

Geographical Variations in the Utilization of Physician Services

The phenomenon of **small area variations** in the delivery and consumption of physician services across geographic regions has been documented by an almost limitless number of studies worldwide. For example, Miller and Holahan (1995) find substantial variation in the utilization of physician services across states, with Florida utilizing physician services at a rate 38 percent above the U.S. mean and Montana 29 percent below the mean. They also find significant variations among urban and rural areas. In another study that examines practice variations in the delivery of primary care physician services in Norway during the late 1990s, Grytten and Sorensen (2003) estimate that variations in physician practice style explain between 47 and 66 percent of the variation in expenditures for laboratory tests, and between 41 and 61 percent of the variation in expenditures for specific procedures.

In addition, an extensive body of literature has suggested that selected medical services are overutilized. The estimates regarding the proportion of inappropriate medical care given range from 15 to 30 percent, with a number of more recent studies putting it at about 4 percent.[10] As a result, the public has become fond of blaming high medical costs on physicians who prescribe needless medical tests or perform unnecessary surgery.

The **physician practice hypothesis** has been used to explain variations in utilization rates across regions. This hypothesis, which is most closely associated with the work of Wennberg (1984, 1985), contends that per capita variations in the use of medical care, particularly surgery, reflect systematic differences in clinical opinions regarding the appropriate amount and type of medical care.

These subjective differences are collectively referred to as "practice style" and exist primarily because of the uncertainty surrounding the practice of medicine. As Eddy (1984) so aptly writes, "Uncertainty creeps into medical practice through every pore. Whether a physician is defining a disease, making a diagnosis, selecting a procedure, observing outcomes, assessing probabilities, assigning preferences or putting it all together, he is walking on very slippery terrain" (p. 75). Physician uncertainty is likely to be greatest when the diagnosis is complicated and the medical procedure is relatively new. As Phelps (1992) writes,

> *When the disease is very easy to diagnose, the consequences of not intervening are well understood, and few alternative interventions exist to treat the disease, then observed variability is quite low. . . . Hernia repair and removal of an inflamed appendix (appendectomy) provide two good examples. Alternatively, when the "indications" for surgery are less clear, or when alternative treatments exist (such as surgery or bed rest plus therapy for low back injuries) variations increase. (p. 25)*

The rate at which medical technology and knowledge are diffused plays a critical role in determining the level of physician uncertainty and degree of practice variations. Other factors also come into play, such as the background and set of beliefs of the individual physician.

Phelps (1992) believes that different local "schools of thought" evolve regarding appropriate practice style. The schools of thought develop as a physician invents a new medical treatment strategy and other doctors in the immediate local community learn and adopt the practice style. Since no property rights are assigned to treatment strategies, the individual physician faces little financial incentive to test and market the new idea on a broader basis. Consequently, the treatment strategy or practice style remains confined to the local area. Phelps claims that "allowing doctors to patent treatment strategies offers a tantalizing step into a market economy where 'professionalism' has previously remained. This would be a two-edged sword, however; doctors who produced and patented a strategy for treatment would reap potential profits, but they would also incur liability for subsequent use of that strategy throughout the country" (p. 41).

Addressing the issue of geographic variations from a slightly different but related angle, Chassin (1993) offers the enthusiasm hypothesis. According to him, geographic differences result primarily because certain physicians, for one reason or another, become "enthusiastic" about a particular medical procedure and therefore use it more frequently than other procedures. When the number of enthusiasts in an area becomes sufficiently large, geographic variations occur. Why

10. Greenspan et al. (1988) estimate that 20 percent of the permanent pacemakers implanted in Philadelphia County in 1983 were unwarranted, while Chassin et al. (1986) note that 17 percent of coronary angiographies for elderly patients had been unnecessary. However, a more recent group of studies found the level of unnecessary care to be much lower. Leape et al. (1993) find that 2 percent of coronary artery bypass surgeries were inappropriate, while Hilborne et al. (1993) find that 4 percent of percutaneous transluminal coronary angioplasties were inappropriate.

the number of enthusiasts differs from area to area is open to conjecture. One explanation offered by the author is that a noteworthy teacher from, say, a teaching hospital in an area becomes enamored with a medical technique and persuades residents and other local practicing physicians of its merits. If he convinces enough physicians in the immediate area, geographic variations occur. This is especially true because, as Phelps notes, the new idea is not patentable.

The most interesting element of the enthusiasm hypothesis is the manner in which it differs from the more conventional physician practice hypothesis. Recall that under the physician practice hypothesis, the uncertainty surrounding the efficacy of a particular medical procedure is a primary reason for geographic variations. This is not the case with the enthusiasm hypothesis. Enthusiasts are anything but uncertain because they are thoroughly convinced of the benefits their patients receive from their medical procedure.

Despite the large number of studies on the physician practice hypothesis, it is difficult to determine the extent to which physician practice style explains geographic variations in the utilization of medical services. This is largely because it is very difficult to quantify practice style. One way to get around this problem is to look at studies that use regression analysis to analyze the consumption of medical care and assume that the unexplained variation, or residual, is partly the result of practice style. Because not all of the residual can be explained by any one factor, we can assume that the unexplained variation represents an upper-bound estimate of the impact of practice style on the consumption of medical services.

Utilizing the residual approach, Folland and Stano (1990) and Stano (1991) review numerous studies and conclude that a significant portion of the variation in the consumption of medical services can be explained by traditional supply and demand factors. Although the authors do not dismiss the role of physician practice style, they suggest that it may not play a large role in explaining differences in the aggregate consumption of medical care across geographic regions.

Other studies have attempted to test directly the impact of practice style on the quantity and type of medical care consumed on a micro level. For example, Roos (1989) developed an index that measures physician hospitalization practice style and tested whether it affected the probability that elderly patients would be hospitalized. The results indicate that practice style cannot be ignored when examining the decision to hospitalize elderly patients.

Because physician practice style is difficult to measure, especially at the aggregate level, its impact on the amount and type of medical care consumed is difficult to judge. There is no doubt, however, that the presence of uncertainty means individual physicians will follow different courses of action when treating patients. Insofar as clinical decisions are based on subjective factors, physician practice style is likely to influence medical care.

The Impact of Utilization Review on the Physician Services Market

Various programs under the heading of managed care have been implemented in recent years to contain the cost of medical care. Most of these programs are directed at altering physician behavior primarily because physicians make most of the clinical decisions. As noted earlier, utilization review (UR) is one of the most frequently used methods to contain costs. Programs such as prospective, concurrent, and retrospective reviews evaluate the medical decisions of hospitals and physicians in an attempt to minimize medical costs by eliminating unnecessary medical care and educating patients and physicians concerning proper medical treatments.

Overall, the cost savings from UR programs have been modest in recent years. For example, while summarizing Wickizer's work and that of colleagues in this area, Wickizer and Lessler (2002) conclude that pre-admission reviews reduce hospital admissions by 10 percent, while concurrent reviews have only a small impact on length of stay. The combined impact of both UR programs has been to decrease hospital inpatient days by about 12 percent. Scheffler et al. (1991) discovered that Blue Cross and Blue Shield utilization review programs decreased hospital patient days by 4.8 percent and inpatient payments by 4.2 percent. Equally important, Feldstein et al. (1988) find that UR programs have a onetime effect on decreasing utilization and costs. The implication is that UR programs may not significantly decrease the growth of medical expenditures over time. In fact, one can argue that any cost savings from UR programs may erode over time as physicians learn to practice in this new environment. Put another way, as physicians eventually learn to "game the system" and present their diagnoses and treatment plans in a manner that will make them more likely to be approved, UR programs may become increasingly unable to control costs by influencing physician behavior over time.

Recently, a number of managed care organizations have questioned the value of UR programs and have significantly altered their approach to utilization review. After interviewing administrators from nearly 50 MCOs, Felt-Lisk and Mays (2002) find that many MCOs have reduced or eliminated their reliance on prospective utilization review. Since few pre-approvals were denied, they were deemed too costly to continue. At the same time, many MCOs have enhanced their concurrent and retrospective utilization review policies. The goal of such changes is to reduce "administration costs of operation and improve relationships with consumer and providers" (p. 212). Other strategies include the establishment or enhancement of **disease management** programs that organize care around the patient with a particular disease or condition in the hopes of improving patient satisfaction and containing costs. Whether such programs have the desired effect is open for question.

Second surgical opinion programs constitute another type of UR aimed directly at altering the behavior of physicians, particularly surgeons. These programs, which can be either voluntary or mandatory in nature, have two major objectives. The first is to increase patient knowledge and thereby reduce the asymmetry-of-information problem. The second is to establish a procedure whereby physicians' decisions are routinely scrutinized by their peers. The ultimate goal is to reduce the number of unnecessary or avoidable operations and thereby reduce medical costs.

Empirical evidence suggests that second-opinion programs have failed to significantly reduce medical costs. For one thing, studies have found that voluntary programs have little or no impact on medical cost savings. The evidence on mandatory programs is not much better. For example, Scheffler et al. (1991) find that mandatory second opinions have no impact on hospital utilization or payments. After reviewing the literature on the subject, Lindsey and Newhouse (1990) conclude that because of design flaws, studies fail to provide any conclusive evidence of cost savings from second opinions. The implication is that cost savings from second surgery opinions are likely to be small.

Several studies have examined the impact of prepaid health plans on the utilization of physician services. The question is whether prepaid health plans lead to fewer or more physician office visits than fee-for-service practices. According to the exhaustive review by Miller and Luft (1994), "Most recent data showed either higher rates or little difference in HMO plan office visits per enrollee" compared to fee-for-service plans (p. 1514). Not enough studies were available to enable Miller and Luft to draw a definitive conclusion about the relation between PPOs and the utilization of physician services, however.

Other efforts to control medical costs have involved the development of clinical practice guidelines for physicians. Numerous medical societies and the Agency for Health Care Policy and Research (AHCPR) are developing and disseminating guidelines that provide physicians and patients with the preferred methods of treating different types of medical conditions. The hope is that guidelines will improve the quality of medical care and at the same time lower costs by providing timely information to physicians concerning the efficacy of various medical procedures.

Rice (1993) argues that practice guidelines may backfire and result in higher medical costs. Any cost savings reaped by preventing a few physicians from using an unacceptable medical procedure may be offset by an increase in costs brought about by the adoption of a new, accepted medical procedure by many physicians. Despite the fact that some medical care providers have begun to implement medical guidelines, it is too early to ascertain their overall effect.

Medical Negligence and Malpractice Insurance

Medical malpractice reform has been one of the most contentious health care issues in recent years, and the issue is complicated by the lack of data measuring the amount of medical negligence in the U.S. health care system. In a book highly critical of the U.S. health care system, Barlett and Steele (2004) cite a number of tragic examples of medical negligence. For example, a man from Texas was diagnosed with lung cancer and entered the hospital for lung cancer surgery. Unfortunately, the surgeons mistakenly removed his healthy lung rather than the cancerous one. The patient died shortly thereafter of lung cancer. Also, a healthy woman from Wisconsin needlessly had her breasts removed because her tissue samples were mixed up with another patient who had breast cancer.

While such cases are well documented in the popular press, they provide little guidance as to the number of patients who are victims of medical negligence each year in the U.S. health care system. One of the most comprehensive studies in the area of medical negligence, commonly referred to as the Harvard study (Weiler et al., 1993, Brennan et al., 1991), reviews more than 30,000 patient records from 51 randomly selected acute care hospitals in New York in 1984. The study find that 3.7 percent of the patients in the study experienced a medical injury, and of that number a little more than 25 percent were the result of medical negligence. Most of the injuries were relatively minor with complete recovery occurring within one month. However, 2.6 percent of the negligent injuries resulted in total disability and another 13.6 percent in death. Extrapolating these results, the researchers estimate that in 1984 medical negligence was responsible for 6,895 deaths and 877 cases of permanent and total disability in the state of New York. The study also found that only 2 percent of those identified as having had sustained a medical injury through negligence filed a malpractice claim, with the ratio of claims to negligent injury increasing for more severe injuries. Evidence also indicates that a large number of claims were filed with little evidence of negligence.

These figures are the root cause of the general frustration that currently exists with our medical malpractice system. When properly designed, malpractice liability law serves two important functions. First, the malpractice legal system, as a type of tort liability law, compensates victims for any damages caused by the negligence of health care providers. Damages include economic losses, pain and suffering costs, and punitive damages (although the latter are rarely awarded). Second, the malpractice system helps deter health care providers from engaging in future acts of negligence. Indeed, the deterrence effect of malpractice liability, by creating incentives for health care providers to offer appropriate medical care, may play a more important role than the compensation function because compensation might be provided more efficiently through other forms of social or private insurance (Danzon, 2000). Stated differently, a malpractice liability system is performing properly when it encourages physicians to provide the socially optimal amount of precautions to guard against medical injuries. That situation occurs when the marginal social benefit derived from the last unit of precautionary care equals the marginal social cost (recall Figure 2–20).

Because of imperfect information and the associated difficulty of establishing properly designed medical liability rules, many people are dissatisfied with the current malpractice system

FIGURE 12–5
Mean Professional Liability Premiums for Self-Employed Physicians, 1988–2000

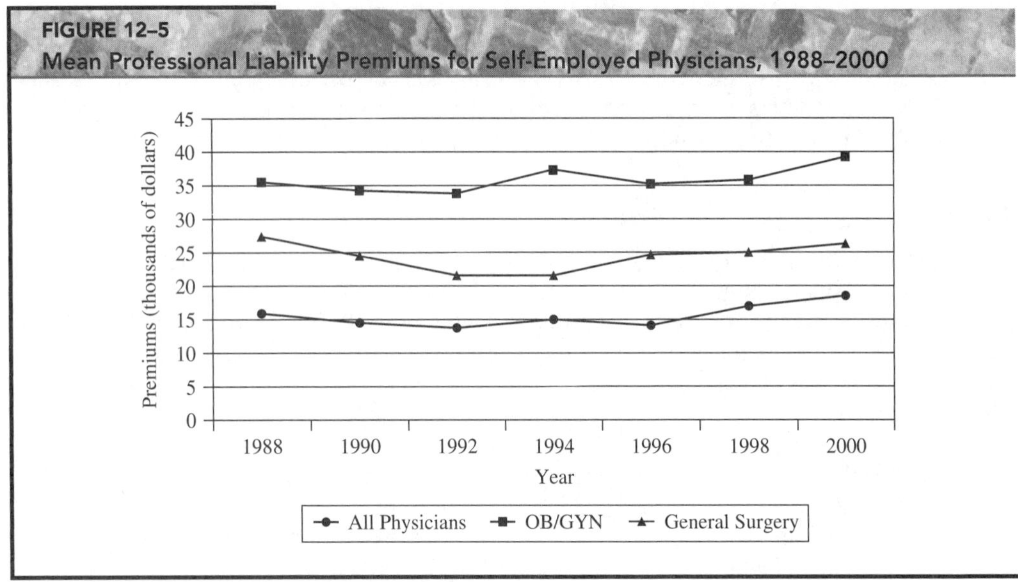

SOURCE: American Medical Association, *Socioeconomic Characteristics of Medical Practice, 2003* (Chicago: AMA, 2003), Table 164.

and have called for various types of reforms. Patient advocates are concerned because so few cases of medical negligence translate into malpractice claims and even fewer result in some type of financial settlement. In addition, there is the frustration that health care providers, particularly physicians, are not held accountable for providing inferior medical care. Health care providers are upset because of the large number of frivolous malpractice claims they must contend with, along with the excessive jury awards that appear to have little relationship to damages incurred. The result is higher liability premiums and higher practice costs. Physicians are also frustrated because they are encouraged by the current malpractice system to overutilize medical services in an attempt to stave off potential malpractice suits. This phenomenon is known as **defensive medicine.**

Any discussion of the implications of medical malpractice on the physician services market must center on the cost of medical malpractice. Physician liability costs generally fall into two categories: medical malpractice insurance costs and defensive medical costs. Figure 12–5 traces out the average liability premiums for self-employed physicians from 1988 through 2000. The graph illustrates that liability premiums stayed relatively constant during the early 1990s and increased steadily since 1996. In 1996 the average liability premium for self-employed physicians equaled $14,100 and increased to $18,400 by 2000. Figure 12–5 also indicates that liability premiums varied widely across specialties, with specialists generally paying more for liability insurance than generalists. For example, in 2000 OB/GYNs paid more than $39,000 per year for liability insurance, while pathologists paid less than $9,000 per year.

Continued increases in malpractice premiums have caused some to say that we have a "physician liability crisis" on our hands. For example, a report by the Department of Health and Human Services (2002) stated that physician liability premiums increased by an average of 10 percent in 2001 and 20 percent in 2002. A number of factors have contributed to this recent rise in medical malpractice premium rates (GAO, 2003a). First and foremost has been the rising severity in malpractice awards. In 1990 the median jury award was $500,000 and the median pretrial settlement was

$350,000. These figures increased to $1 million and $500,000 by 2000 (Roberts, 2002). We learned earlier that insurance providers set premiums equal to the expected benefits to be paid out plus administrative and marketing costs, taxes and profits (recall Equation 11–1). Faced with the prospect of larger payouts on future claims, insurers have been forced to raise premium rates.

Another factor driving up premiums has been the drop in investment income that medical insurers faced beginning in the late 1990s. States generally allow malpractice insurers to invest premiums only in very conservative financial instruments, such as bonds. As a result, when interest rates fell to record lows in the late 1990s, medical insurers suffered a loss in investment income that translated into higher liability premiums. According to the GAO (2003a), a 1.6 percent decrease in rate of return on investments results in an increase in premium rates of about 7.2 percent. Rising reinsurance costs have also contributed to raising premiums. Many small and medium-sized medical insurers generally purchase reinsurance to protect themselves against large unexpected losses. As the severity of malpractice awards increased and became more difficult to predict, reinsurers were forced to increase their premium rates (Thorpe, 2004).

Changes in the structural competitiveness of the malpractice insurance market may have also fueled the recent increase in premiums. A number of medical malpractice insurers across the country have exited the market at the state and national levels in the last few years and that may have impacted the degree of market competitiveness. A case in point is The St. Paul, one of the largest malpractice carriers in the country, which exited the malpractice market in late 2001, leaving a number of health care providers scrambling for insurance coverage (Thorpe, 2004). With less price competition, the remaining firms in the industry have been in a much better position to increase premiums in an attempt to replenish their reserves that were drawn down because of prior losses.

Finally, the underwriting, or profitability, cycle may explain some portion of the increase in liability premiums in recent years. Recall from Chapter 11 that the private health insurance market generally experiences three consecutive years of underwriting gains, followed by three consecutive years of underwriting losses. The concept of adaptive expectations is offered as one explanation for the cycle. If insurers set premiums based on adaptive expectations, then they will systematically overestimate premiums in times of falling claims and underestimate premiums in times of rising claims.

Thorpe (2005) writes that the underwriting cycle may apply to the medical malpractice insurance market with the proviso that the cycle is longer and more substantial. This is primarily because a significant period of time is likely to elapse between when an alleged malpractice event happens and when a monetary settlement occurs. According to Thorpe, during the early 1990s actual medical claim costs were lower than projected, investment income was rising, and profits were increasing. As a result, medical liability premiums remained relatively constant, as illustrated in Figure 12–5. Things began to change in the late 1990s when malpractice claim costs began to rise and investment income fell. Basing their premiums on the payouts of recent past, insurers began to experience losses and, consequently, had to draw down on their reserves. In the last few years, insurers have had to increase premiums in an attempt to cover higher expected payouts and improve profitability.

The issue of state medical malpractice reform has been around since the early 1970s, and the recent rise in premiums has only renewed the call for reform. State tort reforms in recent years have included a variety of measures with the most common including the following (Thorpe, 2004; GAO, 2003a):

- ***Damage caps:*** Involves setting a monetary limit on the amount a plaintiff can be awarded in a malpractice lawsuit.

- ***Joint and several liability:*** Ensures that monetary damages are awarded based on the defendant's degree of responsibility and not on the ability to pay.
- ***Collateral source rule:*** Allows the plaintiff to recover the total amount of any award even if he received funds from other sources such as health insurers or worker's compensation programs.
- ***Limits on attorney fees:*** Limits the fees charged by the plaintiff's attorney.
- ***Installment payments:*** Allows for damages to be paid over time rather than in one lump sum.

Using state-level data from 1985 through 2001, Thorpe (2004) estimates the impact that various state reforms have had on premium levels and loss ratios for insurers. The empirical results indicate that damage caps on awards are related to lower premiums and reduced loss ratios. In particular, he finds that states with caps on awards had premiums that were on average 17 percent lower, and loss ratios that were 12 percent lower, than states without caps. Other types of reforms appear to have no impact on premiums or loss ratios. The exception is states with collateral source rules, which appear to have lower loss ratios. Interestingly, Thorpe also finds that premiums and loss ratios are impacted by the degree of market competition at the state level as measured by a Herfindahl-Hirschman Index. According to his findings, a 10 percent increase in the HHI is related to a 2 percent increase in premiums.

Turning to a discussion of defensive medicine, a number of studies have attempted to estimate the extent to which physicians overutilize medical care to thwart off a malpractice suit. Estimating the cost of defensive medicine poses a unique challenge to researchers because aside from having to precisely define the phenomenon of defensive medicine, they must also distinguish it from the level of clinically justified medical care provided (GAO, 1995). Several studies on the subject find that physicians are encouraged to practice defensive medicine and provide more medical care than is justified. For example, Kessler and McClellan (1996) utilize Medicare data for serious heart disease to estimate whether recent malpractice reforms have reduced medical costs. They find that malpractice reforms have reduced medical expenditures by between 5 and 9 percent without adversely impacting the quality of medical care. Dubay et al. (1999) find that the fear of a malpractice claim, as measured by malpractice premiums, increases the cesarean section rate which is typically less risky to perform than a natural birth delivery. The authors conclude that physicians practice defensive medicine in obstetrics, although the overall cost of that behavior is relatively modest. Consistent with these findings, Grant and McInnes (2004) find that physicians who have experienced a large medical malpractice claim increase their risk-adjusted cesarean rates by approximately one percentage point.

Finally, the practice of defensive medicine may encourage physicians to cut back on certain medical services to avoid the possibility of lawsuits. For example, physicians may avoid treating high-risk patients or providing high-risk procedures when the medical outcome is more in doubt and the likelihood of a lawsuit is greater. This behavior is commonly referred to in the literature as negative defensive medicine because it reduces the availability of medical care.[11] Dubay et al. (2001) studied the impact of malpractice liability on the utilization of prenatal care and infant health, and their results are consistent with the notion of negative defensive medicine. In particular, they find that higher malpractice premiums resulted in an increase in the incidence of late prenatal care among women. Thus, faced with higher premiums, some obstetricians reacted by holding back on high-risk medical services to decrease the probability of being involved in a costly malpractice suit. Dubay et al. also find the impact of increases in malpractice premiums to differ across income groups and other pertinent demographic factors. For example, they find

11. At the other extreme is positive defensive medicine of the type discussed earlier that leads to an increase in the utilization of medical care.

that unmarried women of lower socioeconomic status are more likely to be impacted by negative defensive medicine than married women of more affluent means. Clearly, future work in this area needs to examine more closely the impact of medical malpractice on access to care, particularly among more vulnerable economic groups.

Concerned that rising premiums may cause access problems at local levels by physicians withholding high-risk services and moving or closing practices, the GAO (2003b) examined physician behavior in five states that have reported problems of that kind: Florida, Mississippi, Nevada, Pennsylvania, and West Virginia. The study finds that while there have been isolated incidents in which rising malpractice premiums have affected access to emergency care and newborn delivery, overall the impact has been modest at best. Most of the areas that have been impacted are rural and have the continuing problem of trying to attract and retain qualified health care providers.

The total cost of defensive medicine is particularly hard to determine because most of the research aimed at detecting the prevalence of defensive medicine have been done under specific clinical conditions. As a result, one has to be careful when generalizing about the total cost of defensive medicine in the United States. A study referred to earlier by Kessler and McClellan (1996), which estimates the cost savings from certain tort reforms to be between 5 and 9 percent, is one of the most widely cited studies on the subject. In a more recent study, however, which accounts for the presence of managed care, Kessler and McClellan (2002) estimate the cost savings from tort reform to be a more modest 4 percent.[12] Because these studies apply to limited clinical situations, they should be viewed as an upper bound estimate of the cost of tort reform and defensive medicine.

This rather brief review of issues surrounding medical malpractice indicates that malpractice reform is likely to be on the public agenda for years to come. While the economic costs of malpractice as measured by malpractice premiums and defensive medical costs are not as high as some would believe, they are significant and have prompted a call for serious medical liability reform. The mismatch between the number of medical injuries resulting from negligence and the number of medical claims has also encouraged many to call for reform.

The Performance of the Physician Services Industry

Now that we have reviewed structure and conduct, we are in a position to examine the overall performance of the physician services market. Although the physician services industry appears to be structurally competitive in terms of the actual number of physicians, some evidence concerning practice variations and supplier-induced demand suggests that behaviorally physicians may act with some market power. An analysis of performance in this industry sheds some light on the net effect of these two contradictory perspectives. This section examines measures of physician price, output, and income over time in the United States.

Expenditures on Physician Services

Expenditures on physician and clinical services increased dramatically over the previous decade. According to Table 12–1, expenditures on physician and clinical services equaled $157.5 billion in 1990 and by 2003 grew to $369.7 billion. This represents an overall increase of almost 137 percent. The annual rate of growth topped 10 percent in the early 1990s, and it was not until the mid-1990s

12. Kessler and McClellan (2002) argue that managed care and liability reform are substitutes primarily because the cost containment policies imposed by MCOs limit the use of wasteful precautionary care that results from the practice of defensive medicine.

TABLE 12–1
Expenditures on Physician and Clinical Services for Selected Years (billions of dollars)

Year	Total Expenditures	Annual Rate of Increase	Total Real Expenditures*
1990	$157.5	11.2%	$ 97.9
1995	220.5	4.8	105.6
2000	290.2	7.1	118.6
2001	315.1	8.6	124.3
2002	340.8	8.2	130.8
2003	369.7	8.5	138.1

*Physician expenditures are deflated by the physician services index of the CPI, where 1982–1984 is the base year.

SOURCE: Centers for Medicare and Medicaid Services, http://www.cms.hhs.gov.

that the rate of increase in physician and clinical expenditures began to slow down. Over the period 1990–1995, physician expenditures grew by 4.8 percent per year. By 1997 the rate of growth in physician and clinical expenditures was again on the rise and from 2000 to 2003 physician expenditures grew an average of more than 8 percent a year.

The Physician Services Price Inflation Rate

The most commonly used instrument to measure movements in the average price of physician services is the consumer price index (CPI) for physician services, which is provided for selected years from 1990 to 2004 in Figure 12–6. The data reveal that the average price of physician services increased at an annual rate higher than the general rate of inflation but slightly less than the overall rate of inflation for medical services. From 1990 to 2004 the CPI for physician services increased from 160.8 to 278.3, an increase of almost 73 percent, while the CPI less medical care increased by a little more than 42 percent. Thus it appears the average rate of inflation for physician services was almost twice that of the overall rate of inflation less medical care from 1990 through 2004. Figure 12–6 also indicates that the rate of inflation for physician services was slightly less than the rate of inflation for medical care in general and the disparity appears to have grown in recent years.

Another way to gauge the rate of increase in the price of physician services is to examine data collected by the AMA concerning the average fee for an office visit with established and new patients. In 1986, the average fee for a physician office visit equaled $30.10 for an established patient and $55.57 for a new patient, and these rates increased to $60.63 and $102.46, respectively, by 1997. The average rate of increase from 1990 to 1997 was 6.4 percent for regular patients and 5.3 percent for new patients. It is interesting to note that according to the AMA, the mean fee for both established and new patients actually fell in 1996 by 1.4 percent and 5.3 percent, respectively.

The CPI and AMA data both indicate that although the rate of growth in the average fee for physician services decreased in the 1990s, it still exceeded the general rate of inflation. During the 1990s, physician fees grew at an annual rate of between 4.9 and 6 percent, whereas the overall price level, excluding medical care, grew in the neighborhood of 2 to 3 percent. These

FIGURE 12–6
Consumer Price Index for Physician Services

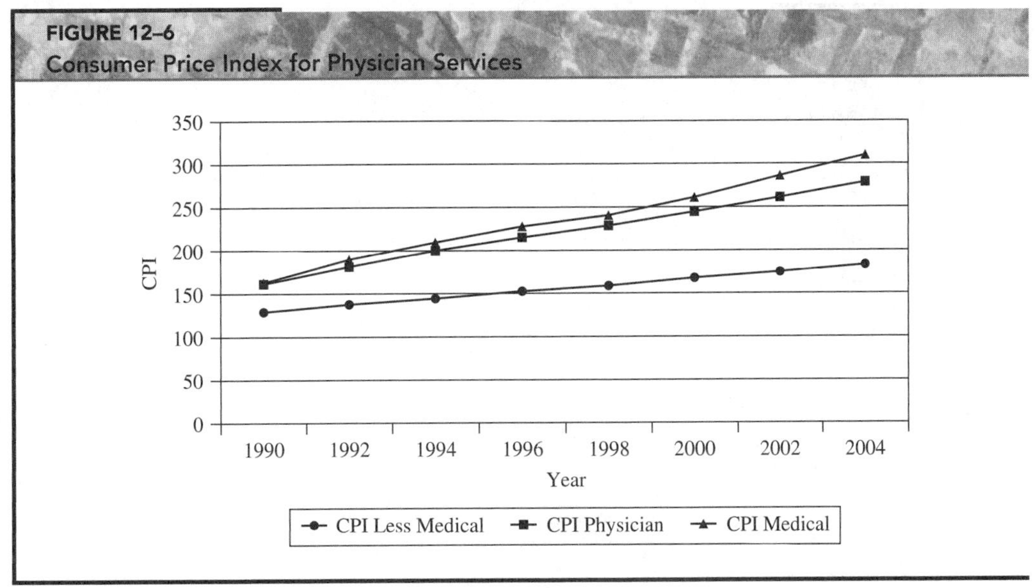

SOURCE: Bureau of Labor Statistics, http://www.bls.gov.

figures overstate the inflation of physician fees for three reasons. First, the fees reported may not adequately reflect any discounts given to patients because they are covered by Medicare or belong to an HMO. Given the expanding role of MCOs, it is safe to assume that the volume and extent of discounts negotiated with physicians increased over time. This means that there may be a significant disparity between the fee reported and the transaction fee. Second, the figures fail to consider any improvements in the quality of physician services that have taken place over time. Finally, the figures do not adequately reflect many of the technological improvements that have taken place in the production of physician services.

The Utilization of Physician Services

Expenditures on physician services increased significantly during the past few decades, with much of that increase occurring early in the 1990s. From 1990 to 2003, physician expenditures increased by 114 percent. Over the same period the CPI for physician services increased by slightly more than 63 percent. Combined, these figures suggest that almost two-thirds of the average annual increase in physician expenditures was the result of price increases, while the remaining one-third was due to increased utilization. The last column in Table 12–1 provides data for real expenditures on physician and clinical services, which is found by dividing nominal values by the relevant CPI. Real expenditures grew by around 3 percent per year on average from 1990 to 2003.

Physician Income

The last item we examine is changes in physician income over time. Data for nominal and real (that is, total physician income deflated by the CPI and in 1988 dollars) income from 1988 to 2000 appear in Figure 12–7. Over the period in question, nominal income increased from \$144.7 thousand to \$205.7 thousand, for an increase of slightly more than 42 percent. The data on real income tell a slightly different story. It appears that while nominal income increased

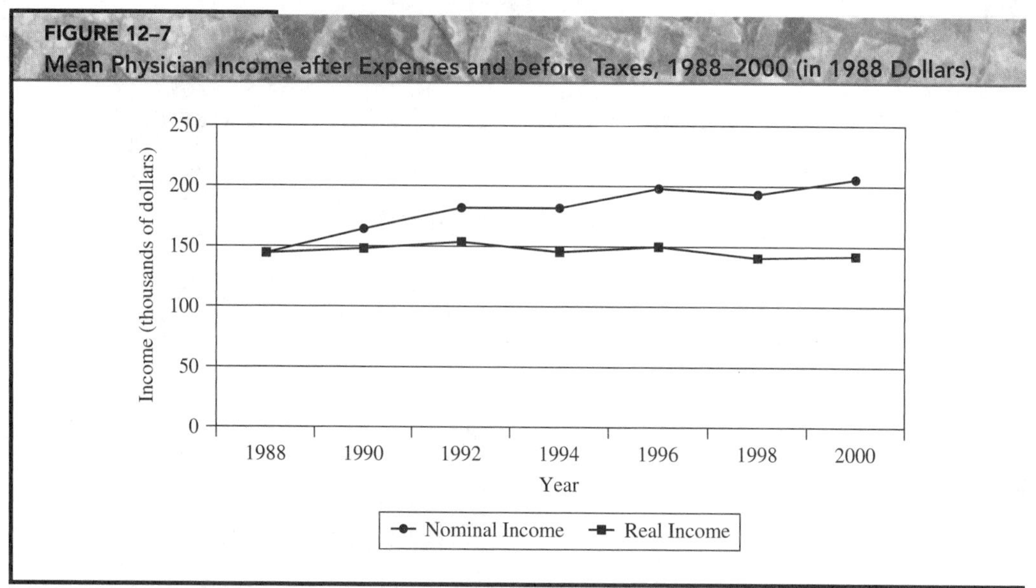

SOURCE: American Medical Association, *Socioeconomic Characteristics of Medical Practice, 2003* (Chicago: AMA, 2003), Table 160.

modestly during the 1990s, real income actually decreased. From 1990 to 2003, real income shrank from $145 thousand to $141 thousand, with the largest decreases taking place between 1992 and 1994, and 1996 and 1998. No doubt these changes can be attributed to the growth in managed care, the increased use of financial incentives directed toward physicians, and the implementation of tighter fee controls by the Medicare and Medicaid programs. For instance, Hadley and Mitchell (2002) find that the growth of managed care, as measured by HMO penetration in the early 1990s, and the employment of financial incentives to restrict services have a negative effect on physicians' earnings. Specifically, they find that a 10 percent increase in HMO enrollments, from 20 to 22 percent, is associated with a 2.6 percent decrease in physician earnings.

To gauge the relative standing of physician income, we can also compare compensation to the growth in real income sustained by other professionals with extensive graduate training. In particular, consider the ratio of total physician income to total compensation of college faculty at doctoral granting institutions. The ratio remained rather stable throughout the early 1990s at around 2.7, indicating that the average physician earned 2.7 times the earnings of the average college professor. By the mid-1990s, however, that ratio began to fall slightly and by 2000 it equaled 2.4. These relative income figures suggest that not only did physicians in general experience a slight decrease in real income throughout the 1990s, they also lost ground relative to other professionals with substantial graduate training.

This conclusion is substantiated by a study that looked at the relative income of physicians from an investment perspective. If expenditures on higher education are treated as an investment in human capital and the increment to earnings received in the job market as a return on that investment, the rate of return received on investments in higher education can be calculated. Utilizing that approach, Weeks et al. (1994) compare the rates of return on educational investments for various professionals, including physicians. According to their results, primary care physicians receive an annual rate of return of 15.9 percent on educational investments over a working life, while specialists receive a 20.9 percent return. As a point of comparison, the authors find that businesspeople and attorneys receive a 29.0 and 25.4 percent rate of return, respectively. These findings imply that physicians receive a rate of return on investments in educational expenditures that is comparable to, if not less than, that of other professionals.

SUMMARY

The physician services market has experienced profound changes in recent years, with both the size and scope of the market increasing substantially. Since 1990 the size of the market has increased, whether measured on the basis of real physician expenditures or the number of practicing physicians. The mode of production has also changed considerably, with economies of scale forcing physicians into large-group practices as opposed to small-group or solo practices. All these changes, coupled with an erosion of barriers to entry, have intensified the level of structural competition in the physician services market. Most of the market power physicians currently possess appears to result primarily from the asymmetry of information that exists between doctor and patient. Although the level of competition varies across regions, overall the market can be classified as being monopolistically competitive. The physician services industry contains a large number of sellers, moderate barriers to entry, a certain amount of product differentiation, and some information imperfections.

The well-publicized geographic variations in physician utilization rates have been the source of much concern for policy analysts and politicians alike. The evidence indicates that much of this concern is uncalled for, since most of the variation can be explained by traditional supply and demand factors.

Without a doubt, the single greatest change in the physician services market has been the growing presence of managed care. Almost 90 percent of all physicians are involved with at least one MCO. All indications suggest that these numbers will increase in the future. Managed care has ushered in a new set of compensation schemes, along with a host of utilization review programs. The evidence on compensation schemes suggests that clinical decisions are sensitive to the method of payment. For example, the utilization of medical resources is inversely related to whether the physician is compensated on a salary or capitation basis rather than the more traditional fee-for-service system. Findings concerning the impact of utilization review programs on utilization and costs have been mixed, however. For example, second-opinion programs appear to have little impact on the level of medical care. There does appear to be a movement toward the development and use of clinical guidelines for physicians. It remains to be seen whether such efforts will affect the amount and cost of physician care.

CASE STUDIES

12-1 One-Stop Shopping[13]

An October 2005 *Wall Street Journal Online*/Harris Interactive health care poll found that many Americans believe that an onsite clinic at a retailer, such as Wal-Mart and CVS, can take the place of a traditional doctor's office visit. Retail chains began providing basic medical services,

13. Source: "Many Americans Open to Care at Retail-Based Health Clinics," *The Wall Street Journal,* October 26, 2005.

including strep throat tests, sports physicals, and flu shots, in response to the rise in consumers' out-of-pocket costs for health care services. The clinics do not require an appointment and services range in price from around $25 to $60 a visit. The majority of those polled were satisfied with the clinics because of their convenient hours—open nights and weekends—and the ability of nurse practitioners to quickly and easily care for patients and write prescriptions. Among the biggest concerns with the clinics were uncertainties about the staff's qualifications and that more serious medical problems might be misdiagnosed or not diagnosed at all.

Questions for Discussion

1. *Are there potential quality implications associated with carving out certain simple tests and services from the typical doctor visit? Does continuity of care matter for these types of services?*
2. *Explain how an electronic medical record might impact "retail health care." Does it make it more feasible? Why or why not?*
3. *Explain the potential economic benefits of retail health care clinics. Who saves—insurers or individuals? Does it matter what type of health plan a consumer has?*

12-2 Physician Referrals[14]

MRI and CT scanning was one of the health care industry's fastest-growing divisions in 2005. Imaging centers were increasingly offering referral deals to physicians in which the physician paid the center a flat fee per procedure and then the physician billed insurers at a higher rate, assuring the physician a profit and significant volume for the imaging centers. Questions arose about the legality of this arrangement, however, because of the potential to violate federal and state laws such as the antikickback law and physician self-referrals. The law against self-referrals has an exception that states that self-referred services are acceptable as long as the doctor performs them in his own office. So imaging companies were structuring referral deals as leases in which each time a doctor sent over a patient, the doctor was essentially renting the scan center's facilities and employees to avoid the self-referral problem. Scanning costs at this time were the fastest-growing sector for Medicare. One reason for this was the medical scans' ability to perceive health conditions, in turn cutting back on the need for diagnostic surgery. However, another potential factor was the incentive for many doctors to order additional scans, either because they had installed a scanning machine in their own offices or because they had a lease contract with another imaging center.

Questions for Discussion

1. *Under the leasing arrangements described in the article, explain how physicians and imaging centers earn revenue. What incentives does this provide for physicians and imaging centers? Are there countervailing forces that may act as controls on those incentives?*
2. *Similar concerns have been recently raised over physician ownership of hospitals and the potential for economic incentives to drive referral decisions. Consider the case in which physicians make referrals to facilities in which they have an ownership stake. Identify and describe some of the important differences between referral to hospitals as opposed to referral to imaging centers.*

14. Source: David Armstrong, "MRI and CT Centers Offer Doctors Way to Profit on Scans," *The Wall Street Journal*, May 2, 2005.

3. *As a lawmaker, what kinds of additional information might you obtain before judging the legal or ethical merits of the contract-lease referral arrangements? Examples: Does the difference in volume reflect inappropriate or unnecessary diagnostic testing? Why or why not? What kinds of information would you need to have to answer that question?*

12-3 Supplier-Induced Demand[15]

According to a *Wall Street Journal Online*/Harris Interactive health care poll, more than half of U.S. adults polled have chosen to go without a doctor-recommended treatment (including filling a prescription, getting a test, or undergoing surgery) or get a second opinion because they felt the treatment was unnecessary or too aggressive. Adult poll respondents also felt that the overly aggressive treatments were the result of misleading information doctors received from drug and medical device companies. Physicians' concerns about malpractice, their desire to earn more, and their desire to meet patients' demands were seen as the main causes of unnecessary care.

Questions for Discussion

1. *Are consumers' perceptions about the motivating forces behind physician treatment decisions reasonable? Why or why not? What kinds of external factors might help explain consumer distrust?*
2. *Describe the ways, if any, in which physician payment methods might influence the treatments that they propose to their patients. Focus on three different kinds of payment mechanisms: fee-for-service ("cost-plus"), prospective fee schedule (that is, price caps), and capitation (in which the physician takes on financial risk).*
3. *Do the results of the survey describe patient uncertainty or improved patient information? What is the likelihood that decisions on the part of consumers might actually affect medical outcomes? In other words, are there benefits to circumspection in seeking treatment, or is postponing or forgoing treatment more likely to have a negative impact on medical outcomes? Explicate your assumptions and support your answers.*

Review Questions and Problems

1. Physician assistants have long argued that they have the ability to provide as much as 70 percent of the medical services provided by primary care physicians at a much lower cost. Yet government regulations limit their ability to work independently of physicians. Explain what would happen to the level of competition in the physician services market if all the statutes limiting the activities of physician assistants were eliminated.
2. Discuss how enhanced competition in the physician services market has affected the ability of physicians to induce the demand for medical services.
3. Analyze the alternative compensation schemes discussed in this chapter that private insurers use to pay physicians. Think in terms of the incentive to provide an excessive amount of medical services.
4. As you know, various medical groups are in the process of developing medical guidelines. Assuming guidelines are developed and widely adopted by physicians, how will this affect the physician services market?

---

15. Source: "Many Ignore Doctor Recommendations on Perception of 'Over Treatment,'" *The Wall Street Journal,* September 13, 2005.

5. Some argue that practice variations exist because information on practice style is disseminated slowly. Phelps (1992) argues that physicians should be allowed to patent and sell their practice strategies. Explain how this policy might affect practice variations.
6. Discuss the theoretical and empirical issues surrounding the supplier-induced demand theory.
7. Discuss the factors that have contributed to the increase in expenditures on physician services over the past decade.
8. Explain the many institutional and structural changes that might make physician licensing obsolete.
9. Why may the physician inflation rate be exaggerated?
10. According to McGuire (2000) the problem of defensive medicine can be analyzed in the context of the supplier-induced demand model because physicians induced the demand for their services to decrease the chances of a medical malpractice suit. Use the supplier-induced demand model to illustrate McGuire's point.
11. Use each of McGuire's quantity setting models to explain how a physician is likely to react to price controls. In particular, explain how the physician continues to earn economic profits despite the implementation of price controls.

CEBS Questions

■ *CEBS Sample Question on Subject Matter from CEBS Course 9 Study Manual*

1. Advocates for the elimination of medical licensure requirements point to which recent changes to advance their position? (pages 346–348)

■ *CEBS Sample Exam Questions*

1. Which statement describes average physician income in recent years?
   A. Gains have been far greater than those of other professionals.
   B. Slight decreases in real income have made physicians lose ground relative to other professionals with graduate training.
   C. Decreases have been substantial.
   D. Specialty physicians have experienced substantial increases while general practitioners have experienced substantial decreases.
   E. Only research physicians have experienced an increase in real income.
2. Which of the following statements regarding the supplier-induced demand (SID) hypothesis regarding physician behavior is (are) correct?
   I. An important element of the hypothesis is the asymmetry of information that exists regarding the various health care options available.
   II. The SID hypothesis suggests that physicians are not motivated by increases in personal income.
   III. Empirical support for the SID hypothesis has been waning in recent years.
   A. III only
   B. I and II only
   C. II and III only
   D. I and III only
   E. I, II, and III

3. All the following statements regarding the structure of the market for physician services are correct EXCEPT:
   A. There has been a significant increase in the physician-to-population ratio over the last three decades.
   B. Almost 90 percent of all physicians have at least one contract with a managed care organization.
   C. Many experts believe there are too many general practitioners and not enough specialists.
   D. The physician services market has become more competitive over time.
   E. There appears to be a movement away from single and two-physician practices toward multiphysician practices.

■ *Answer to Sample Question from Study Manual*

Proponents question the need for medical licensure given: (1) the recent shifts in medical liability from physicians to institution; (2) the growth in for-profit medical care providers; and (3) the growing use of employed rather than self-employed physicians. The growth in for-profit providers and employed physicians has created a greater incentive for institutions to monitor the performance of physicians and, if necessary, to terminate incompetent physicians.

■ *Answers to Sample Exam Questions*

1. B is the answer. See Figure 12–7 and text on pages 367–369.
2. D is the answer. The basic premise of the SID hypothesis is that physicians abuse their role as health care providers to augment their personal income. Therefore, Statement II is false. Statements I and III are correct. See pages 350–353 of the text.
3. C is the answer. It is believed that there are too many specialists in the United States and not enough primary care physicians. The other statements are all true. See pages 340–342 and 345 of the text.

ONLINE RESOURCES

To access Internet links related to the topics in this chapter, please visit our web site at **www.thomsonedu.com/economics/santerre**.

REFERENCES

American Medical Association. *Physician Characteristics and Distribution in the U.S., 1997/98.* Chicago: AMA Center for Health Policy Research, 1998.

______. *Physician Characteristics and Distribution in the U.S., 2005.* Chicago: AMA, 2005.

______. *Socioeconomic Characteristics of Medical Practice, 2003.* Chicago: AMA, 2003.

Barlett, Donald L., and James B. Steele. *Critical Condition.* New York: Doubleday, 2004.

Brennan, Troyen, et al. "Incidence of Adverse Events and Negligence in Hospitalized Patients." *New England Journal of Medicine* 324 (February 7, 1991), pp. 370–76.

Brown, Douglas M. "Do Physicians Underutilize Aides?" *Journal of Human Resources* 23 (summer 1988), pp. 342–55.

Bureau of Labor Statistics, http://www.bls.gov.

Carlsen, Fredrick, and Jostein Grytten. "More Physicians: Improved Availability or Induced Demand?" *Health Economics* 7 (1998), pp. 495–508.

Carpenter, Bruce, and Stephen Neun. "An Analysis of the Location Decision of Young Primary Care

Physicians." *Atlantic Economic Journal* 27 (June 1999), pp. 135–49.

Centers for Medicare & Medicaid Services, http://www.cms.hhs.gov.

Chassin, Mark R. "Explaining Geographic Variations: The Enthusiasm Hypothesis." *Medical Care* 31 (supplement 1993), pp. YS37–YS44.

Chassin, Mark R., et al. "Variations in the Use of Medical and Surgical Services by the Medicare Population." *New England Journal of Medicine* 314 (January 30, 1986), pp. 285–90.

Cooper, Richard A. "Weighing the Evidence for Expanding Physician Supply." *Annals of Internal Medicine* 141 (November, 2004), pp. 705–14.

Cooper, Richard A., Thomas E. Getzen, Heather J. McKee, and Prakash Laud. "Economic and Demographic Trends Signal an Impeding Physician Shortage." *Health Affairs* 21 (January/February 2002), pp. 140–54.

Cromwell, Jerry, and Janet B. Mitchell. "Physician-Induced Demand for Surgery." *Journal of Health Economics* 5 (1986), pp. 293–313.

Danzon, Patricia M. "Liability for Medical Malpractice." In *Handbook of Health Economics,* Volume I, eds. A. J. Culyer and J. P. Newhouse. Amsterdam: Elsevier Science, 2000.

Defelice, Lisa C., and W. David Bradford. "Relative Inefficiencies in Production between Solo and Group Practice Physicians." *Health Economics* 6 (1997), pp. 455–65.

Dubay, Lisa, Robert Kaestner, and Timothy Waidmann. "The Impact of Malpractice Fears on Cesarean Sections Rates. " *Journal of Health Economics* 18 (1999), pp. 491–522.

______. "Medical Malpractice Liability and Its Effect on Prenatal Care Utilization and Infant Health." *Journal of Health Economics* 20 (July 2001), pp. 591–611.

Eddy, David M. "Variations in Physician Practice: The Role of Uncertainty." *Health Affairs* 3 (summer 1984), pp. 74–89.

Escarce, Jose J. "Explaining the Association between Surgeon Supply and Utilization." *Inquiry* 29 (winter 1992), pp. 403–15.

Escarce, Jose J., and Mark V. Pauly. "Physician Opportunity Costs in Physician Practice Cost Functions." *Journal of Health Economics* 17 (April 1998), pp. 129–51.

Feldstein, Paul J., Thomas M. Wickizer, and John R. C. Wheeler. "Private Cost Containment: The Effects of Utilization Review Programs on Health Care Use and Expenditures." *New England Journal of Medicine* 318 (May 19, 1988), pp. 1310–14.

Felt-Lisk, Suzanne, and Glen P. Mays. "Back to the Drawing Board: New Directions in Health Plans' Care Management Strategies." *Health Affairs* 21 (September/October 2002), pp. 210–17.

Folland, Sherman T., and Miron Stano. "Small Area Variations: A Critical Review of Propositions, Methods and Evidence." *Medical Care Review* 47 (winter 1990), pp. 419–65.

Frech, H. E., and Paul B. Ginsburg. "Optimal Scale in Medical Practice: A Survivor Analysis." *Journal of Business* 47 (1974), pp. 23–36.

Friedman, Milton. *Capitalism and Freedom*. Chicago: University of Chicago Press, 1962.

______. *Free to Choose*. New York: Harcourt Brace Jovanovich, 1980.

Fuchs, Victor R. "The Supply of Surgeons and the Demand for Operations." *Journal of Human Resources* 13 (supplement 1978), pp. 35–56.

Gamliel, Sandy, et al. "Will Physicians Meet the Managed Care Challenge?" *Health Affairs* 14 (summer 1995), pp. 131–42.

Gold, Marsha R., et al. "A National Survey of the Arrangements Managed-Care Plans Make with Physicians." *New England Journal of Medicine* 333 (December 21, 1995), pp. 1678–83.

Government Accounting Office. *Medical Liability Impact on Hospital and Physician Costs Extends beyond Insurance*. Washington, D.C., September 1995.

______. "Medical Malpractice Implications of Rising Premiums on Access to Health Care." Washington D.C., August 8, 2003a.

______. "Medical Malpractice Insurance Multiple Factors Have Contributed to Premium Rate Increases." Washington D.C., October 1, 2003b.

______. "Physician Workforce: Physician Supply Increase in Metropolitan and Nonmetropolitan Areas but Geographic Disparities Persist" Washington D.C. October 31, 2003c.

______. *Primary Care Physicians Managing Supply in Canada, Germany, Sweden, and the United Kingdom.* Washington, D.C., May 1994.

Grant, Darren, and Melayne Morgan McInnes. "Malpractice Experience and the Incidence of Cesarean Delivery: A Physician-Level Longitudinal Analysis." *Inquiry* 41 (summer 2004), pp. 170–88.

Greenspan, Allan M., et al. "Incidence of Unwarranted Implantation of Permanent Cardiac Pacemakers in a Large Medical Population." *New England Journal of Medicine* 318 (January 21, 1988), pp. 158–63.

Grumbach, Kevin, Dennis Osmond, Karen Vranizan, Deborah Jaffe, and Andrew B. Bindman. "Primary Care Physicians' Experience of Financial Incentives in Managed-Care Systems." *New England Journal of Medicine* 339 (November 19, 1998), pp. 1516–21.

Grytten, Jostein, and Dorthe Holst. "Supplier Inducement: Its Effect on Dental Services in Norway." *Journal of Health Economics* 9 (1990), pp. 483–91.

______. "Type Contract and Supplier-Induced Demand for Primary Physicians in Norway." *Journal of Health Economics* 20 (2001), pp. 379–93.

Grytten, Jostein, and Rune Sorensen. "Practice Variation and Physician-Specific Effects." *Journal of Health Economics* 22 (2003), pp. 403–81.

Hadley, Jack, and Jean M. Mitchell. "The Growth of Managed Care and Changes in Physicians' Incomes, Autonomy, and Satisfaction, 1991–1997." *International Journal of Health Care Finance and Economics* 2 (2002), pp. 37–50.

Hellinger, Fred J. "The Impact of Financial Incentives on Physician Behavior in Managed Care Plans: A Review of the Evidence." *Medical Care Research and Review* 53 (September 1996), pp. 294–314.

Hemenway, David, and Deborah Fallon. "Testing for Physician-Induced Demand with Hypothetical Cases." *Medical Care* 23 (April 1985), pp. 344–49.

Hilborne, Lee H., et al. "The Appropriateness of the Use of Percutaneous Transluminal Coronary Angioplasty in New York State." *Journal of American Medicine* 269 (February 10, 1993), pp. 761–65.

Hillman, Alan L. "Financial Incentives for Physicians in HMOs." *New England Journal of Medicine* 317 (December 31, 1987), pp. 1743–48.

Hillman, Alan L., Mark V. Pauly, and Joseph J. Kerstein. "How Do Financial Incentives Affect Physicians' Clinical Decisions and the Financial Performance of Health Maintenance Organizations?" *New England Journal of Medicine* 321 (July 13, 1989), pp. 86–92.

Kessel, Reuben. "Price Discrimination in Medicine." *Journal of Law and Economics* 1 (1958), pp. 20–53.

Kessler, Daniel, and Mark McClellan. "Do Doctors Practice Defensive Medicine?" *Quarterly Journal of Economics* 111 (May 1996), pp. 353–90.

______. "Malpractice Law and Health Care Reform: Optimal Liability Policy in an Era of Managed Care." *Journal of Public Economics* 84 (2002), pp. 175–97.

Leape, Lucian L., et al. "The Appropriateness of Use of Coronary Artery Bypass Graft Surgery in New York State." *Journal of the American Medical Association* 269 (February 10, 1993), pp. 753–60.

Leffler, Keith B. "Physician Licensure: Competition and Monopoly in American Medicine." *Journal of Law and Economics* 21 (1978), pp. 165–86.

Lindsey, Phoebe A., and Joseph P. Newhouse. "The Cost and Value of Second Surgical Opinion Programs: A Critical Review of the Literature." *Journal of Health Policy, Politics and Law* 15 (fall 1990), pp. 543–70.

Marder, William D., and Stephen Zuckerman. "Competition and Medical Groups." *Journal of Health Economics* 4 (1985), pp. 167–76.

McCarthy, Thomas R. "The Competitive Nature of the Primary-Care Physician Services Market." *Journal of Health Economics* 4 (1985), pp. 93–117.

McGuire, Thomas. "Physician Agency." In *Handbook of Health Economics,* Volume I, eds. A. J. Culyer and J. P. Newhouse. Amsterdam: Elsevier Science, 2000.

Miller, Mark E., and John Holahan. "Geographic Variations in Physician Utilization." *Medical Care Research and Review* 52 (June 1995), pp. 252–78.

Miller, Robert H., and Harold S. Luft. "Managed Care Plan Performance since 1980." *Journal of the American Medical Association* 271 (May 18, 1994), pp. 1512–19.

Mitchell, Jean M., and Tim R. Sass. "Physician Ownership of Ancillary Services: Indirect Demand Inducement or Quality Assurance." *Journal of Health Economics* 14 (1995), pp. 263–89.

Moore, Thomas. "The Purpose of Licensing." *Journal of Law and Economics* 4 (1961), pp. 93–117.

Noether, Monica. "The Growing Supply of Physicians: Has the Market Become More Competitive?" *Journal of Labor Economics* 4 (1986), pp. 503–37.

Phelps, Charles E. "Diffusion of Information in Medical Care." *Journal of Economic Perspectives* 6 (summer 1992), pp. 23–42.

Politzer, Robert M., et al. "Matching Physician Supply and Requirements: Testing Policy Recommendations." *Inquiry* 33 (summer 1996), pp. 181–94.

Pope, Gregory C., and Russel T. Burge. "Economies of Scale in Physician Practice." *Medical Care Research and Review* 53 (December 1996), pp. 417–40.

Raffel, Marshall W., and Norma K. Raffel. *The U.S. Health System: Origins and Functions*, 3rd ed. New York: Wiley, 1989.

Reinhardt, Uwe E. "Manpower Substitution and Productivity in Medical Practices: Review of Research." *Health Services Research* 8 (1973), pp. 200–27.

———. *Physician Productivity and Demand for Health Manpower*. Cambridge, Mass.: Ballinger, 1975.

———. "A Production Function for Physician Services." *Review of Economics and Statistics* 54 (February 1972), pp. 55–66.

Rice, Thomas H. "An Evaluation of Alternative Policies for Controlling Health Care Costs." In *Building Blocks for Change: How Health Care Reform Affects Our Future*, eds. Jack A. Meyer and Sharon Silow-Carrol. Washington, D.C.: Economic and Social Research Institute, 1993.

Roberts, Richard. "Understanding the Physician Liability Insurance Crisis." *Family Practice Journal* 9, no. 9 (October 2002), p. 47, http://www.aafp.org.

Roos, Noralou P. "Predicting Hospital Utilization by the Elderly: The Importance of Patient, Physician, and Hospital Characteristics." *Medical Care* 27 (October 1989), pp. 905–17.

Rosenthal, Meredith B., Alan Zaslavsky, and Joseph P. Newhouse. "The Geographic Distribution of Physicians Revisited." *Health Services Research* 40 (December 2005), pp. 1931–52.

Rosenthal, Meredith B., Richard G. Frank, Joan L. Buchanan, and Arnold M. Epstein. "Transmission of Financial Incentives to Physicians by Intermediary Organizations in California." *Health Affairs* 21 (July/August 2002), pp. 197–205.

Rosenman, Robert, and Daniel Friesner. "Scope and Scale Inefficiences in Physician Practices." *Health Economics* 13 (2004), pp. 1091–1116.

Rossiter, Louis F., and Gail R. Wilensky. "Identification of Physician Induced Demand." *Journal of Human Resources* 19 (spring 1984), pp. 232–44.

Salsberg, Edward, and Gaetano Forte. "Benefits and Pitfalls in Allying the Experience of Prepaid Group Practices to the U.S. Physician Supply." *Health Affairs*, Web Exclusive, February 4, 2004.

Scheffler, Richard M., Sean D. Sullivan, and Timothy Hoachung Ko. "The Impact of Blue Cross and Blue Shield Plan Utilization Management Programs, 1980–88." *Inquiry* 28 (fall 1991), pp. 263–75.

Schroeder, Steven A. "Physician Supply and the U.S. Medical Marketplace." *Health Affairs* 11 (spring 1992), pp. 235–54.

———. "Western European Responses to Physician Oversupply." *Journal of the American Medical Association* 252 (July 20, 1984), pp. 373–84.

Stano, Miron. "Further Issues in Small Area Variations Analysis." *Journal of Health Politics, Policy and Law* 16 (fall 1991), pp. 573–88.

Stoddard, Jeffrey, Joy M. Grossman, and Liza Rudell. "Physicians More Likely to Face Quality Incentives Than Incentives That May Restrain Care." Issue Brief No. 48. Center for studying Health System Change, January 2002, http://www.hschange.org.

Svorny, Shirley. "Should We Reconsider Licensing Physicians?" *Contemporary Policy Issues* 10 (January 1992), pp. 31–38.

Thorpe, Kenneth E. "The Medical Malpractice 'Crisis': Recent Trends and the Impact of State Tort Reform." *Health Affairs,* Web Exclusive, January 21, 2004.

Thurston, Norman K., and Anne M. Libby. "A Production Function for Physician Services Revisited." *Review of Economics and Statistics* 84 (February 2002), pp. 184–91.

Tussing, A. Dale. "Physician-Induced Demand for Medical Care: Irish General Practitioners." *Economic and Social Review* 14 (1983), pp. 225–47.

Tussing, A. Dale, and Martha Wojtowyzc. "Physician-Induced Demand by Irish GPs." *Social Science and Medicine* 23 (1986), pp. 851–60.

U.S. Department of Health and Human Services. "Confronting the New Health Care Crisis: Improving Health Care Quality and Lowering Costs by Fixing Our Medical Liability System." Washington, D.C., July, 25 2002.

Weeks, William B., Amy E. Wallace, Myron M. Wallace, and H. Gilbert Welch. "A Comparison of the Educational Costs and Incomes of Physicians and Other Professionals." *New England Journal of Medicine* 330 (May 5, 1994), pp. 1280–86.

Weiler, Paul C., et al. *A Measure of Malpractice: Medical Injury, Malpractice Litigation and Patient Compensation*. Cambridge, Mass.: Harvard University Press, 1993.

Weiner, Jonathan P. "Prepaid Group Practice Staffing and U.S. Physician Supply: Lessons for Workforce Policy." *Health Affairs*, Web Exclusive, February 4, 2004.

Wennberg, John E. "Dealing with Medical Practice Variations: A Proposal for Action." *Health Affairs* 3 (summer 1984), pp. 6–32.

______. "On Patient Need, Equity, Supplier-Induced Demand, and the Need to Assess the Outcome of Common Medical Practices." *Medical Care* 23 (May 1985), pp. 512–20.

Wickizer, Thomas M., and Daniel Lessler. "Utilization Management: Issues, Effects, and Future Prospects." *Annual Review of Public Health* 23 (2002), pp. 233–54.

Wilson, Florence A., and Duncan Neuhauser. *Health Services in the United States*, 2nd ed. Cambridge, Mass.: Ballinger, 1985.

CHAPTER 13

THE HOSPITAL SERVICES INDUSTRY

Just about everyone, either as a patient, a visitor, or an employee, has had some experience at a hospital. Some people conceive of hospitals as cold, lifeless facilities that spell gloom and doom. Others imagine hospitals as wondrous places where miraculous lifesaving feats, such as human organ transplants, are performed. Regardless of one's view, it is safe to say that the hospital of today bears little resemblance to its early-nineteenth-century predecessor. According to Peter Temin (1988), a noted economic historian,

> Hospitals were primarily nonmedical institutions throughout most of the nineteenth century. They existed for the care of marginal members of society, whether old, poor, or medically or psychologically deviant. Medicine was practiced outside the hospital, and the medical staffs of hospitals were small. Hospitals were charitable institutions, and they looked for moral rather than physical improvement in their patients. . . . In short, the nineteenth century hospital was closer to an almshouse than to a modern hospital. (pp. 78–79)

With the development of the germ theory of disease, the advent of new technologies, and increased urbanization, the "modern" hospital replaced the old-style version in the years following 1880. Hospitals have subsequently evolved into vibrant centers of medical and business activities.

Today's hospital is a technological marvel. The once simple hospital bed can now cost up to $10,000 when it includes customized accessories, such as automatically inflating air mattresses for patients with bedsores, voice-activated adjustments for paraplegics, and in-bed weight scales for bedridden patients (Anders, 1993a). Aided by advances in computer and pharmaceutical technologies, the modern hospital has proven capable of offering numerous therapeutic and diagnostic services that extend and improve the quantity and quality of lives. Indeed, one may point to the success of modern medicine as the culprit behind the ever-rising cost of delivering hospital services. Accounting for expenditures of $516 billion and 36 percent of all personal health care expenditures in 2003, the hospital services industry is the largest of the medical care industries.

This chapter explores the structure, conduct, and performance of the hospital services industry. Specifically, the chapter:

- describes the number, types, and size distribution of U.S. hospitals
- defines the relevant product and geographical markets for hospitals
- examines sources of barriers to entry in the hospital services industry
- discusses the relation between managed care and hospital structure and behavior
- focuses on hospital competition, regulation, and pricing behavior
- assesses the output, pricing, and profit performance of the hospital services industry

The Structure of the Hospital Services Industry

According to the industrial organization triad, as discussed in Chapter 8, the structural competitiveness of an industry can be evaluated based on a number of characteristics affecting the degree of actual and potential competition. **Actual competition** refers to the intensity of the competition that currently coexists among the firms in an industry. Among the more important factors influencing the degree of actual competition are the number and size distribution of the existing firms, the degree of product differentiation, and the amount of information consumers possess. **Potential competition** depends on how easy it is for new firms to enter an industry. The degree of potential competition can be measured by the magnitude of any barriers to entry resulting from economies of scale or legal impediments, such as patents and government restrictions. These and other structural characteristics of the hospital industry are discussed in more detail next.

Number, Types, and Size Distribution of U.S. Hospitals

The last 25 years have witnessed a dramatic and continual decline in the number of hospitals in the United States. Only about 5,800 of the nearly 7,000 hospitals that existed in 1980 still remained in 2003 (Health Care Forum LLC, 2005). The number of hospital beds also fell by nearly 30 percent over the 25-year span. Increased competitive and regulatory forces brought on by managed care health plans and federal cost containment measures have been cited as part of the explanation for the decline in the number of hospitals and hospital beds.

Hospitals are categorized based on ownership, types of services, and length of stay. In terms of ownership, hospitals can be separated into those operated by the federal government and those that are nonfederal hospitals. Federal hospitals are usually based at military institutions or run by the Veterans Administration. Based on service offerings and average length of stay, nonfederal hospitals can be grouped into community, long-term general and special, psychiatric, and tuberculosis hospitals. Community hospitals, the largest category at roughly 85 percent of all hospitals, provide general medical and surgical services and specialty services, such as ear, nose, and throat care; obstetrics and gynecology; or orthopedic services, and offer short-term stays (an average length of stay of less than 30 days).

Community hospitals can be further differentiated based on type of ownership. The dominant ownership type is the not-for-profit hospital, representing about 61 percent of the community hospitals and controlling nearly 71 percent of all community hospital beds as of 2003. The not-for-profit market share in terms of total beds remained fairly stable since 1980. For-profit hospitals currently account for almost 16 percent of all community hospitals. The market share (in beds) of for-profit hospitals rose from 9 percent in 1980 to 14 percent in 2003, with the increase corresponding to a decline in the state and local government market share from 21 to 16 percent.

The typical community hospital operates with 166 beds; almost half of all community hospitals have between 50 and 200 beds. Only 7 percent of community hospitals have less than 25 beds and only 9 percent have more than 400 beds. The same relative size pattern holds for both not-for-profit and for-profit hospitals, except that for-profit hospitals are smaller than not-for-profit hospitals, on average. Specifically, the average not-for-profit hospital holds 193 beds whereas the typical for-profit hospital contains 139 beds. Public hospitals are smaller yet, a typical one possessing only 115 beds. The relatively small size most likely reflects that a large fraction of public hospitals provide county hospital services in sparsely populated rural areas.

Although these data provide some insight into the ownership structure and size distribution of the different types of hospitals, they offer little information about the market power held by individual hospitals in the United States. The geographical market for hospital services is primarily local in scope, whereas the data are summarized at the national level. In addition, although hospitals compete among themselves, they might also be viewed as competing against other types of health care providers, such as freestanding surgical centers or large physician group practices. Before we can draw any behavioral or performance implications from market structure statistics, we must properly define the product and geographical markets and measure the degree of market concentration.

Measuring Market Concentration

Although some hospitals produce specialized services, such as psychiatric or nose, throat, and eye care services, most hospitals can be treated as multiproduct firms that simultaneously offer a multitude of diagnostic and therapeutic services. The large number and variety of services make it difficult to define and measure the relevant product market (RPM). Some health economists, such as Wilder and Jacobs (1987), have proposed that the RPM should be based on specific diagnoses, such as obstetrics, nervous system, tonsillectomy, or hernia repair services. However, Frech (1987) notes that hospitals are potential suppliers of most medical services even if they do not presently produce them, since they are capable of shifting resources from producing one service to producing another. Furthermore, some hospital services, such as X-rays, blood tests, and surgery, are complements to one another, reflecting the joint nature of the hospital production process. The implication is that the hospital RPM should be defined as a cluster of hospital services. As Frech (1987) notes, "The hundreds or thousands of individual procedures or services should not be viewed as individual markets" (p. 266).

One problem associated with a cluster of hospital services approach to defining the relevant product market is that some hospital facilities provide different levels of care in terms of the degree of technical sophistication and quality of services rendered or the seriousness and complexity of illnesses treated. Thus, some hospitals may not be in the same relevant product market because the level of care differs across services. Professionals in the hospital industry generally distinguish among four types of care.

Primary care services involve the prevention, early detection, and treatment of disease. Services of this nature include obstetrics, gynecology, internal medicine, and general surgery. A hospital that limits itself to providing primary care typically has some diagnostic equipment to perform X-ray and laboratory analysis. *Secondary* care involves more sophisticated treatment and may include cardiology, respiratory care, and physical therapy. Equipment and laboratory capabilities are more sophisticated in secondary care hospitals. *Tertiary* care is designed to arrest disease in process, including heart surgery and such cancer treatments as chemotherapy, and requires still more sophisticated equipment than do primary or secondary services. Community hospitals normally provide both primary and secondary care, and some offer tertiary care. Research hospitals associated with university medical schools are argued to provide state-of-the-art *quaternary*-level care.[1]

Another potential problem with the cluster of services approach is that hospital and nonhospital providers offering partial product lines are excluded from the relevant product market. Those excluded include specialized hospitals, physician clinics, and freestanding outpatient surgery centers. The cluster of services approach to the RPM typically excludes outpatient services when determining a hospital's relevant product market, largely because hospitals are considered as uniquely treating patients whose proper care requires overnight stays. In effect, the cluster of hospital services

1. See *U.S. v. Carilion*, 707 F. Supp. 840 (W.D. Va. 1989), 843.

approach treats hospital outpatient services as belonging to a separate market: the market for outpatient or ambulatory care services. Consequently, the size of the hospital market is measured in inpatient terms by either beds, admissions, inpatient days, or inpatient revenues.

Once the RPM is defined as a **cluster of inpatient hospital services,** the next step is to determine the relevant geographical market (RGM). The proper geographical area reflects the willingness and ability of the patients to switch to alternative suppliers when price is raised or quality is reduced by a nontrivial amount as discussed in Chapter 8. Due to data availability and practical concerns, many researchers have based the RGM on geopolitical boundaries, such as counties, metropolitan areas, or cities. Some have used health service areas to define the RGM; others, such as Luft et al. (1986), have used a fixed 5- or 15-mile radius around each hospital as the appropriate RGM. The problem with RGM definitions of these kinds, however, is that they are based on convenience rather than on sound economic principles.

Based on Elzinga and Hogarty (1978), some economists propose that the RGM should be determined by patient flow data. According to the Elzinga and Hogarty (EH) test, an appropriately defined RGM has small percentages of patients flowing into and out of it. This means that geographic markets are defined such that only a small percentage of people leave to purchase hospital services elsewhere and a small fraction of individuals enter from outside the area to buy hospital services. For example, in *U.S. v. Rockford Memorial,* the court ruled that Rockford, Illinois, and the immediate hinterland was the RGM because 87 percent of Rockford Memorial's patients came from the area immediately surrounding Rockford and 90 percent of Rockford residents requiring hospitalization were hospitalized in Rockford itself.

However, other economists also point out several shortcomings associated with the EH test of the RGM. First, patient flow data reveal the current purchasing patterns of consumers and not necessarily the purchasing patterns that may develop if one or a few hospitals raise their prices by nontrivial amounts. Second, a minority of patients who travel long distances for their hospital care may differ significantly from the majority of patients who do not travel very far. The majority of patients may prefer the convenience of local hospitals regardless of their ability to provide quality care. Thus, basing the willingness to switch on a minority imposes their preferences on the majority of consumers. Third, two stages of competition exist in hospital markets. At the first stage, hospitals compete among themselves to be included in the various health insurers' networks of providers. At the second stage, hospitals within the same network compete for patients. Hospitals can acquire market power at both stages but the EH test, at best, only reflects the degree of competition at the second stage.

Consequently, no single flawless way exists to identify the RGM. In antitrust cases, most agree that all available information should be consulted when determining the RGM for hospital services. Evidence concerning the degree of competition at both stages, EH patient flow evidence, expert testimony by competitors and third-party payers, and strategic-planning documents such as marketing plans are some of the materials reviewed.[2] However, most analysts believe that real-world hospital markets are fairly small or local in nature, which is not surprising. As Judge Posner noted in the *Rockford* antitrust case, "For highly exotic or highly elective hospital treatment, patients will sometimes travel long distances, of course. But for the most part hospital services are local. People want to be hospitalized near their families and homes, in hospitals in which their own—local—doctors have hospital privileges."[3]

2. See the July 2004 report by the DOJ and FTC titled "Improving Health Care: A Dose of Competition" at http://www.usdoj.gov/atr/public/health_care/204694.htm#toc (accessed January 10, 2006). Also see http://www.ftc.gov/bc/docs/horismer.htm (accessed January 10, 2006), which contains the 1992 horizontal merger guidelines.

3. *U.S. v. Rockford Memorial,* 898 F.2d 1278; 1284 (1990).

If markets are defined as being local in nature, many hospital services markets already exceed the threshold concentration figure of 1,800 set by the Justice Department (see Chapter 8). For example, only two community hospitals of equal size are necessary in a market area with a population of 100,000 to generate an HHI of 5,000, which is well above the DOJ threshold.

To get some idea about the actual degree of market concentration at the local level, let's suppose that the metropolitan statistical area (MSA) can be used to identify the RGM. We must remember, however, that most MSAs are large geographically and therefore may define the RGM too broadly for practical purposes. Bates and Santerre (2005) provide some data from the American Hospital Association that can be used to assess the degree of concentration in the hospital services industry across 306 MSAs in the United States in 1993 and 1999. Population in these MSAs ranges from 57,000 to 9 million and averages nearly 650,000 as of 1993. According to their data, only one-quarter of the 306 MSAs contained ten or more community hospitals in 1993. Between six and ten hospitals existed in another 21 percent of the MSAs. Finally, more than half of the MSAs possessed fewer than six community hospitals in 1993.

Assuming all hospitals within an MSA possess equal market shares, these three cutoffs of more than ten hospitals, between six and ten hospitals, and less than six hospitals are roughly consistent with HHIs below 1,000, between 1,000 and 1,800, and above 1,800, respectively. The implication is that most hospital markets, even when broadly defined in terms of the RGM, appear to be heavily concentrated or dominated by a few large community hospitals. These figures represent a simple count of the number of community hospitals in each MSA. They do not reflect how many hospitals belong to the same chains or systems within any particular MSA and therefore underestimate the true degree of market concentration.

Data further suggest that hospital services markets have become even more concentrated over time. This resulted from few hospitals entering the market, hospital closures, and hospital consolidations. By 1999, just six years later, only 22 percent of the MSAs contained ten or more community hospitals. In addition, the percentage of MSAs with mild levels of hospital concentration slipped by one percentage point to 20 percent. Even more alarming, perhaps, the data indicate that fewer than six community hospitals operated in 58 percent of the MSAs by 1999.[4]

Clearly these data paint a picture of a highly concentrated hospital services industry that has become more concentrated over time. However, when assessing the overall competitiveness of a market, economists also consider the degree of potential competition as reflected by any barriers to entry into a market. A high degree of potential competition creates an incentive for aggressive price competition even when only a few firms dominate an industry. We take up entry barriers in the next section.

Barriers to Entry

Entry barriers make it difficult for new firms to enter markets and, during periods of excess demand, allow existing firms to make supranormal economic profits. State certificate of need (CON) laws are often cited as a type of entry barrier into the hospital services industry. Schramm and Renn (1984) take issue with this view of CON laws, however. They point out that the hospital industry is usually characterized by excess capacity rather than excess demand. According to them, it would be irrational for new hospitals to enter in the presence of excess capacity because hospitals already in the industry can satisfy any expansion in demand. Therefore, according to their view, excess capacity rather than CON laws deters entry into the industry.

---

4. Health Care Forum LLC (2005) provides 2003 data on the number of community hospitals in each MSA. Although these data do not cover the same MSAs as the 306 discussed previously, the 2003 data indicate further concentration of the health services industry. According to the figures, 64 percent of the MSAs contained fewer than six hospitals and only 21 percent of MSAs had more than ten hospitals.

Noether (1987), however, found that hospital prices were 4.0 to 4.9 percent higher, on average, in areas where CON laws exist. Furthermore, she noted, "In at least two states, a surge in notices of intent to build has been noted since abolition of the entry review program" (p. 37). Both of these findings suggest that CON laws deter entry and allow entrenched firms to raise prices. Thus, it is not surprising that, in 1987, the federal government ended its policy, which began in 1975, of encouraging the development of CON programs. According to Baker (1988), nearly one-quarter of the states abolished their CON laws by the end of 1987.[5]

Baker (1988) argues that even in the absence of CON laws, entry into the hospital industry may be difficult. The technological specifications for modern hospital buildings, including wide corridors and doorways, large elevators, strongly supported flooring, and extensive plumbing, require about four to nine years of planning and construction time. The relatively huge investment in the hospital infrastructure represents a sunk cost that may discourage new hospitals from entering a market in a timely manner.

In addition to sunk costs, other cost conditions may serve as barriers to entry. In particular, economies of scale, learning curve effects, and system affiliation can all make it costlier for new firms to enter markets. The econometric evidence in support of economies of scale in the hospital services industry is mixed, however. For example, hospital cost studies in the 1960s, which simply related hospital costs to measures of output and capacity, generally concluded that "there was evidence of significant economies of scale, at least up to moderately sized hospitals of around 500 beds" (Cowing et al., 1983, p. 264). However, post-1970 hospital cost studies, controlling for other determinants of hospital costs, including case-mix, input prices, and the number of admitting physicians, reveal that "economies of scale may exist for small hospitals but . . . moderate- and large-size hospitals can generally be characterized by constant returns to scale" (Cowing et al., 1983, p. 276). Unfortunately, the econometric evidence for the post-1970 studies is suspect because the cost functions employed are generally not well grounded in neoclassical cost theory, as presented in Chapter 7. In addition, like the hospital cost studies of the 1960s, the 1970 research fails to treat hospitals as multiproduct firms and assumes rather than tests for long-run cost minimization (see Chapter 7).

To overcome the limitations associated with the hospital cost studies of the 1960s and 1970s, econometric analyses by Cowing and Holtmann (1983), Grannemann et al. (1986), Eakin and Kniesner (1988), Vita (1990), and Fournier and Mitchell (1992) rely to a much greater degree on neoclassical cost theory and treat hospitals as multiproduct firms. Generally, these studies fail to provide any strong and consistent econometric evidence for the presence of long-run economies of scale in the production of inpatient services. In fact, the evidence suggests that the production process for inpatient hospital services exhibits long-run diseconomies of scale, at least for the average-size hospital in the various studies (in particular, see Vita [1990], Eakin and Kniesner [1988], and Grannemann et al. [1986]). The implication of the recent econometric studies is that long-run economies of scale are not a serious deterrent to potential entrants.

Given the problems associated with econometric studies, some researchers have relied on the survivor test developed by Stigler (1958) to determine whether economies of scale exist (Bays, 1986). According to the survivor technique, firm or plant sizes that account for an increasing fraction of industry output over time are considered efficient because they have apparently met and survived the market test. Correspondingly, those that provide a declining share are viewed as inefficient. The survivor test provides a broad measure of efficiency, capturing the ability of firms to both produce with least-cost methods and satisfy consumer wants in the long run.

---

5. For a comprehensive review of the empirical literature on the CON program and some additional empirical findings, see Conover and Sloan (1998).

TABLE 13–1
A Comparison of the Size Distribution of Community Hospitals, Selected Years 1970–2003

	Percentage of Hospitals in Each Bed Size Category				
Bed Size Category	**1970**	**1980**	**1990**	**2000**	**2003**
0–24	6.8%	4.4%	4.2%	5.9%	6.7%
25–49	22.6	17.7	17.4	18.5	19.7
50–99	25.4	25.1	23.5	21.5	21.1
100–199	21.8	23.5	24.3	25.1	23.9
200–299	10.1	12.3	13.7	13.3	12.7
300–399	6.1	7.1	7.6	6.9	7.1
400–499	3.2	4.6	4.1	3.7	3.5
500 and over	4.0	5.4	5.3	5.0	5.3

SOURCE: American Hospital Association. *Hospital Statistics,* various years, Table 4.A.

Table 13–1 shows the percentage of community hospitals in various bed size categories for each decennial year since 1970 and for 2003. According to the data, the percentage of hospitals in the four largest bed size categories increased until the 1980s or 1990s and then decreased thereafter. The smallest two bed size categories followed the opposite pattern. Santerre and Pepper (2000) find that removal of CON laws and rate regulations in many states, and increased price sensitivity since the mid-1980s, led to a reduction in the proportion of the very largest hospitals and to an increase in the fraction of the smaller hospitals. They argue that a continuance of increased price competition may favor hospitals with fewer than 200 beds. The data in Table 13–1 indicate that the 100 to 199 bed size category is the only one to experience a continual rise in the share of hospitals, but only up to 2000. Consequently, survivor analysis is unable to offer a definitive conclusion about the most efficient size for a hospital. Instead, survivor theory appears to suggest that the efficient hospital size may have changed considerably over time in response to the net effect of various types of market and regulatory forces.

Considering both the econometric evidence and the survivor test, a best estimate is that the long-run average cost of a short-term community hospital reaches its lowest point at a size of around 200 beds, give or take 100 beds. The long-run average cost curve is probably shallow, with average costs rising only modestly to the left and right of the minimum point(s). It is important to remember, however, that economies of scale are limited by the size of the market; that is, demand conditions and transportation costs limit the economies of scale that can be realized. Thus, hospitals in rural areas operate with fewer beds than the number dictated by economies of scale considerations simply because the market is smaller. Also, some small hospitals may satisfy niche or specialized demands and continue to operate profitably despite their relative size. All in all, it does not appear that economies of scale are a significant deterrent to potential entrants into the hospital services industry.

Recall from Chapter 8 that learning by doing is another characteristic associated with the cost structure the individual hospital faces. Studies focusing on learning economies in the hospital industry usually investigate how the volume of output affects the quality of patient outcomes.

For example, Farley and Ozminkowski (1992) analyze whether patient outcomes improve in hospitals as the volume of admissions increases for specific diagnoses and procedures. They find that over time, greater volume at a hospital leads to significantly lower risk-adjusted in-hospital mortality rates for three types of admissions: acute myocardial infarction, hernia repair, and respiratory distress syndrome in neonates. Providing further evidence for learning economies in hospital care, Stone et al. (1992) discover that the relative risk of death for AIDS patients is more than twice as great in low-experience hospitals. Their results further indicate that the better outcome at high-AIDS-experienced hospitals is not associated with greater use of medical services. For example, AIDS patients in low-experience hospitals are more likely to be placed in an ICU, have longer ICU stays, and tend to have longer overall lengths of stay and higher costs.[6]

Most empirical studies have offered evidence to support learning by doing for various hospital services and surgical procedures, but the magnitude varies greatly (Halm et al., 2002). One of the exceptions worth mentioning is a study by Ho (2002) that uses longitudinal data on patients receiving coronary angioplasty, a procedure to widen narrowed arteries, to empirically examine changes in outcomes and costs. Because a panel data set of patient outcomes over a relatively long period of time (1984–1996) is used in the empirical test, Ho is able to differentiate between scale economies (more output at a point in time), learning by doing (greater cumulative output over time), and "learning by watching" on health outcomes and costs. **Learning by watching** refers to productivity or quality improvements that occur over time regardless of production volume. It arises from knowledge or technological change that can be easily transferred across hospitals.

Based on data from California hospitals, Ho shows that all hospitals achieved substantial improvements in patient outcomes with respect to coronary angioplasty over time. However, when empirically explaining those improvements using multiple regression analysis and controlling for factors such as case-mix, quality, and hospital characteristics, she finds no evidence that learning by doing improves patient outcomes. Rather, evidence is found to support mild scale economies and learning by watching. In terms of cost reductions, Ho's empirical findings cannot rule out lower costs of performing coronary angioplasties because of learning by doing. Overall she points out that efforts to regionalize the production of coronary angioplasties may lead to lower costs per patient but only small outcome improvements.

If "practice makes perfect," as most studies suggest, hospitals with greater volume may tend to attract an even larger market share over time. The learning economies, combined with limit-pricing techniques, may discourage new firms from entering the industry. Thus, most evidence suggests that learning by doing may act as a barrier to entry into hospital markets and provide existing firms with some market power to raise price.

Membership in a **multihospital system** or chain may also provide an existing hospital with a cost advantage relative to a potential freestanding hospital that is contemplating whether to enter the market. The American Hospital Association defines a multihospital system as two or more hospitals that are owned, leased, sponsored, or managed by a single corporate entity. According to Morrisey and Alexander (1987), a member of a multihospital system may possess four general advantages over an independent hospital, which may result in lower average costs at any given level of output:

(1) economic benefits *such as economies of scale and access to capital;*

(2) improved personnel and management benefits *such as ability to recruit, train and retain high-quality medical and administrative staffs, expand patient referral networks,*

6. However, unlike Farley and Ozminkowski (1992), Stone et al. (1992) does not correct for the likelihood of reverse causation—the so-called selective referral bias. It is entirely possible that AIDS patients flock to hospitals that provide higher-quality care; that is, higher quality leads to higher admissions rather than the reverse.

and provide access to specialists to assist in coping with increasingly complex environments;

(3) organizational benefits *due to expansion of the service area, increased market penetration, and organizational survival through reduced financial deficits, manpower shortages, and facilities problems; and*

(4) community benefits *such as improved access and quality of care through enhanced resources, lower costs, and improved regional planning. (p. 61)*

With these four potential advantages in mind, several empirical studies have examined whether system affiliation actually confers any significant performance differential. While some minor differences have been found, statistical studies have generally established that system affiliation does not lead to lower costs of production. For example, the eighteen studies reviewed by Ermann and Gabel (1984) reveal contradictory evidence regarding cost differences between multihospital and independent hospitals. In addition, Renn et al. (1985) find no significant differences in costs between investor-owned chains and freestanding for-profit hospitals or between system-affiliated and freestanding not-for-profit hospitals. Finally, Wilcox-Gok (2002) finds that system affiliation has no isolated impact on hospital costs when proper controls are made for other hospital characteristics. Thus, available studies suggest empirically that system affiliation offers no major cost advantage to established hospitals.[7]

In sum, learning by doing appears to be the only significant cost structure basis for barriers to entry. Evidence suggests that more experience is associated with lower costs and higher quality, implying that potential entrants may be deterred from entering markets when the existing hospitals possess considerable expertise. Thus, learning economies may give existing firms the potential to raise price above the competitive level and earn excess economic profits. In contrast, economies of scale and system affiliation seem to have little impact on the relative long-run costs of existing and new hospitals.

Number, Types, and Size Distribution of the Buyers of Hospital Services

Another important aspect of the market structure of an industry is the number, types, and size distribution of the buyers. For example, an influential buyer who purchases a sizeable amount of a product from several different sellers may be able to negotiate significant price discounts by playing one seller against the others. Table 13–2 shows the main sources of hospital funds in 2003. Of the $515.9 billion spent on hospital services, governments at all levels are collectively responsible for 58 percent, with the federal government being the main purchaser at 47 percent. The relatively high percentage implies that the federal government may wield considerable power concerning how resources are allocated in the hospital services sector given its large share of spending in both national and local markets. In particular, the DRG system for Medicare reimbursement places many hospitals "at risk" for a sizeable proportion of their operating costs. Similarly, some state governments may be able to influence resource allocation in local markets, where they purchase a large fraction of hospital services under the Medicaid program.

About 42 percent of hospital care spending originates in the private sector. Individual consumers, accounting for only 3.2 percent of all hospital payments, are most often price insensitive and therefore have little impact on the market price of hospital care. The private insurance category, representing commercial insurance companies, Blue Cross plans, and independent

7. But compare Menke (1997), who found that system-affiliated hospitals have lower costs.

TABLE 13–2
Sources of Hospital Funds, 2003

	Dollars (billions)	Percent
Total hospital care expenses	$515.9	100.0%
All private funds	215.0	41.7
Out-of-pocket	16.3	3.2
Private insurance	177.4	34.4
Other	21.3	4.1
Government	300.8	58.3
Federal	242.1	46.9
State and local	58.7	11.4

SOURCE: Centers for Medicare & Medicaid Services, http://www.cms.gov (accessed January 10, 2006).

managed care organizations, directly accounts for slightly more than 34 percent of all spending on hospital services. Whether these buyers have the willingness and ability to bargain successfully for low prices and thereby affect the allocation of resources to hospital services depends on a host of considerations, including their goals (profit or not-for-profit objectives), the competitiveness of the health insurance market, and their individual market penetration rates. For example, an individual private health insurance plan is more able to negotiate favorable hospital prices when it represents a relatively large market share of subscribers in a local hospital market and thereby possesses some bargaining power.

How buyers reimburse hospitals may also affect the way in which resources are allocated to hospital care. Third-party payers contracting with hospital providers choose among a variety of hospital reimbursement plans, including usual and customary charges, discounted usual and customary charges, per diem payments, DRG payments, and capitation payments. Some of these reimbursement schemes shift a greater amount of financial risk onto hospital care providers. For example, DRG payments and capitation fees shift much more risk onto hospital care providers than do usual and customary charges. "At-risk" charges generally create more incentives for cost-effective practices because the health care providers are responsible for absorbing any cost overruns.

Comparative data are unavailable for the different hospital reimbursement practices adopted by various third-party payers. Hoy et al. (1991), however, provide some information regarding the hospital reimbursement practices of HMO and PPO plans sponsored by commercial insurance companies. Although the data on hospital reimbursement methods are limited to the managed care plans owned by commercial insurers, they are nonetheless interesting, fairly representative, and deserving of discussion.

Hoy et al. find that fewer than 20 percent of the PPOs and HMOs owned by commercial insurers reimburse hospital providers on the basis of usual and customary charges, with the most popular reimbursement method being the discounted charge. They also find that PPO plans are much more likely to use per diem payments than HMOs. Specifically, nearly 25 percent of insurer-owned PPOs reimburse by per diem payments, whereas the comparable figure for insurer-owned HMOs is only 5.3 percent.

Data also suggest that the reimbursement schemes of insurer-owned HMOs are generally less oriented toward hospital risk sharing than are those of PPOs. Almost 22 percent of the insurer-owned PPOs reimburse hospitals with either DRG or capitation payments, whereas only 11.5 percent of insurer-owned HMOs reimburse with these at-risk charges. Hoy et al. provide a rationale for this finding by noting that physician gatekeepers and the strong orientation toward avoiding hospitalization make hospital risk sharing less critical to HMOs.

Due to the large variety of reimbursement practices suggested by their study, it is evident that not all HMOs or PPOs should be treated or expected to behave similarly with respect to the buying of hospital services. Indeed, Feldman et al. ("Effects of HMOs," 1990) find that IPA/HMOs are less likely than the more tightly organized staff-network (S/N) HMOs to switch hospitals and concentrate patients at specific hospitals on the basis of price. They argue that a strong and ongoing physician affiliation is more important to IPA physicians than is price. This view is substantiated by the fact that the elasticity of demand for hospital admissions was found to be more elastic for S/N HMOs (−3.044) than IPAs (−1.024). Moreover, Feldman et al. ("Contracts between Hospitals," 1990) show that S/N HMOs secure larger discounts for inpatient services than IPAs. They find that the average discount is 26 percent for general medical and surgery care services at S/N HMOs but only 4 percent at IPAs. The authors also determine that S/N HMOs are more likely to use per diem charges than IPAs, which tend to employ discounted charges.

In sum, the number, size distribution, and types of buyers are important structural features of local hospital markets. Government is responsible for a majority of all hospital purchases and, with the associated purchasing power, has some ability to influence hospital prices and costs through the Medicare and Medicaid programs at the national or state level. The private sector, composed of a large number of different types of insurer/buyers, may be able to influence hospital prices at the local level. The ultimate success of private insurers in negotiating low prices and controlling costs in local hospital markets depends on a host of factors, including the chosen hospital reimbursement strategy, the competitiveness of the hospital and insurance markets, and the goals of the insurer.

Type of Product

Whether the hospitals in a market offer a differentiated or standardized product is another determinant of market structure. According to the anticompetitive view, product differentiation causes the demand curve to become less price elastic and enables the firm to restrict output below and raise price above the competitive level. Hospital choice studies confirm that product differences matter in the hospital services industry. For example, from their review of the literature, Lane and Lindquist (1988) cite seven categories of factors—care, staff, physical facilities, clientele, experience, convenience, and institutional—that strongly affect the choice of hospital. Of these factors, quality of care and staff, equipment and technology, and convenient location were found to be among the more important determinants of choice of hospital.

Marketing and advertising also play important roles in the hospital services industry. The typical hospital engaging in promotion activities spends nearly $120,000 annually on marketing, amounting to approximately 0.1 to 0.2 percent of sales (Barro and Chu, 2002). While that percentage figure pales in comparison to the advertising-to-sales ratios of 10 percent or more observed in the pharmaceutical, cosmetics, soft drink, cereal, and other industries, Gray (1986) notes that hospitals devote as much as 5 percent of gross sales to advertising in some highly competitive areas of the country. Gray notes, "Hospitals plug such things as Saturday surgery (a convenience for patients), referral services, gourmet food, depression clinics—even free transportation" (p. 183).

Of the total marketing budget at hospitals, about 50 percent is spent on advertising (Japsen, 1997). About 43 percent of the advertising budget is devoted to print advertisements in newspapers and magazines. The rest of the advertising budget is directed to radio (14 percent), direct mail (12 percent), Yellow Pages (11 percent), television (11 percent), bus/billboards (4 percent), and other media (5 percent).

Dorfman and Steiner (1954) offer a model that provides a useful starting point for thinking about the determinants of hospital advertising expenditures. While the Dorfman-Steiner theory refers to a monopolist, we simply have to consider other strategic aspects of advertising when applying the model to the hospital services industry. As we discussed previously, the hospital services industry more closely conforms to the characteristics of an oligopolistic market structure in many areas. Following the Dorfman-Steiner approach, we begin by supposing that a hospital faces the following market demand for its services:

(13–1) $$Q = Q(P, A),$$

where Q stands for quantity demanded and P and A represent price and advertising expenditures, respectively.

The quantity demanded of hospital services is expected to decline with an increase in price, as the law of demand suggests, and rise with greater advertising expenditures, *ceteris paribus*. The latter variable affects the quantity demanded of hospital services through a shift in the demand curve to the right. According to theory, demand increases (and may rotate) because of the information signal provided or the brand loyalty created by the advertising message.

Dorfman and Steiner show mathematically that the profit-maximizing amount of advertising relative to total revenues (A/TR), or advertising intensity, results when the following condition holds:

(13–2) $$\frac{A}{TR} = \frac{E_A}{E_P}.$$

E_A represents the advertising elasticity of demand and identifies the percentage change in quantity demanded resulting from a one-percentage-point change in advertising expenditures. It measures the responsiveness of consumer demand to a change in advertising expenditures. For example, if $E_A = 2.0$, then a 1 percent increase in advertising expenditures results in a 2 percent increase in quantity demanded. E_P represents the price elasticity of market demand in absolute terms.

According to this Dorfman-Steiner condition, the profit-maximizing level of advertising intensity equals the ratio of the two elasticities. For instance, if E_A and E_P equal 1.5 and 4.5, respectively, then the profit-maximizing ratio of advertising to sales equals 0.33. That is, the profit-maximizing hospital spends one-third of its revenues on advertising expenditures. One implication of the analysis is that a profit-maximizing hospital advertises more intensely when the advertising elasticity is higher. As one would expect, hospitals spend more on advertising when consumers are more responsive to the messages financed with the advertising expenditures.

Another implication of the model is that advertising expenditures are greater when demand is less elastic with respect to price. That relation holds in part because increased advertising expenditures generally lead to higher per-unit costs and prices. When demand is less elastic with respect to price, the higher price resulting from the increased advertising expenditures leads to a smaller percentage reduction in quantity demanded.

Using the expression for the Lerner index of monopoly power developed in Chapter 11, the price-cost margin can be substituted for the price elasticity of demand facing a monopolist. Thus, Equation 13–2 can be restated as

(13–3) $$\frac{A}{TR} = E_A \frac{(P - MC)}{P}.$$

As a result, Equation 13–3 offers the interpretation that advertising intensity is larger when quantity demanded is more responsive to advertising and also when the gap between price and marginal cost is greater. Thus, a third implication of the Dorfman-Steiner condition is that firms with greater market power tend to advertise their products more aggressively, all other factors held constant. In fact, a perfectly competitive firm may not advertise at all, according to Equation 13–3, because the price-cost margin equals zero in the long run.

Recall that the Dorfman-Steiner model is based on a monopolist and that most hospital services markets are oligopolistic in nature. Within an oligopoly setting, previous research suggests that we must consider that advertising could have both an *industry expansion* and a *market share expansion* effect. That is, advertising by a single hospital may expand the size of the entire industry by informing consumers about the general availability of a product or procedure (such as an MRI) or why one product (such as hospital outpatient care) is superior to a substitute product (outpatient care in physician clinics). Notice that all of the hospitals in an area stand to gain from a single hospital's advertising when it leads to industry expansion. In fact, if all of the hospitals in an industry offer fairly standardized products and each individual hospital attempts to free-ride the advertising efforts of others to gain from the industry expansion without incurring costs, economic theory suggests that little advertising may actually take place. This free-rider argument provides another reason why firms in a perfectly competitive market are not likely to spend much on advertisements. In contrast, one of a few hospitals in an oligopolistic market may be able to internalize more of the gains from the industry expansion effect. Hence advertising expenditures are likely to be greater in an oligopolistic setting than in a perfectly competitive market.

Another consideration is that an individual hospital may gain from the market share effect in an oligopolistic setting. Persuasive advertising may allow a hospital to attract some of its rivals' customers. Using advertising as a nonprice means of competing is further reinforced by the fact that rival hospitals can quickly and easily respond to a price cut by a competitor. Consequently, price competition often does not provide a sustainable method of enlarging market share in an oligopolistic market. A clever advertising campaign, in contrast, can catch rivals off guard and sometimes lead to a sizeable increase in market share for a longer duration than the short-lived market share increase that develops from the initiation of a price war.

The market share expansion effect also implies that diminishing returns may set in with respect to additional advertising expenditures at some point. For example, an oligopolistic hospital with a 65 percent market share may have to spend considerably more on advertising to attract an additional 1 percent of the market from its rivals than was required to capture any previous increments of 1 percent. In addition, the market share effect holds no value for a monopolist, so it may not hold much value for a firm already in possession of 95, 90, or 80 percent of the market. For these reasons, advertising intensity may level off or decline at some level of industry concentration.

Based on the Dorfman-Steiner model, Town and Currim (2002) examine the advertising behavior of a sample of California hospitals from 1991 to 1997. The authors find that the percentage of California hospitals that advertised increased from 16 to 45 percent over the six-year period. These figures compare very closely to those of Barro and Chu (2002), who report that the percentage of hospitals advertising in the nation increased from 36 percent in 1995 to more than 50 percent in 1998. In addition, among hospitals that advertised, Town and Currim explain that inflation-adjusted hospital advertising expenditures in California grew more than sixfold over the period. However, at the national level over the shorter three-year period from 1995 to 1998, hospital expenditures on advertising increased by only 10 percent in real terms according to Barro and Chu.

Following the Dorfman-Steiner model, Town and Currim specify various variables in their multiple regression equation that affect either the advertising or price elasticity of demand. Among the variables specified are the HHI of market concentration, composition of patients by payer type, ownership type, size, teaching status, and system affiliation. Their analysis offers a number of interesting insights. First, the empirical findings support the Dorfman-Steiner theory by indicating that hospital advertising intensity is greater in more concentrated market areas. Specifically, they find that an increase in the HHI from about 1470 to 3310 produces a 72 percent increase in advertising expenditures.

Second, the findings imply that for-profit hospitals did not advertise any differently than their not-for-profit counterparts. We will see later in this chapter that for-profit and not-for-profit hospitals share a lot of behavioral similarities. Finally, their results also suggest that hospitals spend more on advertising in an attempt to attract a greater share of the more profitable Medicare and HMO patients as compared to the less profitable Medicaid or charity care patients. The direct empirical relation between the percentage of HMO patients and advertising intensity may also reflect a hypothesis offered by Barro and Chu. They argue that HMOs achieve market power by threatening to leave hospitals out of their networks. Advertising helps hospitals differentiate their products and make themselves indispensable in the eyes of the consumer and thereby reduce the threat and market power of HMOs.

In summary, data suggest that advertising is beginning to play a greater role in the hospital services industry. The Dorfman-Steiner theory suggests that growing market concentration in the hospital services industry may be one reason for this growing dependence on hospital advertising. Moreover, hospitals may be using advertising to differentiate their products so as to improve their standing with HMO networks for negotiation purposes. Differentiated products, in turn, lower the price elasticity of demand facing an individual hospital and thereby create an additional incentive to spend more on hospital advertising.

If, in the future, hospitals rely more on nonprice methods of competition, such as advertising, price competition may become less aggressive. That is, hospital prices may become relatively rigid as hospitals compete on the basis of advertising, quality, and convenience, for example. The net effect of this trend on consumer welfare is uncertain and depends on a variety of considerations, including whether the nonprice methods promote real or illusory gains for consumers. It also on depends on whether oligopolistic hospitals agree to collude on a number of dimensions, including advertising, at some point. For example, five of the six hospitals in Des Moines, Iowa, were accused of agreeing to limit their advertising, an action in violation of antitrust laws. The hospitals involved in the suit eventually settled with the Justice Department (Burda, 1993).

Summary of the Structure of the Hospital Services Industry

For all practical purposes, the market for hospital services is best defined as hospitals offering a similar cluster of inpatient services within the same geographical area. The geographical market area of most primary and secondary care hospitals tends to be local in nature. The structural competitiveness of the hospital services market is determined by the number, types, and size distribution of hospitals; number, types, and size distribution of buyers/insurers; barriers to entry; type of product; and the extent of any asymmetry of information between patients and hospitals. In terms of the supply side, most local hospital markets are characterized by a relatively few competing hospitals except in major metropolitan areas, where hospitals are more numerous. For example, cities with populations of 100,000 can generally support only two or three hospitals. In addition to the degree of actual competition, the behavior of hospitals depends on the ease of potential entry or the magnitude of any barriers to entry. Learning by doing rather than long-run economies of scale or multihospital systems appears to be the major reason for barriers to entry into the hospital services industry. More experienced hospitals tend to have lower costs and higher quality than newer ones. Hence, based on the number of competitors and barriers to entry in most areas, the supply side of the hospital services industry can be characterized as oligopolistic.

Another important structural factor affecting hospital behavior from the demand side of the market is buyer concentration. Simply put, buyer concentration has the ability to negate seller concentration. The federal government, state governments, and some private insurers may possess the appropriate size on the demand side of the market necessary to influence hospital pricing and output behavior. Also, reimbursement policies that place hospitals at risk for high costs have the potential to promote cost-effective medicine.

The Conduct of the Hospital Services Industry

The industrial organization triad predicts that market structure influences the conduct of the hospitals within a given market area. According to traditional microeconomic theory, a large number of sellers and low barriers to entry promote competition. More intense competition usually shows up in increased output, higher quality, and lower prices. The general conduct of real-world hospitals is difficult to predict on a market or an aggregate basis, however. Hospitals pursue different objectives, operate in various market settings, face alternative types of reimbursement methods from third-party payers, and are subject to a variety of government regulations. Ideally, from a societal point of view, we hope that incentives exist such that hospitals act independently and strive to minimize costs and satisfy consumer wants. However, some structural features of the hospital services industry, such as barriers to entry, product complexity, and asymmetry of information, suggest that such incentives may be lacking in many local markets across the nation. Also, a substantial body of empirical evidence indicates that hospitals sometimes compete on the basis of cost-enhancing quality instead of price in many markets. In this section, we focus on the pricing behavior of hospitals, particularly not-for-profit hospitals. We also discuss what is known empirically about the relation between hospital market structure and various measures of conduct, such as price, costs, and quality. We also examine the effects of ownership structure, managed care, and government regulations on the conduct of hospitals. The section closes with a discussion of the economics of integrated delivery systems.

Pricing Behavior of Not-for-Profit Hospitals

In Chapter 8, we developed several market models, including perfect competition and monopoly, to analyze the pricing behavior of for-profit organizations. However, we just learned that for-profit hospitals make up only 16 percent of all community hospitals. Therefore, the previously discussed market models may be inappropriate for analyzing the conduct of not-for-profit hospitals, which because of their nondistribution constraint may pursue goals other than profit maximization.

Over the years, a number of utility maximization models have been developed to explain the behavior of not-for-profit organizations. In general, utility maximization models assume that the manager of a not-for-profit hospital attempts to maximize his or her own personal utility. Although debate exists over what variables belong in the manager's utility function, most analysts have assumed that the manager derives utility either directly or indirectly from things such as organizational size, quality of services, and discretionary profits. We next discuss the managerial utility maximization models most commonly discussed in the literature about the pricing behavior of not-for-profit hospitals.

Quantity Maximization. Baumol (1967) argues that rather than pursuing profit maximization, large firms with a substantial amount of market power tend to maximize output subject to a break-even level of profits. Because executive salaries and prestige are more strongly correlated with firm size than with profits, managers try to expand sales at the expense of profits. Figure 13–1 depicts the situation for a hospital where Q stands for the number of patient-days. An output- or quantity-maximizing hospital produces output up to the point where the average cost of production equals average revenue, or at Q_0 patient-days in the figure. At that point, the hospital is servicing the maximum number of patient-days without incurring an economic loss. If it expanded services beyond Q_0, the hospital would operate with an economic loss, since AC exceeds AR. A profit-maximizing hospital with the same cost curves produces up to the point where MR = MC and provides Q_1 patient-days and charges P_1. It follows that an output-maximizing hospital produces more output and charges a lower price than a profit-maximizing hospital, *ceteris paribus*.

Davis (1972) points out that most hospitals offer a wide array of services, each with its own price, and it is logical to assume that an output-maximizing hospital follows a pricing strategy that increases the number of patients admitted. The chosen pricing strategy involves a certain degree of cross-subsidization. Specifically, the hospital may charge a price below cost on services for which demand is more elastic to generate more admissions, and then make up for the loss by charging a much higher price for services for which demand is less inelastic. For example, the hospital may charge a price below cost for basic room services to attract more patients and cover the loss by charging a higher price for ancillary services such as pharmaceutical products. The

FIGURE 13–1
The Output Maximization Model

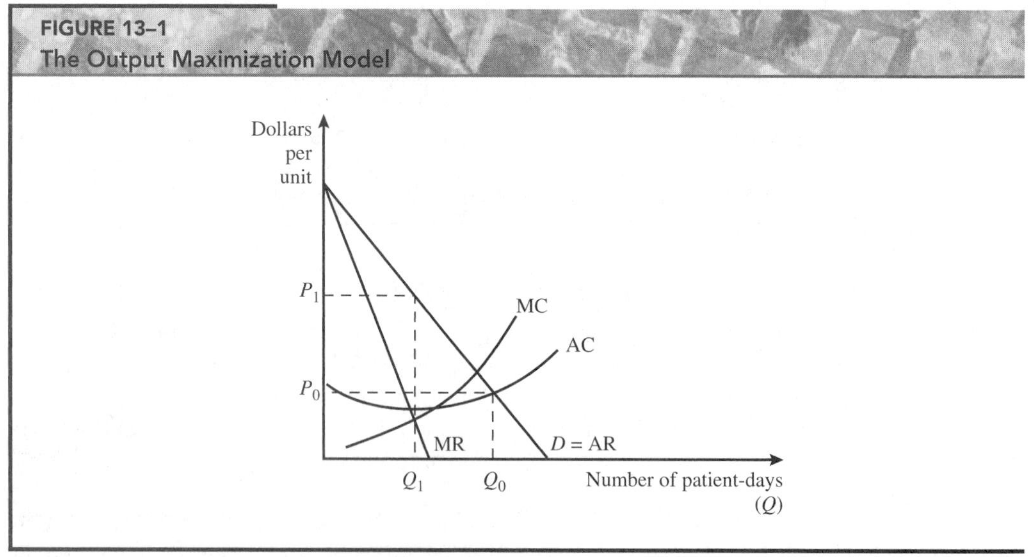

Suppose the typical not-for-profit hospital faces a downward-sloping demand curve and the usually shaped average and marginal cost curves and attempts to maximize the quantity of hospital services subject to a break-even constraint (P = AC). If so, the not-for-profit firm produces more services (Q_0) but charges a lower price (P_0) than an otherwise comparable for-profit hospital (P_1, Q_1).

net effect is that the hospital breaks even. In the process, however, the hospital services more patients through cross-subsidization.

The long-run implications of the model are interesting. In the long run, an output-maximizing hospital may generate some profits to acquire the funds it needs for expansion. It obtains the profits by charging a price that is slightly above the average cost of production. As a result, an output-maximizing hospital should not only provide more output than a profit-maximizing hospital at any point in time but should also have a higher rate of expansion over time.

The quantity maximization model can be used to explain the behavior of a not-for-profit organization. Since such a firm is restricted by law from distributing profits, managers may opt to maximize quantity to increase the firm's market share and enhance its prestige in the community. Economists have pointed out that the assumption of output maximization is consistent with the public's perception concerning how a not-for-profit hospital should operate (Newhouse, 1970). From the public's point of view, hospitals are given not-for-profit status because they are expected to provide care to some people in the community who otherwise might not receive care due to profit considerations. If the managers of a not-for-profit hospital maximize quantity, they validate the public's view that their firm plays an important role in the provision of health care to the community at large. That may make it much easier for the hospital to gather community support for such activities as fund-raising.

In the case of a quantity-maximizing not-for-profit hospital, the interests of the managers may also be aligned with the board of trustees, or board of directors, which oversees the general operation of the hospital. Board members, who generally are leading citizens, may also want to maximize quantity to increase their presence in the community. They may wish to be perceived as taking a leading role in the provision of health care to the community.

The quantity maximization model can also explain why in a given community there might be a certain degree of excess capacity in hospital services. A quantity-maximizing hospital may acquire an additional piece of medical equipment even if it does not generate a profit, provided it may attract a sufficient number of additional admittances. Such buying behavior may lead to a duplication of resources and overcapacity as each hospital expands its facility beyond the profit-maximizing point. The quantity maximization model, however, cannot explain why the cost of hospital services has been rising so rapidly over time in recent decades, because it offers only a static rather than a dynamic view of hospital behavior.[8] The other models, discussed next, set quality of services as an attainable goal. Because quality of services is heavily dependent on technology and because medical technology has changed dramatically over time, these models may provide a partial explanation for rising health care costs.

Quality Maximization. It has been argued that managers derive utility from the quality of hospital care provided. As you know, quality is difficult to measure but can appear in the structure, procedures, or outcomes of a medical care organization. For example, the quality of care is enhanced every time the hospital purchases new equipment, widens the spectrum of services to patients, or retains more specialists on staff. Any increase in the quality of care is also likely to drive up the cost of producing medical services.

Lee's (1971) model of hospital behavior is consistent with the quality maximization argument. The basic premise of the model is that managers of not-for-profit hospitals maximize utility by attempting to enhance the status, or prestige, of their institutions. Since status is defined to be positively related to the "range of services available and the extent to which expensive and

8. A static view analyzes behavior or performance at a point in time. Dynamic analysis considers behavior or performance over time.

highly specialized equipment and personnel (including M.D.'s) are available" (p. 49), the only way managers can achieve their goal is to maximize quality. This quest for status is the force driving the behavior of managers.

According to Lee's theory, the hospital has a desired level of status that it will attempt to achieve. The desired status depends on the mission of the hospital and the hospital's relative standing in the medical community. Because the actual level of status tends to be below the desired level, managers are constantly attempting to improve on status by increasing the quality of care. The hospital must provide the level of quality of care that is consistent with the desired level of status the managers are trying to achieve. For example, a large teaching hospital with a prestigious reputation is obligated to possess the most technologically sophisticated equipment and have a large number of specialists on staff because the managers view their organization as being on the forefront of medical development. In other words, the reputation and status of the hospital demand that it offers the highest-quality care. A small nonteaching hospital, on the other hand, will try to achieve a much more modest status level. The small nonteaching hospital will offer a quality of care below that of a larger hospital but on a par with hospitals of similar status.

Given a relatively inelastic demand for hospital services, managers can pursue a policy of quality maximization with little concern for costs. Any increase in the cost of hospital services associated with an enhancement in quality can be passed on to the payer through a higher price with minimal impact on output. The quest for status through quality maximization may provide one explanation for rising hospital costs in the years prior to managed care and the Medicare prospective payment system.

Because the physicians on staff at the hospital are also likely to receive utility from any increase in the quality of care, the interests of the managers and medical staff are likely to be aligned in this instance. As the hospital acquires more advanced medical inputs, physicians are given the opportunity to provide more varied and sophisticated medical treatment to their patients. The more sophisticated medical inputs may allow physicians on staff to expand their practices. In addition, the hospital is likely to find it easier to recruit and retain medical personnel if it improves the quality of care. The same argument may apply to the board of trustees. Board members may also receive utility from enhanced hospital status.

The quality maximization model suggests that new technology is diffused in a tiered fashion. Any new piece of equipment or medical technology is likely to be adopted first by the most status-conscious institutions, such as research and teaching hospitals. Their lofty status requires that research and teaching hospitals be on the cutting edge of medical technology. Hospitals of lesser status acquire the technology only after it has become a more accepted part of medical treatment and some of the hospitals in that status group have begun to acquire it. The implication is that most hospitals acquire new technology not because it is a prudent investment but because managers do not want to jeopardize the institution's status or relative standing in the medical community. Thus, new technology is acquired primarily for defensive purposes. The quality maximization model may explain why the hospital sector tends toward duplication of resources and overspecialization. Hospitals constantly attempt to expand services to enhance their status, not because profit maximization or efficiency calls for the expansion of services.

Quality and Quantity Maximization. Feldstein (1971) and Newhouse (1970) extend the quality maximization model by combining it with the quantity maximization model. According to Newhouse, management jointly determines the quantity and quality of output and produces the levels that maximize utility. Since any increase in quality comes at the expense of quantity, and vice versa, managers face an important trade-off and must jointly determine the optimal levels of quality and quantity to produce. Figure 13–2 illustrates this trade-off.

FIGURE 13–2
The Impact of Changes in Quality on Costs

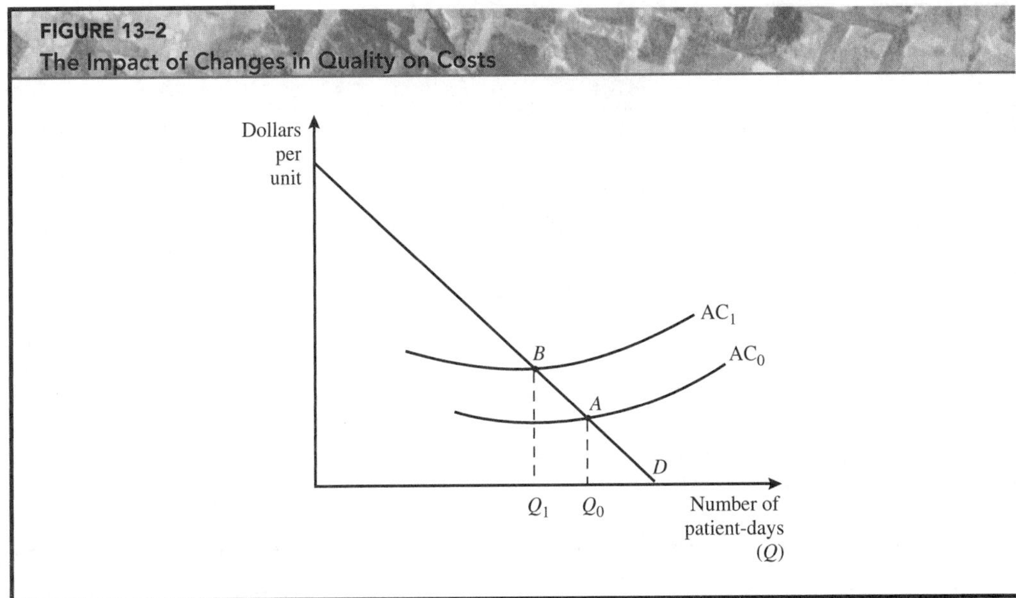

A not-for-profit hospital that chooses to produce with higher quality faces increased costs of AC_1. As a result, the hospital must produce fewer services (Q_1) when faced with a break-even constraint.

Given that quality can be enhanced only by increasing the cost of production (see Chapter 7), every time a hospital attempts to increase quality, its cost curves shift upward. This situation is depicted in Figure 13–2, where initially an output-maximizing hospital produces at point *A*. If management decides to increase quality, that decision causes the average cost curve to shift upward from AC_0 to AC_1. With no change in demand, the output-maximizing level of output equals Q_1 (point *B*), and the increase in quality is associated with a decrease in output. If quality is adjusted further, a trade-off curve between quality and quantity can be derived.[9] The trade-off curve appears in Figure 13–3. Points *A* and *B* on the graph correspond to points *A* and *B* in Figure 13–2. The curve is downward sloping, indicating the trade-off between the quality and quantity of medical care produced.

The quality/quantity maximization model indicates that the managers of not-for-profit hospitals face the dilemma of trying to maximize the level of services provided to the public while at the same time increasing the quality of care to improve the status of the hospital. Because a trade-off exists between the two, managers must choose that mixture of quantity and quality that maximizes their personal utility.

The Managerial Expense Preference Model. The final model discussed in this section is the managerial expense preference model (Williamson, 1963). The model was developed to explain the behavior of large firms that are not directly managed by major stockholders. The basic tenet

9. In all likelihood, any increase in quality will lead to an increase in the demand for hospital services. Consumers may be more willing to purchase medical services of higher quality at a higher price. This does not change the analysis, however, provided the increase in demand is relatively small. In terms of Figure 13–2, a trade-off between quantity and quality still exists if the AC curve shifts upward by more than the demand curve shifts to the right with any increase in quality.

FIGURE 13–3
The Quality/Quantity Maximization Model

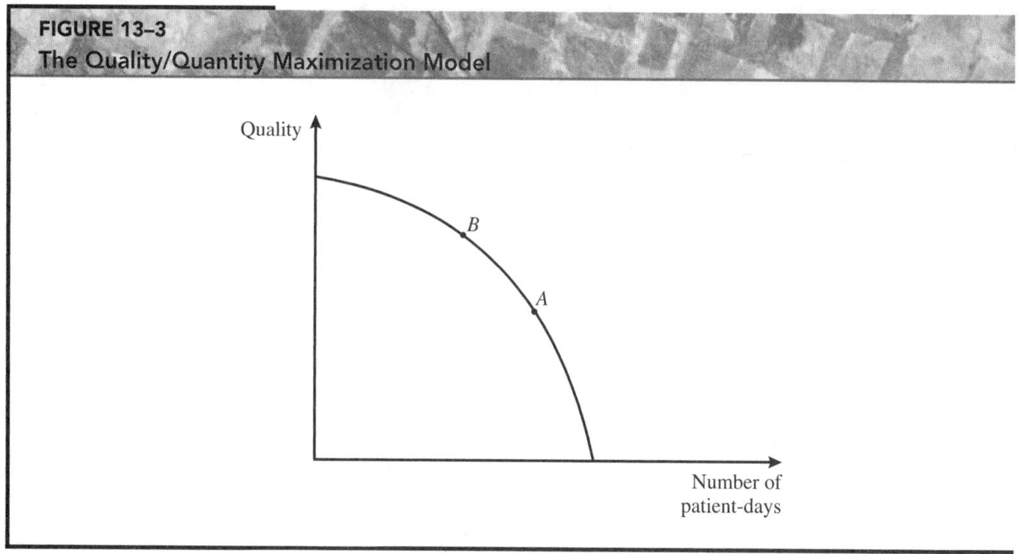

This figure shows the various combinations of quality and quantity of hospital services that can be produced given a fixed budget constraint. To maximize their utility and given the trade-off, decision makers at a not-for-profit hospital must choose a specific point such as *A* or *B*, given their preference weights for the two goods.

of the model is that managers use their authority to divert funds away from profits to serve their own self-interests—that is, to enhance their own utility. Among other things, the funds are used to pursue the five *P*s of increased pay, perquisites, power, prestige, and patronage. In a sense, managers absorb profits in the process of increasing their own utility by maximizing the amount of discretionary expenditures.

The ability of managers to provide stockholders with less than the maximum amount of profits stems from the existence of an asymmetry of information between the stockholders and the managers regarding firm performance. Stockholders do not always have the means to fully monitor activities of managers and ensure that they are providing the maximum amount of profits. Managers are afforded a certain amount of freedom to run the firm, provided stockholders receive what they consider an acceptable level of profits.

In the context of the model we have been working with, managerial expense preference behavior suggests that managers maximize discretionary expenditures by choosing the profit-maximizing level of output and price and then absorbing the profits through discretionary expenditures. The pursuit of discretionary expenditures can be treated as a kind of rent-seeking behavior because the manager is attempting to obtain a bigger slice of the pie for herself rather than trying to enlarge the size of the pie. Figure 13–4 illustrates this rent-seeking process. For simplicity's sake, assume marginal cost is constant and equals average cost. As such, the marginal and average cost curves are the same and horizontal and represented by MC_{true} in Figure 13–4. The MC_{true} curve reflects the true costs that exhibit production efficiency.

To maximize discretionary expenditures, the difference between revenue and the true cost of production, the firm follows the typical profit maximization rule, producing at the Q_0 level of output and charging P_0. However, instead of reflecting excess profits, the rectangle P_0AEC_{EXP} represents the amount of profits managers absorb as discretionary expenditures or income. In the process of enhancing their own utility, managers drive up the cost of production in the form of

FIGURE 13–4
The Managerial Expense Preference Model

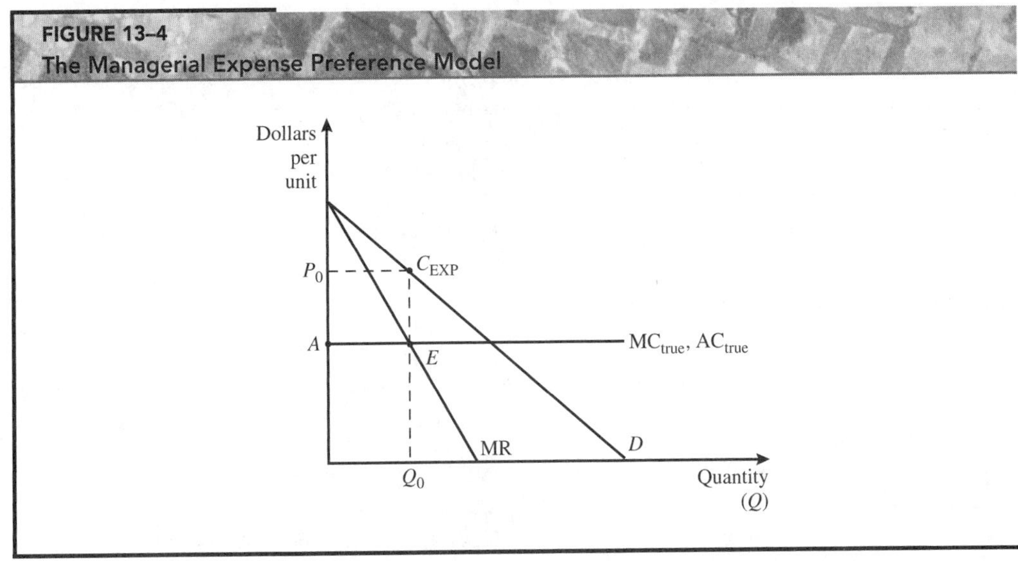

A not-for-profit hospital that maximizes discretionary profits will choose to produce at Q_0 where MR = MC just like an otherwise comparable for-profit hospital. The difference is that the not-for-profit hospital uses the discretionary profits to finance unnecessary expenditures and thereby raises the costs of production to C_{EXP}, a point above the true costs of production. The not-for-profit hospital reports the same price and quantity of services as the for-profit hospital but shows no economic profit.

discretionary expenditures. The point C_{EXP} represents the average cost of production after the expense preference behavior of managers has been taken into account. The vertical distance between points E and C_{EXP} (or that between A and P_0) represents the inefficiencies brought about by expense preference behavior.[10] The firm reports a normal profit rather than excess profits.

The managerial expense preference model has some interesting implications. The model suggests that managers consciously drive up the cost of production in an attempt to further their own self-interests. The model can also help explain the behavior of not-for-profit firms. Surprisingly, the expense preference model suggests that managers of not-for-profit firms act much like their counterparts at for-profit firms; that is, they maximize profits. The difference lies in the extent to which managers absorb profits as discretionary income. Since not-for-profit providers are prohibited by law from distributing profits to external parties, all the profits can be diverted by managers. As a result, we should observe not-for-profit firms having higher costs than for-profit firms that are closely controlled by profit-conscious owners, *ceteris paribus*. The cost differential reflects the wider latitude that not-for-profit managers are given to absorb profits. The fact that some of these profits are spent on additional personnel and equipment may help explain the duplication of resources in the health care sector.

In conclusion, utility maximization models have many positive attributes. First, they explain how firm behavior is affected when managers address their own utility functions rather than attempting to maximize profits. Behavior other than profit maximization is especially important to

10. In a different context, the inefficiency has been referred to as *X*-inefficiency. The inefficiency exists because managers of firms with some market power do not have the incentive to employ inputs efficiently. Inputs are either overemployed or are not used to their fullest potential. In addition, managers may pay input prices beyond the necessary amount.

address when we consider that a significant proportion of health care providers function in not-for-profit settings. Second, the models explain why the health care sector may tend toward duplication of resources and overspecialization, as in the case of the market for hospital services. Third, utility maximization models help explain why health care costs have increased over the years, at least until most recently. Managers who seek to advance their personal goals, such as maximizing the quality of output at the expense of profits, are not likely to be overly concerned with the impact any policy change may have on the financial "bottom line." A lack of concern for the bottom line naturally causes the cost of medical care to increase.

Inside the Black Box of the Hospital

We have introduced a number of economic models describing how the price and quantity of hospital services are determined in a not-for-profit setting based on various assumptions about the objectives of the ultimate decision maker. Harris (1977), however, criticizes these models for failing to capture the internal organization and institutional details of real-world hospitals and offers an alternative model. While his model is not designed to predict the price and quantity of hospital services, it does provide a rich and insightful description of the internal workings of actual hospitals with respect to economic decision making and resource allocation. To give you a flavor of his paper, we provide a brief synopsis. However, we strongly encourage you to read the entire article.

Harris treats the hospital as a firm designed to solve a complicated decision problem—the diagnosis and treatment of illness, which typically involves a "complicated sequence of adaptive responses in the face of uncertainty" (p. 469). He notes that when people become hospitalized they do not really buy the various inputs used during the hospitalization period but, instead, purchase a general guarantee to be given appropriate medical care. And because of the guarantee purchased, it becomes impossible to cease the delivery of care once some cost limit is achieved, especially because medical problems often have numerous idiosyncrasies and therefore each patient receives customized attention. Consequently, any hospital organization must have a certain amount of standby capacity.

Harris goes on to treat the hospital as a split organization resulting from an internal market composed of demanders and suppliers. On the supply side, administrators offer various ancillary services, such as pharmaceuticals, operating rooms, and blood banks, standing ready to deliver a particular medical input. On the demand side, various physicians decide which patients need which ancillary inputs and when.

An important consideration, as Harris notes, is that administration does not make patient care decisions and physicians do not hire the medical inputs. The separation is intended, however, because it eliminates the necessity of the physician to perform repeated cost calculations during an episode of care. The physician is supposed to do everything scientifically indicated for the welfare of his patient without reference to costs. The role of the administrator, however, is to manage the costs of the hospital but at the same time provide necessary inputs for the physician.

Harris relates his split organization theory of the hospital firm to the capacity problem hospitals often face. He recognizes that the medical staff and administration each have their own objectives and constraints. When excess capacity exists and resources are relatively abundant, the system seems to allocate resources reasonably well. However, when capacity limits are neared, physicians, "fearing they will lose access to necessary inputs, grab their own exclusive shares to keep themselves protected" (p. 476). Each physician engages in rent-seeking behavior vying for her own separate empire.

Another aspect of the capacity problem relates to the conflict between physicians and administrators. For the most part administrators want to keep the hospital full because revenues are greater. Physicians, however, desire excess capacity because it assures a continuous supply of resources and reflects higher levels of quality. Internal conflict emerges between physicians and administrators about the hospital's short-run policies regarding capacity. Because price does not serve as an allocation device within the hospital, nonprice methods must be used to allocate resources when capacity constraints exist, such as "loosely enforced standards, rules of thumb, side bargains, cajoling, negotiations, special contingency plans, and in some cases literally shouting and screaming" (p. 478). Physicians may also hedge against shortages by ordering inputs well in advance, or various groups of physicians may form exclusive clubs along clinical lines to better control their share of the hospital inputs. For example, orthopedic beds may become differentiated from general surgical beds and operating rooms may be held for specific uses.

Because conflict ensues when capacity constraints set in, physicians will want to expand capacity in the long run. Administration, on the other hand, will expand capacity only if the resulting beds are full. Physicians are faced with an incentive to expand utilization and increase quality to obtain their share. Administration, as a result, tolerates the creation and perpetuation of the separate clubs or empires even though it negates the risk reduction advantages of sharing resources within the hospital. Interestingly, this model, like the ones developed earlier, can be used to predict the widespread adoption and dispersion of new technologies in the past. Physicians embrace new technologies to expand capacity instead of replacing the existing capacity as a way of at least preserving their share of hospital resources and to improve quality. Indeed, the innovations may have little to do with reducing the intensity of resources used per illness episode and thereby raise the costs of providing medical care.

Market Concentration and Hospital Behavior

Another conduct issue of interest to economists concerns the impact of market concentration on the price, cost, and quality of hospital care. The issue is whether lower prices and higher levels of quality result in a market where output is concentrated among a few large firms or dispersed among a relatively large number of smaller firms. In hospital services markets characterized by insured consumers, not-for-profit entities, government-regulated prices, managed care organizations, and informational asymmetries, economic theory alone cannot predict the impact of increased concentration on societal welfare, so we must turn our attention to empirical studies on the relationship.

Economists investigating the impact of market concentration on hospital behavior tend to examine the periods before and after the mid-1980s. The mid-1980s acts as the cutoff because after that period prospective payment systems like the DRG system began to replace cost-based systems, the market share of for-profit hospital increased in many areas, and enrollments in MCOs started to explode. In simple terms, health care payers became more price conscious, and hospital competition changed from being patient driven to being payer driven (Dranove et al., 1993).

Studies using data prior to the mid-1980s found evidence to support a "medical arms race" among hospitals in more competitive areas (Robinson and Luft, 1985). According to the medical arms race hypothesis, hospitals in more competitive areas provide physicians with greater levels of hospital quality in the form of advanced medical technologies, excess bed capacity, and amenities in return for admitting their patients. The higher quality shows up as increased costs of producing hospital services. In support of the medical arms race hypothesis, many studies using data prior to the mid-1980s find empirical evidence linking increased competition (a lower value for the HHI) with increased hospital costs (Hersch, 1984; Robinson and Luft, 1985; White,

1987; Noether, 1988; Fournier and Mitchell, 1992), lower levels of technical efficiency (Wilson and Jadlow, 1982), greater excess bed capacity (Joskow, 1980; Farley, 1985), and a larger number of duplicate specialized services in local markets (Dranove et al., 1992; Farley, 1985).

Beginning after the mid-1980s with heightened payer-driven competition, empirical studies no longer find support for the medical arms race. The earliest studies find that after the mid-1980s increased competition had no impact on hospital costs (Zwanziger and Melnick, 1988), lowered the hospital inflation rate (Robinson and Phibbs, 1990), or increased costs of not-for-profit hospitals but not the costs of public and for-profit hospitals (Santerre and Bennett, 1992). Studies using more recent data uncover even stronger evidence in support of payer-driven competition. For example, using data for 1987, Melnick et al. (1992) determine that more hospital competition resulted in a lower Blue Cross PPO negotiated price for hospital services in California. Further studies using data after 1990 find that increased hospital competition improves technical efficiency (Rosko, 2001), reduces excess capacity (Santerre and Adams, 2002), lowers hospital prices (Town and Vistnes, 2001) and hospital costs, and results in lower rates of adverse outcomes (Kessler and McClellan, 2000).

By analyzing the impact of hospital consolidations during the 1990s, we can obtain further information about the effects of market structure on hospital prices, costs, and quality of care. Recall from Chapter 9 that hospital consolidations can have procompetitive or anticompetitive impacts on consumer welfare. Using the estimated parameters from their empirical model determining HMO negotiated prices with hospitals during the period 1990–1993, Town and Vistnes (2001) simulate hospital mergers in the Los Angeles region, where competition is relatively fierce, and find that a significant number of the simulated mergers led to predicted price increases in excess of 5 percent.

Spang et al. (2001) analyzed changes in cost and prices from 1989 to 1997 for merging and nonmerging rival hospitals in various metropolitan statistical areas of the United States. The authors find that consolidating hospitals generally had lower growth in costs and prices compared with their rivals but find the cost savings to be very modest and nearly identical price growth in markets with high HMO penetration rates.

Dranove and Lindrooth (2003) take the analysis on consolidations a step further by distinguishing between hospital acquisitions and mergers. In the case of an acquisition, two hospitals become commonly owned within the same system but have separate licenses for reporting and regulatory purposes. Acquisitions involve hospitals in different areas so clinical consolidations do not take place. In contrast, hospital mergers involve the combination of separate facility licenses into a single license. The merged organization issues a single financial or utilization report and is regulated as a single entity for CON and other purposes. Hospitals that merge together are generally in close geographical proximity and therefore may gain from reorganization and clinical consolidations.

Dranove and Lindrooth compare the costs of real hospital consolidations to equivalent hypothetical consolidations from one year prior to the consolidation to four years after the consolidation. The hypothetical consolidations reflect hospitals that did not combine but had similar characteristics to those that actually did combine over the same period. These researchers use national data for independent hospitals that consolidated some time during 1989–1996. They find that consolidation into systems does not generate savings even after four years. Mergers, in contrast, result in savings for two or more years after consolidation. Dranove and Lindrooth argue that system consolidations do "not yield synergistic cost savings, perhaps reflecting the difficulty of achieving efficiencies without combining operations. An actual merger is a big step, requiring giving up a license (with the high cost of going back) and usually a CEO. Hospitals do not merge unless they could confidently pull it off" (p. 996).

But are the cost savings from mergers passed on to the buyers of hospital care? To answer that question, Capps and Dranove (2004) examine the before and after effects of hospital consolidations on actual negotiated PPO prices in four market areas of the United States during the period 1997–2001. The results of their multiple regression analysis, which controls for quality of care, patient case-mix, and other factors, suggest that most consolidating hospitals raise price by more than the median price increase in their markets. Overall, they report that their findings do not support the argument that efficiencies from consolidations among competing hospitals lead to lower prices. Rather, their results are broadly consistent with consolidations among competing hospitals leading to higher prices because of enhanced market power.

The empirical literature concerning the impact of hospital consolidations on the quality of care is less extensive. Ho and Hamilton (2000) compare the quality of medical care before and after hospital mergers and acquisitions in California between 1992 and 1995. They determine empirically that consolidation has no measurable impact on the inpatient mortality of heart attack and stroke patients but find some evidence linking consolidation to higher hospital readmission rates and early discharges. Cuellar and Gertler (2005) use a national panel data set of hospitals over the period 1995–2000 to study the effect of consolidation on three types of quality: (1) rates of inpatient mortality following certain hospital conditions and procedures; (2) rates of procedures considered overused; and (3) patient safety indicators. They find that rates of avoidable inpatient mortality and inadequate safety did not change after consolidation for either indemnity or managed care patients. However, for managed care patients, consolidation did reduce the rate of overutilized procedures. Thus, the few existing studies do not find evidence suggesting that hospital consolidation significantly improves the quality of care.

Without a doubt, the hospital services industry has undergone a tremendous economic transformation over the last 20 years. Most important, payer-driven competition has replaced patient-driven competition and, as a result, the degree of price competition among hospitals has greatly intensified. From this brief review of the literature it appears that hospitals are now forced to consider the cost implications of many of their decisions in competitive areas. If society values low hospital prices for a given level of quality, available evidence for the most part suggests that competition among hospitals has the ability to improve consumer welfare.

Hospital Ownership and Hospital Behavior

Recall that property rights theory argues that for-profit hospitals behave differently from not-for-profit hospitals because the latter face a nondistribution constraint. That is, it is illegal for a not-for-profit hospital to distribute any residual of revenues over costs, which represent profits to a for-profit hospital, to outside parties. The residual must be retained and used to support the purpose for which the not-for-profit hospital was formed. For example, the residual might be used to expand the facilities of the hospital, purchase new equipment, or pay for the hospital care of indigent individuals.

Because of the nondistribution constraint, it is sometimes argued that not-for-profit and government hospitals face less of an incentive than for-profit hospitals to behave efficiently because of the absence of outside owners or residual claimants who face a strong, direct financial incentive to monitor activities and who are able to discipline management when deviations from cost minimization occur. Thus the property rights theory suggests that not-for-profit hospitals may operate with higher costs than otherwise similar for-profit hospitals, as the previously discussed expense preference model predicts.

Also, public choice theorists point out that public hospitals lack a further incentive to minimize the cost of production. Unlike private hospitals (both for-profit and not-for-profit), public hospitals can rely to some extent on direct funding from the government in addition to patient-driven revenues. As a result, public hospitals are not at the complete mercy of the marketplace to minimize costs, unlike private hospitals. Keep in mind, however, that public hospitals are typically monitored directly by elected or appointed committees and those participating on the committees may wish to be reelected or reappointed to their positions. The threat of losing their position on the committee may give them a stakeholder (rather than stockholder) interest in the efficient operation of the hospital. If so, one type of incentive system and disciplining mechanism simply replaces the other.

Property rights theory also suggests that the quality of care might be lower in for-profit hospitals than otherwise similar not-for-profit and public hospitals. To make greater profits, for-profit hospitals may face an incentive to skimp or cut corners on quality, especially quality of care that cannot be easily monitored by outside individuals. In contrast, not-for-profit hospitals, because of the attenuation of property rights, face less of an incentive to sacrifice quality for the sake of profits. This would be particularly true for situations where quality of care enters the utility function of the managers running the not-for-profit hospitals.

Given the theoretical discussion, it should not be too surprising that a relatively large amount of research has examined whether ownership status affects price, costs, and quality of care. Studies tend not to find any systematically large efficiency differences across hospitals with different ownership types. The cost differences that are sometimes observed can usually be explained by unmeasurable variations in quality. Although for-profit hospitals tend to charge higher prices, the price differences can often be explained by the fact that not-for-profit hospitals do not pay most taxes, borrow at lower interest rates because interest on their bonds is tax exempt, and receive donations from outside parties.[11]

There are other explanations for the cost and price similarity. Sloan (1988) argues that physicians on the medical staff may act as residual claimants in not-for-profit hospitals and thus "have a financial stake in keeping such hospitals efficient. Inefficient hospitals are candidates for acquisition by for-profit hospitals" (p. 138). Pauly (1987) claims there is little theoretical justification to assert that not-for-profit hospitals do not minimize production costs. Consider a not-for-profit hospital that maximizes output. Although the managers are not maximizing profits, they still face an incentive to produce output as cheaply as possible. An incentive to minimize costs exists because more output can be produced from a given budget if managers keep per-unit costs to a minimum. The similarity of outcomes may also be explained by the fact that hospitals, regardless of ownership, are actually organized as physician cooperatives with the (for-profit) objective of maximizing the combined incomes of staff physicians (Pauly and Redish, 1973). Finally, various analysts note that market competition forces hospitals of all ownership forms to produce as cheaply as possible and charge reasonable prices. High-cost, high priced hospitals do not survive in competitive markets.

Economists have conducted much less research on quality-of-care differences across hospitals of different ownership types.[12] Representative of the few conducted, in terms of the empirical results, Sloan et al. (2001) compare probability of death at one month, six months, and one year following admission into public, for-profit, and not-for-profit hospitals. The authors use patient data drawn from the National Long Term Care Survey for various years from 1982 to 1994.

11. But see Sloan et al. (2001), who find that payments on behalf of Medicare patients admitted to for-profit hospitals during the first six months following a health shock were higher than those admitted to not-for-profit and public hospitals. They argue that the higher payment to for-profits "plausibly reflects their greater incentive to maximize reimbursements from payers by various means including formal and informal contractual relationships with other suppliers of health care services" (p. 18).

12. See Sloan (2000) for a review of the other studies.

Individuals selected for analysis were admitted to the hospital with primary diagnoses of hip fracture, stroke, coronary heart disease, or congestive heart failure. After holding constant other determinants of mortality, the authors find no discernible difference in mortality rates between hospitals with different ownership forms.

While costs, prices, and quality of care tend to be reasonably similar across differently owned hospitals, most studies find that public hospitals are much more likely to provide greater amounts of uncompensated care. Uncompensated care is usually defined as bad debts and charity and is measured as a percent of total hospital expenses. As evidence, Mann et al. (1997) estimate that uncompensated care as a percentage of expenses was 15.4 and 6.3 percent for urban public and rural public hospitals, respectively, in 1994. The comparable figures for not-for-profit and for-profit were 5.0 and 4.2 percent, respectively. Not surprisingly, public hospitals have been dubbed the "hospital provider of last resort" or "safety net" because of their charitable nature. In fact, one study finds that private hospitals provide less uncompensated care when a public general hospital exists in the area (Thorpe and Brecher, 1987).

These figures on uncompensated care help motivate two other interesting questions. First, why do for-profit hospitals provide any uncompensated care? Supposedly, the business of for-profit hospitals is business and therefore the maximization of profits or stockholder wealth. Providing care to the indigent subtracts from maximum profits and reduces the return to owners. However, Herzlinger and Krasker (1987) point out that for-profit hospitals may provide some uncompensated care because "hospital costs are mostly fixed and the marginal costs of an additional patient day, generally low. Even an indigent patient contributes somewhat to covering the hospital's fixed costs" (p. 103). In addition, providing uncompensated care may favorably impact a for-profit hospital's relationship with regulatory agencies and the community at large.

The second question deals with not-for-profit hospitals. One reason not-for-profit hospitals are granted tax-exempt status is because they are supposed to apply any unused revenues (or profits) toward the express purpose for which they were formed. Not-for-profit hospitals are formed to provide medical care to the sick and needy and are responsible to the community at large. Therefore, not-for-profit hospitals are expected to provide charitable care. The fact that their uncompensated care is only 5 percent of expenses and quite close to that of for-profit hospitals raises the question whether the tax-exempt status of not-for-profit hospitals should be revoked. In fact, state and local governments in Texas, Pennsylvania, and Utah, among others, have introduced legislation intended to pressure not-for-profit hospitals into providing more charity care. Not-for-profit hospitals would be required to prove that they benefit their areas or lose their tax exemption (Lutz, 1993). Morrisey et al. (1996) demonstrate that the concern about the tax-exempt status of not-for-profit hospitals may be warranted. Using 1988 and 1991 data for 189 not-for-profit hospitals in California, they compare the amount of uncompensated care to the estimated tax subsidy that each not-for-profit hospital receives. While not as widespread as commonly believed, the researchers find that nearly 20 percent of all not-for-profit hospitals do not provide uncompensated care sufficient to compensate for the tax subsidies they receive.

Taking the analysis a step further, Nicholson et al. (2000) argue that the dollar value of the tax exemption to not-for-profit hospitals should be compared to total community benefits rather than to the value of uncompensated care. Since not-for-profit hospitals do not have to return profits to residual claimants as for-profits do, the authors note that not-for-profits should be expected to provide community benefits equal to those provided by for-profit hospitals plus the profits these hospitals earn. Based on data for the three largest for-profit hospital systems over the period 1996–1998, they find that community benefits (taxes plus estimated cost of uncompensated care) and profits as a percentage of equity and assets equaled 30 and 10 percent, respectively. When applied to the equity and assets of an average not-for-profit hospital, these percentages imply that a not-for-profit would be expected to spend $9.1 to $13.2 million on community benefits per year, yet uncompensated care accounts for only about $3.3 million. Even after accounting for a host of other public benefits the typical not-for-profit might provide, such as subsidized medical research and price discounts, the authors write that "not-for-profit hospitals appear to fall far short of providing the expected level of community benefit that would justify current levels of investment" (p. 176).

Managed-Care Buyers and Hospital Behavior

Another interesting aspect of hospital conduct is the relation between managed care institutions, such as HMOs, PPOs, and utilization review organizations, and hospital behavior. The question is whether managed care provides the proper incentives for efficiency without seriously sacrificing quality. Most of the research on the relation between MCOs and hospital behavior has examined the effect of HMOs on hospital costs, utilization rates, or the quality of health outcomes. In general, studies suggest that HMO hospitalization rates are about 15 to 20 percent lower than those of traditional insurance plans after controlling for a host of health-related factors, including ages of the patients, case-mix, severity of illnesses, and hospital-specific influences (Luft, 1981; Manning et al., 1984; Dowd et al., 1991; Miller and Luft, 1994). Moreover, studies imply that the lower hospitalization rates tend to hold for both staff and IPA/HMOs (Dowd et al., 1991; Bradbury et al., 1991). Even among intensive care patients, a setting that appears to allow very little room for discretion in treatment decisions, some evidence indicates that managed care results in cost savings when compared to traditional insurance (Rapoport et al., 1992).

Another line of research investigates the effect of MCOs on the degree of technical inefficiency practiced by hospitals. Technical inefficiency occurs when hospitals use more inputs than technically necessary to produce their products, such as inpatient and outpatient care, or fail to produce the maximum amount of products with a given amount of inputs. As mentioned previously, MCOs are supposed to emphasize cost-effective methods of production and use various management strategies and financial incentives to align health care provider interests, such as hospitals, with technical efficiency. Assuming hospitals otherwise face some organizational slack, these cost-effective practices and strategies of MCOs are expected to improve technical efficiency.

Rosko (2001) examines the impact of HMO penetration on technical inefficiency using a national sample of nearly 2,000 urban hospitals in 1997. Rosko finds empirically that increased HMO penetration is associated with less technical inefficiency at the hospital level. Brown (2003) examines the effects of enrollments in both HMOs and preferred provider organizations (PPOs) on technical inefficiency using a production function approach and a panel data set of 613 hospitals over the five-year period from 1992 to 1996. Brown shows overall that greater enrollment in both HMOs and PPOs is associated with increased hospital efficiency at the margin.

Finally, Bates et al. (forthcoming) use a production function format and a national sample of 306 metropolitan hospital services industries in 1999. They find evidence of increased technical efficiency at the industry level in states characterized by more HMO activity and increased health insurer concentration. Taken together, these three studies suggest that greater pressure from HMOs improves the degree of technical efficiency experienced by hospitals.

Research also indicates that inpatient outcomes are not systematically worse (Retchin et al., 1992; Retchin and Brown, 1991; Carlisle et al., 1992; Miller and Luft, 1994; Miller and Luft, 2002) for HMOs compared to traditional insurance coverage, although some disagreement remains about the care of low-income patients in HMOs (compare Ware et al. [1986] and Greenwald and Henke [1992]). Most studies do report worse results on many measures of access to care and lower levels of satisfaction for HMO enrollees (Miller and Luft, 2002). The relatively comparable level of quality has surprised some critics of HMOs because they suspected that the scope and mission of these institutions creates an incentive for an underproduction of care. A number of empirical and theoretical factors may account for the quality-of-care similarity in MCO and non-MCO plans. First, empirically it is very difficult to distinguish among health plans in practice, especially when health insurers have multiple plans and health care providers treat patients belonging to a number of alternative plans. Quality of care may appear similar because the observations are wrongly assigned into MCO and non-MCO plans.

Second, some MCOs are structured as not-for-profit institutions. For example, 42 percent of all HMO enrollees received their care from organizations that were structured as not-for-profit in 1994 (Corrigan et al., 1997). Many researchers argue that not-for-profit institutions pursue goals other than profit maximization, as we discussed earlier in this chapter. If not-for-profit MCOs attempt to maximize some other objective rather than the "bottom line," it is not theoretically apparent why the quality of care in those MCOs should differ from that of traditional indemnity insurers.

Third, like traditional plans, MCOs often invest huge sums of money establishing brand names that can be tarnished by offering inferior care. The prospect of losing repeat buyers and not receiving a proper return on investment can place a considerable amount of pressure on MCOs to provide the proper level of care. Of course, well-informed consumers are necessary for that kind of pressure to materialize. In this regard, it would be interesting to know whether the constant attention given MCOs in the popular press and political arena has had any effect on the behavior and performance of MCOs.

Fourth, physicians that contract with MCOs very likely subscribe to the same basic ethical code of conduct (such as the Hippocratic Oath) as the doctors that deal with traditional insurers. In fact, many physicians simultaneously contract with both types of insurers. Although doctors may find themselves pressured by the financial incentives and management strategies of MCOs at the margin, it is not clear theoretically whether these pressures dominate over ethical concerns, on average.

In contrast to HMOs, only a few studies assess the effect of PPOs on hospital utilization rates and expenditures. They fail to reach a consensus on the *overall* cost-containment effectiveness of PPOs. While Zwanziger and Auerbach (1991) report that PPOs lead to a reduction in inpatient expenditures, the increased expenditures stemming from expansions in outpatient benefits tend to swamp these cost savings (Hester et al., 1987; Garnick et al., 1990; Diehr et al., 1990).[13] According to Fielding and Rice (1993), PPOs are ineffective in controlling overall costs because the typical participating physician has only eleven enrollees from a particular PPO. Consequently, an individual PPO has limited ability to exert any buyer power over the prices and utilization practices of physicians.

Another aspect of managed care is utilization review (UR).[14] According to Ermann (1988), UR "programs seek to determine whether specific services are medically necessary and whether they are delivered at an appropriate level of intensity and cost" (p. 683). Utilization management began in 1972 in the public sector when the federal government established professional standards review organizations (PSROs) to provide UR services for Medicare and Medicaid patients as a result of the concern over unnecessary and low-quality care. However, the PSROs proved to

13. But see Smith (1997/1998), who finds that, on average, PPOs were associated with cost savings of 12 percent per covered life as compared to traditional plans with utilization review. The cost savings result primarily from lower rates of physician visits and hospital admissions.

14. The following discussion borrows heavily from Bailit and Sennett (1991).

be ineffective. For example, the Congressional Budget Office (1981) reports that "for every dollar spent on PSRO review of Medicare patients, only $.40 in resources were recouped, for a net loss of $.60" (p. xiii). As a result, PSROs were terminated in 1982 and, in the following year, replaced by peer review organizations (PROs). PROs are regionally based organizations that compete for government contracts and are responsible for ensuring the quality of services and eliminating unnecessary care through UR.

The first privately sponsored UR programs began in the mid-1960s and focused on hospital utilization. Private UR programs covered very few employees until the middle to late 1980s, but over the last ten years the UR industry has developed rapidly, covering about 90 percent of individuals with private medical insurance. In addition to large national commercial health insurers, such as Aetna, and HMO companies that provide a full spectrum of managed care services, about two hundred companies offer only UR services. Some of these companies are national in scope, but most are regionally or locally based. These companies usually specialize in one area of UR (such as medical and surgical or psychiatric and substance abuse); thus, it is not unusual for an employer to contract simultaneously with several UR companies.

There are three types of UR services, based on time of review. **Prospective** UR addresses the necessity of hospital care while it is still being planned and consequently has the capacity to change or avert planned treatments. Prior authorization and second opinions are examples of prospective UR. **Concurrent** review programs focus on the necessity of continual care for patients and thus intervenes to change planned treatments. For hospitalized patients, review organizations monitor by telephone or through onsite nurses to determine whether patients need certain types of hospital-level care. Finally, **retrospective** programs review care after the fact from records and claims that have little potential to directly affect care provided to patients, except by altering the practice patterns of providers that face retrospective denial of reimbursement.

Although studies on the effectiveness of private UR services in containing hospital costs are relatively limited, the available literature indicates that hospital admissions and length-of-stay prospective review programs have led to a significant reduction in beds per 1,000 employees. In addition, a few studies of hospital review programs report net total health care savings of 4.5 to 8 percent at the individual plan level (for example, Feldstein et al., 1988). Likewise, at the system level, Schwartz and Mendelson (1991) claim that UR programs were associated with a significant reduction in the rate of hospital costs during the 1980s. No evidence yet exists on the relation between UR services and the quality of patient care.

In sum, research has shown that HMOs, PPOs, and UR can contain inpatient hospital costs to some degree. Research further indicates that HMOs contain inpatient care costs without seriously sacrificing health care quality, but timely access and consumer satisfaction remain concerns. Evidence on the quality implications of PPOs and UR programs is unavailable. The ability of PPOs to contain *overall* health care costs appears to be limited due to the small number of PPO patients assigned to the typical physician.

Price Regulations and Hospital Behavior[15]

Public policies may also affect the conduct of hospitals. In 1972, Congress passed Section 222 of the Social Security Amendments, giving states the authority to establish rate-setting programs. By the late 1970s, more than 30 states had adopted some form of hospital rate-setting program (Coelen and Sullivan, 1981). However, only three of the states had a mandatory "all-payer" program that controlled rates for all patient groups, including private payers, commercially insured

15. The following discussion is based largely on Anderson (1991).

patients, patients with public insurance, and Blue Cross plans. By 1996 only one state, Maryland, still had an all-payer rate-setting program.

Proponents of rate-setting programs have argued that these programs can contain health care costs with no concomitant reduction in the quality of care because they view hospitals as operating with organizational slack. The organizational slack, taking form in such factors as higher than necessary hospital salaries, duplication of facilities, and unnecessary hospital amenities, results from imperfect markets or hospital objectives other than cost minimization. When slack is present, price regulations or ceilings may promote lower expenditures without an associated reduction in patient care.

Empirical studies have almost unanimously supported the view that state regulation of hospital fees can lower health care costs. For example, Lanning et al. (1991), whose study correctly controlled for the endogenous nature of state programs, find that states with mature rate-setting programs have 14.6 percent lower per capita health care expenditures than otherwise comparable states without such policies.[16] The reduction in medical costs includes both hospital and nonhospital expenditures, which tends to refute the hypothesis of Morrisey et al. (1984) that rate setting results in an unbundling of services. *Unbundling* refers to the practice whereby decision makers shift the production of services from the regulated (hospital) to the unregulated (physician) sector in response to rate setting.

More recently, Schneider (2003) investigates the impact of mandatory rate regulation on hospital costs over the period 1980–1996. Specifically, he estimates a cost function for a panel of 1,144 hospitals that are located in either regulated or unregulated states and controls for different types of outputs (such as Medicare and Medicaid), average length of stay, input prices, and various hospital organizational and market characteristics. Schneider finds lower hospital operating costs in states with all payer price regulations but that the effect of rate regulation on hospital costs tended to decline after 1991. He points out that rate regulation may have accomplished its cost-control objective in the early years but the gains were not sustainable over time. At the same time, he discovers that hospitals in more concentrated markets tend to have increasingly higher operating costs over time. Overall, Schneider's results indicate "that the opportunity costs of hospital rate regulation increased as the cost-control effects of regulation lessened and the cost-control effects of a feasible organizational alternative—competitive contracting—increased" (p. 310). As a result, many states abandoned their rate regulation programs and turned to managed care as a method of controlling hospital costs in the 1990s.

The findings of empirical studies focusing on the relation between rate setting and quality of care have been mixed, however. For example, Shortell and Hughes (1988) find a strong association between the stringency of state rate review programs and higher mortality rates among inpatients after holding other determinants of health status constant. Gaumer et al. (1989) report a small adverse impact of the presence of rate-setting policies on mortality at the national level but inconsistent effects at the individual state level and no effect of program stringency on mortality. Conversely, a study by Smith et al. (1993) indicates that regulated states had lower mortality rates among Medicare beneficiaries than unregulated states. Finally, a RAND study (for example, Kahn et al., 1990; Draper et al., 1990) concludes that the Medicare PPS, which can be considered a federal rate-setting program, has contained hospital costs without generally lowering the quality of care for Medicare patients. However, a comparable study by Fitzgerald et al. (1988) finds that the overall care for Medicare patients with hip fracture has worsened since the

16. But see Antel et al. (1995). Earlier studies that did not control for the endogeneity of rate setting suggest that the percentage effect is much smaller, at about 2.0 to 4.1 percentage points (see Morrisey et al., 1984). Some empirical evidence (for example, Romeo et al., 1984) has also linked states' prospective payment systems to a slower diffusion of new medical technologies, although the results are too limited to generalize.

implementation of PPS. Clearly, more studies are needed before we can make any generalizations about the relation between government rate-setting programs and the quality of care.

Cost Shifting Behavior

Because the federal government and various state governments are responsible for setting (rather than negotiating) reimbursement rates under the Medicare and Medicaid programs, some individuals believe that lower reimbursement rates for these public programs lead to higher prices paid by private payers. This practice is referred to as **cost shifting**. Ginsburg (2003) defines cost shifting "as the phenomenon in which changes in administered prices of one payer lead to compensating changes in prices charged to other payers" (p. 473). For example, hospitals raising prices paid by commercial insurers in response to a Medicare payment reduction provides an example of cost shifting.

Not all policy analysts, particularly economists, are convinced that cost shifting actually takes place. That's because private prices are normally set to maximize economic profits. As a result, raising private prices in response to public price cuts produces even lower profits because the quantity demanded for medical services falls as prices increases. The theory behind this view is provided in Figure 13–5. In the figure, the private-pay and public-pay submarkets of a

FIGURE 13–5
Analysis of Hospital Cost Shifting

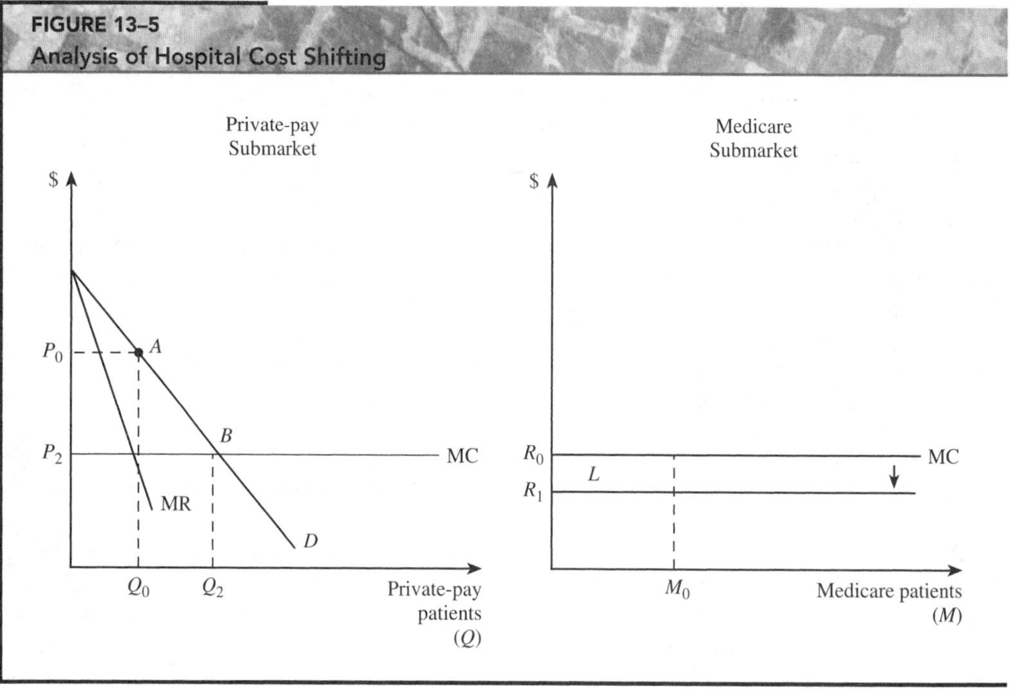

Suppose the two submarkets are in an initial equilibrium represented by R_0, the Medicare reimbursement rate, and point *A*. The latter point reflects that the hospital is initially operating at the profit-maximizing number of private-pay patients. If the government lowers the Medicare reimbursement rate to R_1, the hospital will not raise private price to finance the Medicare loss, *L*, because price is already at the profit-maximizing level in the private submarket. Hence cost shifting does not occur in this case. However, if the hospital is initially operating with some unexploited market power, as at point *B*, where the number of private-pay patients is maximized (rather than profits), hospitals may raise price in response to the Medicare loss. Thus cost shifting can occur. The ability to raise price in this case depends on the magnitude of the price elasticity of demand.

local hospital industry are shown. For simplicity, we suppose that only Medicare patients constitute the public pay category and the marginal (and average) costs, MC, are constant and the same for treating both private-pay and Medicare patients.

In the graphical model on the right, the hospital is treated as a price taker with respect to Medicare patients. It is supposed that the federal government initially sets the fixed administered price, R_0, equal to the marginal costs of treating Medicare patients. The hospital is assumed to treat M_0 Medicare patients during the period. The graph on the left shows the initial equilibrium in the private-pay submarket (before cost shifting presumably takes place). It is assumed that the hospital has (or hospitals collectively have) some degree of market power, as reflected in the downward-sloping demand curve, D. It is further assumed (initially) that the hospital maximizes economic profits. As a result, the hospital treats the number of patients indicated by Q_0 where marginal revenue, MR, equals marginal cost, MC, and charges a price of P_0. Equilibrium in the private-pay submarket is thus represented by point A.

Now suppose the federal government lowers the Medicare reimbursement rate from R_0 to R_1 in the hopes of containing costs. Notice that when the Medicare payment rate declines to R_1, the hospital suffers a loss, L, equal to the rectangular area formed by the difference in per-unit costs and the reimbursement rate and bounded by the number of Medicare patients treated.[17] It is this loss that the hospital may prefer to shift elsewhere. But notice that the hospital faces no incentive to raise price for private payers because profits have already been maximized. That's because a price above P_0 results in fewer private patients treated and lower profits because MR $>$ MC. Hence cost shifting is irrational under this situation.

To successfully practice cost shifting, Morrisey (2003) explains that hospitals must "have market power that heretofore [they] had not exploited." He goes on to note, "If providers have market power and, indeed, have not charged private insurers "what the traffic will bear," then cost shifting can exist—even as a matter of theory" (p. 490). The downward-sloping private-pay demand curve in Figure 13–5 fulfills the first condition that the hospital possesses market power. Now rather than maximizing economic profits, assume that the hospital, as a not-for-profit organization, maximizes the number of patients treated subject to a break-even level of profits. As we saw earlier in this chapter, maximizing an objective other than profits is consistent with the view that not-for-profit organizations face a nondistribution constraint and cannot legally distribute any excess earnings to residual claimants. Maximization of the number of patients is also consistent with the view that not-for-profit hospital administrators and board members may derive personal utility from directing large enterprises.

Point B represents the equilibrium at which the hospital maximizes the number of patients treated subject to a break-even level of profits and therefore initially operates with some unexploited market power. In this case, the hospital treats Q_2 private-pay patients where demand intersects marginal cost and charges a price of P_2. Notice that at Q_2, the chosen number of patients exceeds the number that maximizes economic profits where marginal revenue, MR, equals marginal costs. At point B, the hospital initially earns a normal profit on both private-pay and Medicare patients.

Now suppose the government lowers the Medicare reimbursement rate from R_0 to R_1. In this case, because the hospital initially operates with some unexploited market power, it might respond to the lower Medicare reimbursement rate by raising price above P_2 but not greater than P_0, the price that maximizes profits. It follows theoretically that cost shifting can take place if hospitals initially operate with some amount of unexploited market power.

17. However, we cannot rule out the possibility that hospitals respond to the lower Medicare reimbursement rate by releasing Medicare patients quicker and sicker or by dumping these patients onto other hospitals (although this practice is illegal).

Curious about the degree to which the practice actually occurs in the United States, researchers have subjected the theory of cost shifting to empirical testing. At best, the empirical evidence regarding hospital cost shifting behavior has been mixed. Two papers by Hadley and Feder (1985) and Zwanziger et al. (2000) attest to the ongoing nature of the cost shifting discussion (from 1985 to 2000) and the general inconclusiveness of the empirical findings. Specifically, Hadley and Feder compare 128 private not-for-profit community hospitals in the early 1980s and found that hospital markups on private payers did not vary systematically with revenue pressure in the United States. Instead, hospitals responded to revenue pressure by taking several actions to reduce costs, including reducing personnel, postponing employee pay increases, and limiting charity care. Zwanziger et al. use California data for 1983–1991 and find empirically that both for-profit and not-for-profit hospitals increased private pay prices in response to Medicare payment rate reductions.[18]

Thus economic theory suggests that hospital cost shifting can take place under certain limited conditions, and at least some empirical evidence suggests that it may have occurred in practice. We must remember, however, that hospitals can engage in cost shifting behavior only when they possess a sufficient amount of market power. That is, hospitals must be able to raise price above the competitive level when confronted with losses from treating public-pay patients. When private buyers of medical services, such as individual managed care organizations, also possess market power on the demand side of the market, hospitals may be unable to negotiate higher prices. Thus many economists believe that cost shifting is less likely to occur in today's health economy because the buying clout of many managed care organizations. In fact, Lagnado (2003) points out that hospitals now rank among America's most aggressive debt collectors, as they put pressure on the poor and uninsured to pay their bills. Hospitals would simply raise private-pay prices rather than aggressively collect debts if they could easily shift costs.

Integrated Delivery Systems

As mentioned in Chapter 12, the autonomous, solo-physician clinic, once the mainstay organization in the physician industry, is being gradually replaced by the multiphysician group practice. Interestingly, the hospital industry is undergoing a similar transformation as many formerly independent hospitals are now becoming part of multihospital chains or systems. These horizontal mergers among individual physician practices and among individual hospitals take place largely because increased market power is sought or because of economies of scale, economies of scope, and the other cost advantages associated with health care systems, as previously discussed.

Another organizational arrangement that takes place in the health care sector that involves both the hospital and physician industries is the integration of physician practices with hospitals. According to Robinson (1997, p. 6), "The **integrated delivery system (IDS)** combines physicians and hospitals into a vertically integrated organization with a single ownership and structure, a single chain of authority, and a single bottom line." There are basically four types of IDSs: the physician-hospital organization, the management service organization, the foundation model, and the integrated health organization, although other hybrid organizational forms also exist. These alternative physician-hospital arrangements differ in the degree to which risk, governance, revenue and capital, planning, and management are shared (Burns and Thorpe, 1993). An IDS may include nursing homes, home health care units, and an insurance component in addition to physicians and hospitals.

---

18. See Dranove and White (1998) for the most recent study providing strong evidence to support the absence of meaningful cost shifting. Like Zwanziger et al. (2000), they use California data for 1983 and the early 1990s in their empirical analysis.

IDSs have developed in large part due to the financial pressure from MCOs, which in recent years have exercised their growing power to control costs. A movement by the government toward fixed payment systems, such as the prospective payment system for hospitals and the resource-based relative value scale system for physicians, also served as an impetus for change (Burns and Thorpe, 1993; Morrisey et al., 1996).

Why vertically integrated systems are formed is a question that interests economists, among others. Economists generally analyze organizational arrangements through the "conceptual lens" of agency theory and transaction cost economics (Robinson, 1997; Shortell, 1997). **Agency theory** considers the contractual relationships among parties. According to agency theory, the principal, or owner(s), of the firm enters into a multitude of contracts, either implicitly or formally, with other firms or agents who are the suppliers of inputs. Each contract stipulates the input or product that will be provided, the price that will be paid, and other terms of the agreement, such as product quality and time of delivery. Consequently, agency theory regards the firm as a nexus of many contracts. Within the agency model, the firm essentially serves as a facilitator and coordinator of the many contracts and is responsible for transforming the resulting inputs into an output or multiple outputs. The contractual relationships provide the firm with considerable flexibility to switch among input suppliers when better terms of exchange, such as a lower price or better product quality, become available.

But if agency theory perfectly describes the firm, why do we observe some firms producing inputs internally rather than contracting out for them? For example, why do some hospitals possess their own maintenance staffs, MRI facilities, or nursing home units while others contract out for these same services?

Transaction costs economics provides a reason why firms choose to produce inputs or services internally rather than contracting out. Transaction costs refer to the costs associated with the negotiating, writing, and enforcing of contracts and includes the costs of searching out the best price and quality. Transaction cost theory considers that many contracts are incomplete because not all possible contingencies can be written into a contract. Bounded rationality, especially in the face of uncertainty, is one reason for incomplete contracts. Bounded rationality refers to the limited capacity of the human mind to formulate and solve problems (Williamson, 1985). When contracts are incomplete, some stipulations require renegotiation. During the renegotiation process, one of the parties may have an advantage and the advantage can lead to **opportunistic behavior.** Opportunistic behavior involves self-interest seeking with guile and allows for strategic behavior or deception. The potential for opportunistic behavior increases the cost of contractual relationships.

As an example, suppose a hospital contracts with a company to repair the masonry around the bricks on the exterior of its buildings for $17,000. The company rents and installs the necessary scaffolding and begins the repairs. Upon closer inspection, however, the repair crew realizes that a good proportion of the repair is unnecessary and informs the hospital administrator. Naturally, the hospital administrator asks how much of the $17,000 will be returned. The contractor relates that the scaffolding must be rented for a minimum of one month. The contractor also mentions that transporting, installing, and disassembling the scaffolding is very costly. As you can see, the contractor is in a good position to practice opportunistic behavior by inflating the cost figures. Who would have thought to stipulate a contingency of that kind in the contract?

Transaction cost theory suggests that firms sometimes find internal production more efficient than outsourcing due to the relatively high cost of contracting. The theory by itself, however, suggests that firms should continually find it optimal to vertically integrate through greater internal production or by merging with suppliers. Obviously there must be some limiting factors; otherwise, only one firm would exist in every industry.

The same agency relationship discussed earlier places a limiting factor on the size of firms. Like outside contractors, employees and management are bound to the firm through implicit or formal contracts. For example, employees are expected to show up for work on time and perform well; otherwise, their jobs may be in jeopardy. While ownership of the nonhuman assets gives the firm more control over internal negotiations than external ones (Hart, 1995), greater firm size may lead to higher production costs at some point. As a firm grows physically larger, it becomes increasingly more complex and costly for the owners to monitor the behavior of management and employees. Inefficient behavior may arise as a result of the high monitoring costs.

For example, consider a large corporation in which the principal is represented by the stockholders, and the chief executive officer (CEO) serves as the primary agent. Stockholders, wishing high dividends and stock value appreciation, want the CEO to maximize profits. The CEO, however, may attempt to pursue goals other than maximum profits, especially when he is paid a fixed salary. For example, the CEO may use some of the firm's profit to pay for plush office accommodations, a limousine, or various other expensive perquisites. Alternatively, the CEO may be more interested in empire building and, therefore, may acquire several other unprofitable companies rather than maximize profits. As a result, the corporation may perform poorly because of the CEO's actions. The CEO, however, may blame general economic conditions, and, therefore, the unknowing stockholders may not punish the CEO for the unprofitable behavior.[19]

As another example, salaried employees, particularly when they work as a team, may shirk their responsibilities, engage in on-the-job leisure time, and free-ride on the productive efforts of others. If a sufficient number of those on the team behave similarly, team output suffers and profits decline. The larger the organization, the greater the cost of monitoring the efforts of management and employees because of the proportionately greater interactions among workers (Carlton and Perloff, 1994).

To prevent internal agents, such as CEOs or employees, from operating in an unproductive manner, agency theory suggests that compensation might be tied to performance or profits so as to align the interests of the principal and agents. For example, the CEO's pay may be linked to the profits or stock value of the company. CEOs often receive bonus pay and stock options as part of their total compensation for that reason. The contracts help align the interests of the principal and agents so the interests of the principal are better served. It is important to note, however, that employment contracts are not always complete, so inefficient behavior may result as the firm continues to produce increasingly more services internally rather than purchasing them in the marketplace. Organizational independence, in contrast to internal production, preserves the risk and rewards for efficient performance (Robinson, 1997).

As another limit on firm size, managerial diseconomies may set in as the firm gets too large because of bounded rationality. Managers at the top may lose sight of the production process taking place at the floor level. Communication flows from top to bottom may break down. Bureaucratic inertia may also set in as regimentation replaces innovation and risk taking is not properly rewarded. The loss of control, breakdowns in communication, and loss of innovativeness may all place limits on the size of the firm.

As long as decision makers act rationally, each firm can be expected to choose the size where marginal benefit equals marginal cost. A greater amount of internal production creates benefits because of reduced transaction costs but also may come at a cost as larger firms become more costly and complex to monitor and innovation suffers. The costs of contracting and monitoring

---

19. This possibility was alluded to when we discussed the implications of the utility maximization models. When the ownership constraint is weak, managers may maximize their own personal utilities, which are partly derived from the five *P*s of increased pay, perquisites, power, prestige, and patronage.

differ from firm to firm and from industry to industry. Some firms find market exchange more efficient than internal production at the margin. Transaction costs depend on various factors, such as the degree of market uncertainty, the number of suppliers in the market, and how often the service or input must be obtained. In general, when market conditions are more uncertain, the number of suppliers is fewer and frequency of use is greater, transaction costs are greater, and internal production becomes more efficient than contracting out.

You are probably asking yourself how the discussion of agency theory and transaction cost economics relates to physician-hospital integration. Hospitals and physician practices vertically integrate or fail to vertically integrate for the same reasons as other organizations do. Vertical integration leads to lower transaction costs but can impose incentive problems in large organizations. Robinson (1997) expands on this theme by noting that a contractual relationship between a hospital and physicians can be thought of as **virtual integration.** The term *virtual integration* is just a convenient way of stating that a combination of two or more organizations takes place through contractual relationships rather than through unified ownership. Robinson goes on to compare the relative advantages of vertical and virtual integration with regard to coordination, governance, and clinical innovation, three key activities in a hospital-physician relationship.

Coordination deals with how the individual parts are woven into an overall productive unit. For example, are the various services that combine to form medical care, such as lab tests, imaging, physician care, and inpatient hospital services, all coordinated through one large, unified structure or through two or perhaps more contractual relationships? At the extreme, authority and induced loyalty and commitment might be used to coordinate care in a unified model, while negotiation may be relied on in a purely contractual network (Robinson, 1997; Shortell, 1997). For example, a hospital may offer to process the bills of a physician or purchase and then rent a medical facility to a physician as a way of achieving better coordination through contracting. As another example, hospital and physician services might be better coordinated by allowing more physicians to serve on the hospital's board of trustees.

Governance considers who controls the firm's policies and how much flexibility the firm has to adapt and modify its policies when confronted with changing external events. An important aspect of governance is whether the decision-making process is centralized or decentralized and whether it is dependent on for-profit or not-for-profit objectives. Decentralized governance tends to provide more flexibility, but vertical arrangements between decentralized for-profit and not-for-profit organizations may not last because of a clash of missions (for example, the virtual integration of a Catholic hospital with a physician practice providing abortion services).

Clinical innovation is a function of the entrepreneurial, risk-taking spirit. At the one extreme, virtual integration involves arm's-length agreements with little sharing of financial risks. At the other extreme, vertical integration, hospitals and physician groups might jointly share in the financial risks of the organization through an ownership stake. One issue here is how the resulting organizational arrangement affects the incentive of the firm to minimize costs and undertake innovative activities. For example, Robinson (1997) notes that when "physicians sell their practices and merge into larger systems, they risk losing the entrepreneurial, risk-taking spirit and developing the civil service mentality of the hospital employee" (p. 17). The incentive attenuation might be overcome, however, by providing the physician with an ownership stake in the larger system or by paying performance-based compensation.

Shortell (1997) points out that vertical and virtual arrangements can be thought of as a continuum with respect to the essential activities of coordination, governance, and clinical innovation. In the real world integration is rarely at either extreme but instead is somewhere along the virtual-vertical continuum. Along the coordination continuum, for example, a corporate joint venture falls somewhere in the middle of contracts and unified ownership. Under a joint venture, a hospital and physician group might remain legally separated but agree to jointly coordinate some single type of patient care, for example. A joint task force or committee represents an intermediate governance structure. A Physician Hospital Organization, in which a hospital and physicians jointly own and operate ambulatory care projects or jointly act as an agent for managed care contracts, provides an example of an organizational structure that falls halfway along the clinical innovation continuum.

Shortell further notes that organizations position themselves along the various continuums depending on the demands of the local marketplace for a coordinated health care system, the organization's own capabilities, and the historical context of the organization. For example, if the local market demands a perfectly seamless, coordinated health care system, the unified ownership of vertical integration will be favored over the contractual relationship.

Many analysts initially anticipated that IDSs would lead to improved financial performance for hospitals as well as encourage greater quality of care through coordinated delivery systems. But only about 23 percent of all hospitals participated in some kind of physician-hospital arrangement in 1993 and much vertical disintegration has occurred since that date (Morrisey et al. 1996; Burns and Pauly, 2002). Vertical disintegration most likely occurred because studies failed to find any systematic evidence linking IDSs with greater financial performance (Goes and Zhan, 1995). Burns and Pauly (2002) argue that hospitals and physicians entered into vertical arrangements for reasons that conflict with economic logic.

Summary of the Conduct of the Hospital Services Market

A number of structural and related factors simultaneously influence the conduct of hospitals in the marketplace. The degree of actual competition, barriers to entry, reimbursement practices of third-party payers, and hospital objectives jointly affect how an individual hospital behaves, and therefore only carefully conceived studies can sort out how any individual factor influences hospital conduct. Most empirical studies using data prior to 1983 have found that hospitals competed on the basis of quality rather than price, but recent evidence suggests that the growing price consciousness among health care payers may be causing increased price competition among hospitals.

Empirical evidence also suggests that efficiency differences are quite small among not-for-profit, public, and for-profit hospitals after controlling for quality and case-mix differences. The reason cited for the similarity is that physicians act as residual claimants in not-for-profit hospitals and thus ensure that the hospitals behave as efficiently as possible. The provision of indigent care has been found to be considerably higher in public hospitals than in otherwise identical not-for-profit and for-profit hospitals. In addition, the amount of indigent care has been found to be quite similar for not-for-profit and for-profit hospitals, raising doubt about the desirability of the tax-exempt status generally conferred on not-for-profit hospitals.

MCOs appear to offer modest hospital cost savings without reducing the quality of patient outcomes compared to traditional fee-for-service medicine. HMOs and UR appear to provide more consistent cost savings than PPOs, however. As consumers become more price conscious and the hospital market becomes more competitive, increased cost savings may result from a managed care environment. State rate review programs have also proven effective in containing hospital care costs. However, studies investigating the effect of state rate review policies on the quality of hospital outcomes have failed to reach a definitive conclusion. In addition, the cost containment effects of rate programs appear to have waned in recent years, at least compared to the same effects from MCOs.

Finally, MCOs and fixed reimbursement methods have motivated some hospitals and physician practices to form integrated delivery systems. IDSs involve either vertical or virtual (contractual) integration. Vertical integration may offer cost savings by reducing the transaction costs associated with external market exchanges. Vertical integration can lead to higher operating costs as monitoring costs rise, communication flows breakdown, or innovation suffers in large corporations. To date, empirical studies have uncovered mixed results regarding improved financial performance in IDSs.

The Performance of the Hospital Services Industry

This final section focuses on the overall performance of the hospital services industry by assessing the growth of hospital expenditures, the hospital inflation rate, and hospital input utilization in the aggregate. While it might be best to analyze the performance of the hospital industry in each state or, perhaps, in each metropolitan area in the United States given the structural diversity of hospital markets, the analysis would be unwieldy and the necessary data are less widely available at a disaggregated level. As a result, we examine and discuss various hospital pricing, utilization, and profit trends over time to get some idea about the overall or aggregate performance of the hospital services industry in the United States.

The Growth in Hospital Expenditures

Over the years, expenditures on hospital services, which include spending on both inpatient and outpatient services, have tended to comprise about 30 to 40 percent of all health care spending, making it the dominant expense of most health care payers. The big-ticket aspect of hospital spending should not be surprising given the fact that the severely ill typically receive hospital care and also the technologically intensive method of delivering most types of hospital care. Table 13–3 reveals that nominal hospital care expenditures in the United States rose dramatically

TABLE 13–3
Hospital Expenditures in the United States, Selected Years, 1960–2003

Year	Total Hospital Expenditures (billions of dollars)	Spending as a Percentage of Gross Domestic Product
1960	$ 9.2	1.7%
1970	27.6	2.7
1980	101.5	3.6
1990	253.9	4.4
1995	343.6	4.6
2000	413.1	4.2
2003	515.9	4.7

SOURCE: Center for Medicare & Medicaid Services, http://www.cms.gov (accessed January 10, 2006).

from $9.2 billion in 1960 to $515.9 billion in 2003. As a fraction of gross domestic product, hospital care spending also increased but not steadily throughout the 43-year period. In particular, notice in the table that hospital care spending spurted upward from 1.7 to 4.6 percent of the nation's income over the period from 1960 to the mid-1990s.

However, after that period, hospital care spending declined as a percentage of GDP to 4.2 percent in 2000. As mentioned previously, the middle to late 1990s represents the heyday of managed care. The success of managed care at controlling hospital costs during the heyday shows up in the lower percentage of GDP allocated to health care. But the lower hospital spending could also reflect overall changes in the production of medical care. For example, the push to outpatient care services may have resulted in lost hospital revenues as physician practices have attempted to take over some of this business. Also, the greater use of skilled nursing homes, rather than hospitals, for rehabilitative care may have reduced the revenues of hospitals.

After 1999, hospital care costs as a percentage of GDP began their upward trend once again, rising to 4.7 percent by 2003. The upward trend may reflect the backlash against restrictive managed care plans as insured individuals moved into less restrictive plans with looser networks of physician and hospital providers. Alternatively, the relative increase in hospital spending may reflect that restrictive managed care plans were only able to squeeze out some short-run inefficiencies and that new medical technologies eventually set in motion a long-term increase in hospital spending.

As you are well aware, hospital expenditures equal the product of the price and quantity of hospital services. As yet, we do not know whether the change in hospital expenditures over time is attributable to higher price changes, an increased quantity of services, or a combination of the two factors. This is an important consideration because, first, a greater quantity of hospital services makes people better off, whereas price increases have the opposite effect of reducing real incomes and consumer welfare. Second, as mentioned earlier, various structural elements of health care markets, such as extensive third-party coverage, may give rise to the overproduction of hospital services at the expense of all other goods and services and thereby result in allocative inefficiency. Thus, to get a better understanding of hospital expenditure growth, we next examine trends in various measures of hospital price and output.

The Hospital Services Price Inflation Rate

Expenditures on many types of products can be easily broken down into their price and quantity components. The decomposition of hospital care expenditures into its quantity and price components is much more complicated because of the intangible and heterogeneous nature of hospital services. Yet conceptually we know that an implicit price and an implicit quantity of services exist for every amount of hospital care spending.

When the Bureau of Labor Statistics (BLS) collects data from hospitals to construct a "hospital and related services" price index, the pricing unit is the hospital visit, defined by a date of admission, a date of discharge as documented on a hospital bill, and the specific diagnosis or medical condition.[20] BLS staff members select a sample of hospital bills based on revenues generated by eligible payers (that is, privately insured and uninsured patients). Then the field staff describes the item in terms of the bundle of goods and services consumed during that visit. The goal of the hospital services index is to follow the transaction prices of selected services over

20. See the description of the medical price index and its components at the BLS web site, http://www.bls.gov/cpi/cpifact4.htm (accessed January 10, 2006).

time while keeping constant price-determining characteristics such as length of stay and the medical reason for the visit. The transaction price is the actual amount the hospital receives from the insurance carrier and/or the patient's out-of-pocket payments.

Be aware that adjustments in the price index from one year to the next may be misstated if the quality of goods and services also changes over time. For instance, health outcomes may improve over time as medical care becomes more effective at saving lives, perhaps as health care production moves down the learning curve. The inability to control for quality of outcomes raises concern about the reliability of medical price indices. Nevertheless, the medical price indices reported by BLS continue to be used for private and public policy purposes because they are the best currently available on a systematic basis.

Figure 13–6 shows the general price inflation rate as measured by the percentage change in the urban consumer price index and the hospital services price index over the period 1979 to 2004. The data have several implications. First, the data suggest that the hospital services inflation rate exceeded the general price inflation rate in every year but one over the 25-year span. Second, the hospital sector experienced double-digit inflation rates eight times throughout the time span, unlike the entire economy, which faced double-digit inflation only twice. The recession of the early 1980s helped bring inflationary pressures down in both the health sector and the macroeconomy. Third, despite the introduction of the Medicare PPS system and other public and private cost containment practices after 1983, hospital prices continued to rise more quickly than the prices of other goods. Finally, the data indicate that increased managed care enrollments may have had a disinflationary impact on hospital service prices during the early to late 1990s. Specifically, the rate of growth of hospital prices slowed from a high of 12.2 percent in 1989 to a low of 3.0 percent in 1997. However, the data also suggest that the effects of managed care may be weakening as the gap between the hospital services inflation rate and the general price inflation rate has widened since 1999 for the most part.

FIGURE 13–6
General and Hospital Services Price Inflation, 1979–2004

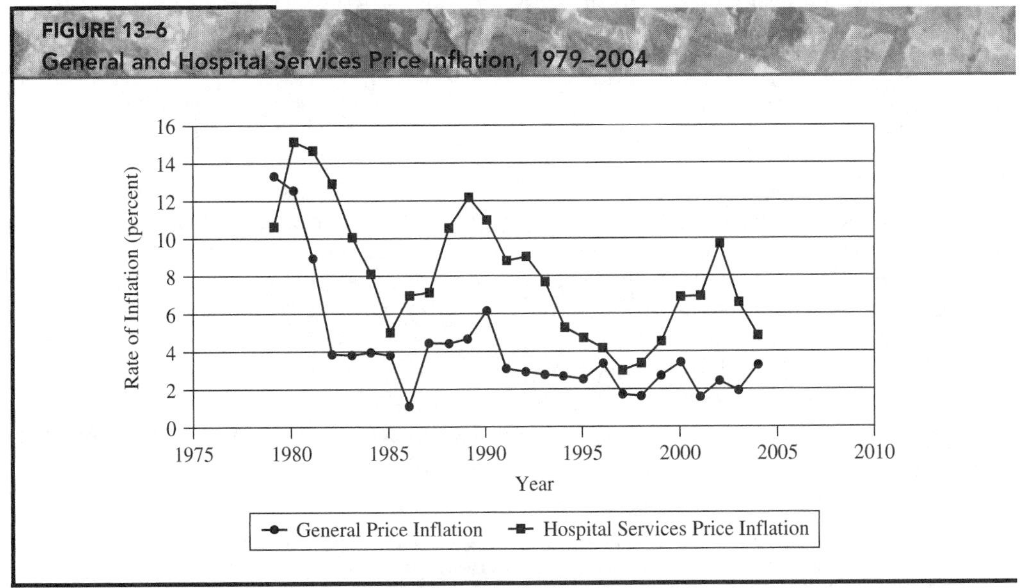

SOURCE: U.S. Department of Labor, Bureau of Labor Statistics, http://www.bls.gov (accessed January 10, 2006).

Overall, the time-series data for the hospital services inflation rate suggest that hospital prices have risen more quickly than most other prices in the U.S. economy over the last several decades. Unfortunately, the data cannot identify the source of the relative price increase in the hospital sector. Lack of a profit motive, fee-for-service medicine, generous insurance coverage, quality competition, and unbridled hospital pricing power could all conceivably contribute to the relatively high and rising hospital inflation rate in the United States.

However, the normal functioning of a market economy can also explain rising hospital prices. That is, relative prices normally rise for goods and services that become more highly valued or more costly to produce than others. Information on marginal social benefit and cost is needed before one can determine whether hospital services are efficiently produced. Unfortunately, the marginal benefit and cost of hospital services are difficult to estimate. Therefore, we must resort to analyzing information such as input usage and the utilization of hospital care to indirectly identify trends in the output performance of hospitals. We do so in the next section.

Hospital Input Usage and Utilization

Some of the more commonly discussed hospital performance indicators include the hospital staffing ratio (number of full-time equivalent personnel per weighted sum of outpatients and inpatients), occupancy rate (average daily inpatients per bed), admission rate per 100 population, average length of stay (average days per patient), and outpatient visits per 100 population. The first two indicators are intended to represent input usage, and the last three are proxy measures for the quantity or utilization of hospital services.

Data for these variables are drawn from Health Care Forum LLC (2005) and show a number of systematic trends. For one, the hospital staffing ratio increased throughout the period 1975–2003, rising from approximately three to nearly five full-time equivalent employees per patient. The higher staffing ratio may reflect the more severely ill patients resulting from the Medicare PPS, since less-sickly patients are now unlikely to be admitted to hospitals. Or the greater staffing ratio may represent the expense preferences of hospital administrators. Alternatively, the higher staffing ratio may signify the continuing ability of hospitals to generate revenues to support their not-for-profit, human service orientation toward providing more services to patients (Pope and Menke, 1990).

Figures for the hospital occupancy rate point to a similar conclusion regarding rising input usage. While fluctuating around 75 percent in the late 1970s and early 1980s, the average occupancy rate at U.S. hospitals declined from its highest level of around 76 percent in 1981 to slightly under 62 percent in 1996. The decline in the occupancy rate began one year before the Medicare PPS in 1983. The implication is one of excess beds at the typical American hospital. According to Anders (1993b), these beds are not cheap; each costs about $30,000 to $40,000 a year in maintenance, staffing, and depreciation charges. With about 200,000 unnecessary beds in the nation, the aggregate cost of excess bed capacity runs about $6 billion to $8 billion a year.[21] Although it is too early to draw any meaningful conclusions, the encouraging news is that the occupancy rate has risen slightly to roughly 66 percent in 2003. The recent rise in the occupancy rate might reflect the increased pressure hospitals face from competitive forces and MCOs to better manage their excess capacity (Santerre and Adams, 2002).

---

21. However, see Friedman and Pauly (1981), who estimate that the excess bed cost is about one-tenth of those figures. Gaynor and Anderson (1995) find evidence supporting the preceding figures, whereas Keeler and Ying (1996) indicate that the cost of excess bed capacity is much greater, at about $25 billion in 1993. Also see Carey (1998), who estimates the implied benefit of an empty bed in the range of $25,000–$35,000 for the period 1987–1992, again suggesting a high cost associated with unoccupied beds in the United States.

Data for the hospital admission rate show an interesting trend. The hospital admission rate hovered near 16 per 100 population from 1975 to 1982. Thereafter the rate fell and equaled 11.8 admissions per 100 population in 2003. The decline in the admission rate has surprised some health policy analysts who expected an increase in the admission rate with the advent of the Medicare PPS because reimbursement under this system is based on a per-case charge. Others argue that the reduced hospital admission rate was inevitable as health care providers substituted for inpatient care with less regulated outpatient and nursing home care.

Figures for the average length of stay (ALOS) show a pattern similar to that for the admission rate, roughly constant at 7.6 days in the years preceding the Medicare PPS. After that point, the ALOS fell precipitously to 7.1 days in 1985 and then leveled off through 1990. From 1991 to 2003, the ALOS fell further from 7.2 to 5.7 days. The reduction in length of stay was predicted as hospitals responded to the per-case charge of the Medicare PPS. A portion of the reduction in the hospital admission rate and length of stay shows up in the higher outpatient visit rate over time in the United States. The outpatient visit rate has continually increased since 1985 from nearly 66 to 190 outpatient visits per 100 population in 2003, a growth of about 10 percent per year.

In sum, since the mid-1980s, a smaller percentage of people have been admitted into hospitals, and those admitted typically stay for a shorter duration. Also, hospital occupancy rates have fallen but staffing ratios continue to climb, in part to provide more services to more severely ill inpatients and to provide increased outpatient services. Health policy analysts have questioned whether the increased services provided to inpatients and outpatients are inappropriately supplied. Let us examine that question in more detail.

Do Hospitals Provide Inappropriate Care or Flat-of-the-Curve Medicine? The supplier-induced demand theory and McGuire's model, as discussed in Chapter 12, predict that health care providers may unnecessarily provide various diagnostic and therapeutic services to patients due to the associated financial gain. With those theories and rising health care costs in mind, a number of studies have attempted to determine whether various types of medical services are inappropriately provided to patients. One of the first studies, by Chassin et al. (1987), measured how appropriately physicians performed coronary angiography, carotid endarterectomy, and upper gastrointestinal (GI) tract endoscopy for the Medicare population in 1981 in several areas of the United States.[22] A panel of physicians was selected to rate a number of indications or clinical settings, each consisting of a unique combination of clinical information and other factors considered in recommending treatment, with respect to the appropriateness of each procedure.[23] *Appropriateness* was defined to mean that the expected health benefits (prolonged life, relief of pain, and cure of disease) of a procedure exceed its expected negative consequences (operative mortality, complications, pain, and anxiety) by a sufficiently wide margin. Only medical appropriateness was considered; the monetary costs of the procedure were ignored.

The authors found significant levels of inappropriate use: 17 percent of the cases for coronary angiography, 32 percent for carotid endarterectomy, and 17 percent for upper GI tract endoscopy. Uncertain use rates for these three services were 9, 32, and 11 percent, respectively. Similarly, Winslow et al. (1988), using data for 1979, 1980, and 1982, found an inappropriate rate of 14 percent and an uncertain rate of 30 percent for coronary artery bypass graft surgery. These

22. The areas studied were Arkansas, Colorado, Iowa, Massachusetts, Montana, Pennsylvania, South Carolina, and northern California. Coronary angiography is an X-ray study of the inside of the heart. Carotid endarterectomy is the removal of the core of the carotid artery, a blood vessel beginning at the large artery of the heart (aorta) and running straight up through the neck, that has become thickened by fatty deposits. Upper gastrointestinal tract endoscopy is an examination of the inside of the body from the mouth to the stomach with a lighting device.

23. An *indication* is a reason to prescribe a medication or perform a treatment.

two studies have been widely cited as offering concrete evidence that a large number of medical services are provided unnecessarily in U.S. hospitals.

Three studies using data for 1990 have raised serious doubt about whether medical services are inappropriately provided. Specifically, Leape et al. (1993), Hilborne et al. (1993), and Bernstein et al. (1993) find very low inappropriate rates for coronary bypass graft surgery (2.4 percent), coronary angioplasty (4 percent), and coronary angiography (4 percent) in a sample of New York hospitals. While the uncertain rate was also low for coronary artery bypass surgery (7 percent), the authors express some concern that the uncertain rates for coronary angioplasty and angiography were quite high at 38 and 20 percent, respectively. The authors of these three studies point to changing practice patterns and the regulatory environment in New York as possible reasons for the large differences in the two sets of studies.

Two recent studies essentially examine the marginal productivity of additional Medicare spending on health outcomes. More specifically, Fisher et al. (2003a, 2003b) examine whether regions with higher Medicare spending are characterized by better quality of care, better survival chances, improved functional status, or greater satisfaction with care. They do that by analyzing patient outcomes across 306 referral areas of the United States between 1993 and 1999. Using end-of-life spending as an indicator of Medicare spending, the researchers classify regions into five quintiles of spending and examine costs and outcomes of care differences separately for hip fracture, colorectal cancer, and myocardial infarction.

End-of-life spending on a reference cohort is used as an indicator of Medicare spending because it is unrelated to underlying illness levels or prices. Medicare spending differs across regions, because people are sicker and the government pays more for services in some areas than others, so it could not be used to categorize areas. Thus residing in hospital referral regions with different end-of-life spending can be treated as a random event and achieves the goal of a natural experiment. Alternatively stated, the results are less likely to be biased by less healthy Medicare beneficiaries choosing to live in high Medicare spending areas because of this randomization process.

To isolate the relation between spending and the various health outcomes measures, Fisher et al. adjust for a number of factors including age, gender, race, income, baseline health, HMO enrollment, region, hospital volume, metropolitan living status, and the teaching status of hospitals. The two studies by Fisher et al. offer a number of valuable insights into the relation between Medicare spending and health outcomes.

First, the authors find that greater regional spending on Medicare can be largely explained by practice patterns that involve more inpatient services and specialty care. That is, differences in spending primarily result from more frequent physician visits, specialist consultations, tests, and minor procedures, and greater use of the hospital and intensive care units. Second, they note that Medicare enrollees in higher-spending regions tend to receive more care than those in lower-spending regions but do not have better health outcomes or satisfaction with care. Three, neither quality of care nor access to care appear to be better for Medicare enrollees in higher-spending regions, all other factors held constant.

The authors conclude their study (2003a) by writing: “These findings call into question the notion that additional growth in health care spending is primarily driven by advances in science and technology and that spending more will inevitably result in improved quality of care” (p. 286). Hence, the authors find some evidence to support “flat-of-the-curve” medicine in the case of additional Medicare spending. The implication is that additional medical care services may not provide important benefits to the population served. As the authors note, the results of their studies underscore the need for research to determine how to safely reduce Medicare spending levels.

The Concentration of Health Care Expenditures. Related to the concern over the provision of unnecessary medical care is the concentration of health care spending among a small minority of the U.S. population. According to data provided by Berk and Monheit (2001), 1 percent of the U.S. population accounted for 27 percent of all health care spending in 1996. The top 5 percent was responsible for more than half of all health care spending in the United States in that same year. The authors also found that the distribution of health care spending remained remarkably stable over the period from 1970 to 1996 despite the increased presence of MCOs in more recent times. The fact that the distribution of health care expenditures is concentrated among a small fraction of people should not be surprising given that the major users of health care services are severely ill patients receiving high-cost critical care in hospitals. In fact, it has been estimated that one in every seven health care dollars is spent during the last six months of someone's life (Clark, 1992). Data also suggest that 18.8 percent of Medicare patients accounted for 81 percent of all Medicare expenditures in 1991 (Iglehart, 1992). The dilemma, as Aaron (1991) notes, is that successful cost containment may "require rationing of services to the very ill"[24] (p. 53).

Hospital Profit Margins

In addition to measures of price and output, economic profitability also provides information about the performance of an industry, as discussed in earlier chapters. Persistent economic profits typically signal an inefficient allocation of resources. That's because, when entry barriers are absent, additional resources are drawn to markets with economic profits until price equals average costs. In addition, negative economic profits indicate that suppliers are not receiving sufficient revenues to cover costs and therefore may exit the industry if the losses persist. Both of these situations are associated with reductions in consumer welfare.

Figure 13-7 shows the total, private payer, overall Medicare, and Medicare inpatient margins experienced by the typical hospital for each year from 1992 to 2003. Figures for the overall Medicare margin are shown only for illustrative purposes (and track the inpatient Medicare margin) because data are limited to the period after 1996. Recall from our discussion in Chapter 11 that profit margins are calculated by subtracting costs from revenues and dividing by revenues. For the total hospital margin, revenues include payments received for inpatient and outpatient care services from all types of payers (Medicare, Medicaid, private insurers, self-pay, and so on) plus any nonpatient revenues (interest earnings, cafeteria revenues, and so on). The other hospital margins reflect only the revenues received from and costs incurred by a particular funding source. Note that all of these margins represent accounting rates of return because, following standard accounting practices, a normal rate of return on capital has not been included as a cost item.[25]

Figure 13-7 shows that the total hospital profit margin hovered around 5 percent over the twelve-year period, ranging from a low of 3.6 percent in 1999 to a high of 6.4 percent in 1997. During the three-year period from 2000 to 2002, the total hospital margin averaged roughly 3.7 percent, which interestingly, corresponds fairly closely to the average health insurer profit margin of 3.6 percent over that same period, as reported in Table 11-1. Notice that the private payer hospital margin declines after 1992 until 2000 and then rises thereafter. That trend in the private payer hospital margin in part reflects the effectiveness of managed care at holding down

---

24. However, Emanuel and Emanuel (1994) estimate that greater use of advance directives (such as living wills), hospice care, and less aggressive interventions at the end of life will save only 3.3 percent of health care costs. Among the reasons they cite: even less aggressive humane care at the end of life is labor intensive and costly to produce.

25. Assigning hospital costs to different payers is difficult in practice because a significant portion of hospital costs are fixed cost and not all payers allow all costs to be reimbursed (such as advertising). See Friedman et al. (2004) for further discussion.

FIGURE 13–7
Total, Private Payer, Medicare, and Medicare Inpatient Hospital Margins, 1992–2003

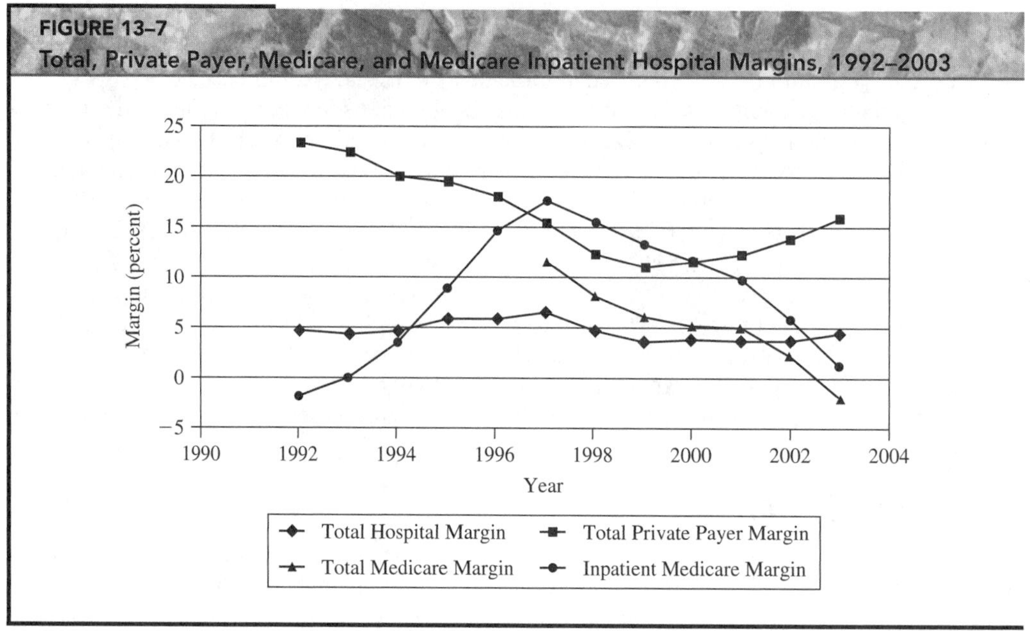

SOURCE: Medicare Payment Advisory Council (MedPAC) at http://www.medpac.gov.

hospital prices during 1993–1999. Notice that the cost containment success of managed care is not reflected in the total hospital margin, maybe because private payers reimburse for only 34 percent of all hospital expenditures (see Table 13–2).

Also notice that the Medicare inpatient hospital margin varied widely over that same period, reaching a low of −1.8 in 1992 and a high of 17.6 percent in 1997. In fact, the data in the figure seem to suggest that the Medicare inpatient hospital margin drives changes in the total hospital margin. Specifically, the rising Medicare inpatient margin from 1992 to 1997 pulls the total margin up slightly and then the Medicare inpatient margin faintly pushes down the total margin as it declines for the years thereafter. This relation holds despite the fact that the Medicare PPS program funds less than 30 percent of all hospital care spending.

From a pricing perspective, the hospital services industry can be viewed as possessing unregulated and regulated segments or submarkets. In the unregulated segment, the private payer price is established through many independent negotiations between individual private insurers and individual hospitals in various local hospital services markets throughout the United States. The private payer price, along with costs, determines the private payer hospital margin. In the regulated segment of the industry, individual price negotiations do not take place. Instead, the federal government simply administers the selected Medicare reimbursement rates at every hospital throughout the United States. The Medicare hospital margin reflects the prices set by the federal government relative to the costs of treating Medicare patients.[26]

Some interaction likely exists between the unregulated and regulated portions of the hospital services industry. The interaction results because Medicare reimbursement rates set by the

26. Bear in mind that the analysis actually becomes more complicated once Medicaid insurance coverage, self-paying patients, and uncompensated care are considered.

government are not completely independent of private payer rates (and vice versa). Since 1997, the Medicare Payment Advisory Commission (MedPAC) has recommended to Congress how Medicare prices should be adjusted in upcoming years.[27] When establishing the Medicare reimbursement rate adjustments, MedPAC considers whether previous Medicare rates are adequate. Adequacy is judged by a number of factors including access to care, volume of care, access to capital, and quality of care.

In addition, MedPAC considers how the costs of treating Medicare patients change from one period to the next and assesses whether cost increases are justified on clinical grounds or reflect general inefficiencies. In terms of inefficiency, hospital cost increases may reflect that unions have negotiated wage increases for their workers that exceed the competitive rate. Wages that exceed the competitive level are referred to as **monopoly rents.** Or the cost increases may capture the fact that not-for-profit hospitals are constructing new buildings, buying new equipment, and funding quality-enhancing but unprofitable services to satisfy the preferences of managers rather than patients.

MedPAC establishes Medicare payment adjustments relative to the hospital market basket index, which measures price inflation for the goods and services that hospitals use to produce inpatient and outpatient care. Specifically, MedPAC recommends a payment adjustment that includes the hospital market basket index plus or minus an additional percentage depending on the adequacy of previous rates and the previous growth of Medicare hospital costs. For example, in its March 2005 report, MedPAC recommends that Congress increases payment rates for the outpatient PPS and the inpatient care PPS by the projected increase in the hospital market basket index less 0.4 percent for fiscal year 2006.[28]

Because MedPAC considers the adequacy of current Medicare reimbursement rates and the growth of Medicare hospital costs in its deliberations, private payer rates indirectly influence its recommendations in a couple of ways. First, fixed costs (such as salaries, facility costs, and the costs of any diagnostic and therapeutic equipment; see Chapter 7) comprise a large share of overall hospital costs and therefore are commonly incurred in some amount by all types of payers. Private payer prices that cover variable costs and some portion of fixed costs help indirectly finance hospital services for Medicare beneficiaries in the short run. Thus, access-to-care and quality-of-care indicators under the Medicare program may be influenced by private payer prices. Quickly rising private payer prices imply lower recommended Medicare price increases, all other factors held constant.

Second, MedPAC explains that the costs of treating Medicare patients tend to grow less (more) rapidly when the financial pressure from private payers is more (less) severe. For example, MedPAC's analysis shows that the average change in Medicare costs per discharge was only 0.8 percent during 1993–1999 but 8.3 percent from 1986 to 1992 and 5.6 percent from 2000 to 2003. As mentioned previously, aggressive managed care pricing took place during 1993–1999. Thus, for another reason, quickly rising private payer prices may translate into lower recommended Medicare price increases, *ceteris paribus*.[29]

In sum, economic profits serve as another indicator of industry performance. Economic profits in the hospital services industry, with its unregulated and regulated segments, are determined by the interplay between market and regulatory forces. Over the period 1992–2003, the hospital

---

27. Check out the following link to learn more about the organization and responsibilities of MedPAC: http://www.medpac.gov/about_medpac/index.cfm?section=about_medpac (accessed January 10, 2006).

28. See http://www.medpac.gov/publications/congressional_reports/Mar05_TOC.pdf (accessed January 10, 2006).

29. Cost shifting involves the reverse scenario that lower Medicare prices result in higher private prices. This possibility was discussed in the conduct section of this chapter.

accounting margin averaged about 4.6 percent and equaled the health insurer margin during 2000–2003. As a result, hospital margins do not appear to be particularly high or low. However, margins vary considerably among rural and metropolitan hospitals, nonteaching and teaching hospitals, and hospitals with different payer mixes. The government faces a formidable task when setting Medicare rates because it must provide incentives for cost containment without seriously compromising other goals of health policy such as ensuring access to and quality of care. Further complications arise because changes in private prices influence the state of the operating environment from which information is used to determine Medicare price adjustments.

Summary

Hospital expenditures represent the largest component of health care spending, accounting for nearly 5 percent of U.S. gross domestic product. Without a doubt, any realistic cost containment policies must be directed at the hospital sector of the health economy. The hospital services industry is best characterized as oligopolistic in nature. Most markets have a few competing hospitals, with existing hospitals generally having a cost advantage over new ones due to learning curve economies. Because of limited actual and potential competition, hospitals may have some ability to raise price above the competitive level, reduce quality, and produce with inefficient methods.

Countervailing the ability of hospitals to raise price is the dominance of some third-party payers in the hospital services market. The federal government sets fixed prices for nearly 30 percent of all hospital revenues under the Medicare program. In addition, large private insurers sometimes have sufficient buyer clout to negotiate sizeable hospital price discounts. Private insurers can also influence production decisions through utilization review mechanisms and by adopting various at-risk reimbursement methods.

Despite these changes, some evidence suggests that Medicare beneficiaries in regions with high levels of Medicare spending are not better off in terms of health outcomes. In addition, hospital care prices and costs continue to rise in the aggregate. Whether the aggregate hospital price and expenditure increases are due to imperfect hospital markets or normal market forces remains to be determined. Some health policy analysts want the federal government to encourage increased competition in the entire hospital sector so that macro-level cost savings are realizable. Others look to government to adopt blanket regulations, such as an "all-payer" Medicare PPS, as a way to contain aggregate hospital care costs. The merits of market-based and government-based solutions continue to be debated by health policy analysts.

Case Studies

13-1 Hospital Quality[30]

Researchers at Harvard University's School of Public Health conducted one of the largest analyses yet of federal hospital practice data and found significant differences in quality of care across American hospitals. Their study analyzed nationwide data from the government-sponsored Hospital Quality Alliance program, which tracks the performance of individual

30. Source: Keith J. Winstein, "How Cities Rate in Hospital Care," *The Wall Street Journal,* July 21, 2005.

hospitals in treating patients for three common health problems: heart attacks, congestive heart failure, and pneumonia. Based on data from 3,500 hospitals reported to the government, the study examined how often facilities followed ten practices with which physicians generally agree—for example, prescribing aspirin to heart attack patients or vaccinating pneumonia patients for the pneumococcal virus. The study then averaged hospital scores to come up with ratings for metropolitan areas. The numbers suggest that where you get sick can make a significant difference in the quality of treatment you receive. For example, you are likely to get better care for certain conditions in Boston, which was the top city for two out of three of the conditions, than you might in San Bernardino, California, which was the bottom city in two of the three illnesses.

Questions for Discussion

1. *In the hospital industry, is there a "business case" for quality? In other words, will higher-quality hospitals be rewarded financially for their efforts? Why or why not?*
2. *Discuss the role of payment mechanisms (used by third-party payers to pay hospitals) in how hospitals may or may not be rewarded for higher quality.*
3. *Why don't all physicians follow the practice guidelines? What can hospitals do to encourage physicians to follow widely accepted practice guidelines?*

13-2 Specialty Hospitals

Hospital specialization has become a controversial topic in recent years, culminating in 2003 when Congress issued a moratorium directing the Centers for Medicare & Medicaid Services (CMS) to cease payments to new physician-owned specialty hospitals for Medicare and Medicaid patients referred by physicians with a financial interest in the facility. The moratorium was mainly a response to concerns that specialized hospitals harm the community by undermining the ability of general hospitals to use excess profits on services such as orthopedic surgery to cross-subsidize unprofitable services considered essential to the community ("cream skimming"). Others argue that specialty hospitals exhibit many of the desirable attributes of "focused factories," offer higher levels of quality and more consumer-responsive products, and provide healthy competition to general hospitals. The moratorium required that CMS and MedPAC complete studies of specialty hospitals, and additional studies were conducted by MedCath and the Health Economics Consulting Group (HECG). At the same time, a study of specialty hospitals published in the *New England Journal of Medicine* found that specialty hospitals were essentially equivalent to or better than their general hospital counterparts in terms of quality, largely due to the higher procedure volumes at specialty hospitals. The CMS study reached similar conclusions regarding quality. With quality concerns effectively off the table, two policy issues remained: (1) is there a conflict of interest when physicians refer patients to facilities in which they have a financial interest, and (2) does competition from specialty hospitals prevent general hospitals from cross-subsidizing unprofitable services? Concerns over the former were allayed by the CMS study, which failed to find a strong relationship between the entry of specialty hospitals and changes in physician referral patterns. Concerns over the latter were addressed by the HECG study, which used econometric models to show that the presence of specialty hospitals was associated with *higher* general hospital operating margins. The moratorium was allowed to expire in June 2005.

Questions for Discussion

1. *The American Hospital Association (AHA) was one of the leading groups that opposed specialty hospitals. It focused primarily on the cross-subsidization issue and the need for a "level playing field." Is there an economic rationale for its argument? Are there any circumstances under which cross-subsidization is the "best" policy (as opposed to direct subsidies)?*
2. *The HECG study found that general hospitals in the same market as one or more specialty hospitals actually had higher operating margins than those in markets without specialty hospitals. The researchers found the same effects after controlling for "endogenous entry"; that is, specialty hospitals may be more likely to enter markets in which prevailing operating margins are higher. Discuss some likely economic explanations for these findings.*

13-3 Business Case for Hospital Quality?[31]

Evidence suggests that quality lapses in the form of hospital-acquired infections add to the high cost of U.S. health care. A study by a Pennsylvania state agency finds that 11,668 hospital-acquired infections were associated with an additional 1,510 deaths, 205,000 extra hospital days, and $2 billion in hospital charges in 2004. In 2005, Pennsylvania was the scene of a nationwide consumer campaign requiring hospitals to publicly report their infection data, motivated by fears that hospitals were underreporting infection rates. The application of simple standardized procedures, it was argued, could have prevented most if not all of these infections. Studies have shown that there was generally poor hospital compliance with known infection control techniques, such as washing hands before seeing a new patient. The data from Pennsylvania was extrapolated to the rest of the country, and suggest that more than 125 people per day die from hospital-acquired infections, resulting in an extra $50 billion in related hospital charges per year.

Questions for Discussion

1. *In addition to improving infection control, hospitals can improve quality and safety in other ways. For example, hospitals can invest in computerized physician order entry systems, which help catch errors before they reach the patient. Discuss how one might measure the rate of return of these kinds of investments.*
2. *Thinking about the previous question, describe the incentives that hospitals have to invest in improvements in quality and safety. In other words, for hospitals, what is the "business case" for quality improvements?*
3. *Assuming that third-party health insurers end up paying for 75 to 90 percent of the estimated $2 billion in costs attributed to hospital-acquired infections, to what extent should health insurers encourage, or even help pay for, improvements in hospital quality and safety?*

Review Questions and Problems

1. Answer the following questions on the number, size distribution, and ownership of American community hospitals.
   A. What has happened to the number of community hospitals and beds since the 1980s? Using the demand theory developed in Chapter 5, what reasons can you think of for that change?

31. Source: Rhonda L. Rundle, "Pennsylvania Finds High Toll in Hospital-Acquired Infections," *The Wall Street Journal*, July 13, 2005.

B. Which is the dominant form of hospital ownership? Rank the average for-profit, not-for-profit, and public hospital in terms of bed size.
C. Within which particular bed size category do most hospitals operate?

2. Explain how the relevant product market is typically defined for community hospitals. Why? How is the relevant geographical market defined? Why?
3. Assume there are ten equally sized hospitals in a market area. Calculate the Herfindahl-Hirschman index. Two hospitals in the market area inform the Department of Justice that they wish to merge. According to the current DOJ merger guidelines, will the merger be contested? Explain.
4. What are some possible sources of barriers to entry into the hospital industry? What has the literature concluded about the severity of these barriers?
5. Compare and contrast the technique and results associated with the econometric and survivor techniques of determining long-run economies of scale in the hospital services industry.
6. Answer the following questions on the buyers of hospital services.
   A. Who is the largest buyer of hospital services?
   B. What percentage of hospital costs are paid directly by the consumer?
   C. What factors affect the willingness and ability of private third-party payers to negotiate for low hospital prices?
7. What are some of the different ways third-party payers have reimbursed hospitals? Which methods are considered to constitute "at-risk" payments?
8. Compare and contrast the various managerial objectives in the quantity maximization, quality maximization, quality/quantity maximization, and managerial expense preference models.
9. In your words, discuss the fundamental difference between the profit maximization and utility maximization models. Also, identify what factors are likely to enter into a manager's utility function.
10. Use the quality maximization model to describe the role not-for-profit hospitals play in the diffusion of new medical technologies.
11. A study by Mark (1996) finds that not-for-profit psychiatric hospitals are no more efficient than their for-profit counterparts after controlling for quality. At the same time, the study finds that not-for-profit psychiatric hospitals provide a higher quality of care as measured by the number of violations and complaints received. Use the quality/quantity maximization model to explain these results.
12. Executives of not-for-profit hospitals have been criticized for being overcompensated (but see Santerre and Thomas, 1993). Use the managerial expense preference model to illustrate the theory behind these accusations.
13. According to Schlesinger et al. (1996), the not-for-profit firm "must engage in activities that generate prestige or otherwise enhance the reputation of those affiliated with the agency" (p. 712). For example, a not-for-profit hospital may conduct medical research in a particular area in order to develop a national reputation and gain what Schlesinger refers to as "prestige from exclusivity" (p. 712). Use the quality maximization model to explain this behavior.
14. Some economists have suggested that the best way to control medical costs is to remove the profit incentive for health care providers, particularly hospitals. This would involve making all hospitals not-for-profit institutions. Use the utility maximization model to explain the likely impact such a policy would have on the cost of producing hospital services. What would happen if instead a policy was instituted that reduced barriers to entry in the hospital sector and therefore made the market more competitive?

15. According to Lutz (1993), the attorney general of Texas challenged the tax-exempt status of the Methodist Hospital of Houston. At the heart of the controversy was a disagreement over the amount of charitable care the hospital had been providing. The attorney general claimed that the hospital provided only $25.9 million in charity care from 1986 through 1990. Using a much broader definition of charity care that included items that were not reimbursed, such as the costs of community service programs and education, the hospital claimed it had provided $191.9 million of charity care from 1986 through 1990. In addition, the hospital was criticized for adding in 1989 an extravagant, nine-story building called the John S. Dunn Tower that included a spacious, two-story lobby, a health club, and a gourmet restaurant. Use the economic theory developed in this chapter to put the debate between the attorney general of Texas and Methodist Hospital in a broader context.
16. Studies using data prior to 1983 found that increased hospital competition led to higher hospital prices. How do researchers explain that result? What have more recent studies concluded about the relation between competition and prices in the hospital industry? Why has this change occurred?
17. Explain the property rights and public choice theories concerning how differences in ownership affect the costs of producing hospital services. Why do empirical studies tend to find few cost differences among the various hospital ownership types?
18. According to empirical studies, what effect do managed care programs have on the costs of producing hospital services? How has managed care affected the quality of care according to studies?
19. According to empirical studies, what effect do state rate review regulations have on the costs of producing hospital services? How have state rate review regulations affected the quality of care?
20. Why may vertically integrated delivery systems lead to lower production costs? Why may these systems lead to higher costs? Use agency theory and transaction cost economics in your explanations.
21. Answer the following questions on the aggregate performance of the hospital sector by filling in the blanks.
    A. Hospital expenditures as a fraction of GDP were ________ in 1960 and increased to ________ by 2003.
    B. Since 1980, the hospital inflation rate has ________ the general inflation rate in nearly every year.
    C. Since 1982, the hospital occupancy rate, admission rate, and average length of stay have tended to ________. The hospital staffing ratio has tended to ________. (Why?)
22. Discuss the general conclusions researchers have reached concerning the provision of inappropriate hospital services.
23. Explain what studies have found concerning the concentration of health care expenditures. What may that finding mean in terms of serious cost containment efforts?
24. Explain how the total hospital margin is calculated. Would you say that the hospital margin has been excessive in the recent past?
25. Explain the two ways that private payer prices may influence the rates set under the Medicare PPS.
26. What does cost shifting involve? Why do many economists suspect that cost shifting may not occur in practice? Theoretically, what conditions are necessary for hospitals to practice cost shifting?

CEBS QUESTIONS

■ *CEBS Sample Question on Subject Matter from CEBS Course 9 Study Manual*

1. Discuss the property rights theory as it applies to not-for-profit hospitals. (pages 403–406)

■ *CEBS Sample Exam Questions*

1. The supply side of the hospital services industry can be characterized as:
   A. Perfect competition
   B. Oligopoly
   C. Monopolistic competition
   D. Static dynamism
   E. Pure monopoly
2. Which of the following statements describe(s) insights revealed by recent studies examining the relationship between Medicare spending and health outcomes?
   I. Greater regional spending on Medicare can be attributed to greater access to the latest medical technological innovations.
   II. Medicare enrollees in higher spending regions tend to be more satisfied with their care and have better health outcomes.
   III. Evidence exists that increasing Medicare expenditures may provide important benefits to the population being served.
   A. None
   B. I only
   C. III only
   D. I and II only
   E. II and III only
3. All the following statements regarding the utilization of hospital services in recent years are correct EXCEPT:
   A. A smaller percentage of the population has been admitted to hospitals.
   B. Hospital admissions typically are for a shorter duration.
   C. Hospital occupancy rates have risen slightly in recent years.
   D. Outpatient visits (per 100 population) have decreased.
   E. Staffing ratios in hospitals have increased.

■ *Answer to Sample Question from Study Manual*

The property right theory suggests that not-for-profit hospitals may operate with higher costs than otherwise similar for-profit hospitals because of the absence of outside owners or residual claimants. The theory also suggests that not-for-profit hospitals, because of the attenuation of property rights, face less of an incentive to sacrifice quality for the sake of profits. This is particularly true for situations where quality of care enters the utility function of the managers running the not-for-profit hospitals.

■ *Answers to Sample Exam Questions*

1. B is the answer. Oligopoly is the market term that best describes the hospital services industry. See pages 392–393 of the text.
2. A is the answer. All three statements are not true. The studies actually showed that greater regional spending on Medicare could be largely explained by practice patterns, Medicare enrollees in higher spending regions did not have better health outcomes or satisfaction with care, and increases in Medicare spending are not likely to result in improved quality of care. See page 422 of the text.
3. D is the answer. With the decrease in inpatient admissions and shorter length of hospital stays, outpatient visits have increased. See pages 420–421.

Online Resources

To access Internet links related to the topics in this chapter, please visit our web site at **www.thomsonedu.com/economics/santerre**.

References

Aaron, Henry J. *Serious and Unstable Condition: Financing America's Health Care*. Washington, D.C.: The Brookings Institution, 1991.

Anders, George. "Medical Luxury: Hospital Beds Go High-Tech, and Some Cost as Much as a Car." *The Wall Street Journal*, May 6, 1993a, p. A1.

_____. "As Outpatient Care Gains, Communities Need to Trim Their Excess Hospital Beds." *The Wall Street Journal*, February 22, 1993b, p. B1.

Anderson, Gerard F. "All-Payer Ratesetting: Down but Not Out." *Health Care Financing Review* (annual supplement, 1991), pp. 35–41.

Antel, John J., Robert L. Ohsfeldt, and Edmund R. Becker. "State Regulation and Hospital Costs." *Review of Economics and Statistics* 77 (August 1995), pp. 416–22.

Bailit, Howard L., and Cary Sennett. "Utilization Management as a Cost-Containment Strategy." *Health Care Financing Review* (annual supplement, 1991), pp. 87–93.

Baker, Jonathan B. "The Antitrust Analysis of Hospital Mergers and the Transformation of the Hospital Industry." *Law and Contemporary Problems* 51 (spring 1988), pp. 93–164.

Barro, Jason R., and Michael Chu. "HMO Penetration, Ownership Status, and the Rise of Hospital Advertising." NBER Working Paper No. 8899. Cambridge, Mass.: National Bureau of Economic Research, April 2002.

Bates, Laurie J., Kankana Mukherjee, and Rexford E. Santerre. "Market Structure and Technical Efficiency in the Hospital Services Industry: A DEA Approach." *Medical Care Research and Review*, August 2006.

Bates, Laurie J., and Rexford E. Santerre. "Do Agglomeration Economies Exist in the Hospital Services Industry?" *Eastern Economic Journal* (fall 2005).

Baumol, William. *Business Behavior, Value and Growth*. Englewood Cliffs, N.J.: Prentice Hall, 1967.

Bays, Carson W. "The Determinants of Hospital Size: A Survivor Analysis." *Applied Economics* 18 (1986), pp. 359–77.

Berk, Marc L., and Alan C. Monheit. "The Concentration of Health Expenditures: Revisited." *Health Affairs* 20 (March/April 2001), pp. 9–18.

Bernstein, Steven J., et al. "The Appropriateness of Use of Coronary Angiography in New York State." *Journal of the American Medical Association* 269 (February 10, 1993), pp. 766–69.

Bradbury, R. C., Joseph H. Golec, and Frank E. Stearns. "Comparing Hospital Length of Stay in Independent Practice Association HMOs and Traditional Insurance Programs." *Inquiry* 28 (spring 1991), pp. 87–93.

Brown, H. S. "Managed Care and Technical Efficiency." *Health Economics* 12 (2003), pp. 149–58.

Burda, David. "Flurry of Merger Plans Has Eyes Focused on Iowa." *Modern Healthcare* (April 12, 1993), p. 24.

Burns, Lawton R., and Mark V. Pauly. "Integrated Delivery Networks: A Detour on the Road to Integrated Health Care?" *Health Affairs* 21 (July/August 2002), pp. 128–43.

Burns, Lawton R., and Darrell P. Thorpe. "Trends and Models in Physician-Hospital Organization." *Health Care Management Review* 18 (fall 1993), pp. 7–20.

Capps, Cory, and David Dranove. "Hospital Consolidation and Negotiated PPO Prices." *Health Affairs* 23 (March/April 2004), pp. 175–81.

Carlisle, David M., et al. "HMO vs. Fee-for-Service Care of Older Persons with Acute Myocardial Infarction." *American Journal of Public Health* 82 (December 1992), pp. 1626–30.

Carlton, Dennis W., and Jeffrey M. Perloff. *Modern Industrial Organization*. Reading, Mass.: Addison-Wesley, 1994.

Carey, Kathleen. "Stochastic Demand for Hospitals and Optimizing 'Excess' Bed Capacity." *Journal of Regulatory Economics* 14 (1998), pp. 165–87.

Chassin, Mark R., et al. "Does Inappropriate Use Explain Geographic Variations in the Use of Health Care Services?" *Journal of the American Medical Association* 258 (November 13, 1987), pp. 2533–37.

Clark, Nicola. "The High Costs of Dying." *The Wall Street Journal*, February 22, 1992, p. A16.

Coelen, C., and D. Sullivan. "An Analysis of the Effects of Prospective Reimbursement Programs on Hospital Expenditures." *Health Care Financing Review* 2, no. 3 (1981), pp. 1–40.

Congressional Budget Office. *Impact of PSROs on Health-Care Costs: Update of CBO's 1979 Evaluation*. Washington, D.C.: U.S. Government Printing Office, 1981.

Conover, Christopher J., and Frank A. Sloan. "Does Removing Certificate of Need Regulations Lead to a Surge in Health Care Spending?" *Journal of Health Politics, Policy, and Law* 23 (June 1998), pp. 456–81.

Corrigan, Janet M., Jill S. Eden, Marsha R. Gold, and Jeremy D. Pickreign. "Trends toward a National Health Care Marketplace." *Inquiry* 34 (spring 1997), pp. 11–28.

Cowing, Thomas G., and Alphonse G. Holtmann. "Multiproduct Short-Run Hospital Cost Functions: Empirical Evidence and Policy Implications from Cross-Section Data." *Southern Economic Journal* (January 1983), pp. 637–53.

Cowing, Thomas G., Alphonse G. Holtmann, and S. Powers. "Hospital Cost Analysis: A Survey and Evaluation of Recent Studies." In *Advances in Health Economics and Health Services Research*, vol. 4, eds. Richard M. Scheffler and Louis F. Rossiter. Greenwich, Conn.: JAI Press, 1983, pp. 257–303.

Cuellar, Alison E., and Paul J. Gertler. "How the Expansion of Hospital Systems has affected Consumers." *Health Affairs*, 24 (January/February 2005), pp. 213–19.

Davis, Karen. "Economic Theories of Behavior in Not-for-profit, Private Hospitals." *Economic and Business Bulletin* (winter 1972), pp. 1–13.

Diehr, Paula, et al. "Use of a Preferred Provider Plan by Employees of the City of Seattle." *Medical Care* 28 (November 1990), pp. 1073–88.

Dorfman, Robert, and Peter O. Steiner. "Optimal Advertising and Optimal Quality." *American Economic Review* 44 (1954), pp. 826–36.

Dowd, B. R., Roger Feldman, Stephen Cassou, and Michael Finch. "Health Plan Choice and the Utilization of Health Care Services." *Review of Economics and Statistics* 73 (February 1991), pp. 85–93.

Dranove, David, Mark Shanley, and Carol Simon. "Is Hospital Competition Wasteful?" *RAND Journal of Economics* 23 (summer 1992), pp. 247–62.

Dranove, David, Mark Shanley, and William D. White. "Price and Concentration in Hospital Markets: The Switch from Patient-Driven to Payer-Driven Competition." *Journal of Law and Economics* 36 (April 1993), pp. 179–204.

Dranove, David, and Richard Lindrooth. "Hospital Consolidation and Costs: Another Look at the Evidence." *Journal of Health Economics* 22 (2003), pp. 983–97.

Dranove, David, and William D. White. "Medicaid-Dependent Hospitals and Their Patients: How Have They Fared? *Health Services Research* 33 (1998), pp. 163–86.

Draper, D., et al. "Studying the Effects of the DRG-Based Prospective Payment System on the Quality of Care: Design, Sampling, and Fieldwork." *Journal of the American Medical Association* 264 (October 17, 1990), pp. 1956–61.

Eakin, B. Kelly, and Thomas J. Kniesner. "Estimating a Non-Minimum Cost Function for Hospitals." *Southern Economic Journal* (January 1988), pp. 583–97.

Elzinga, K. G., and T. F. Hogarty. "The Problem of Geographic Market Definition Revisited: The Case of Coal." *Antitrust Bulletin* 23 (1978), pp. 1–18.

Emanuel, Ezekiel J., and Linda L. Emanuel. "The Economics of Dying: The Illusion of Cost Savings at the End of Life." *New England Journal of Medicine* 330 (February 24, 1994), pp. 540–44.

Ermann, Dan. "Hospital Utilization Review: Past Experience, Future Directions." *Journal of Health Politics, Policy and Law* 13 (winter 1988), pp. 683–704.

Ermann, Dan, and Jon Gabel. "Multihospital Systems: Issues and Empirical Findings." *Health Affairs* 3 (spring 1984), pp. 50–64.

Farley, Dean E. *Competition among Hospitals: Market Structure and Its Relation to Utilization, Costs and Financial Position*. Research note 7, Hospital Studies Program, National Center for Health Services Research and Health Care Technology Assessment, 1985.

Farley, Dean E., and Ronald J. Ozminkowski. "Volume-Outcome Relationships and Inhospital Mortality: The Effect of Changes in Volume over Time." *Medical Care* 30 (January 1992), pp. 77–94.

Feldman, R., et al. "Effects of HMOs on the Creation of Competitive Markets for Hospital Services." *Journal of Health Economics* 9 (September 1990), pp. 207–22.

Feldman, Roger, John Kralewski, Janet Shapiro, and Hung-Ching Chan. "Contracts between Hospitals and Health Maintenance Organizations." *Health Care Management Review* 15, no. 1 (winter 1990), pp. 47–60.

Feldstein, Martin S. "Hospital Cost Inflation: A Study of Not-for-profit Price Dynamics." *American Economic Review* 61 (December 1971), pp. 853–72.

Feldstein, Paul J., T. M. Wickizer, and J. R. Wheeler. "Private Cost Containment: The Effects of Utilization Review Programs on Health Care Use and Expenditures." *New England Journal of Medicine* 318 (May 19, 1988), pp. 1310–14.

Fielding, Jonathan E., and Thomas Rice. "Can Managed Competition Solve the Problems of Market Failure?" *Health Affairs* 12 (supplement, 1993), pp. 216–28.

Fisher, Charles R. "Trends in Total Hospital Financial Performance under the Prospective Payment System." *Health Care Financing Review* 13 (spring 1992), pp. 1–16.

Fisher, Elliott S., David E. Wennberg, Therese A. Stukel, Daniel J. Gottlieb, F. L. Lucas, and Etoile L. Pinder. "The Implications of Regional Variations in Medicare Spending. Part 1: The Content, Quality, and Accessibility of Care." *Annals of Internal Medicine* 138 (February 18, 2003a), pp. 273–87.

_____. "The Implications of Regional Variations in Medicare Spending. Part 2: Health Outcomes and Satisfaction of Care." *Annals of Internal Medicine* 138 (February 18, 2003b), pp. 288–99.

Fitzgerald, John F., Patricia S. Moore, and Robert S. Dittus. "The Care of Elderly Patients with Hip Fracture: Changes since Implementation of the Prospective Payment System." *New England Journal of Medicine* (November 24, 1988), pp. 1392–97.

Fournier, Gary M., and Jean M. Mitchell. "Hospital Costs and Competition for Services: A Multiproduct Analysis." *Review of Economics and Statistics* (November 1992), pp. 627–34.

Frech, H. E., III. "Comments on Antitrust Issues." In *Advances in Health Economics and Health Services Research*, vol. 7, eds. Richard M. Scheffler and Louis F. Rossiter. Greenwich, Conn.: JAI Press, 1987, pp. 263–67.

Friedman, Bernard, and Mark Pauly. "Cost Functions for a Service Firm with Variable Quality and Stochastic Demand: The Case of Hospitals." *Review of Economics and Statistics* 63 (November 1981), pp. 620–24.

Friedman, Bernard, Neeraj Sood, Kelly Engstrom, and Diane McKenzie. "New Evidence on Hospital Profitability by Payer Group and the Effects of Payer Generosity." *International Journal of Health Care Finance and Economics* 4 (2004), pp. 231–46.

Garnick, Deborah W., et al. "Services and Charges by PPO Physicians for PPO and Indemnity Patients: An Episode of Care Comparison." *Medical Care* 28 (October 1990), pp. 894–906.

Gaumer, Gary L., et al. "Effects of State Prospective Reimbursement Programs on Hospital Mortality." *Medical Care* 27 (July 1989), pp. 724–36.

Gaynor, Martin, and Gerard F. Anderson. "Uncertain Demand, the Structure of Hospital Costs, and the Cost of Empty Hospital Beds." *Journal of Health Economics* 14 (1995), pp. 291–317.

Ginsburg, Paul B. "Can Hospitals and Physicians Shift the Effects of Cuts in Medicare Reimbursement to Private Payers?" *Health Affairs,* Web Exclusive http://www.healthaffairs.org (October 8, 2003), pp. 472–9.

Goes, James B., and Chun Liu Zhan. "The Effects of Hospital-Physician Integration Strategies on Hospital Financial Performance." *Health Services Research* 30 (October 1995), pp. 507–30.

Grannemann, Thomas W., Randall S. Brown, and Mark V. Pauly. "Estimating Hospital Costs: A Multiple-Output Analysis." *Journal of Health Economics* 5 (1986), pp. 107–27.

Gray, James. "The Selling of Medicine, 1986." *Medical Economics* (January 20, 1986), pp. 180–94.

Greenwald, Howard P., and Curtis J. Henke. "HMO Membership, Treatment, and Mortality Risk among Prostatic Cancer Patients." *American Journal of Public Health* 82 (August 1992), pp. 1099–1104.

Hadley, Jack, and Judith, Feder. "Hospital Cost Shifting and Care for the Uninsured." *Health Affairs* 4 (1985), pp. 67–80.

Halm, Ethan A., Clara Lee, and Mark R. Chassin. "Is Volume Related to Outcome in Health Care? A Systematic Review and Methodologic Critique of the Literature." *Annals of Internal Medicine* 137 (September 2002), pp. 511–20.

Harris, Jeffrey E. "The Internal Organization of Hospitals: Some Economic Implications." *Bell Journal of Economics* 8 (1977), pp. 467–82.

Hart, Oliver. *Firms, Contracts, and Financial Structure.* Oxford: Clarendon Press, 1995.

Health Care Forum LLC. *Hospital Statistics*. Chicago: American Hospital Association, 2005.

Hersch, Philip L. "Competition and the Performance of Hospital Markets." *Review of Industrial Organization* 1 (winter 1984), pp. 324–40.

Herzlinger, Regina E., and William S. Krasker. "Who Profits from Not-for-profits?" *Harvard Business Review* (January–February 1987), pp. 93–106.

Hester, James A., Anne Marie Wouters, and Norman Wright. "Evaluation of a Preferred Provider Organization." *Milbank Quarterly* 65 (1987), pp. 575–613.

Hilborne, Lee H., et al. "The Appropriateness of Use of Percutaneous Transluminal Coronary Angioplasty in New York State." *Journal of the American Medical Association* 269 (February 10, 1993), pp. 761–65.

Ho, Vivian. "Learning and the Evolution of Medical Technologies: The Diffusion of Coronary Angioplasty." *Journal of Health Economics* 21 (2002), pp. 873–85.

Ho, Vivian, and Barton H. Hamilton. "Hospital Mergers and Acquisitions: Does Market Consolidation Harm Patients?" *Journal of Health Economics* 19 (2000), pp. 767–91.

Hoy, Elizabeth W., Richard E. Curtis, and Thomas Rice. "Change and Growth in Managed Care." *Health Affairs* 10 (winter 1991), pp. 18–36.

Iglehart, John. "The American Health Care System—Medicare Program." *New England Journal of Medicine* 327 (November 12, 1992), pp. 1467–72.

Japsen, Bruce. "Ad Budget Drop." *Modern Healthcare* 27 (February 17, 1997), pp. 70–71.

Joskow, Paul L. "The Effects of Competition and Regulation on Hospital Bed Supply and the Reservation Quality of Hospitals." *Bell Journal of Economics* (autumn 1980), pp. 421–47.

Kahn, K. L., et al. "Comparing Outcomes of Care before and after Implementation of the DRG-Based Prospective Payment System." *Journal of the American Medical Association* 264 (October 17, 1990), pp. 1984–88.

Keeler, Theodore E., and John S. Ying. "Hospital Costs and Excess Bed Capacity: A Statistical Analysis." *Review of Economics and Statistics* 78 (August 1996), pp. 470–81.

Kessler, Daniel P., and Mark B. McClellan. "Is Hospital Competition Socially Wasteful?" *Quarterly Journal of Economics* (May 2000), pp. 577–615.

Lagnado, L. "Hospitals Try Extreme Measures to Collect Their Overdue Debts." *The Wall Street Journal,* October 30, 2003, p. A1.

Lane, Paul M., and Jay D. Lindquist. "Hospital Choice: A Summary of the Key Empirical and Hypothetical Findings of the 1980s." *Journal of Health Care Marketing* 8 (December 1988), pp. 5–20.

Lanning, Joyce A., Michael A. Morrisey, and Robert L. Ohsfeldt. "Endogenous Hospital Regulation and Its Effects on Hospital and Non-Hospital Expenditures." *Journal of Regulatory Economics* 3 (1991), pp. 137–54.

Leape, Lucian L., et al. "The Appropriateness of Use of Coronary Artery Bypass Graft Surgery in New York State." *Journal of the American Medical Association* 269 (February 10, 1993), pp. 753–60.

Lee, Maw Lin. "A Conspicuous Production Theory of Hospital Behavior." *Southern Economic Journal* 38 (July 1971), pp. 48–58.

Luft, Harold S. *Health Maintenance Organizations: Dimensions of Performance*. New York: Wiley-Interscience, 1981.

Luft, Harold S., et al. "The Role of Specialized Clinical Services in Competition among Hospitals." *Inquiry* 23 (spring 1986), pp. 83–94.

Lutz, Sandy. "Charity Care and the Law: Case Is Far from Closed." *Modern Healthcare* (March 8, 1993), pp. 26–28.

Mann, Joyce M., Glenn A. Melnick, Anil Bamezai, and Jack Zwanziger. "A Profile of Uncompensated Hospital Care, 1983–1995." *Health Affairs* 16 (July/August 1997), pp. 223–32.

Manning, Willard G., et al. "A Controlled Trial of the Effect of a Prepaid Group Practice on Use of Services." *New England Journal of Medicine* 310 (June 7, 1984), pp. 1505–10.

Mark, Tami L. "Psychiatric Hospital Ownership and Performance." *Journal of Human Resources* 31 (summer 1996), pp. 631–49.

Melnick, Glenn A., Jack Zwanziger, Anil Bamezai, and Robert Pattison. "The Effects of Market Structure and Bargaining Position on Hospital Prices." *Journal of Health Economics* 11 (1992), pp. 217–33.

Menke, Terri J. "The Effect of Chain Membership on Hospital Costs." *Health Services Research* 32 (June 1997), pp. 177–96.

Miller, Robert H., and Harold S. Luft. "Managed Care Performance since 1980: A Literature Analysis." *Journal of the American Medical Association* 271 (May 18, 1994), pp. 1512–19.

_____. "HMO Plan Performance Update: An Analysis of the Literature, 1997–2000." *Health Affairs* 21 (July/August 2002), pp. 63–86.

Morrisey, M. A. "Cost Shifting: New Myths, Old Confusion, and Enduring Reality." *Health Affairs*, Web Exclusive http://www.healthaffairs.org (October 8, 2003), pp. 489–91.

Morrisey, Michael A., and Jeffrey A. Alexander. "Hospital Participation in Multihospital Systems." In *Advances in Health Economics and Health Services Research*, vol. 7, eds. Richard M. Scheffler and Louis F. Rossiter. Greenwich, Conn.: JAI Press, 1987, pp. 59–82.

Morrisey, Michael A., Jeffrey Alexander, Lawton R. Burns, and Victoria Johnson. "Managed Care and Physician/Hospital Integration." *Health Affairs* 15 (winter 1996), pp. 62–73.

Morrisey, Michael A., Douglas A. Conrad, Stephen M. Shortell, and Karen S. Cook. "Hospital Rate Review: A Theory and an Empirical Review." *Journal of Health Economics* 3 (September 1984), pp. 25–47.

Morrisey, Michael A., Gerald J. Wedig, and Mahmud Hassan. "Do Not-for-profit Hospitals Pay Their Way?" *Health Affairs* 15 (winter 1996), pp. 132–44.

Newhouse, Joseph. "Toward a Theory of Not-for-profit Institutions: An Economic Model of a Hospital." *American Economic Review* 60 (March 1970), pp. 64–74.

Nicholson, Sean, Mark V. Pauly, Lawton R. Burns, Agnieska Baumritter, and David A. Asch. "Measuring Community Benefits Provided by For-Profit and Not-for-profit Hospitals." *Health Affairs* 19 (November/December 2000), pp. 168–77.

Noether, Monica. "Competition among Hospitals." *Journal of Health Economics* 7 (1988), pp. 259–84.

_____. *Competition among Hospitals*. Washington, D.C.: Federal Trade Commission, 1987.

Pauly, M., and M. Redish. "The Not-for-Profit Hospital as a Physicians' Cooperative." *American Economic Review* 63 (1973), pp. 87–99.

Pauly, Mark V. "Not-for-profit Firms in Medical Markets." *American Economic Review Proceedings* 77 (May 1987), pp. 257–62.

Pope, Gregory C., and Terri Menke. "Hospital Labor Markets in the 1980s." *Health Affairs* 9 (winter 1990), pp. 127–37.

Rapoport, John, Stephen Gehlbach, Stanley Lemeshow, and Daniel Teres. "Resource Utilization among Intensive Care Patients: Managed Care vs.

Traditional Insurance." *Archives of Internal Medicine* 152 (November 1992), pp. 2207–12.

Renn, Steven C., Carl J. Schramm, J. Michael Watt, and Robert A. Derzon. "The Effects of Ownership and System Affiliation on the Economic Performance of Hospitals." *Inquiry* 22 (fall 1985), pp. 219–36.

Retchin, Sheldon M., and Barbara Brown. "Elderly Patients with Congestive Heart Failure under Prepaid Care." *American Journal of Medicine* 90 (February 1991), pp. 236–42.

Retchin, Sheldon M., et al. "How the Elderly Fare in HMOs: Outcomes from the Medicare Competition Demonstrations." *Health Services Research* 27 (December 1992), pp. 651–69.

Robinson, James C. "Physician-Hospital Integration and the Economic Theory of the Firm." *Medical Care Research and Review* 54 (March 1997), pp. 3–24.

Robinson, James C., and Harold S. Luft. "The Impact of Hospital Market Structure on Patient Volume, Average Length of Stay, and the Cost of Care." *Journal of Health Economics* 4 (December 1985), pp. 333–56.

Robinson, James C., and Ciaran S. Phibbs. "An Evaluation of Medicaid Selective Contracting in California." *Journal of Health Economics* 8 (February 1990), pp. 437–55.

Romeo, Anthony A., Judith L. Wagner, and Robert H. Lee. "Prospective Reimbursement and the Diffusion of New Technologies in Hospitals." *Journal of Health Economics* 3 (1984), pp. 1–24.

Rosko, Michael D. "Impact of HMO Penetration and Other Environmental Factors on Hospital X-Inefficiency." *Medical Care Research and Review* 58 (December 2001), pp. 430–54.

Santerre, Rexford E., and Ammon S. Adams. "The Effect of Competition on Reserve Capacity: The Case of California Hospitals in the Late 1990s." *International Journal of Health Care Finance and Economics* 2(2002), pp. 205–18.

Santerre, Rexford E., and Dana C. Bennett. "Hospital Market Structure and Cost Performance: A Case Study." *Eastern Economic Journal* 18 (spring 1992), pp. 209–19.

Santerre, Rexford E., and Debra Pepper. "Survivorship in the US Hospital Services Industry." *Managerial and Decision Economics* 21 (2000), pp. 181–89.

Santerre, Rexford E., and Janet M. Thomas. "The Determinants of Hospital CEO Compensation," *Health Care Management Review* 18 (summer 1993), pp. 31–40.

Scherer, F. M., and David Ross. *Industrial Market Structure and Economic Performance*. Boston: Houghton Mifflin, 1990.

Schlesinger, Mark, Bradford Gary, and Elizabeth Bradley. "Charity and Community: The Role of Not-for-profit Ownership in a Managed Care System." *Journal of Health Politics, Policy and Law* 21 (winter 1996), pp. 697–752.

Schneider, John E. "Changes in the Effects of Mandatory Rate Regulation on Growth in Hospital Operating Costs, 1980–1996." *Review of Industrial Organization* 22 (2003), pp. 297–312.

Schramm, Carl J., and Steven C. Renn. "Hospital Mergers, Market Concentration and the Herfindahl-Hirschman Index." *Emory Law Journal* 33 (fall 1984), pp. 869–88.

Schwartz, William B., and D. N. Mendelson "Hospital Cost Containment in the 1980s—Hard Lessons Learned and Prospects for the 1990s" *New England Journal of Medicine* 324 (April 11, 1991), pp. 1037–41.

Shortell, Stephen M. "Physician-Hospital Integration and the Economic Theory of the Firm: Comment." *Medical Care Research and Review* 54 (March 1997), pp. 25–31.

Shortell, Stephen M., and Edward F. X. Hughes. "The Effects of Regulation, Competition, and Ownership on Mortality Rates among Hospital Inpatients." *New England Journal of Medicine* 318 (April 28, 1988), pp. 1100–7.

Sloan, Frank A., Gabriel A. Picone, Donald H. Taylor, Jr., and Shin-Yi Chou. "Hospital Ownership and Cost and Quality of Care: Is There a Dime's Worth of Difference?" *Journal of Health Economics* 20 (2001), pp. 1–21.

Sloan, Frank A. "Property Rights in the Hospital Industry." In *Health Care in America*, ed. H. E. Frech III. San Francisco: Pacific Research Institute for Public Policy, 1988, pp. 103–41.

Sloan, Frank A. "Not-for-Profit Ownership and Hospital Behavior." In *Handbook of Health Economics, Vol. 1B*, eds. A. J. Culyer and J. P. Newhouse. Amsterdam: Elsevier Science, 2000, pp. 1141–74.

Smith, David W., Stephanie L. McFall, and Michael B. Pine. "State Rate Regulation and Inpatient Mortality Rates." *Inquiry* 30 (spring 1993), pp. 23–33.

Smith, Dean. "The Effects of Preferred Provider Organizations on Health Care Use and Costs." *Inquiry* 34 (winter 1997/1998), pp. 278–87.

Spang, Heather R., Gloria J. Bazzoli, and Richard J. Arnould. "Hospital Mergers and Savings for Consumers: Exploring New Evidence." *Health Affairs* 20 (July/August 2001), pp. 150–58.

Stigler, George J. "The Economies of Scale." *Journal of Law and Economics* 1 (October 1958), pp. 54–71.

Stone, Valerie E., George R. Seage, Thomas Hertz, and Arnold M. Epstein. "The Relation between Hospital Experience and Mortality for Patients with AIDS." *Journal of the American Medical Association* 268 (November 18, 1992), pp. 2655–61.

Temin, Peter. "An Economic History of American Hospitals." In *Health Care in America*, ed. H. E. Frech III. San Francisco: Pacific Research Institute for Public Policy, 1988, pp. 75–102.

Thorpe, Kenneth E., and Charles E. Brecher. "Improved Access for the Uninsured Poor in Large Cities: Do Public Hospitals Make a Difference?" *Journal of Health Politics, Policy and Law* (summer 1987), pp. 313–24.

Town, Robert, and Gregory Vistnes. "Hospital Competition in HMO Networks." *Journal of Health Economics* 20 (2001), pp. 733–53.

Town, Robert J., and Imran Currim. "Hospital Advertising in California, 1991–1997." *Inquiry* 39 (fall 2002), pp. 298–313.

Vita, Michael G. "Exploring Hospital Production Relationships with Flexible Functional Forms." *Journal of Health Economics* 9 (June 1990), pp. 1–21.

Ware, John E., et al. "Comparison of Health Outcomes at a Health Maintenance Organization with Those of Fee-for-Service Care." *Lancet* (May 3, 1986), pp. 1017–22.

White, Stephen L. "The Effects of Competition on Hospital Costs in Florida." *Policy Studies Journal* 15 (March 1987), pp. 375–93.

Wilcox-Gok, Virginia. "The Effects of For-Profit Status and System Membership on the Financial Performance of Hospitals." *Applied Economics* 34 (2002), pp. 479–89.

Wilder, R. P., and P. Jacobs. "Antitrust Considerations for Hospital Mergers: Market Definition and Market Concentration." In *Advances in Health Economics and Health Services Research*, eds. Richard M. Scheffler and Louis F. Rossiter. Greenwich, Conn.: JAI Press, 1987, pp. 245–62.

Williamson, Oliver E. "Managerial Discretion and Business Behavior." *American Economic Review* 53 (December 1963), pp. 1032–57.

Williamson, Oliver E. *The Economic Institutions of Capitalism*. New York: Free Press, 1985.

Wilson, George W., and Joseph M. Jadlow. "Competition, Profit Incentives, and Technical Efficiency in the Provision of Nuclear Medicine Services." *Bell Journal of Economics* (autumn 1982), pp. 472–82.

Winslow, Constance Monroe, et al. "The Appropriateness of Performing Coronary Artery Bypass Surgery." *Journal of the American Medical Association* 260 (July 22–29, 1988), pp. 505–9.

Zwanziger, Jack, and Rebecca R. Auerbach. "Evaluating PPO Performance Using Prior Expenditure Data." *Medical Care* 29 (February 1991), pp. 142–51.

Zwanziger, Jack, and Glenn A. Melnick. "The Effects of Hospital Competition and the Medicare PPS Program on Hospital Cost Behavior in California." *Journal of Health Economics* 7 (1988), pp. 301–20.

Zwanziger Jack, Glenn A. Melnick, and Anil Bamezai. "Can Cost Shifting Continue in a Price Competitive Environment." *Health Economics* 9 (2000), pp. 211–255.

THE PHARMACEUTICAL INDUSTRY

CHAPTER 14

The research-based pharmaceutical industry as it is known today began with the development of sulfanilamide in the mid-1930s and penicillin in 1938.[1] With World War II came an increased demand for sulfa drugs and penicillin to protect soldiers from infection. The pharmaceutical industry quickly responded by replacing handicraft methods of preparing drugs, traditionally required for individual prescriptions, with mass production techniques (Egan et al., 1982). Chemical firms, such as Lederle and Merck, found ways to produce drugs in bulk form, which were then transformed into dosage form (such as powders and tablets) by drug companies, such as Upjohn. Pfizer developed a fermentation process to allow penicillin to be produced in large quantities. Penicillin was soon followed by other antibiotics, and research was stimulated in other therapeutic fields as well (Statman, 1983).

Following the war, high potential profits generated further innovation and drew other companies into the pharmaceutical industry. Many drug firms expanded and acquired sales forces to market their drugs in finished form. Research and development efforts in the pharmaceutical industry continually expanded during the postwar period.

This chapter provides a contemporary analysis of the pharmaceutical industry. Although the pharmaceutical industry of today closely resembles its postwar antecedent in terms of many supply-side characteristics, we will see that several institutional changes on the demand side of the market have had wide-sweeping effects on the conduct of the industry. The chapter studies the structure, conduct, and performance of the pharmaceutical industry. Specifically, it:

- discusses seller concentration, buyer concentration, barriers to entry, and product differentiation to see whether existing drug firms are endowed with some market power
- examines some topics pertaining to the conduct of the pharmaceutical industry, including price competition, promotional strategies, and product innovation. The important question concerns the actual degree of price and product competition that presently takes place in this industry
- assesses the performance of the contemporary pharmaceutical industry in terms of aggregate prices, output, and profits. The main query here is whether firms in the pharmaceutical industry have tended to charge high prices and earn excess profits

1. Statman (1983) points out that the drug trade is very old. The Ebers Papyrus lists 811 prescriptions used in Egypt in 550 BC.

The Structure of the Pharmaceutical Industry

Number and Size Distribution of Sellers

When one thinks about the pharmaceutical industry, the names of a few large companies, such as Pfizer, Johnson & Johnson, and Merck, normally come to mind. But actually a sizeable number of large companies coexist in the drug industry. Table 14–1 lists the total sales and market share of the 20 largest companies selling pharmaceutical products in the United States as of June 2005. Pfizer, the leader with a 12 percent market share, sells $10 billion more of pharmaceuticals than GlaxoSmithKline, the next largest domestic seller of drug products. Pfizer, GlaxoSmithKline, and many of the other companies listed produce brand-name pharmaceuticals, although they may manufacture and sell generic versions of these drugs as well. Some of the companies listed, such as Hoffman–La Roche and Boehringer Ingelheim, are headquartered outside the United States.

TABLE 14–1
Largest Pharmaceutical Companies by U.S. Sales, June 2005

Corporation	Total Sales (U.S. $Billions)	Market Share (percent)
Pfizer	$29.4	12%
GlaxoSmithKline	19.2	7.8
Johnson & Johnson	16.5	6.7
Merck & Co.	14.8	6.0
AstraZeneca	12.4	5.0
Novartis	11.0	4.5
Amgen	10.9	4.4
Sanofi-Aventis	10.8	4.4
Bristol-Myers Squibb	8.7	3.5
Lilly	8.5	3.4
Wyeth	8.4	3.4
Abbott	7.0	2.9
Hoffman–La Roche	6.8	2.8
TAP Pharmaceutical	4.8	2.0
Boehringer Ingelheim	4.5	1.8
Teva	3.9	1.6
Schering-Plough	3.4	1.4
Forest Lab	3.3	1.3
Eisai	2.6	1.1
Watson	2.5	1.0

SOURCE: IMS Health, http://www.imshealth.com (accessed November 30, 2005).

Other companies such as Teva, Forest Lab, and Watson you may not have heard of because they deal primarily in generic drug products.

Also, a multitude of lesser-known, smaller firms exist in the pharmaceutical industry. These drug firms primarily manufacture and retail generic drugs and place little, if any, emphasis on new drug discovery. In fact, government statistics indicate that a relatively large number of firms operate in the domestic drug industry. Table 14–2 displays some information on the number and size distribution of pharmaceutical companies in 1997. To put the pharmaceutical industry in some perspective, the table also gives comparative information on some other industries. These industries are chosen because the industry description is fairly straightforward and most people have some familiarity with them.

Based on the six-digit North American Industry Classification System (NAICS) of 325412 for pharmaceutical preparations, the data show that the U.S. pharmaceutical industry contained 707 firms in 1997. The four largest drug firms account for 36 percent of all industry output, and the largest eight are responsible for 50 percent. The Herfindahl-Hirschman index of market concentration (HHI) is very low at 462. Interestingly, these figures for 1997 correspond very closely to the CR_4, CR_8, and HHI that can be calculated from the figures in Table 14–1 for 2005. Both sets of figures imply that the pharmaceutical industry contains a considerable number of equally sized firms, and therefore appears to be reasonably competitive from a structural perspective.

Census estimates of market concentration in the pharmaceutical industry are based on an assumption that the market for all pharmaceuticals, despite the intended use of the many individual drugs, properly constitutes the relevant product market (RPM). A fairly broad definition of

TABLE 14–2
Concentration Ratios for Selected Industries, 1997

NAICS Code	Industry Description	Four-Firm Ratio	Eight-Firm Ratio	Number of Firms	HHI Index
325412	Pharmaceutical Preparations	36	50	707	462
311511	Fluid Milk	21	31	402	205
311230	Cereal Breakfast Foods	83	94	48	2,446
312111	Soft Drinks	47	56	388	800
325611	Soap and Detergents	66	78	738	1,619
324110	Petroleum Refining	29	49	122	422
326211	Tires	72	91	110	1,690
327213	Glass Containers	91	98	11	2,960
327320	Ready-Mixed Concrete	7	11	2,888	29
331312	Primary Aluminum	59	82	13	1,231
332431	Metal Cans	58	87	107	1,180
333292	Textile Machinery	24	36	454	269
336111	Automobile	80	96	173	2,350

SOURCE: U.S. Bureau of the Census, "Concentration Ratios in Manufacturing," *1997 Census of Manufacturers,* June 2001, Table 4, http://www.census.gov.

the RPM may be desirable if firms can allocate resources to new drug development or expand existing developments in a timely manner without substantial retraining or new hiring of personnel (DiMasi, 2000). That is, the aggregated approach of measuring the RPM captures the threat that drug firms face from the possibility that another drug company may develop a substitute product when more independent companies exist in the overall pharmaceutical industry.

If barriers to new development within a specific product line exist, therapeutic markets offer a narrower approach to defining the relevant product market for drugs. Given that most drugs are not substitutes in consumption because they have different intended uses, therapeutic markets are defined to include only drugs that treat common diseases or illnesses. For example, a physician looking to relieve a patient's ulcer condition does not choose among various brands of antidepressants and antiulcer drugs. However, the doctor may choose among Tagamet, Zantac, or Pepcid, which are all antiulcer drugs.

Data for concentration ratios based on therapeutic markets typically suggest a more concentrated market environment in the drug industry. For example, Figure 14–1 shows how many therapeutic classes out of 66 fall into different ranges of the three-firm concentration ratio during 1994. In particular, the data show that the top three drug companies are responsible for less than 30 percent of all sales in only 3 of the 66 therapeutic markets. Moreover, the figures indicate that the top three drug firms account for less than 50 percent of sales in only 9 of the 66 therapeutic markets. Clearly, the data imply that only a few drug manufacturers tend to dominate most therapeutic markets.

However, DiMasi (2000) reminds us that concentration measures of any type at a point in time are only rough static indicators of industry structure. Consistent measures of market concentration at different points in time often serve as an accurate indicator of the trend in concentration, although even then the particular reason for the trend (such as mergers for market power or

FIGURE 14–1
Market Share of the Top Three Innovator Drugs in 66 Therapeutic Classes, 1994

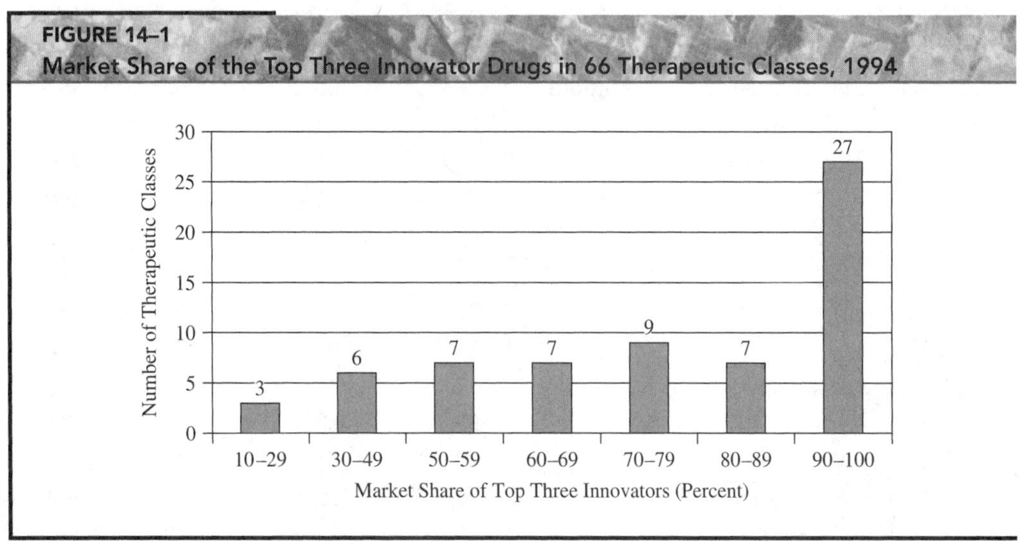

SOURCE: Congressional Budget Office (1998). Market shares are calculated as the total sales (valued at retail prices) of the top three innovator drugs in a therapeutic class divided by the total sales of all drugs (both brand-name and generic) in the class. Congressional Budget Office, *How Increased Competition from Generic Drugs has affected Prices and Returns in the Pharmaceutical Industry.* (July 1998) at http://www.cbo.gov.

efficiency) may not be apparent. Data for earlier editions of the *Census of Manufacturers*, based on the broad definition of the RPM, suggest that the degree of seller concentration in the pharmaceutical industry, while relatively stable in earlier years, may have started to increase in more recent years. For example, the four-firm concentration ratio was approximately 28 percent in 1947, 22 percent in 1963, and 22 percent in 1992. However, note in Table 14–2 (or Table 14–1 for 2005) that the four-firm concentration ratio equals 36 percent in 1997. The upward spike in the aggregate level of concentration since 1992 may have resulted from the many mergers involving relatively large drug companies. Some examples of the mergers taking place since 1992 include Pfizer with Warner-Lambert and Pharmacia; Glaxo Wellcome and SmithKline Beecham, and Ciba-Geigy with Sandoz (to form Novartis).

Sales data are unavailable to analyze changes over time in market concentration at the therapeutic level. However, DiMasi (2000) offers some information on the percentage of new chemical entities (NCEs) produced by the largest drug firms over time. New chemical entities contain active ingredients that have not been previously marketed in the United States. and thereby provide a measure of innovation. In fact, since innovations represent the lifeblood of the pharmaceutical industry, as discussed later in this chapter, it seems only fitting to use a measure of innovation when examining the relative importance of a few dominant drug firms.

In his study, DiMasi measures the four-firm concentration ratio and HHI of the number of NCEs in different therapeutic classes for the 1960s, 1970s, 1980s, and 1990s. Among his findings, he shows that the four-firm concentration ratios for cardiovascular NCEs are 61.6, 44.5, 27.7, and 23.3 percent during the various periods, respectively. These figures mean that the top four drug manufacturers accounted for nearly 62 percent of all new cardiovascular drugs during the 1960s but only 23 percent during the 1990s. Similarly, he reports HHIs of 1243, 864, 412, and 328 for cardiovascular NCEs for the four consecutive periods. He notes that other therapeutic classes generally exhibit a downward trend in concentration, although the specific period at which deconcentration occurred varied by therapeutic class.

Taking all of the information together, today's pharmaceutical industry comes across as being mildly concentrated. A few drug companies account for nearly 40 percent of all sales in the aggregate market and tend to dominate most therapeutic markets. However, evidence also indicates that dominant positions may not be very permanent in the pharmaceutical industry. Market shares are reasonably close among the top ten drug companies, and significant deconcentration has taken place at the therapeutic level for new chemical entities. Consequently, information on market concentration cannot by itself identify whether drug companies possess significant market power. Information on other market structure elements and the market behavior of drug firms must be considered before drawing conclusions about the market power of firms in the pharmaceutical industry.

The Buyer Side of the Pharmaceutical Market

The degree of buyer concentration is another important element that makes up market structure. For example, we discussed in Chapter 11 that a single buyer may exert monopsony power and force the reimbursement price below the competitive level. As another example, a powerful buyer may be able to offset any market power otherwise existing on the seller side of the market. Consequently, it is worthwhile to also examine the demand side of the pharmaceutical market in terms of the number and size distribution of buyers.

Data in Table 14–3 show that the buyer side of the market is relatively fragmented. Unlike spending on hospital and physician services, consumers directly pay for a relatively large percentage of drug costs. In particular, out-of-pocket expenses amount to $53 billion and represent

TABLE 14–3
Buyers of Prescription Drugs, 2003

Source	Expenditures (billions of dollars)	Percentage of Total
Total	$179.2	100.0%
All private	136.0	75.9
Out-of-pocket	53.2	29.7
Private insurance	82.9	46.3
All government	48.2	24.1
Federal	25.2	14.1
State	18.0	10.0

Note: Includes spending on drugs and other medical nondurables. Percentages do not sum to 100 percent due to rounding.

SOURCE: Centers for Medicare and Medicaid Services, http://www.cms.gov (accessed January, 2006).

nearly 30 percent of all prescription drug expenses in 2003. Interestingly, that same percentage figure was 63 percent just ten years earlier. Beginning in the early 1990s, many managed care companies attracted enrollees by offering them prescription drug coverage. Not surprisingly, the percentage of prescription drug costs reimbursed by insurers rose from 24.5 percent in 1993 to 46.3 percent in 2003.

The government, at all levels, currently accounts for 24 percent of all spending on prescription drugs. Eighteen percent of all pharmaceutical spending falls under the Medicaid program, which is funded by both federal and state governments. The Medicare program currently accounts for only 1.6 percent of all prescription drug spending. Most of this spending reflects drugs administered by hospital-based physicians to Medicare recipients receiving inpatient care.

As was pointed out in Chapter 10, the buyer side of the pharmaceutical market changed dramatically as of January 2006 because of the Medicare Prescription Drug Improvement and Modernization Act of 2003 (MMA). The act allows Medicare beneficiaries to enroll in private drug benefit plans that contract with the government. Beneficiaries who join a Medicare drug plan pay a monthly premium equal to 25 percent of the cost of a standard drug plan. As mentioned earlier, the drug benefit is designed with an annual deductible, benefit limits, and a catastrophic threshold, which are all indexed to grow over time. Most Medicare beneficiaries are also responsible for paying a coinsurance amount or a copayment. Medicare provides additional premium and cost-sharing assistance to beneficiaries with limited incomes and financial resources.

Of an estimated 43.1 million Medicare beneficiaries in 2006, about 29.3 million are expected to enroll in Medicare drug plans, with 10.9 million receiving low-income subsidies.[2] While Medicare funds most of the program, the increased pharmaceutical expenditures will show up as private insurance payments because private insurers are responsible for negotiating prices and

2. "Fact Sheet: The Medicare Prescription Drug Benefit," http://www.kff.org (accessed January 11, 2006).

paying for drugs under the MMA. It is too early to speculate on how the MMA may lead to a transformation of the buyer side of the pharmaceutical industry and thereby influence the pricing behavior of drug manufacturers.

The Realized Demand for Pharmaceutical Products. Although consumers are responsible for footing a relatively large portion of the drug bill, they generally are not responsible for choosing which specific drug to buy. Since the passage of the Federal Food, Drug and Cosmetic Act of 1938, consumer access to powerful drugs has been severely restricted (Temin, 1992). The 1938 act gave drug manufacturers the responsibility to assign new drugs to either of two classes: over-the-counter (OTC) or prescription (Rx).[3] Directions for use on the label make a drug available for self-medication. A prescription-only warning makes a drug available only by a physician's prescription. The Food and Drug Administration has to approve the manufacturer's proposed label.

Because prescription drugs remain the dominant type sold today, the "realized demands for pharmaceuticals depend not only on ultimate consumer tastes but also on the behavior of physicians who prescribe these drugs and the retail and hospital pharmacists who dispense the prescriptions" (Caves et al., 1991, p. 4). Physicians are not always in a position to serve the best financial interests of consumers, primarily because they are unaffected financially by the choice of prescription and often lack suitable information about the price, effectiveness, and risk of substitute drug products (Temin, 1980). Moreover, customary prescribing behavior minimizes effort and also provides a legal defense if a malpractice suit arises. Custom tends to favor high-priced, brand-name pharmaceutical products, especially because the "trademarked *brandname* attached to a pioneering product by the innovator is short, and easier to remember than its *generic name*, which in turn is a shorter, simpler version of the *chemical name* that describes the molecular structure of the active chemical entity to scientists" (Caves et al., 1991, p. 5).

The point is that physicians are responsible for prescribing medicines, yet lack a financial incentive to make cost-effective choices. The result is often the selection of a high-priced, brand-name drug when an equally effective lower-priced generic is available. Back in the 1950s, cost-effective buying was even less common than it is today because states had enacted antisubstitution laws that prevented pharmacists from substituting lower-priced but therapeutically equivalent generics for brand-name drugs. Antisubstitution laws required pharmacists to fill prescriptions as written, precluding the dispensing of a lower-priced substitute when the physician had specified a brand-name product.

By 1984, the last of the antisubstitution laws was repealed (Caves et al., 1991). Pharmacists are now permitted to substitute generic products on prescriptions written for brand-name drugs. According to Carroll and Wolfgang (1991), "while consumers and prescribers have the legal right to request or deny substitution, for the great majority of prescriptions they leave choice to the pharmacists. Thus, for the most part, pharmacists determine the extent to which generic substitution will occur"(p. 110). Grabowski and Vernon (1986) point out that generic products generally provide higher profit margins to pharmacists, suggesting that pharmacists face a financial incentive to substitute bioequivalent generic drugs for brand-name drugs. According to Caves et al. (1991), generic substitution increased remarkably from 5 to 29 percent of brand-written, multisource prescriptions over the period 1980–1989.[4] Estimates indicate that the generics' share of the U.S. pharmaceutical market is now about 47 percent (PhRMA, 2002).

---

3. According to the *Henry Holt Encyclopedia of Word and Phrase Origins*, "Rx. The Latin 'recipere,' 'take this,' provides the R in the symbol Rx used by pharmacists for centuries, while the slant across the R's leg is a sign of the Roman god Jupiter, patron of medicine. The symbol looks like Rx and is pronounced that way."

4. A **single-source drug** is normally covered by a patent. A **multisource drug** is available from a number of suppliers.

Third-Party Influences on the Demand for Pharmaceutical Products. Many third-party payers have turned to formularies, drug utilization review, and required generic substitution as ways to control the decisions of prescription-writing physicians or pharmacists and rein in pharmaceutical costs. A formulary is a list of selected pharmaceutical products that physicians are required to prescribe. The listed drugs are thought to be medically effective and reasonably priced. Virtually all hospitals use formularies. A majority of MCOs and many state Medicaid programs also employ formularies.

Like hospital utilization review, **drug utilization review** is designed to monitor the actions of physicians. By monitoring, third-party payers can ensure that physicians follow the formulary and can single out physicians who inappropriately prescribe medicines. Some third-party payers also require that pharmacists substitute lower-priced generic products for higher-priced brand-name products whenever medically possible. Many MCOs have adopted drug utilization review programs and generic substitution requirements.

The federal Maximum Allowable Cost (MAC) program, which began in 1974, also mandates drug substitution in government health programs, such as Medicare and Medicaid. The MAC program limits reimbursement for multiple-source drugs to the lowest cost at which chemically equivalent drugs are generally available, plus a reasonable fee for dispensing a drug (Schwartzman, 1976). If a doctor prescribes a specified drug whose price exceeds the MAC price, the pharmacist can obtain reimbursement only for the MAC price unless the doctor certifies in writing that the drug is medically necessary. Such certification entitles the pharmacist to full reimbursement. Otherwise, the pharmacist must bill the patient for the difference between the price of the drug and MAC reimbursement (Schwartzman, 1976).

Two laws enacted during the 1990s by the federal government effectively impose price controls on drugs sold to Medicaid patients and federal agencies (Price Waterhouse, 1993). First, under the Omnibus Budget Reconciliation Act of 1990, federal matching subsidies are granted to state Medicaid programs only for drugs covered by a manufacturer rebate agreement. The rebate agreement normally contains both a basic and an additional component. The basic rebate per unit dispensed is the difference between the average manufacturer price and the "best price" for a drug, the latter being the lowest price charged to any other private or government buyer. There is also a minimum basic rebate equaling about 15 percent of the average manufacturer price. The additional rebate per unit dispensed equals the excess of the increase in the average manufacturer price over the increase in the urban consumer price index since September 1990.

The second federal law affecting pharmaceutical prices is the Veterans Health Care Act of 1992, which influences the price federal agencies, such as the Veterans Administration and the Department of Defense, pay for pharmaceutical goods. The act mandates that drug manufacturers enter into pricing agreements with the Federal Supply Schedule, the Veterans Administration depot, and the Department of Defense depot as a condition for conducting business with the federal government. The price of a branded drug purchased under these agreements must be no higher than 76 percent of the nonfederal average manufacturer's price during the most recent year. In addition, any increase in the price of a prescription drug is limited to the increase in the urban consumer price index.

The intent behind both the Medicaid rebate scheme and the Veterans Health Care Act is to reduce the prices the federal government pays for pharmaceutical goods as a way to control drug costs. One unintended consequence of these laws is that drug manufacturers may be forced to raise their private prices to maintain profits. Because these two public programs reimburse at a fixed fraction of private drug prices the argument is that an increase in private prices leads to higher public prices as well. If so, the federal government may merely shift part of the public drug cost burden to private payers.

In sum, consumers pay relatively high out-of-pocket costs for pharmaceutical products, yet exert only a very small influence over the choice and prices of prescription products. Physicians, pharmacists, and third-party payers have more control over the ultimate choice and price paid. Changes, such as required substitution, formulary restrictions, and drug utilization review, suggest that the buyer side of the market has become more cost conscious for those drugs paid for by a third-party payer. Changes such as these most likely increase the elasticity of demand for any one company's pharmaceutical product and make the seller side of the market more price competitive, especially as more individuals enroll in MCOs.

Pharmacy Benefit Management Companies. Another influential player in pharmaceutical markets, in addition to the consumer, third-party payer/health plan, physician, manufacturer, and pharmacist, is the pharmacy benefit management company (PBM). In fact, more than 200 million Americans currently obtain their drugs through a PBM (PricewaterhouseCoopers, 2001). PBMs never physically handle prescription drugs, only serving as intermediaries between health plans and both drug manufacturers and pharmacies. Health plans pay a fee to PBMs. The fee paid to the PBM may be based on the number of covered lives or on a fee-for-service basis whereby the health plan pays the PBM the (reduced) cost of the prescription plus an administration fee. In return, the PBM negotiates rebates from drug manufacturers by offering to include their products on a formulary. PBMs also arrange price discounts from pharmacies by channeling a relatively large volume of consumers/patients to them.

PBMs promote generic substitution through their formularies and also through their interactions with pharmacies. Many PBMs use lower copayments as a financial inducement for consumers to purchase generic as opposed to brand-name drugs and formulary versus nonformulary drugs. In addition to focusing on cost containment, some PBMs have turned their attention to disease management. Disease management involves the assembly of comprehensive databases on current prescribing practices and health outcomes to determine cost-effective methods of treating various diseases. As Cohen (2000) writes:

> *Diabetes is a prime candidate for PBM-led disease management, as it is a chronic high-cost illness with multiple symptoms covering a wide range of therapeutic classes, and whose treatment relies heavily on the extended delivery of pharmacotherapy. With the current claims databases at their disposal, PBMs already can identify a number of factors leading to above-average treatment costs and lower-than-average quality of care (for example, inappropriate drug treatment and/or poor patient compliance). (p. 317)*

In the early 1990s, several drug manufacturers acquired large PBMs. For example, Eli Lilly purchased PCS in 1994, Merck purchased Medco in 1993, and Smithkline Beecham bought Diversified Pharmaceutical Services in 1994.[5] If a drug company acquires a PBM, the antitrust concern is that the newly created vertically integrated pharmaceutical organization may give unwarranted favorable treatment to its own drugs and may not include competitor drugs, perhaps some that are even more cost effective, on its formulary. The foreclosure of competitors from the market might thereby lessen competition and lead to higher prices and lower quality. Another antitrust concern is that the PBM may share information on drug prices with rival manufacturers and the PBM could be used to facilitate a collusive arrangement among drug manufacturers. These concerns may be valid. According to PricewaterhouseCoopers (2001), the market for pharmacy benefit management is relatively concentrated, with four PBMs accounting for more than 80 percent of the market in 2001.

5. Both Eli Lilly and Smithkline Beecham later divested their PBMs.

But recall that economic theory also offers an efficiency justification for vertically integrated organizations like PBMs. In the chapter on the hospital services industry, we learned that a supplier might merge with a buyer to minimize the transaction costs associated with market transactions. By producing internally, the combined firm avoids the transaction costs of negotiating, writing, and enforcing contracts. In addition, the combined firm can avoid the opportunistic behavior that results from incomplete contracts. If a vertical arrangement like a PBM results in efficiencies and adequate market competition exists, consumers benefit from the resulting lower prices.

It follows that both the potential benefits and costs must be considered when determining the economic desirability of PBMs owned by drug manufacturers. It is interesting to note that the Federal Trade Commission imposed conditions on both of the Medco and Eli Lilly acquisitions of PBMs. Among the conditions, the FTC required that companies maintain "open formularies" that include drugs selected and approved by an independent Pharmacy and Therapeutics committee. Also, the vertically integrated organizations were not allowed to share proprietary and nonproprietary information they received from competitors, such as prices (FTC, 1998).

Barriers to Entry

Economic theory suggests that barriers to entry may prevent potential competition and confer market power on pharmaceutical companies. Three types of barriers to entry into the pharmaceutical industry are typically cited. The first and most effective source is a *government patent* that gives the innovating firm the right to be the sole producer of a drug product for a legal maximum of 20 years.[6] The argument is that a patent is necessary to protect the economic profits of the innovating firm over some time period. Otherwise, easy imitation, lower prices, and smaller profits reduce the financial incentive for firms to undertake risky and costly, but socially valuable, research and development activities. The economic rationale underlying the patent system is that even though the patent confers monopoly power on the innovator, the monopoly restriction of output is better than having no product at all. That is, the new drug might not be introduced on the market if not for the patent protection; thus, some of the drug is better than none.

Patent protection does not guarantee that the company will remain perfectly insulated from competition. Lu and Comanor (1994) observe that a pharmaceutical patent is granted for a new drug's *chemical composition*, not its *therapeutic novelty*. This means a new drug may receive patent protection because of a different chemical composition even though it treats the same disease that an established, already patented drug does. For example, SmithKline held a patent on its antiulcer drug, Tagamet, until May 1994. Prior to patent expiration, SmithKline faced competition from Glaxo's Zantac and Merck's Pepcid, which are also antiulcer drugs but have different chemical compositions. In fact, while Tagamet was first to market and was the world's biggest-selling drug at one point, Glaxo's Zantac took over as drug leader for more than six years. While Zantac was considered less of a scientific breakthrough, it was marketed more aggressively (Moore, 1993). Thus, a legal patent does not guarantee a monopoly position. The entry of new brand-name drugs expands the choices of physicians and provides competition for an established drug with a similar indication.[7]

---

6. The legal patent period was changed from 17 to 20 years in 1996.

7. According to the *Mosby Medical Encyclopedia* (1992), "an indication is a reason to prescribe a medication or perform a treatment, as a bacterial infection may be an indication for prescribing a specific antibiotic or as appendicitis is an indication for appendectomy" (p. 411).

Another point concerning a legal patent is that its effective duration is often less than 20 years because the FDA takes a number of years to approve a product for commercial introduction. With the passage of the Drug Price Competition and Patent Term Restoration Act of 1984 (Hatch-Waxman Act), the effective life of a new drug patent is extended by a maximum of 5 years, but not beyond 14 years of effective life, if it can be shown that the FDA delayed its introduction into the market by at least that amount of time.

The Hatch-Waxman Act not only increased the effective patent life of new drugs but also quickened the approval process for generic drugs. No longer must producers of generic drugs prove safety and effectiveness; they need only show that the generic is bioequivalent to a brand-name drug (that is, it contains the same active ingredient[s]). Consequently, the act has made it easier for generics to enter pharmaceutical product markets once the patent period expires. Partly in response to this act and to third-party pressure for drug cost control, the generic share of prescriptions increased sharply from 19 percent in 1984 to 47 percent by 2000 (PhRMA, 2002). Overall, the impact of the Hatch-Waxman Act is interesting. On the one hand, it increased the market power of the drug innovator by extending the effective patent life. On the other hand, the act enhanced postpatent competition by reducing the cost of generic entry.

The second type of barrier to entry into the pharmaceutical industry is a **first-mover** or **brand loyalty advantage** (Schmalensee, 1982). A drug innovator can usually acquire and maintain a first-mover advantage because the quality of a substitute generic product is generally unknown and requires one to experience it. Generic drugs can be considered experience goods because consumers normally lack the knowledge they need to judge or experience the drugs' quality. Physicians have little time or financial incentive to seek out information about the efficacy and risk of new generic products. Furthermore, the cost of a bad consumption experience can be particularly harmful in terms of a prolonged illness, adverse side effect, or malpractice suit when switching from a known brand name to an unknown generic drug (Scherer and Ross, 1990). Therefore, unless a generic drug offers different and important therapeutic advantages or a very large discount, physicians and consumers, when faced with the choice, are reluctant to choose generic over brand-name drugs after the patents expire.

Many industrial organization economists believe that a first-mover advantage confers market power on the innovator of a new product. A first-mover advantage allows pioneer firms to charge high prices and maintain a dominant market share even after the expiration of a patent. McRae and Tapon (1985) write,

> *Being first on the market with a new product or process enhances a firm's image; in many industries, this enhanced image may be further exploited after patent expiry through the continued promotion of brand names. To the extent that consumer preference schemes give a market advantage to pioneering brands, it appears that the trademark protection of brand names effectively replaces patent protection after 17 years.* De facto, *the combination of patent and trademark protection may produce a composite entry barrier which extends indefinitely into the future. (p. 44)*

It is because of a first-mover advantage that McRae and Tapon found that compulsory licensing of patented pharmaceuticals was not sufficient to induce more competition in the Canadian pharmaceutical industry. **Compulsory licensing** means that a firm is given legal permission to import or manufacture a patented drug if it pays a stipulated royalty rate (of 4 percent in Canada) to the patent holder. Despite the effective elimination of the patent barrier through the compulsory licensing program, the market power of first entrants, in terms of high prices and market shares, declined only modestly over a six-year period in Quebec. The authors attribute that finding to the high postpatent barrier associated with first-mover brand loyalty.

Finally, *control over a key input*, such as a specific chemical or active ingredient, can also make it difficult for new firms to enter a drug market. New competitors require access to the input, and the originating firm may sell it to the new entrants only if it is profitable to do so. If it is not, and replication is difficult or costly, new firms may find it unprofitable to enter the industry.

In sum, significant barriers to entry exist in the pharmaceutical industry. Legal patents and brand names may give entrenched firms an advantage over potential entrants. Theoretically, the advantage translates into market power and the ability to maintain market share despite high prices. FDA approval lags reduce the effective patent life, but brand-name recognition typically increases the effective monopoly period for a drug product.[8]

Consumer Information and the Role of the FDA

As with most medical goods and services, a substantial amount of technical knowledge is necessary to judge a pharmaceutical product. Because pharmaceutical products are experience goods, or in some cases credence goods that require repeated use, they are difficult to evaluate on an a priori basis. Consumers therefore face some risk when directly purchasing pharmaceutical products. Temin (1980) points to three types of risk. First, there is the risk associated with overpaying or receiving a pharmaceutical product of inferior quality. Second, an adverse reaction to a drug may lead to sickness or death. Third, a consumer may purchase the wrong drug or take the wrong dosage and therefore fail to recover from an illness or injury.

In the early 1930s, before prescription-only pharmaceuticals became the norm, drug products were less complex and were limited mainly to anti-infection drugs. Thus, self-medication was more feasible during that time period. Today, however, many substitute drugs are available to treat any given disease, and some are associated with adverse side effects for certain patients. Others cannot be used in conjunction with other drugs or alcoholic beverages. It is not surprising that physicians, as experts, are assigned the role of prescribing most medicines to consumers as a way to reduce consumer risks.

The FDA also plays an important role in protecting consumers from the risks associated with drug purchases. In addition to determining whether drugs should be assigned over-the-counter or prescription status, the FDA must approve a new drug before it can be sold in the marketplace. Government approval is necessary, it is argued, because drug firms may otherwise perform insufficient testing in an attempt to gain a first-mover advantage or to avoid high costs. The elixir sulfanilamide and thalidomide tragedies in the 1930s and 1960s are two examples where people have either died or become harmed by unsafe drug products.[9]

Because the market may fail in the absence of government intervention and provide either unsafe or ineffective drugs, the FDA has been assigned the role of approving new drugs. Many critics (such as Grabowski and Vernon, 1983) argue that the stringent regulations of the FDA since 1962 have led to higher R&D costs and a lower number of new chemical entities introduced into the marketplace. We explicitly address this notion later in the chapter. Grabowski and Vernon point out that the FDA tends to err on the side of conservatism, resulting in long FDA approval times and a slower rate of pharmaceutical innovations. The economic argument goes like the following.

8. Schwartzman (1976) also examined economies of scale in pharmaceutical manufacturing, promotion, and research and development as barriers to entry. While Schwartzman found no evidence supporting manufacturing economies, he noted that larger firms tend to be associated with promotion and R&D economies. These two economies make it harder for small potential competitors, but not large ones, to compete with entrenched pharmaceutical companies. This and other studies on research economies are taken up in the conduct section.

9. The elixir sulfanilamide disaster occurred when Massengill Company used diethylene glycol as a solvent to formulate a liquid form of sulfanilamide without testing it for toxicity. More than 100 children died from the poisonous chemical. The other tragedy happened in Germany and other European countries when thalidomide, a sleeping pill, caused babies to be born without hands or feet (phocomelia).

Suppose the safety and effectiveness of a new drug submitted to the FDA for approval are associated with some uncertainty. An all-knowing FDA approves the drug application when the therapeutic benefits of the drug outweigh its risk. Thus, a correct decision means the FDA approves a safe and effective product or rejects an unsafe or ineffective one. Due to uncertainty, however, the FDA may make two types of errors.

The first error, called *type 1* error, occurs when the FDA rejects the application for a new drug that is truly safe and effective. In contrast, a *type 2* error occurs when the FDA approves a drug that is unsafe or ineffective. As Grabowski and Vernon (1983) write, "Both types of error influence patients' health and well-being since consuming a 'bad' drug or not having access to a 'good' drug can have deleterious effects on health" (p. 10). One would think either type of error is random and therefore equally likely to occur in an uncertain world. However, that is not the case. An FDA member who unknowingly approves an unsafe drug faces personal losses: job loss and political indignation. Moreover, the outcome from approving an unsafe drug is eventually known and highly visible.

The cost associated with rejecting a safe and effective drug, a type 1 error, on the other hand, is borne by a third party (the drug manufacturer or a sick patient) rather than by an FDA member and therefore is less visible. The rejection of a good drug may never be known. Thus, according to this view, the FDA faces an incentive to reject rather than accept, or at least delay the approval of, a drug more often than is necessary in a perfect world.

Interestingly, an unconstrained market faces incentives to accept "bad" drugs and commit a type 2 error. Profit-seeking drug firms wishing to be the first to market with a new drug may skimp on necessary testing. The FDA faces an incentive to reject or delay "good" drugs and commit a type 1 error. Longer approval periods translate into further testing, higher R&D costs, lower expected profitability, and fewer drug innovations. Thus, both the market and the government potentially make mistakes. The gnawing question is which institution, the market or the government, makes fewer and less costly ones.[10]

The Structure of the Pharmaceutical Industry: A Summary

The structure of an industry reflects whether certain markets conditions hold such that firms can, either unilaterally or collectively, exploit their market power and operate inefficiently. Competitive market conditions such as a large number of sellers and buyers, low entry barriers, perfect information, and homogeneous products all point to a situation in which sellers are unable to exert market power. The degree of structural competition in the pharmaceutical industry is not easy to assess, because measures of concentration are sensitive to the definition of the relevant product market and have tended to change significantly over time. Moreover, patents and brand loyalty make it more difficult for new firms to enter various therapeutic markets by establishing an entry barrier. Established brand-name firms, however, may not face these obstacles if they have sufficient resources to produce similar drugs but with slightly different chemical compositions.

The demand side of the market remains fairly fragmented, so any market power that drug manufacturers possess is not automatically offset by influential buyers. However, the use of formularies, drug utilization programs, mandated generic substitution, and third-party payer contracts with informed pharmaceutical benefit management companies places greater emphasis on cost-effective medicines, which counteracts seller market power to some extent. In addition, government pays for

10. The Prescription Drug User Fee Act of 1992 and the Food and Drug Administration Modernization Act of 1997 included provisions designed to improve the efficiency of FDA review procedures and the clinical development process. See Reichert et al. (2001) for more information on these laws and their effectiveness in achieving their goals.

18 percent of all prescription drug expenses under the Medicaid program, which, we learned, involves the implementation of various types of drug price controls. Given this ambiguity about the degree of structural competitiveness, we now turn to a discussion of the conduct of firms in the pharmaceutical industry.

THE CONDUCT OF THE PHARMACEUTICAL INDUSTRY

In this section, we analyze evidence regarding the behavior of pharmaceutical companies in recent years. Three practices of drug firms are examined: pricing, promotion, and product innovation. The basic question is whether evidence exists for competitive or noncompetitive behavior in the pharmaceutical industry. For example, we ask the following four questions, among others:

1. Are drug prices lower when drug firms face more intense competition?
2. Are newcomers more likely to enter pharmaceutical markets when existing firms' profits are high during the postpatent period, or do postpatent barriers prevent entry?
3. Is drug promotion informative or persuasive? Do the promotion expenditures of established firms impede the entry of new firms?
4. Is a large firm size necessary for product innovation in the pharmaceutical industry?

Pricing Behavior

The relatively high concentration of sales among a few firms and substantial barriers to entry in many therapeutic markets imply that pharmaceutical companies possess the ability to price their drug products above the marginal costs of production and generate economic profits. In addition, first-mover advantages may mean that leading firms have the power to maintain brand-name prices above costs and still dominate the market over generic companies even after patent expiration. Promotion expenditures by the leading pharmaceutical firms may help reinforce the habit-buying practices of many buyers, especially physicians.

The potential for noncompetitive pricing has motivated several researchers to examine the pricing practices of pharmaceutical companies. One of the first studies on pharmaceutical competition, by Hurwitz and Caves (1988), analyzes how generic competition affected the post-patent pricing practices of 56 leading brand-name pharmaceuticals during 1978 and 1983. In particular, they develop a sample of 56 observations by drawing from a list of drug products that had eventually become available as generics but were originally subject to patents held by the pharmaceutical firms that developed them.

Next, the authors estimate a multiple regression equation relating the leading firm's market share (in terms of pills sold) during 1978 and 1983 to the relative drug prices of the leader and follower firms, sales promotion spending by the leader and follower firms, and several variables reflecting the degree of brand loyalty to the leading firm's product. The relative difference in the prices of drugs offered by the leading firm and follower firms is calculated as $(P_L - P_F)/P_F$, where P_L and P_F reflect the weighted average drug prices of the leading firm and those of the follower firms, respectively. The expectation is that the relative drug price ratio inversely affects the market share of the leading firm, as the law of demand suggests.

The logarithm of the leading firm's and follower firms' sales promotion expenditures are also specified to capture own- and cross-promotion effects. Sales promotion outlays are calculated to include spending on detailing (that is, personal promotion by pharmaceutical salespeople), medical journal advertising, and direct-mail advertising. The expectation is that own-promotion causes the market share of the leading firm to increase, whereas cross-promotion causes the leader's market share to decline.

Several variables are also included to capture the brand loyalty built up by the leader during the patent period. One such variable is the number of years the leader's brand was marketed exclusively under a patent (that is, the effective patent life). The market share of the leading firm is expected to increase with the effective patent life given the greater opportunity to establish goodwill and entrench buying habits. However, because goodwill and buying habits might also erode as health professionals gain some experience with generic substitutes, Hurwitz and Caves also specify the number of years since the entry of the first generic competitor and the total number of generic suppliers. The hypothesis is that the market share of the leading firm decreases with respect to both of these variables as health professionals and consumers gain more information about the availability of generic brands.

Hurwitz and Caves obtain some interesting results and are able to explain about 66 percent of the variation in the leading firm's market share. The results generally support the various hypotheses. First, as expected, a higher positive price differential between the leader and follower firms is associated with a reduction in the leading firm's market share, *ceteris paribus*. Specifically, the authors calculate that a 10 percent increase in the average leader's price differential resulted in a market share loss of less than 0.5 percent. This result suggests that the leader's market share declined by very little when price was raised above the followers' average prices—not too surprising, the authors argue, when one considers that the average price differential was 127 percent, yet the average leader commanded a 63.4 percent market share.

The regression results associated with the other variables prove interesting, as well. First, the own- and cross-promotion effects are found to positively and inversely affect the leader's share, as expected. Thus one implication of the analysis is that producers of generic brands are able to penetrate the leader's market share through their promotional outlays and pricing policies. Second, the results indicate that a longer "monopoly" marketing period helps build brand loyalty and prevent generic entry from chipping away at the leader's share. Third, the regression analysis shows that the leader's market share falls with a greater number of generic firms as health care professionals become more experienced with generic brands. The arrival of an additional supplier is estimated to reduce the leader's market share by about 1.25 percentage points, on average.

In sum, Hurwitz and Caves find that price differentials affect the choice between brand-name and generic products, but buyers are relatively insensitive to relative price changes. Goodwill established during the patent period extends the effective patent life of a pharmaceutical product as buyers continue to pay a substantial premium after the patent has expired. Finally, promotion by the leader firms helps protect market share from eroding, but promotion by followers tends to reduce the leader's market share.

In another study, Caves et al. (1991) examine the effect of generic entry on both brand-name and generic pricing practices. The study covered the postpatent competition between 30 brand-name drugs and a number of generic drugs over the period 1976–1987 and reached a number of interesting conclusions. First, the authors found that the innovator's (the leading brand-name firm's) price initially rises after patent expiration up until the point where a generic competitor enters the market. That finding implies that leading pharmaceutical firms do not engage in limit pricing because they would otherwise set a low price to discourage or limit entry.[11] Second, the

11. Recall that limit pricing occurs when the dominant or innovator firm prices its product just below the break-even price of a potential entrant as a way to discourage entry. The price of a dominant firm tends to decline over time if limit pricing is practiced.

authors discover that the innovator's price declines with a greater number of generic entrants, but by only 4.5 percent, on average. Third, they find some evidence indicating that innovators' prices were more sensitive to entry during the 1980s compared to past periods, most likely reflecting the growing price consciousness of pharmaceutical buyers. Fourth, Caves et al. find that generic producers enter markets offering prices much lower than the brand-name price. Generic prices also fall with further generic competitor entry, potentially declining to 17 percent of the brand-name producer's preentry price. Despite the huge discount, generic producers were found to gain a relatively small market share.

Grabowski and Vernon (1992) examine the pricing patterns associated with seventeen major pharmaceutical products that were first exposed to generic competition from 1983 to 1987. The 1980s are a particularly interesting period, because barriers to entry by generic companies had been lowered by the Hatch-Waxman Act. Among their results, Grabowski and Vernon find that a 10 percent increase in the brand-name profit margin at time of entry resulted in a 6 percent increase in the number of entrants by the end of the first year. Thus, the entry of new generic products is sensitive to expected profits in the product market, as economic theory suggests, when barriers to entry are low.

In addition, the authors find that price accounts for most of the variation in a generic company's market share but note that other factors, such as first- (or second-) mover advantages and perceptions of quality differences among generic suppliers, may also be important in specific circumstances. As far as pricing patterns are concerned, their evidence, like that of Caves et al. (1991), suggests that generics offer significant discounts and that their prices decline substantially over time.

One seemingly inconsistent finding of Grabowski and Vernon's study was that branded drugs' prices increase in nominal terms by 11 percent after two years of entry. One suspects that innovator firms react to competition by lowering price. But Grabowski and Vernon note that the higher branded drug price occurs in response to the dynamics of a segmented market. That is, as generics enter the market and satisfy price-sensitive buyers with lower prices, brand-name firms are left with buyers who are relatively price insensitive. As a result, brand-name companies are able to raise price, at least in the short run, because they now effectively face a less elastic demand for their pharmaceutical products. Although the innovator's price increases, the average market price of a drug is found to decline to 79 percent of the preentry price after two years as generics attain a greater share of the market. On average, brand-name drugs lose half of the market to generics after two years, according to Grabowski and Vernon.

A study by Lu and Comanor (1994) is particularly interesting because it examines price competition among the brand-name producers of 148 new molecular entities between 1978 and 1987. Prior studies have not examined price competition among rival patented products.

Lu and Comanor argue that an innovator's pricing decision is influenced by several factors, including the drug's therapeutic properties, physician brand loyalty, adoption rate by demanders, and the reactions of rivals. As a result, their empirical model links a measure reflecting a drug's relative price to its FDA rating as an indicator of therapeutic novelty, a dummy variable indicating whether the drug treats an acute or a chronic illness as a measure of frequency of buying, and the number of branded substitute suppliers as an indicator of rivalry. According to the authors, therapeutic novelty should lead to a higher relative price, while the number of substitute suppliers should result in a lower relative price.

Lu and Comanor discover that a greater number of substitute branded products results in lower prices, as expected. In addition, they find that the therapeutic novelty of a drug influences pricing strategy over time. In particular, the authors note that therapeutically innovative drugs are generally introduced under a modified price-skimming strategy. A modified price-skimming strategy means that therapeutically innovative drug prices are initially set high and then held relatively constant over time. Imitative drugs, on the other hand, are introduced under a market penetration strategy. The prices of imitative drugs are low at first to enlarge market share, but are then increased over time as information about their availability spreads.

Wiggins and Maness (2004) examines price competition among 98 anti-infective products (such as penicillins, tetracyclines, erythromycins, and cephalosporins) from 1984 to 1990. Their analysis provides two major conclusions. First, in contrast to the studies previously cited, they find that prices fall sharply with initial entry. Second, they find that subsequent entry continued to reduce prices, although at a much smaller rate, even when there were a relatively large number of competitors. The authors argue that the increased price sensitivity may result from the easier entry of generics brought on by the Hatch-Waxman Act of 1984 and/or because anti-infectives may be more price sensitive than other segments of the pharmaceutical industry.[12]

Finally, Reiffen and Ward (2005) examine competition among the generic sellers of 31 drugs that went off patent in the late 1980s or early 1990s. Their study offers a number of valuable insights about generic drug industry dynamics. First, consistent with the preceding studies, they find that generic drug prices fall with an increase in the number of competitors. They show that the initial generic company's price-cost margin equals approximately 20 to 30 percent but declines with an increase in the number of producers and approaches zero when ten or more competitors exist. Second, they show that more generic firms enter a given market, and enter it more quickly, when expected profits are greater. This result implies that generic competition grows faster in markets characterized by a large number of users and a greater willingness to pay for the drugs.

Taken together, these six studies suggest that both prepatent and postpatent price competition often exist in pharmaceutical markets. The prices of both brand-name and generic products are found to be lower when a greater number of substitute products are available. Pioneer firms sometimes raise the prices of their branded products upon entry in response to a less elastic demand. The goodwill established during the patent period plays an important role, allowing established firms to maintain a large market share despite the huge discounts offered by generic companies.

Promotion of Pharmaceutical Products

Medicines are cited as one of the first products advertised in printed form (Leffler, 1981). Timely product information is especially valuable in the pharmaceutical industry due to the continual introduction of new lifesaving drugs. With about 22,000 different drugs on the market, doctors have a great deal to learn and remember (Schwartzman, 1976). Before prescribing, doctors must know the appropriate drug, the correct dosage, and the properties of the drug for different patients, classified by various characteristics, such as age, weight, and general health status. Thus, it is not surprising that promotion expenditures can run as high as 20 to 30 percent of sales for many research-based pharmaceutical companies. Nearly 70 percent of the promotional budget is spent on personal promotion by detailers (pharmaceutical salespeople), and another 27 percent is spent on journal advertising. Direct-mail advertising accounts for the rest of the promotional budget (Hurwitz and Caves, 1988).

12. Also see Ellison et al. (1997), who find relatively high elasticities between generic substitutes and also significant elasticities between therapeutic substitutes at both the prescribing and dispensing stages.

It is unclear to economists whether pharmaceutical promotion strategies enhance or reduce societal welfare. As we saw in Chapter 8, advertising may promote or impede competition depending on whether informed or habit-buying behavior results. Studies on this topic by Leffler (1981), Hurwitz and Caves (1988), and Caves et al. (1991) find evidence supporting both the informational and persuasion effects of pharmaceutical promotion.

In terms of informative advertising, Leffler find that advertising intensity is greater for newer and more important pharmaceutical products, which, he argues, reflects the informational content of the promotion message. Leffler, as well as Hurwitz and Caves, discovers that the new entrants' promotion expenditures helped them expand their market shares. Caves et al. conclude that increased generic competition results in less advertising by the innovator, which, they argue, must reflect the informational rather than persuasive content of the innovator's pharmaceutical advertising during the preentry period.

The evidence for persuasive advertising is equally strong. In particular, Leffler find that less detailing of younger physicians occurs for older products. That is, advertisers tend to direct their advertisements to the physician age group that was in medical school when the drug product was originally introduced. Thus, the creation of brand loyalty and reinforcement of habit buying must be the real purpose behind advertising. Hurwitz and Caves find that the leading firms' promotion expenditures preserved their market share from new generic entrants. Finally, the study by Caves et al. notes that generic firms gain relatively small shares despite their huge discounts, perhaps reflecting the goodwill built up by the innovator's promotion expenditures during the patent period.

Given the inconsistent findings in the literature, Rizzo (1999) investigates the informative versus persuasive aspects of promotional activities in an entirely different manner by examining the impact of promotional expenditures on price elasticity of demand. According to economic theory, demand becomes more elastic and price declines when buyers are more fully informed because of promotional activities. In contrast, persuasive promotional activities cause habit buying, less elastic demand, and higher prices according to economic theory. Therefore, we can infer whether promotional activities are persuasive or informative by empirically studying how such activities influence price elasticity of demand.

In his empirical study, Rizzo considers how detailing expenditures influenced the price elasticity of demand for antihypertensive drug products. There are several major classes within the group of drugs used to treat hypertension, including ACE inhibitors, calcium channel blockers, beta-blockers, diuretics, and other types. These broad classes of antihypertensive drugs, as well as the drugs within each class, can be considered differentiated competitors. Rizzo estimates the yearly demand for 46 different antihypertensive drugs over the period 1988–1993. The demand for each drug is estimated as a function of its price, detailing expenses, average competitor price within the same drug class, average detailing expenditures within the same drug class, and other factors.

Of interest to us, Rizzo allows the detailing expenses of each drug to interact with its price in the estimation equation so the impact of detailing on price elasticity could be isolated. Both stock and flow measures of detailing expenses are included in the empirical model. The stock measure captures past detailing efforts to allow the effects of promotional activities to accumulate over time. The flow measure represents detailing expenditures in the current period so the short-run impact of promotional activities on price elasticity can also be studied.

In support of the persuasive view of promotional activities, Rizzo find that greater detailing efforts led to a lower price elasticity of demand for antihypertensive drugs. As an example of his findings, Rizzo reports that price elasticity with no detailing equaled −1.98 for one of his models. For that same model, price elasticity of demand equaled −1.46 when the stock of detailing was considered. Notice that the accumulated effects of past promotional activities caused price elasticity to decline as the persuasive view of advertising suggests. Finally, price elasticity of demand equaled −.48 in the short run as a result of increased current detailing activities. Thus, Rizzo provides direct empirical evidence "that product promotion inhibits price competition in the pharmaceutical industry, lowering price elasticities and leading to higher equilibrium prices" (pp. 112–13). It will be interesting to learn whether future studies find similar results about the relation between promotional activities and price elasticity of demand for other types of drugs.

Product Innovation

The most important contribution associated with the pharmaceutical industry is the timely introduction of new drug products that can extend or improve lives. New drug discoveries require research and development activities. In this section, we look at several issues relating to the R&D process, including the various stages of the R&D process, determinants of R&D, and the relation between firm size and innovative activity.

Stages of the R&D Process. Product innovation in the pharmaceutical industry is argued to be both very risky and time consuming. The research and development (R&D) process for new chemical entities is normally spread over many years, and only a small fraction of new drug discoveries are eventually approved for marketing. Research and development costs constitute a sizeable proportion of sales revenues. For example, Figure 14–2 shows that R&D expenditures for research-based pharmaceutical companies ranged from a low of 10.9 percent of sales in 1974 and 1978 to a high of 20.4 percent of sales in 1994.

Due to the high cost and risk associated with R&D, the decision-making process underlying new drug development tends to unfold sequentially. At several points in the R&D process, a company reviews the development status of a drug and makes a decision about continuing or abandoning the project. The decision rests on the expected net profitability of the proposed drug and thus

FIGURE 14–2
R&D Intensity of Major Pharmaceutical Companies, 1970–2004

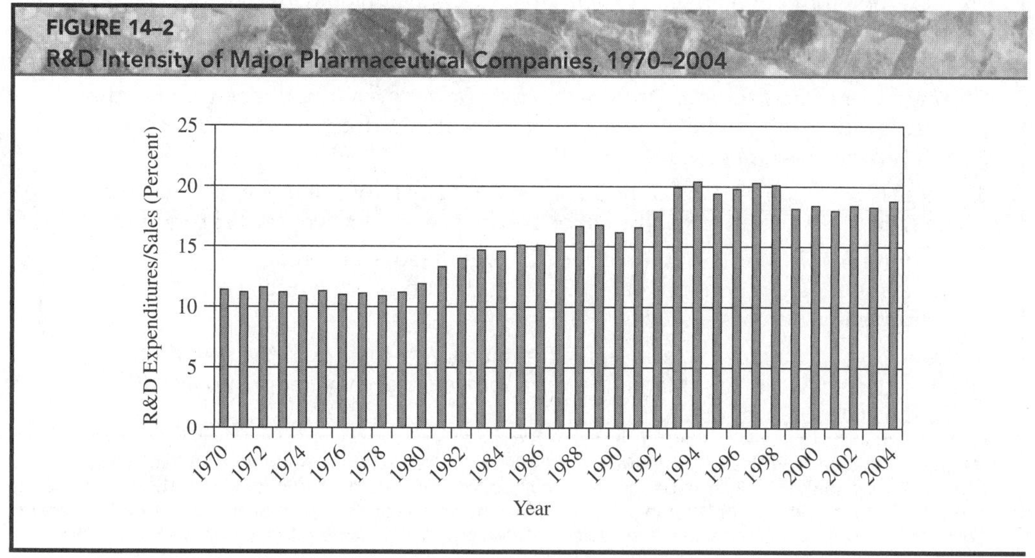

SOURCE: PhRMA, *Industry Profile 2005*, http://www.phrma.org (accessed December 1, 2005).

considers both expected revenues and costs. Expected revenues depend in part on the therapeutic properties of the drug, the size of the target market, and the number of substitute drugs. Anticipated costs depend on the frequency and severity of adverse reactions to the drug and the projected additional development, marketing, distribution, and production costs (DiMasi et al., 1991).

Researchers generally identify eight stages in the R&D process; these stages are summarized in Table 14–4, including the duration of each stage, in months. DiMasi et al. (1991) estimate that the preclinical period of discovery, animal testing, and investigational exemption for new drug (IND) filing lasts about 42.6 months. Almost 58 percent of the (uncapitalized) expected costs per marketed new chemical entity (NCE) are incurred during this period, most likely reflecting the huge number of misses before a pharmaceutical company discovers a drug that warrants further testing at the clinical stage.

TABLE 14–4
Stages of the Drug Development Process

1. *Discovery stage.* Basic research synthesis of new chemicals and early studies of chemical properties. Identification of a specific new chemical entity worthy of further testing.
2. *Preclinical animal testing.* Short-term animal toxicity testing for evidence of safety in the short run in preparation for human testing.
3. *IND filing.* A request is made for authorization to begin human testing by filing a notice of claimed investigational exemption for new drug (IND). If there is no hold on the application, the firm begins clinical testing 30 days after filing. (42.6 months for the first three stages)
4. *Phase I of clinical testing.* Dosage administered to a small number of healthy volunteers for information on toxicity and safe dose ranges in humans. Data are gathered on the drug's absorption and distribution in the body, its metabolic effects, and the rate and manner in which the drug is eliminated from the body. (15.5 months)
5. *Phase II of clinical testing.* Drug is used on a larger number of people whom the drug is intended to benefit. Evidence of therapeutic effectiveness and additional safety data are obtained. (24.3 months)
6. *Phase III of clinical testing.* Large-scale tests on humans over a longer period to uncover unanticipated side effects and additional evidence of effectiveness. (36.0 months)
7. *Long-term animal studies.* The effects of prolonged exposures and the effects on subsequent generations are determined. Such studies are typically conducted concurrently with other studies. (33.6 months)
8. *New drug approval.* Application for commercial marketing of the new drug. Review of evidence by the FDA. Marketing for approved uses may begin upon notification by the FDA. (30.3 months)

SOURCES: Adapted from Joseph A. DiMasi, Ronald W. Hansen, Henry G. Grabowski, and Louis Lasagna, "Cost of Innovation in the Pharmaceutical Industry," *Journal of Health Economics* 10, (1991), pp. 107–42; and John R. Virts and J. Fred Weston, "Expectations and the Allocation of Research and Development Resources," in *Drugs and Health,* ed. Robert Helms (Washington, D.C.: American Enterprise Institute, 1981), pp. 21–45.

DiMasi et al. estimate that the clinical period from the initiation of Phase I testing to drug approval lasts about 98.9 months, with the FDA approval process taking about 2½ years, on average. The average time needed to complete the entire process from synthesis to marketing approval is estimated at twelve years.[13] About 75 percent of the NCEs in Phase I testing enter Phase II testing, and about 36 percent eventually enter Phase III testing. Only 18.3 percent of the drugs that entered clinical trials during 1980–1984 are now marketed (DiMasi, 1995).

Determinants of R&D Spending.[14] As with any investment, the optimal amount of R&D spending depends on the expected future streams of revenues less costs or economic profits. Expected marginal revenues, MR, decline with respect to R&D expenditures due to the law of diminishing marginal productivity.[15] The marginal or opportunity cost, MC, is likely to rise or remain constant with respect to R&D spending. The expected net profits from R&D are maximized when MR is set equal to MC. In mathematical terms, the firm finds the optimal amount of R&D spending, R^*, by solving the following equation:

$$\text{MR}(R, X) = \text{MC}(R, Z), \tag{14–1}$$

where R equals investment expenditures on R&D, X stands for a vector of exogenous factors influencing the rate of return from new drug R&D, and Z represents a vector of exogenous variables influencing the marginal cost associated with new drug R&D.

Solving Equation 14–1 for R yields a reduced-form equation for the optimal level of R&D spending in terms of X and Z:

$$R^* = f(X, Z). \tag{14–2}$$

Variables that increase the rate of return, X, lead to increased spending on R&D. Similarly, variables that raise the opportunity cost, Z, lead to lower R&D expenditures.

Grabowski and Vernon (1981) were among the first to estimate an R&D regression equation based on Equation 14–2 for a pooled sample of ten pharmaceutical companies taken over the entire fourteen-year period from 1962 to 1975. For a factor influencing the firm's expected rate of return in each time period, they use an indicator of past R&D success, measured by the number of NCEs per dollar of R&D spending in the previous five years. The expectation is that R&D spending increases with greater past success. They also specify an index of firm diversification as a revenue-influencing factor. The argument is that a more diversified firm is better able to exploit R&D spending on a number of different drugs and thus is more inclined to undertake R&D.

To control for factors influencing the opportunity cost of R&D, Z, the authors specify a variable measuring each firm's cash flow margin in each year. The opportunity cost of internal funds is less than that of external funds. That is, because of transaction costs, the cost of borrowing external funds (that is, loans from banks or sales of stocks and bonds), is generally higher than that of using internal funds. Thus R&D spending is expected to increase with the cash flow margin. Following convention, R&D spending is deflated by sales to get a measure of R&D intensity.

Their regression results provide important insights. As expected, R&D investment spending is found to be influenced by variables affecting marginal benefit and cost. In particular, R&D spending is observed to increase with a greater degree of past R&D success and, more important, with a

13. Some overlap occurs across the various stages.

14. This section is based on Grabowski and Vernon (1981).

15. R&D can be considered as an input in the discovery of new drugs. Thus, the marginal revenue—or, more correctly, the marginal revenue product of R&D—is equal to the market price of the resulting new drug, P, times the marginal productivity of R&D, MP, in the innovation process.

larger cash flow margin. This latter result represents a critical finding because it suggests that a ceiling on drug prices, by reducing cash flows, could result in a reduction in pharmaceutical R&D.

Building on this earlier work by Grabowski and Vernon (1981), Giaccotto et al. (2005) use national time-series data in the United States to explore the relation between real drug prices and the R&D spending of major pharmaceutical companies from 1952 to 2001. They argue theoretically that changes in real drug prices capture the cash flow effect, previously discussed, and also the impact of changing price expectations on R&D spending behavior. Specifically, these researchers hypothesize that pharmaceutical R&D spending rises with real drug prices because of greater cash flows and also because of more favorable expectations regarding the prices of new drug products.

Based on their multiple regression analysis, Giaccotto et al. determine that the elasticity of R&D intensity with respect to the real drug price equals 0.583. This estimate suggests that a 10 percent decrease in real drug prices is associated with a 5.83 percent reduction in pharmaceutical R&D intensity, assuming all other factors remain constant. Using this elasticity estimate, they estimate that pharmaceutical expenditures would have been about 30 percent lower if the federal government had limited drug prices to the same rate of growth as the general price inflation rate during the 1980–2001 period. This policy scenario, while hypothetical in nature, corresponds to the previously discussed Veterans Health Care Act of 1992, which limits drug price increases for federal agency purchases to the general price inflation rate. In addition, their simulations show that a drug price control policy of that kind would have resulted in 300 to 365 fewer new drugs in the global economy because of reduced R&D spending. Consequently, these researchers estimate that more than one-third of all new drugs actually brought to market would have been lost if the price control had been adopted during that time period.[16]

Santerre and Vernon (2006) extend the study by Giaccotto et al. by comparing the long-term costs, in terms of new drugs and value of lives lost, to the short-run benefits, in terms of consumer drug cost savings, resulting from the hypothetical price control policy just discussed. Specifically, they use national data for the period from 1960 to 2000 to estimate an aggregate consumer demand for pharmaceuticals in the United States. Parameters from the estimated demand curve are then used to simulate the value of the consumer surplus gains that would have resulted from a lower controlled drug price (that is, holding drug price increases to the same rate of growth as the general consumer price level) over the 1981–2000 period.

Based on simulations involving a variety of likely values for the real interest rate, coinsurance rate, and own-price elasticity of demand, Santerre and Vernon estimate that the future value of consumer surplus gains from this (hypothetical) drug price control policy would range between $176 and $767 billion by the end of 2000. They then compare this range of figures to the value of lives that would have been lost because of fewer new drugs brought to the U.S. market over this period because of the drug price control. They approximate that the long-term cost of the hypothetical price control policy lies between $19.7 trillion and $21.8 trillion in terms of value of lives lost. Thus, the long-term costs of the drug price control policy are estimated to be more than 25 times greater than short-run benefits. These results lead Santerre and Vernon to conclude that a drug price control policy of that nature would have done much more harm than good from a social welfare perspective. Regardless of the results, these two papers remind us that society should consider both the long-term costs and the short-run benefits when evaluating the relative merits of a drug price control policy.

16. Interested readers may also want to consult Vernon (2005) for further evidence on drug price controls and pharmaceutical R&D behavior.

Firm Size and Innovation. Another important issue regarding the conduct of pharmaceutical firms is the relation between firm size and innovative activities. The question is whether large pharmaceutical firms are more likely than small firms to engage in successful innovative ventures. Given the importance of product innovation in this industry, antitrust laws concerning mergers may not be enforced so strictly if larger firms are found to be more innovative than smaller ones.

Economic theory by itself offers only limited insight on the relation between firm size and innovation. Schumpeter (1950) is among the first economists to propose that larger firms may be more successful at innovation than smaller firms because they have the resources necessary to engage in modern large-scale R&D activities. Modern and commercially successful innovations are very expensive to undertake, and therefore small firms may lack the necessary physical and financial resources. In addition, larger firms diversify their R&D efforts among various projects and thus can better absorb the risks associated with innovative activities. Finally, many analysts believe that economies of scale exist in research such that per-unit costs fall with a greater production of R&D activities because more efficient, specialized research inputs are used.

These three factors—resource capability, risk absorption, and research economies—suggest that larger firms tend to face a greater incentive to undertake successful R&D activities than smaller firms. Opposing this tendency, however, is the argument that greater bureaucratic red tape in larger organizations stifles creativity. Since important decisions are normally made at a centralized level in a large, bureaucratic firm, communication flows ultimately break down and decisions take longer to execute. The resulting time lags delay or discourage new product ideas from being pursued or continued.

Because theory cannot offer a definitive answer, various researchers have empirically questioned whether larger drug firms are more innovative than smaller ones. Schwartzman (1976) summarizes the pre-1960s empirical research on firm size and innovation as follows:[17]

> *According to Edwin Mansfield and Henry Grabowski, large drug companies do not spend proportionately more money on research than smaller ones. W. S. Comanor observes diseconomies of scale in research. Jerome Schnee concludes that leading companies do not produce proportionately more innovations than other firms. (p. 83)*

Thus, the pre-1960s research suggests that larger drug firms are not more innovative than smaller ones. Close examination of these studies by Schwartzman, however, reveals poor data for the measurement of firm size or faulty analysis of the data.

Schwartzman's own empirical work, using data for the late 1960s, reaches three separate conclusions supporting the premise that large firm size encourages greater innovation in the pharmaceutical industry. First, he finds that research effort, as measured by laboratory employment, increases more than proportionately with the size of the drug firm. Second, his study reveals that research output, as measured by either the number of new chemical entities or the number of patents, increases more than proportionately with research effort, indicating economies of scale in research. Third, Schwartzman shows that larger firms discover relatively more new drugs per employee than do smaller firms.

The general conclusions reached by Schwartzman have recently come under attack. Using data for 1982, Acs and Audretsch (1988) analyze the innovative contributions of small and large firms, defined as firms having fewer or more than five hundred employees, respectively. The Small Business Administration constructed the innovation database by examining more than a hundred technology, engineering, and trade journals covering a number of different manufacturing industries

17. See Mansfield (1968), Grabowski (1968), Comanor (1965), and Schnee (1971).

for evidence of new-product innovations. For the pharmaceutical industry, the authors find that larger firms had 9.23 times the innovations of smaller firms in 1982. However, larger pharmaceutical firms also had 19.41 times the employment of smaller drug firms. Together these results indicate that larger firms generate only half the number of pharmaceutical innovations that smaller firms do on a per-employee basis. Thus, according to their empirical results, large firm size may not be necessary for pharmaceutical innovation. Taking all the manufacturing industries in their entire sample into consideration, Acs and Audretsch conclude that small firms are about 43 percent more innovative than their larger counterparts.

In a related study, Acs and Audretsch (1987) analyze the specific characteristics affecting the differential innovation rates of large and small firms across different industries. The authors determine that large firms tend to have an innovative advantage in industries that are capital intensive, advertising intensive, and relatively concentrated at the aggregate level. In contrast, small firms are more innovative in industries in which total innovation and the use of skilled labor play a large role and some, but not many, large firms exist.

We mentioned earlier that the pharmaceutical industry is characterized by high advertising intensity. This industry characteristic tends to favor the innovation of large pharmaceutical firms. However, most of the characteristics described previously suggest that small pharmaceutical companies may be more innovative. First, total innovation plays a very important role in the pharmaceutical industry. In fact, Acs and Audretsch (1988) cite the pharmaceutical industry as the fourth most innovative out of 247 industries in 1982. Second, the skilled labor of pharmacologists, biochemists, and immunologists, among others, is necessary in the drug industry given the high technical sophistication of pharmaceutical R&D. Third, casual empiricism suggests that a number of large, highly visible firms coexist with a much larger number of smaller firms in the pharmaceutical industry. Fourth, Schwartzman (1976) notes that capital requirements for manufacturing are relatively low in the pharmaceutical industry. Finally, we saw that the pharmaceutical industry is characterized by relatively low aggregate seller concentration.

Thus, the safest conclusion to draw is that a mixture of firm sizes is most favorable for fostering pharmaceutical innovation.[18] While smaller drug firms seem to hold a decisive advantage, the preceding results suggest that the innovativeness of smaller firms is greatest when large firms dominate in an industry. Encouraging innovation through a diversity of firm sizes should not be too surprising. Many researchers note that new ideas are relatively cheap to conceive, but the commercial development and successful marketing of new products are costly and risky. Small firms might have the edge at the discovery stage, but large firms possess development and marketing advantages. Greer (1992) contrasts the innovativeness of large and small firms as follows:

> *The foot-dragging behavior of leading firms is so common that theorists have dubbed it "the fast-second strategy." Briefly the idea is that, for a large firm,* innovation *is often costlier, riskier, and less profitable than* imitation. *A large firm can lie back, let others gamble, then respond quickly with a "fast second" if anything started by their smaller rivals catches fire. (p. 669)*

Greer notes that Genentech, an infant firm in the late 1970s, founded biotechnology. Larger pharmaceutical firms, such as Eli Lilly, followed Genentech's lead into biotechnology in the mid-1980s.

---

18. Like studies in the past, recent empirical analyses uncover mixed evidence concerning the relation between firm size and innovation. On the one hand, studies by DiMasi et al. (1995) and Henderson and Cockburn (1996) find that research efforts are proportionately more productive in larger firms. Langowitz and Graves (1992), on the other hand, find that research output is subject to diminishing returns with respect to both R&D expenditures and firm size.

The Conduct of the Pharmaceutical Industry: A Summary

The studies discussed in this section show that a considerable amount of competition takes place in the pharmaceutical industry. Drug firms sometimes face price competition during the patent period from other branded products, and prices are lower when more branded competition exists. Branded drugs also compete with generics on the basis of price during the postpatent period. Generics offer huge discounts relative to branded products. Also, product competition is particularly important in the pharmaceutical industry. Incentives for new product development exist because a new drug product, especially a therapeutically important one, can easily supplant others in the market.

However, the degree of competition in the pharmaceutical industry is not perfect. Firms offering single-source drugs are able to raise price above the marginal cost of production because substitutes are unavailable. Furthermore, evidence shows that pharmaceutical marketing is used partly to reinforce the habit-buying practices of physicians. Hence, some drug buyers still remain price insensitive due to brand loyalty.

The Performance of the Pharmaceutical Industry

In this section, we appraise the performance of the contemporary pharmaceutical industry. Competitive market impediments, such as patents, trademarks, and high promotion expenditures, characterize the pharmaceutical industry and suggest that entrenched companies may possess enough market power to restrict output, raise prices, and earn excessive profits.

First, we compare the prescription drug price inflation rate to the general inflation rate in the United States and identify trends and measurement problems. Second, since product innovation is the true output of the pharmaceutical industry, we discuss studies analyzing the benefits of new drugs and examine historical data on the number of new chemical entities. Finally, we look at some comparative data on the aggregate profitability of pharmaceutical companies.

The Relative Price Inflation Rate of Pharmaceutical Products

To gauge performance, policy makers often examine how the price of a product changes over time. While the price of a good or service most likely changes over time because of imbalances in supply and demand, policy makers feel that continually rising prices harm consumers by reducing consumer surplus, especially if their incomes are relatively fixed. With that in mind, let's study how drug prices have tended to change over time.

Figure 14–3 compares the prescription drug price and general price inflation rates in the United States for the period 1970–2004. The figure indicates that throughout most of the 1970s, the general price inflation rate outpaced the prescription drug inflation rate. Specifically, prices in general increased at an average annual rate of 7.4 percent—almost twice the rate of 3.9 percent at which drug prices grew. Thus, real or relative drug prices declined throughout most of the 1970s.

During the 1980s there was a reversal in the relative price trend. According to Figure 14–3, real drug prices continuously surged as the drug price inflation rate outstripped the general price inflation rate. In particular, drug prices grew at an average annual rate of 9.6 percent compared to an average annual increase of 5.1 percent for prices in general during the 1980s.

The quick rise of real drug prices of the 1980s came to a halt in the middle of the 1990s. During the 1990s, the drug price inflation rate averaged 5.03 percent whereas the general price inflation rate averaged 2.94 percent. In fact, the drug price inflation rate tended to track the general

FIGURE 14–3
Drug and General Price Inflation, 1970–2004

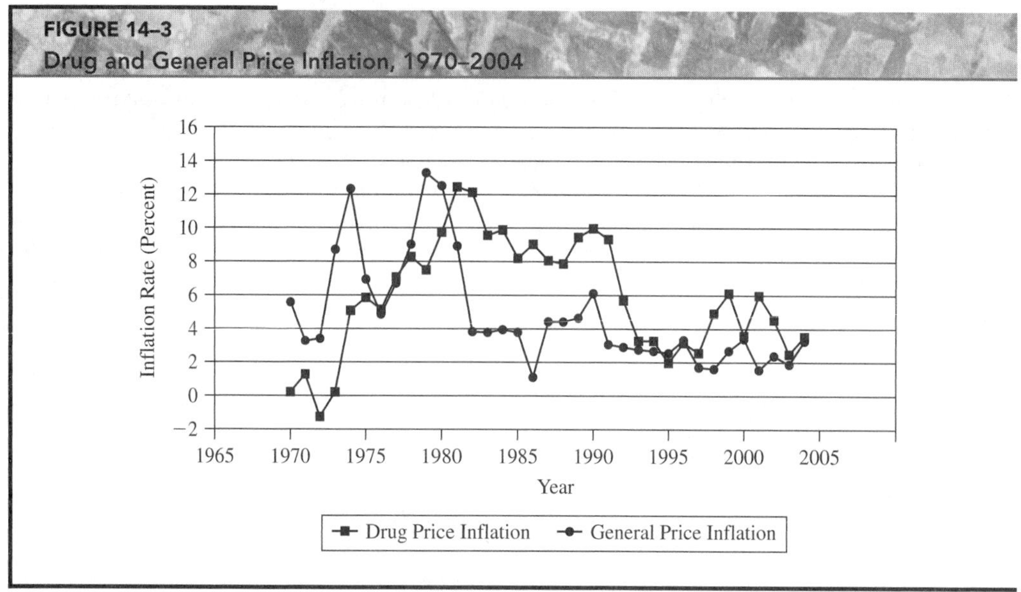

SOURCE: Bureau of Labor Statistics, http://www.bls.gov (accessed December 1, 2005).

price inflation rate during 1993–1996. Pharmaceutical companies may have been reluctant to raise prices during that particular period because of the intense scrutiny directed toward the drug industry by the Clinton administration (Pear, 1993). However, since 1996, real drug prices have tended to increase faster than the general price level. Over the period from 2000 to 2004, the drug price inflation rate averaged 4.03 percent and the general price inflation rate averaged 2.49 percent. The two rates differed by less than a percentage point in 2003 and 2004.

Before moving on to the next section, it should be noted that the price indices used to calculate inflation rates are not flawless measures. Hence, reported rates may be under- or overstated. Of relevance to pharmaceutical products, the Bureau of Labor Statistics (BLS), the government agency responsible for determining price indices, faces a difficult task when measuring changes in the quality of products over time. Yet as Scherer (1993) has noted, "some new drugs, by improving the quality of life or making expensive surgery unnecessary, plainly yield enormous increments of consumer surplus" (p. 103). Because new pharmaceutical products are introduced and utilized at such a rapid rate, quality-adjusted price inflation rates may be lower than the BLS reported rates. If pharmaceutical manufacturers adjust new drug prices to compensate for the higher quality, however, no overstating of the true drug price inflation rate occurs.

Output of New Pharmaceutical Products

Another measure of an industry's performance is output. According to theory, societal welfare is enhanced when goods are produced up to the point where marginal social benefit equals marginal social cost (see Chapter 3). Empirically, costs and benefits are hard to measure, so we must often rely on information regarding industrial structure and conduct, as well as sound judgment, to determine whether the right incentives exist for efficient output levels. Because of some noncompetitive structural conditions (patents, trademarks, promotion) existing in the pharmaceutical industry, one might expect some restrictions on output. The question is whether evidence supports this expectation.

New chemical entities (NCEs) probably represent the single most important measure of pharmaceutical output. New drugs improve quality of life by relieving pain and have significantly reduced deaths from many diseases including tuberculosis, kidney infection, and hypertension. Pharmaceutical innovations have virtually eliminated diseases such as whooping cough and polio. In addition, drugs often reduce the cost of treating diseases. For example, the use of tranquilizers has substantially reduced the hospitalization of mental patients (Peltzman, 1974). Weidenbaum (1993) notes that "the cost of treating ulcers with H-2 antagonist drug therapy runs about $900 per year. The cost of ulcer surgery, by contrast, averages $28,900" (p. 87).

Academic research also provides empirical evidence that new drug products extend and/or improve the quality of lives and often substitute for expensive types of invasive surgery. For example, Lichtenberg (2005) performs an econometric analysis of the effect of new drugs on longevity using disease-level data from 52 countries during 1982–2001. His empirical analysis allows him to control for other potential determinants of longevity, such as education, income, nutrition, the environment, and lifestyle. He finds that new drugs have a strong positive impact on the probability of survival. More specifically, Lichtenberg discovers that new drugs increase life expectancy of the entire population by an average annual increase of one week (based on conservative assumptions). This means that people in society, on average, can expect to live one week longer each year because of new drugs. He also estimates that new drugs, on average, produce an additional life-year at an incremental cost of about $6,750, which is far lower than most estimates of the value of a statistical life-year ($100,000 to $150,000).

As another example, Frech and Miller (2004) explore the impact of pharmaceutical consumption on life expectancy and disability-adjusted life expectancy using data for a sample of eighteen countries belonging to the Organization of Economic Cooperation and Development. They find empirically that lagged pharmaceutical consumption is associated with a positive impact on life expectancy at ages 40 and 60. Moreover, they discover that increased pharmaceutical consumption relates directly to disability-adjusted life-years at birth and at age 60. Thus, Frech and Miller's study supports the premise that pharmaceuticals help improve the quality and quantity of lives.

Finally, Lichtenberg (2001) uses data from a large-scale survey containing three waves of interviews in 1996. He finds empirically that people consuming newer drugs are less likely to die and miss workdays by the end of the survey period than people who consume older drugs. In addition, he finds that the use of newer drugs lowers all types of nondrug spending on medical care, resulting in a substantial reduction in the costs of treating a given medical condition.

Interesting, both Lichtenberg (2005) and Frech (2002) suggest that the empirical findings from these pharmaceutical studies (and the Cutler and McClellan [2001] study on the benefits of new medical technologies) conflict with the notion developed in Chapter 3 that medical care has only a small marginal impact on health outcomes. You may recall that the low marginal productivity of medical care is referred to as "flat-of-the-curve" medicine.

But a movement along a given total product curve for health should not be confused with a shifting of the total product curve for health. Flat-of-the-curve medicine refers to changes in health that result from marginal changes in medical care at a given point in time, such as a year, and for a given state of technology. An additional day spent in the hospital, an additional visit to a physician's office, and an additional tablet of some medication all provide examples of marginal changes in medical care that result in a movement along a given total product curve for health and are potentially indicative of flat-of-the-curve medicine. New procedures, devices, and

FIGURE 14–4
Annual Number of New Chemical Entities, 1940–2004

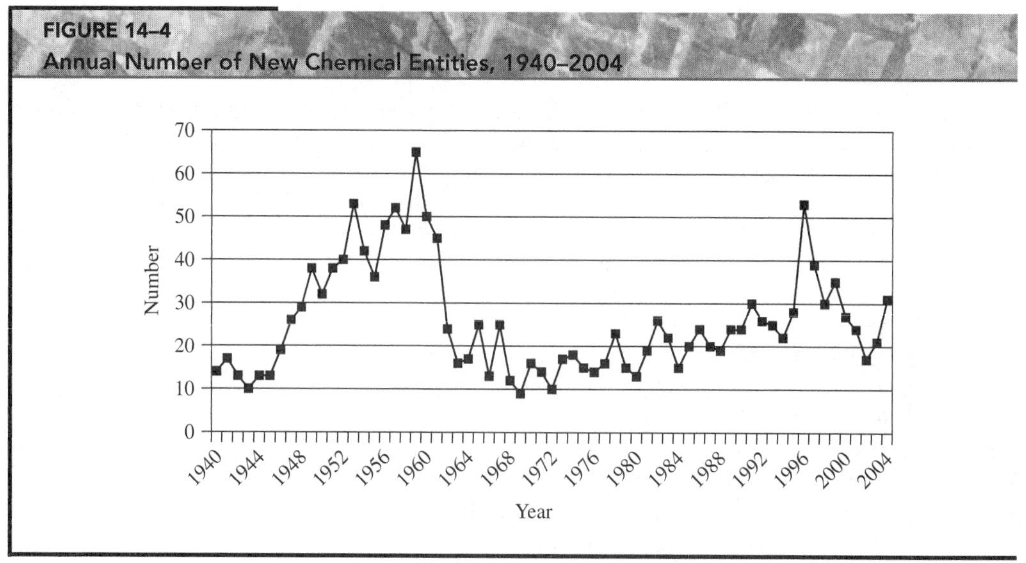

SOURCE: *Statistical Fact Book,* (Washington D.C.: Pharmaceutical Manufacturers Association, various years), as cited by William S. Comanor and Stuart O. Schweitzer, "Pharmaceuticals," in *The Structure of American Industry*, ed. Walter Adams and James Brock (Englewood Cliffs, N J: Prentice Hall, 1995), Table 7–2. Since 1990 the figures represent approvals rather than introductions and are from PhRMA, *Industry profit* (Washington, D.C.: 2002), Figure 3–2 and the Federal and Drug Administration, http://www.FDA.gov.

medicines, however, shift the total product curve upward, implying that better health outcomes can now be attained from the same amount of medical care spending or lifestyle than before. Indeed, both Lichtenberg studies (2001, 2005) find that newer drugs are much more effective than older drugs at improving health.

If new drugs are important to health as studies seem to suggest, it may be useful to learn how the number of NCEs has changed over time. Data on the number of NCEs introduced into the United States appear in Figure 14–4. Until 1960, new drug introductions showed a clear pattern. According to Statman (1983),

> *Sixty-seven new drugs were introduced into the U.S. market during the first half of the 1940s. The drug innovation rate doubled during the second half of the 1940s. It increased to 125 during the late 1940s, then nearly doubled again to 205 in the first half of the 1950s. It increased further to 248 during the second half of the 1950s.* (p. 6)

The tremendous rate at which NCEs were created and introduced during the 1940s and 1950s reflects the birth of the modern pharmaceutical industry in the United States, as pointed out in the introduction to this chapter.

However, the 1960s witnessed a dramatic decline in the number of NCEs. Although 453 drugs were introduced in the 1950s, only 236 new drugs were introduced during the 1960s. The 1970s saw no reversal in the downward trend since the 1960s, with only 158 NCEs introduced in the marketplace by pharmaceutical companies.

Two reasons have been cited for the decline in drug innovations after the early 1960s. First, the decline may have been caused by a "depletion of research opportunities," as early evidence suggests that the innovation slowdown continued worldwide in the 1970s and 1980s

(Grabowski, 1989). Second, the decline may have been the result of the 1962 amendment to the Food, Drug and Cosmetic Act, which significantly increased the costs of pharmaceutical innovations due to safety and efficacy concerns. The so-called Kefauver-Harris Act prompted the FDA to adopt more stringent rules concerning new drug testing and approval. The greater amount of testing and approval time raised drug manufacturers' costs and reduced the effective patent life of a new drug, thereby discouraging new drug discoveries.

Beginning in 1980 and continuing throughout the 1990s, the innovative activities of pharmaceutical companies showed signs of life once again. As Figure 14–4 reflects, the number of NCEs increased from 158 in the 1970s to 202 in the 1980s and then increased even further to 312 in the 1990s. In addition, Figure 14–2 shows that while R&D intensity was relatively flat during the 1970s, an upward trend to R&D intensity emerged during the 1980s and continued throughout most of the 1990s. Several explanations have been offered for the heightened innovativeness of pharmaceutical companies since the beginning of the 1980s.

First, the Hatch-Waxman Act of 1984 was designed in part to correct for the regulatory lag created by the 1962 act. As mentioned previously, the life of a new drug patent can be extended for up to five years (but no more than fourteen years in total) to compensate for any approval delay by the FDA. The longer expected effective patent life for new drugs creates a better opportunity for profits and encourages more innovation.

Second, the faster pace of new drug discoveries has been attributed to the recent revolution in methods of drug discovery and development. Previously, pharmaceutical R&D largely involved **molecule manipulation,** the trial-and-error examination of the therapeutic properties of a large number of chemical entities, especially closely related derivatives of known entities (Duetsch, 1993). Today, technologies such as genetic engineering, monoclonal antibodies, cellular biology, and immunology—all contributing to the creation of biotechnology—enable researchers to better understand the sources of diseases and how the human body potentially reacts to drug treatment. This more scientific approach to R&D is referred to as **discovery by design.** According to the Boston Consulting Group (1993),

> *With knowledge about the relation between the structure and function of the molecule targeted for the drug action, small molecules can be designed that interact very specifically with the target. The target molecule is commonly a receptor on a cell surface—for example, the H_2 receptors that help to regulate acid production in the stomach. Rational drug design promises to supplement the traditional random search for activity and to provide specific guidance to researchers seeking useful drugs for diseases that have largely resisted treatment in the past. (p. 31)*

In fact, as a result of genetic engineering, scientists have recently discovered the gene responsible for Huntington's disease, among others (Boston Consulting Group, 1993).

Third, unlike the 1970s, during which real drug prices were declining, real drug prices were high during the 1980s and for most of the 1990s (review Figure 14–3). The high real drug prices and the resulting sizeable cash flow margins helped fund R&D expenditures, a necessary ingredient for innovation. Recall that Grabowski and Vernon (1981) find empirically that cash flow is a major determinant of R&D expenditures. Thus, the large number of NCEs in both the 1980s and 1990s may be an indirect function of the relatively high drug prices observed during those periods.

Fourth, the Prescription Drug User Fee Act (PDUFA) of 1992, and its extensions in 1997 and 2002, specifies performance goals for the FDA in terms of faster review times of NCEs. The act also allows the FDA to collect fees from pharmaceutical companies when submitting a drug application for approval. In addition, companies pay annual fees for each manufacturing establishment and

TABLE 14–5
Return on Assets and Stockholder Equity for Drug and All Manufacturing Companies, Various Years

	After-Tax Return on Equity						
	1986	1989	1992	1995	1997	2001	2004
All manufacturing	9.6%	13.5%	2.6%	16.2%	16.6%	2.0%	15.7%
Drugs (SIC 283 or NAICS 3254)	24.1	25.3	22.3	27.0	23.2	32.1	14.6
	After-Tax Return on Assets						
	1986	1989	1992	1995	1997	2001	2004
All manufacturing	4.2%	5.5%	0.9%	6.2%	6.6%	.8%	6.4%
Drugs (SIC 283 or NAICS 3254)	11.8	12.5	10.5	10.4	9.5	12.2	7.2

SOURCE: U.S. Bureau of the Census, *Quarterly Financial Report* (various issues), http://www.census.gov (accessed January 11, 2006).

for each prescription drug product marketed. The user fee revenues, rather than general tax revenues, are now used to pay for a substantial portion of the costs associated with FDA review. The FDA has used some of the revenues to speed up approval times by hiring additional staff and making other improvements in the review process. In fact, Philipson et al. (2005) estimate that the original PDUFA and its extension in 1997 accelerated the shortening of review times by 6 to 7 percent and 3 to 4 percent a year, respectively.

The early 2000s continue to show positive signs of innovative activities in the pharmaceutical industry. First, data show that pharmaceutical R&D intensity in the early 2000s remains above the levels observed in the 1970s and the 1980s (see Figure 14–2). Second, the FDA approved 120 NCEs during the first four years of the new millennium, which compare favorably to the NCEs during the first four years of the 1970s (n = 75), 1980s (n = 95), and 1990s (n = 127). The only indicator of less pharmaceutical innovation in the future may be the relatively low real drug prices during the early 2000s as captured in Figure 14–3 (and also the relatively dismal profit performance in 2004; see Table 14–5).

Profits in the Pharmaceutical Industry

Most complaints aimed at the pharmaceutical industry have concerned excessive profits. Patents, brand loyalty, and an inelastic demand for drugs written by physicians are cited as the causes of high pharmaceutical profits. Some comparative data for the after-tax return on equity (ROE) and return on assets (ROA) are shown in Table 14–5 for all manufacturing firms and drug firms for selected years from 1986 to 2004. ROE and ROA are determined by dividing net income (net sales less operating costs and expenses) after taxes by the value of stockholder equity and the firm's assets, respectively. The data illustrate that, for every year shown but 2004, the profitability of drug firms, as measured by either ROE or ROA, is much higher than that of the manufacturing industry average. Specifically, the ROE and ROA for drug firms, on average, were more than twice the manufacturing industry average for the six periods.[19]

Researchers point out that pharmaceutical accounting rates of return may be biased upward due to unusually high R&D and marketing outlays (for example, see Scherer, 1993). Expenditures on these "intangible assets" are expensed, but should be capitalized and then depreciated over an appropriate time period because they ordinarily yield a long-term flow of benefits to drug manufacturers. Studies have found that pharmaceutical returns are 20 to 25 percent lower when R&D and marketing outlays are treated as intangible assets (Office of Technology Assessment, 1993).

Even after accounting biases have been eliminated, pharmaceutical returns generally remain higher than the manufacturing average (Comanor, 1986). Pharmaceutical industry spokespeople point out that research and development is a risky venture. High R&D risks translate into high pharmaceutical returns, because otherwise risk-averse individuals would be unwilling to invest in drug firms. They note that the successful introduction of a pharmaceutical product costs about $802 million or more because a drug firm encounters a large number of misses before finding a commercial hit (DiMasi et al., 2002).

So is it true that pharmaceutical R&D is a risky undertaking? According to the evidence provided in Table 14–5, rates of return in the pharmaceutical industry seem to be more stable than the average return in the manufacturing sector, at least for the seven years reported.

Perhaps focusing on aggregate industry returns masks the variability of returns at the individual firm or product level. Indeed, some evidence suggests that may be the case. A study by Grabowski and Vernon (1990), which analyzes the returns associated with 100 new drug introductions during the 1970s, uncovers evidence indicating that pharmaceutical R&D is very risky and costly. Based on a number of assumptions concerning product duration, cash flow margins, R&D costs, and worldwide sales, the authors find that the variation in returns for new drug introductions is highly skewed, with only the top 30 drugs covering average R&D costs. Moreover, the authors discover that the present value of the cash flow associated with the 10 least profitable of the top 30 drugs just barely covered the present value of their R&D costs.

One implication of Grabowski and Vernon's study is that a successful drug company must have an occasional "blockbuster" to cover the large fixed costs that characterize the R&D process. Another implication is that the real drug price increases of the 1980s, as evidenced by Figure 14–3, may have been necessary for the average new drug innovation to recover its R&D costs. Overall, their study implies that the high rate of profit observed in the pharmaceutical industry may be justified by the significant risk and cost of new product innovations. The authors find that the average return to R&D equaled the 9 percent industry cost of capital, implying a normal rate of return on pharmaceutical R&D investment.

However, another study on the returns to R&D by the Office of Technology Assessment (OTA, 1993) shows that Grabowski and Vernon's results do not hold for drugs introduced from 1981 to 1983. The OTA study found that each NCE, on average, can be expected to return a net present value of at least $36 million more than necessary to bring forth the investment in R&D. The implication is that drug prices could be reduced across the board by at least 4.3 percent without reducing returns below the amount necessary to repay R&D investors. One reason the OTA's results differ from those of Grabowski and Vernon is that the increasing real drug prices and associated greater pharmaceutical revenues during the 1980s were more than adequate to cover R&D costs. The OTA study claims,

19. In addition, the pharmaceutical profit margin (net income/sales) is also more than twice the manufacturing profit margin of 7.0 percent in 2004.

> *Together, the findings on returns on pharmaceutical R&D and to the industry as a whole explain why R&D expenditures have risen so dramatically in real terms throughout the 1980s. Investors have followed the promise of high returns on future innovations. Ultimately investment in research is determined by expected revenues. The dramatic increase in real revenues to new drugs throughout the 1980s has sent signals to the industry that more investment will be rewarded handsomely. The industry has responded as expected, by increasing its commitment to investment, including investment in R&D. (p. 104)*

The Performance of the Pharmaceutical Industry: A Summary

In this section, we reviewed data concerning the prescription drug price inflation rate and profits as measures of industry performance. Drug prices were shown to have increased more rapidly than general prices for all but a few years since 1981. The average profit rate in the pharmaceutical industry was also shown to be higher than the average profit rate in the manufacturing sector during the 1980s and 1990s. By themselves, these two performance measures suggest that society's scarce resources may be misallocated in the pharmaceutical industry.

Data regarding the introduction of NCEs paint a somewhat different picture of the pharmaceutical industry. After slowing during the 1960s and 1970s, the number of new chemical entities by U.S. drug firms actually increased during the 1980s and 1990s. The first four years of the 2000s also compare favorably, in terms of NCEs, to the earlier periods. The R&D spending of U.S. drug firms also increased during the 1980s, and this trend continued through the 1990s. The first four years of the 2000s have also witnessed relatively high levels of R&D intensity in the pharmaceutical industry. Two reasons for the greater innovation of U.S. drug firms in recent years may be rising real drug prices and consistent profitability. As Grabowski and Vernon (1981) and others show major determinants of pharmaceutical innovation are cash flow and future price expectations.

This discussion implies that a trade-off might exist between "static" and "dynamic" efficiency. Static efficiency refers to the efficiency of firms at a point in time and reflects how successfully firms employ a given technology or produce a given product. In contrast, dynamic efficiency relates to the efficiency of firms over time and captures how successful they are at developing new products and processes. As Berndt (2002) writes:

> *Although this conflict between static efficiency (price new drugs low, near short-run marginal cost) versus dynamic efficiency (price new drugs high, maintain incentives for innovation) is a deep and enduring one, as the costs of bringing new drugs to market have increased sharply in recent years, this tradeoff is becoming more severe. The resolution of this static versus dynamic efficiency conflict is likely the single most important issue facing the pharmaceutical industry over the next decade. (p. 45)*

SUMMARY

This chapter assessed the structure, conduct, and performance of the U.S. pharmaceutical industry. Based on the six-digit NAICS, the pharmaceutical industry was shown to contain a relatively large number of equally sized firms, but disaggregation of the pharmaceutical industry into therapeutic markets showed that only a few major drugs typically compete with one another. Legal patents and brand loyalty built up during the patent period are argued to cause substantial barriers to entry into therapeutic markets. Generic drug companies offering huge discounts are particularly ineffective in influencing the loyalty attached to brand-name drugs because physicians are often responsible for selecting drugs. Physicians are not normally price sensitive since they are effectively spending someone else's money.

Further evidence, however, reveals that considerable deconcentration has taken place in the pharmaceutical industry at the therapeutic level. Studies show that price competition takes place among multisource drugs. Price competition sometimes occurs among branded drugs during the patent period and between generic and brand-name drugs during the postpatent period. Drug prices are usually lower when there are more substitute products. Studies show that generic competition causes the brand-name firm's market share to fall by an average of 50 percent two years after entry. The innovator firm's advertising helps preserve its market share, while the follower firms' advertising helps them gain market share.

New product innovation, the major benefit of the pharmaceutical industry, tends to be a risky endeavor and was shown to depend on past R&D success and cash flow. Debate still continues over the relation between firm size and innovation. The safest conclusion to draw from recent studies is that a mixture of firm sizes in the pharmaceutical industry best favors innovation.

Recent data suggest that real drug prices have risen and pharmaceutical firms have experienced relatively high rates of return since the beginning of the 1980s. The resulting cash flow has financed the increase in R&D spending as a percentage of sales and the resulting greater number of new chemical entity introductions during the 1980, 1990s, and early 2000s. All in all, the pharmaceutical industry seems to best fit the model of a "mild to tight differentiated oligopoly." That is, there is some evidence of a few competitors in therapeutic markets, substantial but not perfect barriers to entry based on patents and trademarks, product differentiation, evidence of price and product rivalry rather than cooperation, and evidence of relatively high profits.

The future should witness a continual evolution in the pharmaceutical industry. The demand side of the market will most likely adopt further cost-saving methods, such as formularies, drug review utilization, and generic substitution. Government may be prone to impose price controls if drug prices continue to soar given the greater financial responsibilities of the public sector in pharmaceutical markets as a result of the MMA of 2003. Seller concentration in many therapeutic markets should diminish as many drug patents soon expire and generic competition increases. It will be interesting to follow the effects of these demand- and supply-side changes on new drug innovation.

CASE STUDIES

14-1 Pharmaceuticals and Technology Assessment[20]

In September 2005 the Food and Drug Administration approved Remicade, a drug previously approved for treating diseases such as rheumatoid arthritis and Crohn's disease, for the treatment of ulcerative colitis. The hope is that the drug will save people from having to undergo surgery and possibly allow them to discontinue the use of other drugs that can have dangerous side effects. Ulcerative colitis is a lower digestive system disorder characterized by abdominal pain, bloody diarrhea, fatigue, weight loss, and loss of body fluids and nutrients; about one third of those with the disease end up having their colon surgically removed. As of September 2005, no other drug comparable to Remicade existed for treating ulcerative colitis. Patients taking Remicade were found more likely to go into clinical remission and to stop taking other drugs all together. Side effects of Remicade can include various infections, with tuberculosis being a rare side effect. The cost for a full-year treatment of Remicade ranges from $15,000 to $17,000, but Medicare and private insurance usually cover the drug.

20. Source: Daniel Rosenberg, "Remicade May Prevent Surgery for Ulcerative Colitis Patients," *The Wall Street Journal*, September 26, 2005.

Questions for Discussion

1. *Remicade has the potential to reduce the use of surgery to treat ulcerative colitis. But the cost for a full-year treatment of Remicade is $15,000 to $17,000. Discuss how you might approach a cost effectiveness or cost-benefit analysis of Remicade versus surgical interventions.*
2. *Why do pharmaceutical companies often market and promote products, even with FDA approval, beyond their originally intended purpose? What incentives are at play?*
3. *Should clinical practice guidelines be used to distinguish between candidates for Remicade versus surgery? Why or why not?*

14-2 Marketing the Brand Name[21]

In Germany the health ministry has set up a special commission to decide how much the state will pay for certain drugs. In an attempt to cut health care costs in 2004, the ministry decided that it would no longer cover the high prices of certain brand-name drugs when an appropriate generic drug was available. Since the implementation of this legislation in January 2005, demand for many of the once-popular drugs, such as Pfizer's Lipitor, fell substantially. Pharmaceutical companies viewed Germany, the biggest drug market in Europe, as a key battleground for protecting their brands and sales, in large part because other European countries often considered German drug prices when setting their own. Some of the world's largest pharmaceutical companies decided to fight back. Pfizer took the lead and sent its representatives to appear on talk shows in Germany, sent sales forces to Germany to visit physicians, and contested relevant German legislation.

Questions for Discussion

1. *Similar to Germany, increasing expenditures on prescription drugs has prompted concerns over access and price in the U.S. market. One U.S. proposal has been to "re-import" drugs from Canada, which employs price controls and pooled purchasing systems similar to those in Germany. What are some potential problems with "re-importation"? Explain.*
2. *Identify some of the structural aspects of the German health care system that allows it to control pharmaceutical expenditures. In theory, could the same controls be employed in the United States? Why or why not?*
3. *Regulation and pooled purchasing are two factors listed in this article as contributing to differences in prescription drug costs worldwide. Identify and discuss a third factor.*

14-3 Tiered Copayments for Medicaid[22]

In an effort to slow increases in Medicaid expenditures, a federal commission in September 2005 recommended allowing states to increase copayments on some expensive drugs, particularly when cheaper alternatives are available. The theory is that higher copayments on the expensive drugs will steer patients to less expensive alternatives, saving Medicaid an estimated $2 billion over five years. There is concern that the very sick and minorities in the Medicaid program would suffer most under the proposed changes. Other proposals were aimed at ensuring that the government does not pay too much for prescription drugs for Medicaid patients and allowing

---

21. Source: Jeanne Whalen and Vera Sprothen, "German Curbs on Drug Costs Rile Big Brands," *The Wall Street Journal,* May 2, 2005.
22. Source: "Panel Favors Higher Co-Payments for Certain Drugs in Medicaid," *The Wall Street Journal,* September 2, 2005.

states to negotiate discounted payments for prescription drugs. The commission also wanted to tighten financial eligibility requirements, allowing states to consider a greater portion of a person's assets when determining eligibility. Nationally, the Medicaid program serves 53 million people and costs states and the federal government about $329 billion a year. The commission hoped its recommendations would reduce Medicaid spending by $11 billion.

Questions for Discussion

1. *Critics argue that some Medicaid patients do not have the option to shift to "cheaper alternatives," and will therefore be forced to shoulder the financial burden caused by higher copayments. Is it realistic to assume that some patients will not be able to switch to a different drug?*
2. *Are there meaningful differences between name-brand drugs and generics? What about between name-brand drug A and name-brand drug B, both of the same drug class and designed to treat the same ailments?*
3. *Comment on whether you feel this is a good policy from an economic perspective. What are the trade-offs associated with using price incentives in a low-income population?*

14-4 Direct-to-Consumer Advertising[23]

The verdict against Merck over Vioxx, a painkiller, will worsen a growing negative reaction toward the pharmaceutical industry that has deeply affected the development and marketing of drugs in the United States. Merck took Vioxx off the market back in September 2004 due to its link to a small number of heart attacks and strokes. Vioxx belonged to the class of painkillers called Cox-2 inhibitors, and sales of Cox-2 inhibitors have fallen sharply, while development of others has been delayed. As a result of the verdict, drug makers are being forced to rethink which drugs they pursue. Additionally, the Food and Drug Administration (FDA) has put more pressure on the pharmaceutical industry, which will most likely slow the arrival of new drugs and treatments on the market. The FDA has also become more aggressive about publicizing its concerns *before* the link between a drug and its side effects become clear, and it plans to do even more through a proposed "Drug Watch" web site. The FDA is also calling for tougher warnings on the labels of many drugs. The public concern over pharmaceutical companies and their drugs stemmed from accusations that drug companies were suppressing clinical trials that showed negative results for various drugs. Following these accusations, major medical journals set policies requiring companies to register clinical trials in a public database before they begin if they want the results of the trial to be considered for publication. These and other regulatory initiatives forced the pharmaceutical industry to make public much more information about drug testing that it had previously kept private.

Questions for Discussion

1. *If you read the fine print on the box, you will observe that prescription drugs are associated with nontrivial risks. Indeed, the monitoring, reporting, and control of those risks are an important mission of the FDA. What went wrong in the Vioxx case? Think about the mix of patients that may have been taking Vioxx, and whether the benefit-risk trade-off varies within that distribution.*

---

23. Source: Scott Hensley, Paul Davies, and Barbara Martinez, "Vioxx Verdict Stokes Backlash That Hit FDA, Manufacturers," *The Wall Street Journal*, August 22, 2005.

2. *In the Merck civil case, jurors eschewed scientific arguments in favor of cover-up angles—mainly that Merck covered up evidence on risks while continuing widespread advertising of Vioxx. Merck's argument was more scientific, emphasizing that the overall risks of the drug were very small and the overall benefits very high. Suppose you are the jury foreperson. Discuss how you would critically evaluate each of these arguments.*
3. *Discuss the positive and negative consequences of this ruling from the perspective of the public.*

Review Questions and Problems

1. Describe three benefits associated with pharmaceutical products. Cite one example of each.
2. How do the six-digit NAICS and the therapeutic market definition of the pharmaceutical industry differ in terms of seller concentration? Which is the better measure? Why? Think in terms of actual and potential competition.
3. Explain some of the methods adopted by third-party payers to control drug prices.
4. Cite three reasons why unconstrained physicians tend to purchase brand-name instead of generic products.
5. What benefits and costs do pharmacists face when dispensing generic drugs?
6. Explain the purpose and functioning of a PBM company. What are the antitrust concerns about a drug manufacturer purchasing a PBM company? What is the efficiency justification for such an acquisition?
7. What is the economic rationale behind a patent? Why may the effective patent life of a drug be shorter than the legal life? Why may the effective patent life be longer than the legal life?
8. What two effects did the Hatch-Waxman Act of 1984 have on the supply side of the pharmaceutical market?
9. Why might the FDA tend to delay the drug approval process? Explain in terms of type 1 and type 2 errors.
10. What general conclusions have studies reached concerning drug price competition?
11. What general conclusion have studies reached concerning the promotion of pharmaceutical products? Cite some evidence.
12. What are the two main determinants of R&D spending according to Grabowski and Vernon? What is the relation between firm size and pharmaceutical innovation? Briefly summarize the theoretical considerations and empirical findings.
13. How has the pharmaceutical producer price index compared to the general producer price index since the 1970s?
14. Explain the trend in the number of NCE introductions from after WWII until 2004. What factors account for any changes?
15. What three reasons are claimed to account for the high reported profits of pharmaceutical companies? Do you think drug companies earn excessive profits? Why or why not?

CEBS Questions

■ *CEBS Sample Question on Subject Matter from CEBS Course 9 Study Manual*

1. List and define the methods used by third-party payers to control pharmaceutical costs. (pages 446–447)

■ *CEBS Sample Exam Questions*

1. Which of the following statements is the safest conclusion regarding the relationship between firm size and the innovation process in the pharmaceutical industry?
   A. Large firms are the best innovators because they have the financial resources to conduct effective research and development.
   B. Large firms are the best innovators because they can advertise more effectively.
   C. Small firms are the best innovators because there is less bureaucratic red tape in smaller firms.
   D. Small firms are the best innovators because they have more creative talent.
   E. A mixture of firm sizes is most favorable for fostering pharmaceutical innovation.
2. Which of the following is (are) correct statements regarding the economic performance of the pharmaceutical industry in recent years?
   I. Real drug prices have increased more rapidly than general prices.
   II. The average profit rate is higher than that in the manufacturing sector.
   III. The risk of the pharmaceutical industry is less than that of the manufacturing sector.
      A. I only
      B. II only
      C. I and II only
      D. II and III only
      E. I and III only
3. All the following statements regarding a patent for a pharmaceutical drug are correct EXCEPT:
   A. The legal maximum number of years for a patent is 14 years.
   B. The effective life of a patent is often less than the legal maximum because the FDA takes a number of years to approve a product for commercial introduction.
   C. A pharmaceutical patent is granted for a drug's chemical composition, not its therapeutic novelty.
   D. A legal patent does not guarantee a market position.
   E. The Hatch-Waxman Act quickened the approval process for generic drug.

■ *Answer to Sample Question from Study Manual*

The methods used are formularies, drug utilization review, and required generic substitution. A formulary is a required list of selected pharmaceutical products that physicians are required to prescribe for the third-party payers' patients. A drug utilization review monitors the actions of physicians and identifies physicians who inappropriately prescribe medicines. Generic substitution requires that pharmacists substitute lower-priced generic products for higher priced brand-names whenever possible.

■ *Answers to Sample Exam Questions*

1. E is the answer. See pages 461–462 of the text.
2. C is the answer. Statement III is incorrect. The pharmaceutical industry faces high risks in product innovations and product liability. Statements I and II are correct. See pages 463–464 and 470 of the text.
3. A is the answer. The legal patent maximum period is 20 years. See pages 448–449 of the text.

Online Resources

To access Internet links related to the topics in this chapter, please visit our web site at **www.thomsonedu.com/economics/santerre**.

References

Acs, Zoltan J., and David B. Audretsch. "Innovation in Large and Small Firms: An Empirical Analysis." *American Economic Review* 78 (September 1988), pp. 678–90.

_____. "Innovation, Market Structure, and Firm Size." *Review of Economics and Statistics* 69 (November 1987), pp. 567–74.

Berndt, Ernst B. "Pharmaceuticals in U.S. Health Care: Determinants of Quantity and Price." *Journal of Economic Perspectives* 16 (fall 2002), pp. 45–66.

Boston Consulting Group. *The Changing Environment for U.S. Pharmaceuticals.* Boston: Boston Consulting Group, 1993.

Carroll, Norman V., and Alan P. Wolfgang. "Risks, Benefits, and Generic Substitution." *Journal of Consumer Affairs* 25 (summer 1991), pp. 110–21.

Caves, Richard E., Michael D. Whinston, and Mark A. Hurwitz. "Patent Expiration, Entry, and Competition in the U.S. Pharmaceutical Industry." *Brookings Papers: Microeconomics 1991* (1991), pp. 1–66.

Cohen, Joshua P. "PBMs and a Medicare Prescription Drug Benefit." *Food and Drug Law Journal* 55 (2000), pp. 293–476.

Comanor, William S. "The Political Economy of the Pharmaceutical Industry." *Journal of Economic Literature* (September 1986), pp. 1178–1217.

_____. "Research and Technical Change in the Pharmaceutical Industry." *Review of Economics and Statistics* (May 1965), pp. 182–90.

Comanor, William S., and Stuart O. Schweitzer. "Pharmaceuticals." In *The Structure of American Industry,* eds. Walter Adams and James Brock. Englewood Cliffs, N.J.: Prentice Hall, 1995, pp. 177–96.

Cutler, David M., and Mark McClellan. "Is Technological Change in Medical Care Worth It?" *Health Affairs* 20 (September/October 2001), pp. 11–29.

DiMasi, Joseph A. "Success Rates for New Drugs Entering Clinical Testing in the United States." *Clinical and Pharmacology Therapeutics* 58 (July 1995), pp. 1–14.

_____. "New Drug Innovation and Pharmaceutical Industry Structure: Trends in the Output of Pharmaceutical Firms." *Drug Information Journal* 34 (2000), 1169–94.

DiMasi, Joseph A., Henry G. Grabowski, and John Vernon. "R&D Costs, Innovative Output and Firm Size in the Pharmaceutical Industry." *International Journal of the Economics of Business* 2 (1995), pp. 201–19.

DiMasi, Joseph A., R. W. Hansen and Henry G. Grabowski. "The Price of Innovation: New Estimates of Drug Development Costs." *Journal of Health Economics* 22 (2002), pp. 151–85.

DiMasi, Joseph A., Ronald W. Hansen, Henry G. Grabowski, and Louis Lasagna. "Cost of Innovation in the Pharmaceutical Industry." *Journal of Health Economics* 10 (1991), pp. 107–42.

Duetsch, Larry L. "Pharmaceuticals: The Critical Role of Innovation." In *Industry Studies,* ed. Larry L. Duetsch. Englewood Cliffs, N.J.: Prentice Hall, 1993.

Egan, John W., Harlow N. Higinbotham, and J. Fred Weston. *Economics of the Pharmaceutical Industry.* New York: Praeger, 1982.

Ellison, Sara F., Ian Cockburn, Zvi Griliches, and Jerry Hausman. "Characteristics of Demand for Pharmaceutical Products: An Examination of Four Cephalosporins." *RAND Journal of Economics* 28 (autumn 1997), pp. 426–46.

Federal Trade Commission. "Merck Settles FTC Charges That Its Acquisition of Medco Could Cause Higher Prices and Reduced Quality for Prescription Drugs." Press release (August 27, 1998), http://www.ftc.gov.

Frech, H. E., III. "The Competitive Revolution." *Regulation* (summer 2002), pp. 52–57.

Frech, H. E., III., and Richard D. Miller. "The Effects of Pharmaceutical Consumption and Obesity on the

Quality of Life in the Organization of Economic Cooperation and Development (OECD) Countries." *Pharmacoeconomics* 22 (supplement, 2004), pp. 25–36.

Giaccotto, Carmelo, Rexford E. Santerre, and John A. Vernon. "Drug Prices and Research and Development Investment Behavior in the Pharmaceutical Industry." *Journal of Law and Economics* 48 (April 2005), pp. 195–214.

Grabowski, Henry G. "An Analysis of U.S. International Competitiveness in Pharmaceuticals." *Managerial and Decision Economics* 10 (March 1989), pp. 27–33.

_____. "The Determinants of Industrial Research and Development: A Study of the Chemical, Drug and Petroleum Industries." *Journal of Political Economy* (March–April 1968), pp. 292–305.

Grabowski, Henry G., and John M. Vernon. "Brand Loyalty, Entry, and Price Competition in Pharmaceuticals after the 1984 Drug Act." *Journal of Law and Economics* 35 (October 1992), pp. 331–50.

_____. "A New Look at the Returns and Risks to Pharmaceutical R&D." *Management Science* 36 (July 1990), pp. 804–21.

_____. "Longer Patents for Lower Imitation Barriers: The 1984 Drug Act." *American Economic Review Papers and Proceedings* 76 (May 1986), pp. 195–98.

_____. *The Regulation of Pharmaceuticals: Balancing the Benefits and Risks.* Washington, D.C.: American Enterprise Institute, 1983.

_____. "The Determinants of Research and Development Expenditures in the Pharmaceutical Industry." In *Drugs and Health,* ed. Robert Helms. Washington, D.C.: American Enterprise Institute, 1981, pp. 3–20.

Greer, Douglas F. *Industrial Organization and Public Policy.* New York: Macmillan, 1992.

Henderson, Rebecca, and Ian Cockburn. "Scale, Scope and Spillovers: The Determinants of Research Productivity in Drug Discovery." *RAND Journal* 27 (spring 1996), pp. 32–59.

Hurwitz, Mark A., and Richard E. Caves. "Persuasion or Information? Promotion and the Shares of Brand Name and Generic Pharmaceuticals." *Journal of Law and Economics* 31 (October 1988), pp. 299–320.

Langowitz, Nan S., and Samuel B. Graves. "Innovative Productivity in Pharmaceutical Firms." *Research Technology Management* 35 (March–April 1992), pp. 39–41.

Leffler, Keith B. "Persuasion or Information? The Economics of Prescription Drug Advertising." *Journal of Law and Economics* 24 (April 1981), pp. 45–74.

Lichtenberg, Frank R. "The Impact of New Drug Launches on Longevity: Evidence from Longitudinal, Disease-Level Data from 52 Countries, 1982–2001." *International Journal of Health Care Finance and Economics* 5 (2005), pp. 47–73.

_____. "Are the Benefits of New Drugs Worth Their Cost? Evidence from the 1996 MEPS." *Health Affairs* 20 (September/October 2001), pp. 241–51.

Lu, Z. John, and William S. Comanor. "Strategic Pricing and New Pharmaceuticals." Mimeo, University of California at Santa Barbara, 1994.

Mansfield, Edwin. *Industrial Research and Technological Innovation.* New York: W. W. Norton, 1968.

McRae, James J., and Francis Tapon. "Some Empirical Evidence on Post-Patent Barriers to Entry in the Canadian Pharmaceutical Industry." *Journal of Health Economics* 4 (1985), pp. 43–61.

Moore, Stephen D. "Glaxo, SmithKline Renew Their Rivalry in Medicines Used to Prevent Vomiting." *The Wall Street Journal,* November 19, 1993, p. B4D.

Mosby Medical Encyclopedia. New York: C. V. Mosby, 1992.

Office of Technology Assessment. *Pharmaceutical R and D: Costs, Risks and Rewards.* OTA-11-522. Washington, D.C.: U.S. Government Printing Office, February 1993.

Pear, Robert. "Clinton Backs Off Drug Price Limits." *New York Times,* as printed by *San Jose Mercury News,* May 17, 1993.

Peltzman, Sam. *Regulation of Pharmaceutical Innovation: The 1962 Amendments.* Washington, D.C.: American Enterprise Institute, 1974.

Pharmaceutical Research and Manufacturers of America (PhRMA). *Industry Profile.* Washington, D.C.: PhRMA, 2002.

Philipson, Tomas J., Ernst R. Berndt, Adrian H. B. Gottschalk, and Matthew W. Strobeck. "Assessing the Safety and Efficacy of the FDA: The Case of the Prescription Drug User Fee Acts." NBER Working Paper 11724, National Bureau of Economic Research, October 2005.

Price Waterhouse. *Financial Trends in the Pharmaceutical Industry and Projected Effects of Recent Federal*

Legislation. Report prepared for the Pharmaceutical Manufacturers Association, October 21, 1993.

PricewaterhouseCoopers. "Study of Pharmaceutical Benefit Management." HCFA Contract No. 500-97-0399/0097, June 2001, http://www.pcmanet.org/research/ostudies/hcfastudy.pdf.

Reichert, Janice M., Jennifer Chee, and Claire S. Kotzampaltiris. "The Effects of the Prescription Drug User Fee Act and the Food and Drug Admisistration Modernization Act on the Development and Approval of Therapeutic Medicines." *Drug Information Journal* 32 (2001), pp. 85–94.

Reiffen, David, and Michael R. Ward. "Generic Drug Industry Dynamics." *Review of Economics and Statistics* 87 (February 2005), pp. 37–49.

Rizzo, John A. "Advertising and Competition in the Ethical Pharmaceutical Industry: The Case of Antihypertensive Drugs." *Journal of Law and Economics* 42 (April 1999), pp. 89–116.

Santerre, Rexford E. and John A. Vernon. "Assessing Consumer Gains from a Drug Price Control Policy in the U.S." *Southern Economics Journal* (July 2006).

Scherer, F. M. "Pricing, Profits, and Technological Progress in the Pharmaceutical Industry." *Journal of Economic Perspectives* 7 (summer 1993), pp. 97–115.

Scherer, F. M., and David Ross. *Industrial Market Structure and Economic Performance.* Boston: Houghton Mifflin, 1990.

Schmalensee, Richard. "Product Differentiation Advantages of Pioneering Brands." *American Economic Review* 72 (June 1982), pp. 349–65.

Schnee, Jerome. "Innovation and Discovery in the Ethical Pharmaceutical Industry." Chapter 8 in *Research and Innovation in the Modern Corporation,* eds. Edwin Mansfield, John Rapaport, Jerome Schnee, Samuel Wagner, and Michael Hamburger. New York: W. W. Norton, 1971.

Schumpeter, Joseph. Capitalism, *Socialism and Democracy*. New York: Harper, 1950.

Schwartzman, David. *Innovation in the Pharmaceutical Industry*. Baltimore: Johns Hopkins University Press, 1976.

Statman, Meir. *Competition in the Pharmaceutical Industry: The Declining Profitability of Drug Innovation.* Washington, D.C.: American Enterprise Institute, 1983.

Tanouye, Elyse. "Heartburn Drug Makers Feel Judge's Heat." *The Wall Street Journal,* October 16, 1995, p. B8.

Tanouye, Elyse, and Thomas M. Burton. "More Firms 'Switch' Prescription Drugs to Give Them Over-the-Counter Status." *The Wall Street Journal,* July 29, 1993, p. B1.

Temin, Peter. "Realized Benefits from Switching Drugs." *Journal of Law and Economics* 35 (October 1992), pp. 351–69.

_____. *Taking Your Medicine: Drug Regulation in the United States.* Cambridge, Mass.: Harvard University Press, 1980.

Vernon, John A. "Examining the Link between Price Regulation and Pharmaceutical R&D Investment." *Health Economics* 14 (2005), pp. 1–16.

Virts, John R., and J. Fred Weston. "Expectations and the Allocation of Research and Development Resources." In *Drugs and Health,* ed. Robert Helms. Washington, D.C.: American Enterprise Institute, 1981, pp. 21–45.

Weidenbaum, Murray. "Are Drug Prices Too High?" *Public Interest* 112 (summer 1993), pp. 84–89.

Wiggins, Steven N., and Robert Maness. "Price Competition in Pharmaceuticals: The Case of Anti-Infectives." *Economic Inquiry* 42 (April 2004), pp. 247–63.

CHAPTER 15

THE LONG-TERM CARE INDUSTRY

In a cult movie of the 1970s, Wild in the Streets, *Max Frost, a rock star and newly elected 21-year-old president, created an imaginative solution to what was perceived as an "elderly" problem in the United States. He placed all the elderly people into concentration camps and fed them hallucinogens like LSD. Far away in the concentration camps, elderly people were kept out of sight and out of mind (literally so because of the hallucinogens). You see, Max and his followers despised authority. To Max and friends, if you were 35 or older, you were* elderly. *Elderly people, like parents, teachers, and policemen, possessed authority. Hey! What do you expect from a movie that was designed to appeal to the rebellious young adults growing up during the 1960s?*

Today, one could rightfully argue that we do have a problem concerning the elderly in the United States. The problem has nothing to do with authority, however. The problem pertains to the delivery and financing of long-term care for individuals incapable of caring for themselves. Elderly people make up a majority of the individuals requiring long-term care, and the number of elderly people has grown both in absolute and relative terms over time. In fact, while only one in ten people in the United States was age 65 or older in Max Frost's day (the 1960s), today that number is one in eight. And the population is expected to get even older on average in years to come. Projections suggest that by the year 2050 one out of every five people will be a senior citizen. Indeed, nearly 5 percent of the U.S. population is expected to be age 85 and older by 2050!

We learned earlier in the text that health capital depreciates more rapidly with age. Consequently, the graying of the United States will likely be associated with a more intensive use of medical services for a growing number of elderly, all of which will contribute to rising health care costs in the future. Of particular concern is the increasing cost of caring for the chronically ill elderly on a long-term basis. Finding ways of containing long-term care costs without compromising the quality of care or lives will be a tremendous challenge. Society will have to make hard choices and trade-offs are inevitable unless some truly imaginative solutions are found.

With these choices, trade-offs, and imaginative solutions in mind, this chapter investigates the market for long-term care services. Specifically, this chapter:

- studies the structure of the long-term care industry by analyzing the number and size distribution of the various providers of long-term care services such as nursing homes and home health care agencies. We also look at the buyer side and barriers to entry in the long-term care market, among other structural features.
- discusses the conduct of long-term care providers. In particular, the behavior of long-term care providers, mainly nursing homes, in response to market competition, various pricing methods (such as prospective versus retrospective reimbursement), form of ownership, and regulations are extensively studied. Quality issues pertaining to long-term care are also highlighted.

- examines the performance of the long-term care industry by observing and discussing various indicators such as aggregate price, input usage, output, insurance coverage, and expenditures.

The information obtained will help us better understand the structure, operation, and performance of the contemporary long-term care services industry. The resulting information will be vital in our roles as informed consumers and voters, health care providers, and public policy makers.

The Structure of the Long-Term Care Services Industry

Before we begin our discussion of the industry, it would be useful to define **long-term care.** Long-term care is typically defined as:

> . . . *a set of health care, personal care, and social services delivered over a sustained period of time to persons who have lost, or never acquired, some degree of functional capacity, as measured by an index of functional ability.*

According to the definition, long-term care primarily enhances the quality of life rather than cures a particular medical problem. In many instances, patients in need of long-term care have one or more physical limitations that will be with them for the rest of their lives or, at the very least, for an extended period of time. For example, an elderly man may need help bathing and walking because of a recent stroke. Or a young woman may need continual assistance because of a car accident that left her permanently paralyzed from the neck down. In each instance the need for long-term care is likely to be permanent and the emphasis is on enhancing the quality of life and gaining some measure of independence for the patient. Although hospitals and physicians offer some level of long-term care, they primarily provide short-term treatment aimed at curing rather than caring for or rehabilitating a patient.

Scanlon (1980) points out that, unlike the demand for medical services, the demand for nursing home care reflects a basic rather than a derived demand. He goes on to note that nursing homes are long-term substitutes for independent living and that the function of nursing homes is not to restore health, or "cure," but to provide "care" to those with permanent disabilities. Consequently, physicians play only a minor role in the choice process concerning nursing home care, unlike the choice concerning hospital services where they play a dominant role.

Other elements to keep in mind are that the continuum of care and the organizational settings in which care is provided varies widely. The continuum of care varies from the occasional need for assistance to perform various household chores, such as mowing the lawn or shopping for groceries, to the need for around-the-clock nursing care. Or the continuum of care may include a rehabilitation program that involves physical, occupational, and/or speech therapy. The spectrum of organizational settings that provide long-term care also varies extensively. For example, friends and family members may provide long-term care on an informal basis in the elderly person's own home, or long-term care can be provided in a formal, highly intensive setting such as a skilled nursing home. Intermediate care can be provided by a home health care agency or at an assisted living facility. We begin to analyze the structure of the long-term care industry by examining the need for long-term care. This discussion is followed by a review of the major providers of long-term care services.

TABLE 15–1
A Measurement of the Need for Long-Term Care

Measurement	Examples of Basic Functions
Activities of daily living (ADL)	Bathing
	Dressing
	Eating
	Getting in and out of a chair or bed
Instrumental activities of daily living (IADL)	Going outside the home
	Performing household chores
	Keeping track of household finances
	Cooking and preparing meals
	Using the telephone
	Taking medicine

SOURCE: General Accounting Office, *Long-Term Care, Current Issues and Future Directions.* GAO/HEHS-95-109. Washington, D.C.: GAO, April 1995.

The Need for Long-Term Care

It is generally recognized that an individual needs long-term care when faced with a long-term physical or mental limitation severe enough to impede the ability to carry out the everyday activities of independent living. One of the most frequently used methods to determine whether an individual requires long-term care is to assess whether that individual has the ability to carry out a predetermined list of activities of daily living (ADL), or instrumental activities of daily living (IADL) (see Table 15–1). ADL and IADL are sets of activities used by health care professionals to measure the ability of individuals to perform routine daily living activities. These rating scales are of value because they provide policy analysts with an objective means of establishing the need for long-term health care, both in terms of the number of people who require long-term care and the intensity of care needed.

Using these criteria, the 1999 National Long-Term Care Survey estimates that 19.7 percent of the elderly population, or 7 million people, are chronically disabled and may be in need of some type of long-term care.[1] The elderly are not the only ones in need of long-term care. In 2002, 7.1 percent of the population under age 18 and 6.3 percent of individuals aged 18 to 44 had some limitation in activity based on ADLs, IADLs, or other limitations due to a chronic condition (NCHS, 2004). Clearly, however, the need for long-term care is greatest among the elderly population.

Structure of Informal Care Providers

It is generally agreed that family members and friends provide a substantial amount of long-term care on an informal basis. By its very nature, however, the amount of care provided is difficult to accurately measure. Fortunately, a few recent surveys shed some light on the number of

1. Throughout this chapter, the elderly population is defined as all individuals age 65 and older.

people providing long-term care on an informal basis and the backgrounds of those individuals. According to data from the Commonwealth Fund Biennial Health Insurance Survey (Ho et al., 2005), there were 18 million informed caregivers in the United States in 2003, of which 16 million were between ages 19 and 64 and another 2 million were age 65 or older. A second study (NAC and AARP, 2005), estimates that during the same year there were more than 44 million informed caregivers in the United States, with more than half of those caregivers providing in excess of nine hours a week of care. Finally, AARP (2001) estimates that there were approximately 65 million informal caregivers in the United States in 2000. The wide difference in the survey results can largely be explained by the fact that each survey took a slightly different approach to estimating the amount of informal care. For example, differences exist in terms of the definition of elder care and the timing during which the care was provided.[2]

Despite the wide variation in the estimates concerning the amount of informal care provided, the surveys are in general agreement regarding who is providing the care. According to the NAC and AARP study, the representative informal caregiver tends to be a woman in her forties who is providing more than 20 hours of care per week. She is most likely employed full-time, possesses at least a high school degree, and is of relatively modest means with a median household income of about $38,000 per year. Not surprisingly, most caregivers are related to the recipient, usually a relationship involving a daughter and her mother. Finally, in more than 75 percent of the cases the caregiver does not reside with the recipient of the long-term care.

Thus, the evidence appears to indicate that on a macro level a substantial amount of informal care is being provided on a routine basis throughout the U.S. economy. Whether the amount and intensity of informal care provided has increased or decreased over time, however, is difficult to determine given a lack of time-series data and the absence of consistency among cross-sectional surveys. A comparison of the results from the NAC and AARP studies for 1997 with a study by Wagner (1997) using 1987 data provides some insights. The results indicate that while the demographic makeup of informal health care providers has changed little over time, the overall amount of care provided increased significantly. From 1987 to 1997 the number of households providing informal care increased from approximately 7 million to slightly more than 22 million. A comparison of the 1997 and 2004 NEC and AARP studies, however, suggests that the amount of informal care provided may have planed off recently, as both studies estimate the number of households providing informal care to be around 22 million. At the very least these findings suggest that "caregiving for an elder has become a 'normative' experience for U.S. families" (Wagner, 1997, p. 2).

Structure of the Nursing Home Care Industry

The structure, conduct, and performance paradigm of industrial organization suggests that the structure of an industry matters. In conjunction with the firm's objectives and various government regulations, structure affects how intensely firms compete and ultimately their performance in the health and overall economy. Among the more critical factors influencing market structure are the number and size distribution of firms, the number and size distribution of buyers, and the height of any barriers to entry into the industry. We next assess each of these structural features with respect to the nursing home industry.

---

2. In terms of timing, the person being surveyed could be asked, "Are you currently providing long-term care?" or "Have you provided care to anyone in the last year?" Naturally, the latter survey question will generate much higher estimates regarding the amount of informal care provided.

TABLE 15–2
Characteristics of the Nursing Home Industry

	1995	1997	1999
Nursing Homes	16,700	17,000	18,000
For-profit	66.1%	67.1%	66.5%
Not-for-profit	25.7%	26.1%	26.7%
Government	8.2%	6.8%	6.7%
Nursing Home Beds (1,000)	1,771	1,821	1,879
For-profit	65.0%	70.0%	65.7%
Not-for-profit	26.4%	24.0%	26.6%
Government	8.5%	6.0%	7.7%
Size Distribution			
Fewer than 50 beds	16.8%	12.9%	11.5%
50–99 beds	35.6%	37.2%	38.7%
100–199 beds	40.1%	42.2%	41.8%
200 beds or more	7.5%	7.7%	8.0%
Occupancy	88.4%	87.4%	86.6%

SOURCE: *National Nursing Home Survey: 1995 Summary* (April 2000); *National Nursing Home Survey: 1997 Summary* (July 2000); and *National Nursing Home Survey, 1999 Summary* (June 2002).

Number and Characteristics of Nursing Home Providers. Table 15–2 provides estimates for the number, amount of beds, ownership status, size distribution, and occupancy rate of nursing homes in the United States. According to the data, roughly 18,000 nursing homes function in the United States with approximately 1.9 million beds. These two figures suggest that the typical nursing home facility operates with about 100 beds, roughly half the bed size of the typical hospital in the United States.

Most nursing homes are organized on a for-profit basis although the percentage has declined slightly over time. Data (not shown) also suggest that 80 percent of the nursing homes are Medicare and Medicaid certified and 60 percent of the nursing homes belong to a chain or group. The data in Table 15–2 also indicate the percentage of nursing homes in the smallest bed-size category, fewer than 50 beds, has tended to decline over time while the percentage of nursing homes in the largest bed-size category, 200 or more beds, has only marginally increased over time. Moreover, the percentage of nursing homes with 100 to 199 beds remain fairly constant over time. As a result, the survivorship principle suggests that the 50–99 bed-size category may be the optimal size given that most nursing homes find it best to operate in this bed-size range over time. We will examine later what econometric studies tend to suggest about the existence of scale economies in nursing homes. Finally, the data in Table 15–2 imply that the occupancy rate of the typical nursing home in the United States is roughly 87 percent and that occupancy has declined marginally over time. The 87 percent nursing home occupancy rate is dramatically higher than the 60 to 70 percent occupancy rate observed in the hospital services industry.

Taking all of the information together, we can get a clearer picture of the typical nursing home. The representative nursing home is organized on a for-profit basis and is most likely affiliated with a nursing home chain. It contains approximately 100 beds and 90 of those beds are occupied on a typical day. About 300 nursing homes operate in the typical state in the United States.

Buyers and Users of Nursing Home Services. Nursing home expenditures were slightly more than $110 billion in 2003. According to Figure 15–1, four groups are primarily responsible for paying for nursing home services: the Medicaid program, the Medicare program, consumers, and private health insurers. The single largest payer of nursing home services is the Medicaid program, accounting for approximately 46 percent of nursing home expenditures. The next largest category of government funding is the Medicare program, accounting for about 12 percent of total funding.

Individual consumers represent the second-largest payer group for nursing home care services. Out-of-pocket costs account for 28 percent of nursing home expenditures and largely reflect the amount paid by private payers for long-term care services. Roughly 40 percent of all nursing home residents are private-pay patients. Empirical studies find that the price elasticity of demand for private-pay nursing home care varies widely, ranging from −0.16 to −2.30. Studies also find that the income elasticity of demand for nursing home care varies considerably with estimates ranging from −0.38 to 2.27 (Reschovsky, 1998). As one might expect, price and income elasticities of demand tend to be more elastic for elderly individuals who are either married or less chronically ill (Reschovsky, 1998) because home care represents a viable alternative in these two cases. The availability of informal care is another determinant of the demand for long-term care by private-pay individuals.

FIGURE 15–1
Expenditure Shares for Nursing Home Services, 2003

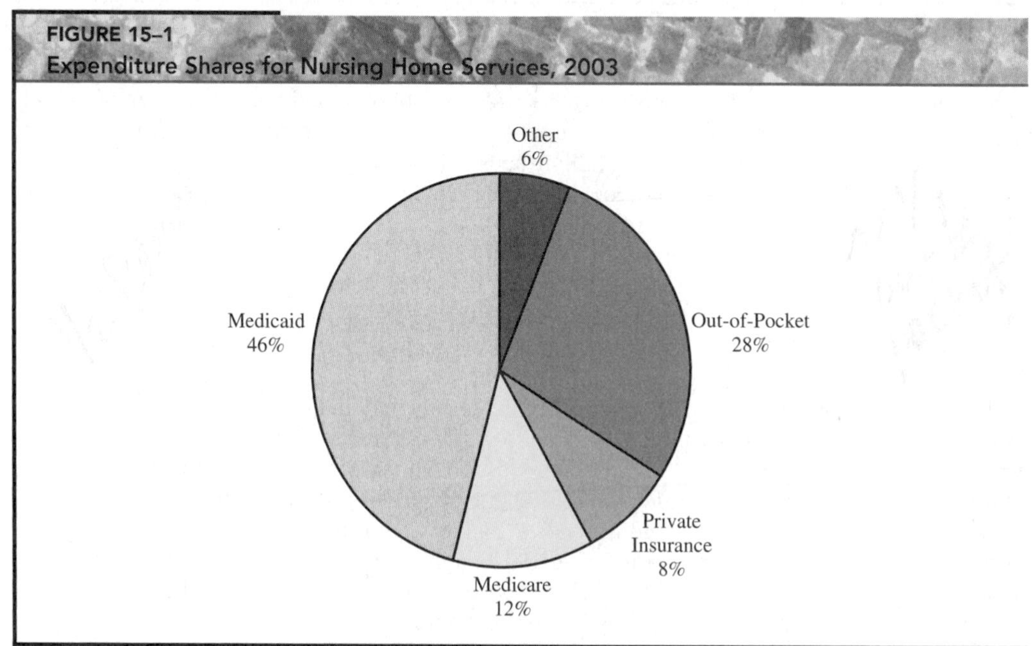

SOURCE: Centers for Medicare & Medicaid Services. National Health Expenditures Tables, Table 7. http://www.cms.gov.

Finally, private insurers represent the next-largest payer for nursing home care at 8 percent of the cost. Most of the reimbursement pays for short-term post-acute nursing home services. Presently, only a small percentage of individuals have private insurance coverage for long-term care. We will take up the reasons for the low long-term care insurance coverage rate later.

In sum, data suggest that most nursing home care is paid for by federal and state governments, reflecting the large amount of short-term services provided to individuals under the Medicare program and long-term services provided to individuals under the Medicaid program. The government, because of its dominance in the market, may exert some influence on the operation and performance of short-term Medicare and long-term Medicaid nursing home services. Out-of-pocket costs remain sizeable for nursing home care. Studies find that the demand for nursing home care by private payers is more elastic with respect to price and income compared to the demand for medical care. The elastic nature of the private demand for nursing home care services may also limit the ability of an individual nursing home to raise price or reduce quality below the competitive level.

Barriers to Entry. As discussed throughout the text, barriers to entry play an important role in the structure, conduct, and performance of an industry. Simply put, barriers to entry reduce the degree of potential competition and thereby may provide existing firms with some market power depending on the degree of actual competition. The market power may show up in high prices and/or reduced quality of care. It was also pointed out in earlier chapters that barriers to entry may be government created (for example, certificate of need programs, government franchises, or patents) or because of technical considerations (such as economies of scale, high sunk costs, learning curve effects, or exclusive control over a necessary input).

As mentioned in earlier chapters, econometric studies examine the existence of scale economies by estimating cost functions for goods or services. The estimated cost function shows the isolated empirical relationship between total operating costs and some measure of output or size after controlling for other determinants of costs such as input prices, quality of care, and patient case-mix. According to Rosko and Broyles (1988), "most research findings suggest that scale economies are minimal in the nursing home industry and that there are no pronounced scale effects beyond 40 beds" (p. 253). More contemporary studies generally confirm the earlier research. Christensen (2004) finds that small nursing homes experience some economies of scale while larger nursing homes experience no significant economies and may face some diseconomies of scale. Chen and Shea (2004) find that economies of scale do not exist in the nursing home industry with the exception of the Medicare post-acute care segment of the market. Therefore, it follows that scale economies do not represent a significant entry barrier into nursing home markets.

Sunk or irretrievable costs may cause a barrier to entry into an industry. Recall that irretrievable costs may involve initial investments or assets that cannot be easily salvaged when a firm exits the industry. Contestability theory suggests that markets are more contestable or potentially competitive when sunk costs are low because new entrants realize they can leave an industry relatively costlessly if economic circumstances do not turn out as initially suspected. Conversely, if sunk costs are significant, firms will be reluctant to enter new markets, *ceteris paribus*. We saw in Chapter 13 that hospitals entail huge sunk costs because of the immense cost and time involved in hospital construction. Nursing homes, however, are much smaller on average than hospitals. In addition, unlike hospitals with numerous floors and wide elevators, nursing homes tend to have one or two floors to minimize access problems of chronically ill residents. Also, unlike hospitals, very little diagnostic and therapeutic equipment is necessary to provide nursing home care. The upshot is that much less sunk costs are involved in nursing home care than hospital care, with the implication that sunk costs most likely do not seriously inhibit entry into the nursing home marketplace.

Certificate of need programs may represent a serious entry barrier in the nursing home industry. Recall that CON laws require that new and existing health care providers, like nursing homes, obtain approval before building new medical facilities or purchasing new capital items. CON laws are designed to control the amount of capital devoted to medical care as a way of controlling health care costs. However, if enforced too stringently, CON laws might result in inefficiency if too much capital is discouraged, competition is stymied as a result, and monopoly pricing ensues. Consequently, the effect of CON laws on the behavior and performance of nursing homes remains an empirical issue.

Unfortunately, only a few studies have examined empirically the impact of CON laws on the provision of nursing home care. After controlling for a host of factors such as income, age composition, and the state Medicaid reimbursement rate, Gulley and Santerre (2003) find that the existence of a state CON law program had no impact on the number of nursing homes or the number of nursing home beds relative to the elderly population across the 3,040 counties of the United States in 1991. Similarly, Grabowski et al. (2003) find that the repeal of CON and moratorium laws had no effect on nursing home or long-term care Medicaid expenditures. That study estimated a number of fixed effects models using state-level data from 1981–1998. As Harrington et al. (1997) note, the ineffectiveness of CON laws in reducing the number of homes and beds may result from the "lack of coordination with other regulatory programs, lack of significant compliance mechanisms, politicized review processes, and high approval rates for most requests" (p. 575).

Focusing on the growth rather than the level of nursing home beds, Harrington et al. (1997) found that the presence of a CON/moratorium program does matter. Specifically, Harrington et al. determined empirically that state regulations measurably slow the growth of nursing home beds. What remains to be determined is whether the reduction in the rate of growth is optimal from a societal perspective. While the reduced growth in nursing home beds may help contain the rising costs from excessive capital creation, it may also provide existing nursing homes with some market power. If so, existing nursing homes may desire CON laws because of the resulting market power. But according to Harrington et al., "the nursing home industry in general has been strongly ideologically opposed to CON and moratorium regulatory controls" (p. 586).

In sum, the nursing home industry contains a relatively large number of nursing homes with low market shares. Barriers to entry are relatively low, especially in areas without binding growth regulations such as CON laws. While the typical nursing home most likely faces a downward-sloping demand curve because most residents prefer locations near friends and relatives, the individual nursing home probably has very little control over price since it faces the countervailing power of government and the highly price elastic demand of private buyers. From a structural perspective, the nursing home industry comes closest to resembling a monopolistically competitive industry.

Structure of the Home Health Care and Hospice Industry

Similar to the nursing home industry, we now analyze the structure of the home health care and hospice industry. Once again, the characteristics of the seller and buyer side of the market are discussed to assess the structural competitiveness of the market. These structural features become important when evaluating the conduct and performance of the industry.

Number and Characteristics of Home Health Care and Hospice Care Providers. Because of its dynamic nature, agencies may provide home health care services, hospice care, or both. Haupt (1998) differentiates between home health care and hospice care in the following manner:

> *Home health care is provided to individuals or families in their place of residence to promote, maintain, or restore health or to maximize the level of independence while minimizing the effects of disability and illness, including terminal illness. Hospice care is defined as a program of palliative care and supportive care services that provides physical, psychological, social, and spiritual care for dying persons, their families, and other loved ones. (1)*

Given that home health care agencies can potentially provide both home health and hospice care, the following information on the number of providers refers to institutions providing either type of care unless noted differently.

The market for home health care and hospice has seen some rather dramatic shifts in recent years, largely because of changes in government funding. About 13,500 home health and hospice care agencies provided services to 2.5 million patients in 1996, a dramatic increase of 70 percent from just four years earlier. The sharp increase in the number of agencies and patients occurred largely in response to the shift away from hospitals and nursing homes in an effort to contain health care costs. Thereafter, the number of agencies and patients dropped significantly and by 2000 there were 11,400 home health and hospice agencies servicing 1.46 million patients. The decline was largely because of the Balanced Budget Act of 1997 that called for the implementation of the Interim Payment System, which placed stricter limits on the Medicare cost-based reimbursement system.

In 2000, the Prospective Payment System for the payment of Medicare home health services was put in place. It pays home health agencies a predetermined rate for each 60-day episode of home health care. At the same time, a prospective payment system for hospice health agencies was also introduced. Since 2000, the number of home health and hospice care agencies has remained relatively stable, suggesting that the fixed Medicare payments have been adequate to at least cover costs. For example, the number of Medicare-certified home health care and hospice agencies changed from 7,099 and 2,267 to 6,813 and 2,275 between 2001 and 2002, respectively. However, there are indications that the number of home health and hospice care agencies is currently on the rise (MedPAC, 2005).

Not-for-profit providers accounted for about one-third of all agencies but half of all patients; comparable government figures were 11 and 9 percent, respectively. In both absolute and relative terms, not-for-profit home care and hospice care agencies treated many more hospice patients than for-profit agencies. Most agencies, 92 percent, are Medicare and Medicaid certified. Nearly half of all agencies were affiliated with a group or chain and slightly over one-quarter were operated by a hospital. Thirty-seven percent of all agencies were freestanding institutions.

In sum, the typical home health care patient is cared for by a not-for-profit agency that is affiliated with either a chain of home care agencies or a hospital. Also, the typical home care agency is likely to be Medicare and Medicaid certified and services approximately 185 patients throughout the year. While not noted previously, there are 220 patients per agency located in a metropolitan area but only 111 patients per agency in nonmetropolitan areas.

Buyers and Users of Home Health Care Services. Home health care costs amounted to approximately $40 billion in 2003. The largest payer for home health care services, amounting to 46.5 percent of all purchases, was the federal government, with the bulk of these funds coming from the Medicare program. Private insurers were responsible for 18.5 percent of total expenditures, while out-of-pocket expenses picked up an additional 16.5 percent. The remaining 18.5 percent came from other public and private sources. It should be pointed out that the Medicaid program does not currently reimburse for long-term care provided in the home. Generally, home health care is demanded because a person is receiving long-term custodial services, recovering from an illness or a surgical procedure, or receiving hospice care. The demand for home health care, both in the short and long term, depends on the out-of-pocket price for home health care, the out-of-pocket price for institutional care, the wealth of the individual, the availability of informal care, and the demographic characteristics of the individual.

Barriers to Entry. Entry barriers are most likely minimal in the home care services industry. Since services are provided in the home, very little capital is necessary. Hence sunk costs play virtually no role. While most home care agencies are Medicaid and Medicare certified, which could cause an entry barrier, some states have as many unlicensed home care agencies as certified.

Economic theory suggests that cost structure characteristics such as scale and scope economies or learning curve effects might prohibit the entry of new firms. Cost characteristics do not appear particularly binding on the entry of new firms, however. For example, Kass (1987), in a study of 1,704 home health agencies using 1982 data, finds that economies of scale and scope are not substantial. For another study on approximately 100 home health agencies in Connecticut over the period from 1987 to 1991, Gonzales (1997) finds similar results, showing that economies of scope are fully exhausted at nine services (skilled nursing care, physical therapy, occupational therapy, and so on). Given that most of the home health agencies in the sample normally provided between seven and eleven services, scope economies do not seem to provide existing home health agencies with a cost advantage over new ones. While Gonzales does provide some evidence for scale economies, the relation between size and total costs does not appear to be particularly sizeable. Specifically, Gonzales finds that a 10 percent increase in size, as measured by home visits, leads to a 7.6 percent increase in costs. Therefore, the average cost curve is relatively flat such that the per-unit cost of production is fairly close for both small- and large-sized home health care agencies, *ceteris paribus*.

The Structure of the Long-Term Care Industry: A Summary

It is difficult to judge the degree of structural competitiveness in the long-term care industry. Long-term care tends to take place in local markets because elderly people wish to remain fairly close to family and friends. Consequently, detailed micro-information on the number and size distribution of nursing home and health care agencies is needed before conclusions can be drawn about the structural competitiveness of the long-term care industry in each local market area.

Having stated this limitation, long-term care most likely can be treated as a monopolistically competitive industry. There appears to be a sufficient number of actual competitors. For example, one nursing home competes against others and also with home health care agencies for patients. Also, for some recipients of long-term care, informal care remains an alternative to formal care. Moreover, most studies find that the demand for private-pay long-term care, particularly nursing home care, is highly elastic with respect to price. In addition, sources of technical barriers to entry such as economies of scale, sunk costs, and chain organizations do not seem to reduce the degree of potential competition. Only CON laws, when binding, and other government-created barriers (such as zoning laws) may limit the entry of new firms. We next assess how the conduct of the long-term care industry is influenced by its monopolistically competitive nature.

THE CONDUCT OF THE LONG-TERM CARE INDUSTRY

In this section of the chapter we discuss how various external circumstances such as government regulations influence the behavior of long-term care providers. The price and quality of long-term care are two of the behavioral issues discussed. Virtually all of the discussion focuses on the nursing home industry because that is where most research has been directed. The monopolistically competitive nature of the nursing home industry, and the resulting downward-sloping demand curve, suggest that individual nursing homes may have some latitude in determining the price charged for private long-term care. Up against this framework, we examine the effect of Medicaid reimbursement, as a type of price regulation, on the behavior of nursing homes. We also examine whether type of ownership matters and the impact of market competition on the behavior of nursing home care providers.

The Dual Market Model of Nursing Home Pricing

The nursing home industry provides an interesting but complex setting to examine the pricing behavior of individual firms. Complexities result because, on a routine basis, nursing home decision makers must question the financial consequences of admitting patients who seek care on either a short- or long-term basis and who may privately pay or receive insurance coverage from public programs such as Medicare or Medicaid. Consequently, decision makers in nursing homes must recognize the trade-offs involved and simultaneously determine the price charged and number of patients for each type of service and payer category. In this chapter we ignore short-term nursing home care because our concern is solely with issues relating to the delivery of long-term nursing home care. Neglecting short-term care is not too problematic because, as we saw when we examined the market structure of long-term care providers, most individuals receive long-term rather than short-term care in nursing homes.

We also saw that the dominant payers for nursing home care are private individuals who pay out of pocket and the Medicaid program. These two purchasers add an interesting twist to the pricing issue. While each state government sets the price paid by its Medicaid program for long-term care, the individual nursing home must still determine how many private-pay and Medicaid patients to treat and the price charged to private payers. Luckily for us, Scanlon (1980) provides an insightful model to investigate this choice-making process of an individual nursing home. A graphical illustration of his dual market model is provided in Figure 15–2.

Dollar values are shown on the vertical axis and the total number of private-pay and Medicaid patients are shown on the horizontal axis. The aggregated demand curve facing the individual health care provider has three distinct segments. The first segment, labeled *AB,* shows the private demand that lies above the Medicaid reimbursement rate of P_M. The second segment, *BC,* represents the Medicaid reimbursement rate of P_M for a particular number of Medicaid-eligible individuals in the market area, as measured by the horizontal distance *BC*. The third segment, CD_P, reflects the remaining portion of the private-pay demand. The curve AMR_P indicates the marginal revenue associated with the first segment of the private-pay demand curve. Given that the Medicaid reimbursement rate is independent of the number of Medicaid patients, P_M also reflects the marginal revenue associated with treating each additional Medicaid patient.

The profit-maximizing nursing home continues to treat additional patients as long as the additional revenues compensate for the added costs, MC. Thus, in equilibrium, the nursing home treats a total of $0Q_T$ patients where P_M = MC. Of the $0Q_T$ patients, $0Q_P$ are private-pay patients because they add more to profits over that range (that is, $MR_P > P_M$). The number of Medicaid patients lies between Q_P and Q_T. The theoretical model indicates that private-pay patients pay a

FIGURE 15–2
The Dual Market Model of Nursing Home Behavior

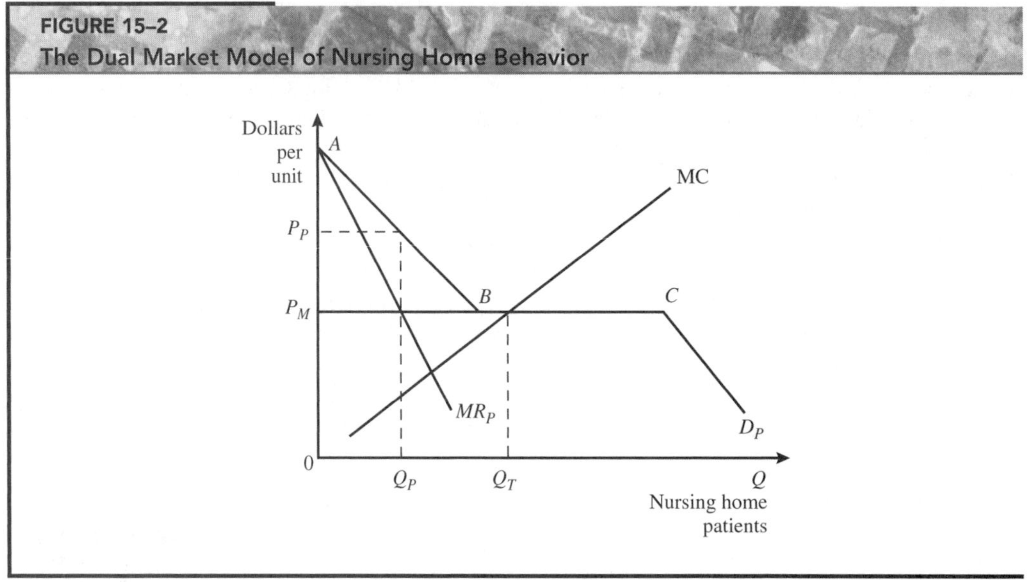

Lines *AB* and AMR_P represent the demand and marginal revenue curves for private-pay patients. Line segment *BC* represents the Medicaid reimbursement rate of P_M for the number of individuals eligible for Medicaid coverage in the market area. Line segment CD_P identifies the remainder of the private demand curve. The nursing home admits $0Q_T$ patients because the marginal revenue of $P_M = MC$. Of the total patients, $0Q_P$ are private pay and the remaining portion, Q_PQ_T, represents the number of Medicaid patients. Private-pay patients pay P_P for nursing home care. Because the horizontal distance Q_PQ_T, representing the number of Medicaid patients admitted, is less than the horizontal distance *BC*, showing the number eligible for Medicaid coverage, an excess demand for Medicaid nursing home care exists in the market area.

higher price than Medicaid patients for the same services. According to the figure, each private-pay patient pays P_P, whereas the health care provider receives P_M for each Medicaid patient. In addition, the figure suggests that excess Medicaid demand exists at the government-established price of P_M because the horizontal distance between Q_P and Q_T, the number of admitted Medicaid patients, is less than the horizontal distance *BC*, reflecting the number of Medicaid eligible individuals in the market area.

An interesting policy question concerns what the government might do to reduce any excess demand for nursing home care. As one option, the government might raise the Medicaid reimbursement rate. As the Medicaid fee increases, the horizontal segment of the MR curve shifts upward along the MC curve and the nursing home expands its number of Medicaid patients relative to the number of private-pay patients. The exact number of additional Medicaid patients depends on the slopes of the private demand and marginal cost curves. Flatter curves imply that more Medicaid patients are admitted in response to a higher Medicaid reimbursement rate.

Notice, according to Figure 15–2, that private-pay patients are required to pay a higher price if the Medicaid reimbursement rate is increased. Gertler (1989) points out another possible consequence of a higher Medicaid reimbursement rate when a capacity constraint exists such as a CON law. Recall from Chapter 5 that higher quality shifts demand upward to the right and lower quality shifts it to the left. In response to a higher Medicaid reimbursement rate, Gertler notes that nursing homes may react by lowering quality instead of, or in addition to, raising the private-pay price. Both actions reduce the quantity demanded of nursing home care by private-pay patients and provide additional rooms for the marginally more profitable Medicaid patients.

Consequently, private-pay patients may pay a higher price and/or receive a lower quality of care as a result of the higher Medicaid reimbursement rate if a capacity constraint exists. It should be pointed out that Medicaid patients also face a lower quality of care because it is illegal and also may not be cost effective for nursing homes to provide different levels of care to private-pay and Medicaid patients. For one reason, complementarities exist with respect to providing various activities such as food and laundry services to both private-pay and Medicaid patients. Although reduced, as long as the resulting quality of care is beyond the level of care provided in private homes, both private-pay and Medicaid patients may find it preferable to remain in the nursing home. Thus, when a capacity constraint and excess Medicaid demand exist, higher Medicaid reimbursement may be associated with reduced quality. Gertler (1989), Nyman (1985), and Zinn (1994) all find that a higher Medicaid reimbursement lowers quality. However, using more recent data, Grabowski (2001) finds that higher Medicaid reimbursement has only a small negative impact on quality, pointing to a lessening of the capacity constraint over time because of the elimination of CON laws in many states and a decline in nursing home utilization.

Raising the Medicaid reimbursement rate is likely to be a costly public policy option. Taxes on the general public must be raised to support the increased subsidy, especially if the higher price causes more individuals to become financially eligible for Medicaid coverage. Also, the nursing home may earn excess economic profits if price increases relative to average cost and entry barriers exist. If entry barriers do not exist, however, the greater profitability may create an incentive for new firms to enter the nursing home industry in the long run. Entry will shift down the private demand curve facing each individual nursing home and could result in a lower price paid by private-pay patients.

Another policy option is for the government to directly subsidize the costs of providing nursing home care. The subsidy reduces the marginal costs of production and shifts the MC curve downward. The lower marginal cost, in turn, creates an incentive for the representative nursing home to admit more Medicaid-eligible patients. Once again, however, this may be a costly alternative, as general taxes must be increased to cover the subsidy to nursing homes.

Policy analysts have long questioned whether an excess demand for Medicaid patients exists in the market for nursing home services. Testing for the existence of excess demand in the nursing home market has proven to be a difficult task for researchers. Nyman (1993) approaches the problem by developing a three-part empirical test and estimating a trio of utilization equations where the dependent variable equaled either the number of total, private-pay, or Medicaid patients. For the first part of the test, Nyman (1993) estimates the extent to which the total number of nursing home patients was positively related to total number of beds available, the idea being that if an excess demand for nursing home services exists, beds would be highly correlated with utilization. Or, put in other terms, a bed built is a bed filled when excess demand exists.

The second part of the test involved examining the empirical relationship between beds and the number of private-pay and Medicaid patients. If an excess demand situation exists, the marginal bed would be filled by a Medicaid patient rather than a private-pay patient, the assumption being that the needs of private-pay patients have already been satisfied, making the additional bed available for a Medicaid patient. The third portion of the test examined whether private patients crowd out Medicaid patients in areas with greater overall need for care.

Using 1988 county-level data, Nyman performs the three-part empirical test for three states: Wisconsin, Minnesota, and Oregon. The empirical results are interesting in that they do not support the proposition that the market for nursing home services is subject to excess demand. In particular, the empirical results find no evidence of excess demand in Wisconsin and Oregon and only limited evidence of excess demand in Minnesota. The implication is that Medicaid patients are not crowded out of the nursing home market by private-pay patients who are willing to pay a higher price for long-term care. These findings are supported by the fact that the overall occupancy rate for nursing homes fell below 90 percent during the 1990s and recent government studies that indicate that most Medicare beneficiaries have access to skilled nursing home care (MedPAC, 2005).

The Effect of Alternative Payment Methods

While useful for predicting the impact of changes in the Medicaid reimbursement rate or marginal costs on the behavior of nursing homes, the static analysis of Figure 15–2 may ignore some dynamic aspects of the reimbursement issue. As discussed in previous chapters, third-party payers may pay health care providers in a number of different ways. For example, the payment from the state government to the nursing home may be based on the actual cost at each nursing facility or some fixed amount based independently on some industry-wide standard. Differences in payment methods matter because they influence how individual nursing homes behave over time in terms of costs, quality of care, and patient case-mix. Some examples may highlight the differences.

First, suppose a state government sets the reimbursement rate for the next period based on the nursing facility's actual costs of servicing Medicaid patients. In fact, many states paid for nursing home care using retrospective cost-based reimbursement systems before 1980 (Coburn et al., 1993). Because of the retrospective and facility-specific nature of the reimbursement method, the nursing home faces less incentive to control costs, realizing it can simply pass on any cost increases to the state government. The higher costs will impose a greater tax burden on the general public. There is a silver lining to this dark cloud, however. If the nursing home can easily pass on any cost increases to the state government, it may be less likely to compromise quality of care and more likely to admit patients in more severe case-mix categories.

Second, suppose a state government sets a flat rate independent of actual facility costs or prospectively sets the reimbursement rate at the industry average projected forward with an automatic annual adjustment for inflation. The important consideration is that no allowance is made for actual costs incurred by the nursing facility for either the flat rate or prospective payment method. Nursing homes are permitted to keep any profits but must also incur losses if actual costs exceed the Medicaid reimbursement, so they are at financial risk for any cost overruns. In this case the nursing facility faces an incentive to control the costs of servicing patients. Lower nursing home costs imply lower taxes for the general public but also mean that nursing homes may control costs by skimping on the quality of care or by practicing cherry-picking behavior. As a result, patients in the heavier case-mix categories may experience admission discrimination, and those that are admitted may not be provided with the proper quality of care.

As we can see, the government faces a policy dilemma not only when establishing the level of reimbursement but also with the method of reimbursement under Medicaid. Some hybrid forms of reimbursement exist that attempt to rectify some of the weaknesses of pure retrospective or prospective systems. One such method is case-mix adjusted reimbursement, which tries to compensate each nursing facility based on its particular patient case-mix and may include financial penalties and/or rewards to encourage efficient behavior. Price regulations like these, while well intended, can be difficult in practice to design correctly and typically involve substantial administrative costs (for example, see Nyman and Connor, 1994).

Empirical studies tend to find that the reimbursement method influences the incentives of nursing homes with respect to costs, quality, and patient case-mix. In terms of costs, an early study by Frech and Ginsburg (1981) used national data for 1973 and 1974 with the number of inpatient days and input prices specified as typical arguments in a cost function and also controlled for the type of reimbursement, among other factors. The authors found that pure cost reimbursement without ceilings was associated with the highest costs. Specifically, compared to simple flat-rate systems, pure cost reimbursement led to costs that were 21 percent higher in the typical home. They also found that prospective reimbursement systems led to costs that were between pure cost and flat-rate reimbursement. The exact outcome depended on whether the prospective rates were established on the basis of the industry or the individual facility's experience in a previous year. When prospective rates are based on a facility's cost experience in the previous period, incentives are diluted and more resemble cost reimbursement. Using cost data for 1978 to 1980, Holahan and Cohen (1987) reach a similar conclusion that prospective and flat-rate systems generally reduced cost growth more than retrospective payment.

In terms of quality, Zinn (1994) finds that both fixed rate and prospective systems led to fewer RNs per resident and worse process quality (a greater percentage of patients restrained and greater percentage not toileted, respectively) when compared to retrospective reimbursement. Case-mix reimbursement was found to increase the number of RNs per resident and improve process quality (lower percentage not toileted) relative to cost reimbursement. Using national data for 1987, Cohen and Spector (1996) find that in states with fixed reimbursement, nursing homes use more lower-skilled and fewer higher-skilled professional nurses than homes in states with cost-based approaches. Finally, for case-mix, based on national data for 1981, Cohen and Dubay (1990) determine that nursing homes respond to flat-rate systems by decreasing the severity of their case-mixes through admission discrimination and also decrease their staffing levels.

Scale Economies with Respect to Quality

Notice in the previous discussion that nursing homes may respond to changing external circumstances by altering the quality of care. Generally a trade-off exists between costs and quality of care. The severity of the trade-off depends on whether scale economies hold with respect to quality. Figure 15–3, where total costs are shown on the vertical axis and the level of quality is depicted

FIGURE 15–3
The Cost Savings from Quality Reductions

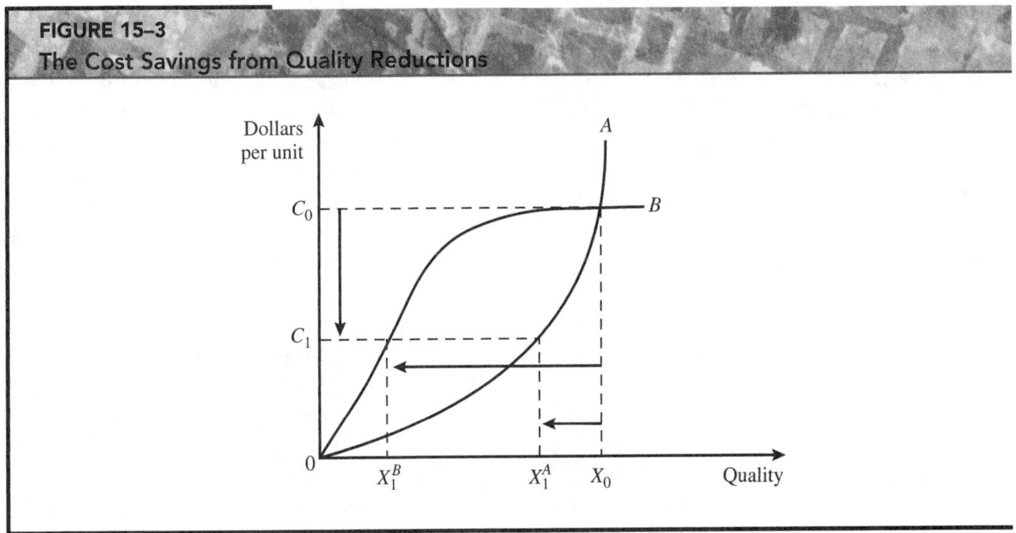

Curve 0*B* depicts scale economies with respect to quality whereas curve 0*A* shows diseconomies of scale with respect to quality. The graphical model suggests that quality must be sacrificed a great deal to achieve a given cost savings of C_0C_1 when scale economies hold. Conversely, the model indicates that quality improvements come at a much larger cost when the quality/cost relation exhibits diseconomies of scale.

on the horizontal axis, helps clarify this point. Notice that two curves, $0A$ and $0B$, are drawn in the figure. Both curves show how much it costs to provide varying levels of quality at a representative nursing home. Suppose we begin with costs of C_0 and, correspondingly, a quality level of X_0 in each case. Now suppose that policy makers wish to reduce nursing home costs to C_1. Notice the degree to which the level of quality must change to accommodate the reduction in costs in the two cases. In the case of curve $0A$, quality declines by a relatively small amount to X_1^A, but for curve $0B$ quality falls by a much larger amount to X_1^B. The difference in the reduction of quality can be explained by scale economies. Curve $0B$ reflects decreasing costs or increasing returns with respect to quality, so costs increase proportionately slower than quality. Consequently it takes a relatively large change in quality to achieve a given level of cost savings. Curve $0A$, in contrast, reflects increasing costs or decreasing returns, so smaller reductions in quality can attain a given level of cost savings.

In an imaginative paper, Gertler and Waldman (1992) measure scale economies with respect to quality in nursing homes. Based on some relatively sophisticated theoretical and empirical modeling techniques, they find that the nursing home cost function exhibits diseconomies of scale in quality. As a result the authors point out that policies aimed at improving quality will be very costly. Policies aimed at cost savings, however, can be achieved with very small reductions in quality. For example, the authors determined that an increase in the Medicaid reimbursement rate lowers quality, as the Scanlon model with a capacity constraint predicts. However, the quality reduction was relatively small at 0.02 percent, whereas the cost savings were relatively larger at 0.2 percent given a one standard deviation increase in Medicaid reimbursement. As another example, the authors find that increased market competition improves quality. More specifically, an increase in competition, as measured by a one standard deviation reduction in the Herfindahl-Hirschmann Index, raised quality by only 2.5 percent but increased costs by a much larger 20 percent.

Ownership and Conduct

According to property rights theory, ownership status may also influence how institutions behave. In for-profit organizations, individuals claim private ownership to any residual profits. In contrast, public and not-for-profit institutions are subject to a nondistribution constraint, meaning that any residual earnings cannot be distributed to those who control the organization like managers, employees, or directors (Hansmann, 1996). As a result, some theorists believe that the lack of property rights to any residual profits provides less of an incentive for public and not-for-profit organizations to operate with least-cost methods of production. However, other theorists point out that although not-for-profit organizations do not maximize profits, they do pursue goals such as quantity and quality maximization. Alternative goals can be more easily realized when costs are held to a minimum.

Although the theory may be suspect, a relatively large number of studies have supported the basic prediction of property rights theory in the case of nursing homes. One of the more cited studies, Nyman and Bricker (1989), compare the technical efficiency of not-for-profit and for-profit nursing homes. Technical efficiency exists when a given amount of output is produced with the fewest inputs. The authors employ a linear programming technique called **data envelopment analysis (DEA)** to determine the factors that influence the technical efficiency of a sample of nursing homes operating in Wisconsin. Briefly, this technique identifies benchmark firms that produce a fixed level of output with the fewest inputs. The inputs used in the Nyman and Bricker study include total nursing hours, total social service worker hours, total therapist hours, and total all other hours in an average day.

The benchmark firms are then used as a reference set to calculate an efficiency score for the remaining firms in the sample. The benchmark or most efficient firms are assigned a score of 1, while the less efficient firms are given scores less than 1 depending on their level of technical inefficiency. The efficiency scores in Nyman and Bricker's sample range from .226 to 1.

The efficiency scores are then regressed on a series of independent variables to determine the factors that influence the extent to which nursing homes efficiently utilize inputs. In their study, the factors used in the regression equation include a dummy variable controlling for the ownership status of the nursing home. The dummy variable equals 1 if the nursing home was a for-profit firm and zero if it is organized on a not-for-profit basis. The hypothesis is that for-profit homes have higher efficiency scores as the basic property rights theory indicates.

Nyman and Bricker's findings indicate that for-profit nursing homes employed 4.5 percent fewer inputs per patient-day than otherwise comparable not-for-profit homes. The authors' findings are consistent with the predictions of the managerial expense preference model, as discussed earlier in the context of not-for-profit hospitals. Because managers of not-for-profit nursing homes are not pressured by owners to operate in an efficient manner, they increase costs by expanding discretionary expenditures and employing more than the minimum amount of inputs. The authors go on to state that if for-profit managers similarly acted in an inefficient manner, the owners would replace them. If the findings of this study are generally indicative of managerial behavior in the nursing home industry, as other studies such as Nyman et al. (1990), Fizel and Nunnikhoven (1992), and Chattopadhyay and Heffley (1994) tend to confirm, ownership status does affect the performance of nursing homes. In the absence of an ownership constraint, managers of not-for-profit nursing homes act in an inefficient manner by overemploying labor inputs and operating at a point above the cost curve of otherwise similar for-profit nursing homes.

In their study, Nyman and Bricker attempt to control for quality differences among nursing homes by specifying the number of Medicaid certification code violations and other indirect measures of quality in the regression equation. Controlling for quality is particularly important when it comes to a service such as nursing home care because fewer labor inputs per patient may reflect a lower level of quality rather than greater efficiency. Their approach to holding quality constant is troublesome, however. Like the number and types of patients and inputs, the level of quality is also a variable decided by nursing home administrators. Stated in econometric terms, the level of quality is endogenous to the individual nursing home—a choice variable decided within the model—and not an exogenous variable, a parameter determined outside the model. The failure to properly specify quality as an endogenous variable could have led to improperly drawn conclusions.

In fact, theory suggests that not-for-profit organizations, because of the attenuation of property rights, may provide better quality of service than for-profits do when asymmetric information exists. Without sufficient consumer information, for-profit organizations may have more incentive to engage in opportunistic behavior in the process of maximizing profits. Not-for-profit institutions, in contrast, have less incentive to take advantage of consumers because of the nondistribution constraint. Consequently, not-for-profit status may signal an interest in quality over profits and serve as a guarantee of quality assurance, much as a trademark does.

Using a large sample of nursing facilities for 1998, Harrington et al. (2001) examine whether the level of quality varied systematically across nursing homes with different ownership structures. As a measure of quality the authors used the number of deficiencies as revealed by state inspections at a total of nearly 14,000 nursing homes. According to their results, investor-owned nursing facilities averaged 5.89 deficiencies per home compared to 4.02 at not-for-profit homes and 4.12 at public nursing homes. After controlling for other determinants of quality such as patient case-mix by an ADL index and the proportion of Medicaid patients, among other factors in a multiple regression model, the authors find that an investor-owned hospital was associated with 0.679 more deficiencies than an otherwise comparable not-for-profit nursing home. Moreover, a nursing home belonging to a chain was associated with 0.633 additional deficiencies than an otherwise comparable freestanding nursing facility, and for-profit nursing homes are more likely to be a member of a chain.

An article by Hillmer et al. (2005) does a nice job of summarizing the research on the relationship between nursing home ownership status and the quality of care provided. A systematic review of the literature generated 81 results from 38 different studies on the subject. Quality measures vary widely and include structure indicators (such as nursing aide turnover), quality indicators (such as inappropriate restraints) and outcome indicators (such as infections). Of the 81 results, only 6 indicate that not-for-profit nursing homes deliver a lower quality of care than for-profit nursing homes, while 33 results find just the opposite, that for-profit nursing homes provide inferior care. The remaining results find no significant difference in the quality of care delivered across ownership type. Overall, the results suggest that "residents of for-profit nursing homes were more likely to be the recipients of poor quality compared with similar residents in not-for-profit facilities" (p. 162).

But showing empirically that not-for-profit nursing homes provide higher quality of care than do for-profits does not necessarily offer evidence supporting the theory that for-profits pursue profits over quality when asymmetric information exists or that for-profits provide inefficiently low quality. Quality is just one of the many attributes that make up a good and service. For a given price, more quality generally means less and lower amounts of other types of attributes. In this case, people who value quality highly will be drawn to institutions offering high levels of quality. Decision makers of not-for-profit nursing homes may maximize quality or quality and quantity rather than profits, as discussed in Chapter 13. As a result quality may be higher in not-for-profit nursing homes not because of asymmetric information but because of differences in the taste for quality and alternative goals of organizations. It is important to understand the theoretical reason for any disparity in quality. If ownership form by itself results in quality differences, public policy might be directed toward encouraging one type of ownership form over another if quality improvement is an issue. However, if asymmetric information is the cause for quality differences, public policy might be aimed at offering improved information to consumers.

Chou (2002) sorts out the differences by comparing the effect of ownership status on the quality of nursing home care in the presence and nonpresence of asymmetric information. For the test, Chou measures quality of care by mortality and several adverse health outcome measures (decubitus ulcers, dehydration, and urinary tract infection). Asymmetric information is defined as existing when nursing residents have no spouse or no child visiting within a month after admission. Chou argues that nursing home residents are usually frail and disabled; therefore, family members often serve as representatives to monitor or evaluate the quality of care.

Chou's empirical findings prove to be very interesting. The results for two of the four quality indicators suggest that not-for-profit nursing homes provide better quality than for-profits when asymmetric information exists. That is, when residents lack family members to monitor the service, for-profit nursing homes face less incentive to maintain the quality of care. Chou's empirical results support the theory that for-profit nursing homes practice opportunistic behavior and sacrifice quality of care for more profits when asymmetric information exists.

Grabowski and Hirth (2003) take the analysis a step further by analyzing whether competitive spillovers from not-for-profits cause for-profit nursing homes to deliver higher quality of care. The authors argue theoretically that patients in for-profit nursing homes will be better informed because not-for-profits attract a greater proportion of uninformed consumers given the quality assurance signal generated by the nondistribution constraint. Grabowski and Hirth test their theory by empirically examining how the market share of not-for-profits affects nursing home quality while holding constant a host of demand and supply side factors. They find that a higher not-for-profit market share improves for-profit and marketwide nursing home quality as measured by several structural, procedural, and outcome indicators. Grabowski and Hirth conclude by noting that if not-for-profits "have a competitive advantage in 'trustworthiness' while for-profits have greater incentives for efficiency, intersectoral competition can yield better outcomes than a market consisting exclusively of one type of firm." That is, competition from not-for-profits raises the quality of nursing home care while competition from for-profits limits inefficiency and the exercise of market power.

Market Concentration and Nursing Home Conduct

Conventional microeconomic theory predicts that more competition results in lower prices and greater quality. Costs of production are unaffected by competition, according to conventional microeconomic theory, because firms are assumed to be motivated by maximum profits. The drive for maximum profits ensures that firms operate on and not purposely above the cost curve.

We have been learning throughout this text that conventional microeconomic theory does not always relate perfectly well to medical markets. Motivations other than profit maximization, third-party reimbursement, low out-of-pocket prices, and rational consumer ignorance are some of the various features of medical markets that point to that conclusion. It is also important to realize that some of these features apply only to specific medical markets and not to all of them. For example, we learned in an earlier chapter that hospitals reacted to increased competition by raising quality, costs, and prices prior to the 1980s because of the so-called medical arms race. But the medical arms race does not apply to the care provided by nursing homes. Furthermore, unlike the market for hospital services, the nursing home market may be characterized by excess demand and not excess capacity. That is why it is so important to carefully consider the theoretical relation and review the empirical findings between conditions such as market structure and the conduct of firms in each specific medical market such as the nursing home industry. To that we now turn our attention.

Market Concentration and the Price of Nursing Home Care. Following in the footsteps of industrial organization (IO) theory, health economists have been interested in the relationship between the degree of competition, as measured by market concentration, and the pricing behavior of medical firms of various kinds of which nursing homes are no exception. Nyman (1994) was among the first to apply IO theory to an analysis of market behavior in the nursing home industry. Nyman begins by deriving and specifying the price markup function or Lerner (1934) index facing the individual nursing home in the following form.

$$\frac{(P_i - C_i)}{P_i} = \frac{1}{[\alpha|E_m| + (1-\alpha)|E_i|]} \tag{15–1}$$

In Equation 15–1, P_i and C_i stand for the price charged by the individual nursing home and marginal cost, respectively, so the expression on the left-hand side of the equality symbol represents the firm's markup of price above marginal cost expressed as a percentage of price. The expressions $|E_m|$ and $|E_i|$ stand for market demand elasticity and the individual nursing home's price elasticity of demand stated in absolute terms. Because of fewer alternatives, the market demand elasticity is less than the price elasticity of demand faced by the individual nursing home and depends on the availability of other substitutes for nursing home care such as home health agencies and informal care provided in the home.

The α parameter reflects the conjectural variations held by nursing homes in the market and captures whether the typical nursing facility expects the others to match or offset its output decision. If nursing homes expect matching or coordinated behavior, α equals 1 and the markup depends on market elasticity alone. The markup is the largest and equals that of a monopoly when firms in a market perfectly collude.[3] If firms compete rather than collude, α equals 0, and the individual nursing home's markup depends on the degree to which the firm can successfully differentiate its product from others in the same market. A less differentiated product means a higher price elasticity of demand facing the individual nursing home and hence a lower markup of price over the costs of production.

Based on Equation 15–1, Nyman uses multiple regression analysis to investigate the determinants of the markup percentage across a sample of nursing homes in Wisconsin using 1988 data. Since Nyman examines the factors affecting the markup on private payers of nursing home care, he uses the Medicaid reimbursement rate instead of marginal cost in the Lerner index, as the analysis surrounding Figure 15–2 suggests. That is, the opportunity cost of caring for a private-pay patient is the additional revenues that would be received from caring for a Medicaid patient. Nyman specifies a Herfindahl-Hirschman index of market concentration with the county defined as the relevant geographical market in the multiple regression equation along with other variables affecting market elasticity and the price elasticity of demand facing the individual firm. Recall from the discussion in Chapter 8 that matching behavior and collusion are more likely to prevail in highly concentrated markets. Thus, one expects a direct relation between the HHI and the markup of private price relative to the Medicaid reimbursement rate.

For his sample, the average markup over the Medicaid fee for a skilled nursing facility was 18.2 percent and the average HHI was 2,240. Although Nyman estimates a positive coefficient on the HHI, the estimate was not statistically different from zero, suggesting that a marginal change in the level of market concentration had no appreciable impact on the price markup charged by the typical nursing home. An insignificant estimate on the HHI might reflect that nursing home markets were highly contestable in Wisconsin because of low entry barriers at that time. The threat of potential competition may have forced nursing homes to charge a price independent of the low degree of actual competition, given that matching behavior was not expected because of low entry barriers.

More recently, Mukamel and Spector (2002) use 1991 data for a sample of for-profit nursing homes in New York to estimate the price elasticity of the private demand facing individual nursing homes to assess their degree of market power. They implicitly assume that the representative nursing home expects offsetting behavior (that is, α equals zero in Equation 15–1) and thus $(P_i - MC_i)/P_i = 1/|E_i|$. As noted earlier, lower price elasticities of demand suggest more power to elevate price above the marginal costs of production. Mukamel and Spector consider that CON laws may or may not be binding, different degrees of patient case-mix severity, and the Medicaid reimbursement rate may replace marginal cost in the Lerner index as noted earlier. The authors calculate that the average price elasticity facing the individual nursing home lies between 3.46 and 3.85, depending on whether estimated marginal costs or the Medicaid rate is used to calculate the Lerner index. The authors note that these elasticities are relatively low and result in comparatively high price markups to private payers. Mukamel and Spector go on to note that the "large price mark ups and the possibility that nursing homes behave as monopolists in the private pay market raise the question of whether this aspect of the market should be regulated" (p. 419).[4]

3. The expression on the right-hand side of the equality symbol can be referred to as a modified Lerner index of monopoly power. The Lerner index of monopoly power holds that the markup of price over marginal cost as a percentage of price equals one divided by the price elasticity of market demand, or $(P - MC)/P = 1/E_m$. For a price-taker facing a perfectly elastic demand curve, E_m equals infinity, so $(P - MC)/P$ equals zero, as perfect competition suggests. The Lerner index suggests that a monopolist's power over price falls with a higher price elasticity of market demand.

4. An elasticity of demand of 5.13 can be inferred from Nyman's (1994) study using his average measures for private price of $66.67 per patient-day and the average Medicaid reimbursement rate of $53.76 per day.

Market Competition and Quality. Another important issue concerns how the degree of market competition influences the quality of nursing home care. From a theoretical perspective, the impact of market concentration, one aspect of competition, on quality is theoretically ambiguous. On the one hand, when a few for-profit firms command a large share of market sales and competition is thereby diminished, traditional IO theory suggests that the few firms may face an incentive to restrict both output and quality in an attempt to earn greater profits. On the other hand, when few firms exist in the market, consumers may be able to gather better information on potential suppliers, which can promote better quality (Pauly and Satterthwaite, 1981).

Zinn (1994) attempts to clear up the theoretical ambiguity by empirically examining the relation between various measures of market competition and alternative structural and process measures of the quality of nursing home care. Process measures of quality include the proportion of residents not toileted, the prevalence of urethral catheterization, and the prevalence of physical restraint usage. The number of registered nurses per nursing home resident represents the structural measure of quality. The unit of analysis is the 2,713 counties in the 48 contiguous states of the United States. Among the measures of competition are market share concentration, measured by the HHI based on bed capacity in the county; the presence of an entry barrier, measured by a statewide moratorium on nursing home bed construction; and the availability of substitutes, measured by home health staff per capita and the percentage of women aged 15 to 64 not in the workforce (that is, availability of informal care).

Control variables included education of the county population, excess bed capacity, proportion of for-profit facilities, and three variables measuring patient case-mix. Data were for 1987. Using multiple regression analysis, Zinn estimates the impact of each independent variable on each of the four quality measures and obtained some insightful results relating to the effects of market competition. First, she finds that increased market concentration, as indicated by a higher HHI, tends to improve the quality of care, particularly process quality. Hence the empirical results suggest that better quality of care results when fewer nursing homes exist in a market, *ceteris paribus,* providing support for the Pauly and Satterthwaite (1981) argument that less providers means more-informed choices and greater competition.

While Zinn finds empirically that more actual competitors results in lower quality of nursing home care, she also finds that entry barriers are associated with reduced quality. That is, registered nurse staffing tends to be lower and the use of physical restraints higher in markets where a moratorium on nursing home bed construction erects barriers to new competitors. Consequently, her empirical results indicate that more actual competition lowers quality, but greater potential competition (that is, no entry barriers) raises quality. The reason for the inconsistent finding is not readily apparent unless it is the size and not the number of nursing homes that really matters. Recall that the HHI increases with fewer firms but also when market shares are less equal among firms. Perhaps quality of care is better when nursing homes produce a greater volume of services. That might be the case if practice makes perfect in the nursing home industry. Unfortunately, Zinn does not control for the average size of the typical nursing home in the market to test whether this hypothesis is valid.

The empirical results regarding the availability of substitutes on the quality of nursing home care were also mixed. The availability of home health resources was found to be associated with higher levels of RN staffing but not with any of the process quality measures. The proportion of women aged 15 to 64 not in the workforce, representing an informal substitute for nursing home care, was found to lower the proportion of residents not toileted but is associated with the greater use of physical restraints and lower RN staffing. Zinn explains that it is possible that fewer women participating in the workforce translates into a smaller labor pool for nursing homes.

Conduct of the Long-Term Care Industry: A Summary

We have examined theoretically and empirically a large number of issues relating to how long-term care providers react to influences such as the level and type of Medicaid reimbursement, form of ownership, and market competition. Because few studies focus on the home health care industry, the analysis focused solely on how these various factors influence the private price of nursing home care, the quality of nursing home care, and patient case-mix. What follows is a brief summary of the findings.

Under normal conditions, the dual market model of nursing home behavior predicts that a greater Medicaid reimbursement rate increases the access of Medicaid recipients to nursing home beds. Interestingly, the dual market model also predicts that the quality of nursing home care suffers if the Medicaid reimbursement rate increases when a capacity constraint exists. According to the model, nursing homes lower quality to reduce the number of private-pay patients and thereby make additional room for the marginally more profitable Medicaid patients. While earlier empirical studies have found an inverse relation between Medicaid reimbursement and nursing home quality, some recent evidence suggests that the relation may no longer hold because an excess demand condition may no longer exist in the nursing home industry. Excess demand may no longer apply because of the elimination of CON laws in some states and a growing availability of alternatives to nursing home care such as home health care and assisted living arrangements.

The method of Medicaid reimbursement was also found to matter in terms of the incentives faced by nursing homes. Nursing homes face less financial risk when Medicaid payments are more flexible and facility specific. Thus, we can think of the degree of financial risk imposed on nursing homes as ascending from retrospective to facility-specific prospective, class prospective, and flat-rate reimbursement systems. Empirical studies clearly suggest that the reimbursement method matters because of financial incentives. Studies tend to suggest that more restrictive methods are associated with lower nursing home costs and reductions in quality and patient case-mix severity. Recently, Chen and Shea (2002) question whether the cost reductions brought on by restrictive payment systems reflect efficiency or simply unwanted cuts in quality. Using a national sample of 4,635 nursing homes and 1994 data, the authors find that costs are unaffected by prospective reimbursement when quality differences among facilities are controlled for and the endogeneity of quality variables is addressed. As a result, like Zinn (1994) and some others, Chen and Shea argue that the level and method of Medicaid reimbursement should be linked to the quality of care.

Next we addressed the efficiency and quality implications of the type of ownership. Property rights theory suggests that for-profit nursing homes may behave more efficiently than not-for-profits although the precise objective of the latter ownership form is theoretically unclear. Empirical studies indicate that for-profit nursing homes are more technically efficient and produce at a lower cost than not-for-profits. However, many question whether the cost savings associated with for-profit nursing homes reflect lower quality when compared to otherwise similar not-for-profits. Indeed, the theory implies that not-for-profit organizations may provide a higher quality of care than for-profits when an asymmetry of information exists. Chou's (2002) study empirically supports the theory.

We then examined the impact of market competition on the price and quality of nursing home care. The Lerner index of monopoly power tells us that the ability of firms to elevate price above the marginal costs of production depends on market elasticity of demand, the individual firm's elasticity of demand, and the conjectural variations formed by the firms in the industry. Using multiple regression analysis, Nyman (1994) was unable to empirically link the Lerner index to a Herfindahl-Hirschman index of market concentration using a sample of nursing homes in Wisconsin in 1975. Directly calculating the Lerner index, Mukamel and Spector (2002) find empirically that the mean price elasticities calculated for nursing homes in New York State in 1991 ranged from 3.46 to 3.85, quite low for an industry professed to be monopolistically competitive. Further evidence is needed on this issue before wide-sweeping conclusions can be drawn about the relative profitability of nursing homes in the private pay segment of the industry.

Finally, we turned our attention to the impact of market competition on the quality of care and relied on Zinn's (1994) study for empirical insights. With respect to market competition, her study analyzes the impact of market concentration, entry barriers, and the availability of substitutes on various structural and process measures of quality. We discussed how the relation between market concentration and quality of care is theoretically unclear and depends on whether less firms in an industry leads to a restriction of quality or means more informed choices. Zinn's results lend empirical support for the latter hypothesis, as greater market concentration is found to improve the quality of nursing home care. Entry barriers were found to be associated with lower levels of quality, and the empirical results concerning the availability of substitutes was mixed. It is unclear what policy implications arise for the proper structure of the nursing home industry given that greater market concentration improves whereas entry barriers lower the quality of care.

The Performance of the Long-Term Care Industry

We conclude the chapter with an examination of the overall performance of the market for long-term care. This presents a number of interesting challenges because the long-term care industry is unique and differs in three important respects from the previous medical industries discussed. First, long-term care is generally associated with chronic care and care for those with disabilities rather than acute care. As a result, care is generally provided on a long-term basis and the cost may be spread out over a number of years, possibly even decades. Second, much of the long-term care provided is informal in nature and provided by family and friends. Since no direct payment is made for the care provided, the cost is indirect and involves forgone wages. Third, the number and type of formal health care providers is diverse and runs the gamut from skilled nursing home facilities to assisted living centers with everything in between, such as meals on wheels programs and senior centers. To keep the discussion manageable, we focus primarily on nursing homes and home health care. The objective of this section is to assess the overall performance of the long-term care industry by examining such measures as expenditures on long-term care; private insurance for long-term care; the price of nursing home care; and the utilization of nursing home, home health care, and hospice services.

Expenditures on Long-Term Care

Informal Expenditures on Long-Term Care. Calculating the cost of informal care poses an interesting challenge to researchers because they must impute the economic cost of the caregiver's time. For example, what is the economic value of a caregiver's time when she spends all day Saturday helping her mother with some household chores and bringing her to the doctor? Or what is the economic value of the time of a semi-retired man who drives every afternoon to his father's house to help him prepare his meals?

A study sponsored by Metropolitan Life (1997) estimates the cost of informal caregivers on U.S. businesses and focuses on the loss in productivity that results when full-time employees provide informal care. According to the report, overall productivity can be negatively impacted in six ways. First, the firm incurs recruitment and training costs when an employee leaves to provide care. Second, the firm experiences absenteeism costs when an employee fails to show up for work because of caregiving responsibilities. Third, productivity diminishes when an employee cuts the workday short to provide care. For example, an employee may show up late for work, leave work early, or take an extended lunch break to attend to caregiving problems or issues. Fourth, the firm bears the cost of workday interruptions when employees address caregiving responsibilities while at work. A case in point would be an employee who spends the better part of the morning at work on the phone with a physician's office straightening out whether her mother received the proper medical treatment during her last visit with the doctor. Fifth, there are the costs associated with an eldercare crisis. Such costs occur when, for example, an employee is forced to take time off from work because his father fell down the stairs at home and fractured his hip. Finally, the authors consider the increase in administration costs that results when supervisors take time during work to accommodate the needs of employees addressing caregiving issues.

The Metropolitan Life study estimates the total cost of lost productivity because of caregiving at approximately $11.4 billion a year, with the replacement and training cost being the largest single component, equaling just under $5 billion a year. This estimate should be considered low because it focuses on only one segment of informal health care providers: full-time workers.

Taking a slightly different approach, White-Means and Chollet (1996) estimate the imputed average wage or value of time for caregivers to equal $6.23 per hour in 1989 dollars. The average imputed wage was estimated to be relatively higher for males, $11.84, and full-time workers, $9.26, and substantially lower for females, $6.01, and caregivers who did not work, $5.26. Overall, these value-of-time estimates are lower than you might expect because, in addition to estimating a wage equation based on a human capital model, the authors corrected the results to control for individuals who were not employed.

Finally, Arno et al. (1999) estimate the cost of informal caregiving using current market wage rates. According to the authors, their main focus is to estimate "the potential cost . . . of informal caregiving if informal caregivers had to be replaced by paid workers" (p. 184). Based on the results generated from the NAC and AARP study (1997) referred to earlier in the chapter, the authors estimate 25.8 million individuals provided almost eighteen hours of informal care per week. Multiplying these by an hourly wage of $8.18, the authors calculate the market value of informal care to equal $196 billion in 1997. More recent estimates by Arno (2002) have the economic value of informal caregiving at $257 billion in 2000, based on 27.3 million informal caregivers and an hourly wage of $8.81.

The astute reader will notice that the economic value of informal caregiving estimated by Arno et al. (1999) is substantially higher than the previous two studies. Three reasons account for the difference. First, they consider the work effort of all informal caregivers and not just full-time workers, as was the case in the Metropolitan Life study. Second, Arno et al. utilize the market wage rate, rather than the imputed wage rate as White-Means and Chollet (1996) do. Third, the authors base their analysis on a more contemporary data set that considers slightly higher nominal wages and a greater prevalence of informal caregiving.

Overall, these studies indicate that a substantial amount of informal care is provided at a significant cost to the U.S. economy. The two estimates by Arno suggest that the economic value of informal care has increased in recent years because of a mild increase in the amount of informal care provided and an increase in the opportunity cost of providing care to caregivers in terms of forgone wages.

Formal Expenditures on Long-Term Care

Data in Table 15–3 examine the extent to which formal expenditures on long-term care have changed over time. The analysis focuses exclusively on expenditures for nursing home care provided by freestanding nursing homes and home health care delivered by freestanding home health facilities.

TABLE 15–3
Nursing Home and Home Health Care Expenditures, Selected Years 1980–2003

	1980	1990	1995	1997	1998	2000	2002	2003
National health expenditures (billions of dollars)	$245.8	$696.0	$990.2	$1,093.1	$1,150.9	$1,309.9	$1,559.0	$1,678.9
Annual rate of increase	11.7%	11.0%	5.7%	5.1%	5.2%	7.2%	9.3%	7.7%
Nursing home expenditures (billions of dollars)	$17.7	$52.7	$74.6	$85.1	$89.5	$95.3	$106.6	$110.8
Annual rate of increase	20.6%	11.5%	9.1%	6.4%	5.2%	5.1%	5.3%	4.0%
Home health care expenditures (billions of dollars)	$2.4	$12.6	$30.5	$34.5	$33.6	$31.6	$36.5	$40.0
Annual rate of increase	16.8%	18.1%	17.1%	2.8%	−2.8%	−2.0%	8.5%	9.5%

For 1980, the average annual rate of growth is between 1960 and 1980; for 1990, it is the average annual rate of growth from 1980.

SOURCE: Centers for Medicare & Medicaid Services, National Health Expenditures Tables, Table 2.

We focus on these two types of facilities for two reasons. First, the data are available and consistent, which provides us with the opportunity to trace expenditures over time. Second, since expenditures on nursing home and home health care represent the bulk of the institutional expenditures on long-term care, they can serve as a proxy for total formal expenditures.

In 1980 expenditures on nursing home care and home health care equaled $17.7 billion and $2.4 billion, respectively, and in total they accounted for only 8 percent of total national health expenditures. The next decade and a half saw a phenomenal growth in expenditures on nursing home and home health care. As a result, by 1995 nursing home expenditures and home health care represented 10.6 percent of national health care expenditures. The largest increase in percentage terms took place in home health care as expenditures on freestanding home health care facilities increased at an annual rate just under 20 percent from 1980 through 1995. This increase was the direct result of an increase in both the number of individuals receiving home health services and an increase in the number of visits per patient (MedPAC, 1999).

As was the case with national health care expenditures, the rate of increase in nursing home and home health care decelerated in the mid-1990s. For example, in 1997 the rate of increase in expenditures on nursing home care fell to 6.4 percent, which was slightly more than the 5.1 percent increase in overall national health expenditures. Much of the decrease in the rate of growth in nursing home care expenditures can be attributed to a more modest growth in medical prices and increased use of alternative forms of long-term care such as home health care and assisted living facilities (Levit et al., 2002). Changes in the rate of growth of home health care expenditures have been much more volatile. The volatility results because home health care is one of the smallest categories in the national health accounts and even modest changes in spending generate significant changes in rates of growth. In 1996 home health care expenditures increased by more than 10 percent and by 1997 they increased by only 2.8 percent.

From 1998 through 2000 expenditures on nursing home and home health care continued to grow, but at a much lower rate. In fact, home health care expenditures actually fell by more than 2.8 percent in 1998 and by almost 4 percent in 1999. Most of this decrease can be attributed to changes in public policy that brought about a decrease in the proportion of medical expenditures financed through public sources in 1998 for the first time in a decade. The most significant change took place in the Medicare program with the passage of the Balanced Budget Act (BBA) of 1997, which called for significant savings by restraining payments to providers. The slight increase in spending in 2000 resulted from the Balanced Budget Refinement Act (BBRA) of 1999. Faced with the criticism that the BBA of 1997 reduced spending too much and too quickly, Congress passed the BBRA of 1999, which limited or delayed some of new payment provisions (MedPAC, 2000). More recently, nursing home expenditures have continued to increase at a relatively modest pace while home health care expenditures have increased at a much higher rate. In 2003, nursing home expenditures equaled $110.8 billion while home health expenditures reached the $40 billion mark.

Taken together, these figures indicate that the economic cost of long-term care is substantial, with informal caregivers paying for the bulk of the care measured in terms of forgone wages. Using 2000 as a benchmark, it appears that two-thirds of all long-term care provided in the United States is on an informal basis.[5] Extending the analysis one step further, expenditures for long-term care (both informal and formal) account for about 30 percent of all health care

5. This figure was arrived at by dividing the total dollar amount of formal and informal care provided in 2000 into the cost of informal care as estimated by Arno (2002), or [$257 billion/($257 billion + $126.9 billion)] = 67 percent. The amount of formal long-term care provided was assumed to equal the combined value of nursing home expenditures ($95.3 billion) and home health care expenditures ($31.6 billion).

expenditures in the United States and represent the second-largest spending category behind hospital care. While these percentages can only be considered "ballpark" at best, they do underscore the importance of long-term care and illustrate that informal caregivers are the mainstay of the U.S. long-term care health system.

Private Insurance for Long-Term Care

Given the high cost of long-term care, researchers have long wondered why so few individuals, particularly those at or approaching retirement age, have not purchased long-term care insurance. According to the America's Health Insurance Plans, more than 9.1 million long-term care policies had been sold by the end of 2002. Although this is an impressive number, one has to keep in mind that at the same point in time there were 102 million people age 45 or older in the United States. Among the factors contributing to the relatively small number of long-term insurance policies purchased are adverse selection, moral hazard, Medicaid crowding out, and intertemporal risk (Norton, 2000; Cutler, 1996).

Adverse selection occurs because there is an asymmetry of information concerning the health status of potential consumers. When this situation develops, high-risk individuals have the incentive to withhold information concerning their true health status from insurers and purchase long-term care insurance at premiums based on a pool of subscribers with better health. Over time premiums are driven upward as the high-risk subscribers consume more custodial care than their healthier counterparts. Faced with the choice of paying high premiums, low-risk subscribers may elect not to renew their long-term care policies while potential new customers' may decide to self-insure and not purchase any long-term care insurance. The problem of adverse selection is particularly difficult in the market for long-term care because the potential population is heterogeneous and a relative lack of claims data makes it difficult for insurance companies to accurately assess risk.

For example, Temkin-Greener et al. (2000/2001) estimate that at least one out of seven individuals age 65 or older who have been rejected for long-term care insurance because of poor health pose no greater financial risk to the insurer than those who have been accepted. Adverse selection also appears to be impacting the demand side of the long-term care market. For example, Sloan and Norton (1997) find that individuals who reported a high probability that they would need nursing home services in five years were more likely to purchase long-term care insurance, while Mellor (2001) finds self-reported poor health to have a significant, yet marginal, impact on the probability of having long-term care insurance.

Moral hazard has also been offered as an explanation for the lack of demand for private long-term care insurance. In a now classic article, Pauly (1990) argues that the elderly prefer to receive care from family in their own homes rather than from a staff of health care professionals in a nursing home, all else held constant. As a result, the elderly may shy away from purchasing private health insurance because it lowers the out-of-pocket price of formal care and provides their children with an inducement to institutionalize them if and when they need long-term care, or perhaps even prematurely. The incentive to substitute child-provided informal care with formal care results from the relative decrease in the price of formal care that occurs when long-term care insurance is present.

While the preference for informal care on the part of the elderly may decrease the demand for long-term care insurance, the desire to protect bequests to family and friends may have just the opposite effect. Long-term care can be quite expensive and even a relatively short stay in a nursing home can wipe out a family's savings. To guard against the potential loss of a desired bequest, a risk-averse individual may purchase long-term health insurance. Thus, the desire to leave a specific bequest in a world where long-term care costs are difficult to project should increase the demand for long-term care insurance.

There is little empirical evidence supporting the notion that the elderly substitute child-provided care for long-term care insurance. For example, Mellor (2001) finds that the availability of informal caregivers had no statistical impact on whether an elderly person purchased a long-term care insurance policy or intended to purchase one. Sloan and Norton (1997) find that the existence of children had no impact on the likelihood of purchasing long-term health insurance. In addition, Sloan and Norton also find that the bequest motive had no impact on the decision to purchase long-term care insurance. Specifically, elderly people who responded that leaving an inheritance was somewhat or very important are no more likely to purchase long-term care insurance than the rest of the sample.

Public support for long-term care through the Medicaid program may also dampen the incentive to purchase private long-term care insurance. Faced with the reduced risk of having to privately pay for long-term care because of the Medicaid program, some consumers may elect to forgo the purchase of long-term care insurance. The basic question from an economic perspective is, therefore, whether private long-term care insurance and Medicaid can be considered substitutes. Sloan and Norton (1997) are careful to point out that private insurance and Medicaid can be considered only imperfect substitutes at best. Strict eligibility requirements necessitate that individuals deplete most of their financial assets before becoming eligible for Medicaid coverage. As a result, the Medicaid program offers little opportunity to protect assets that may be consumed in the future or bequeathed to loved ones. Coupled with this, elderly individuals on Medicaid coverage have to contend with the stigma of "going on public assistance."

The empirical evidence appears to support the notion that the demand for long-term care insurance is experiencing at least some degree of crowding out from the Medicaid program. Sloan and Norton (1997) find Medicaid crowding out for individuals over age 70 but not for those between ages 51 and 64. However, the marginal effects appear rather small, suggesting that we need to look elsewhere for an explanation as to why few people purchase long-term care insurance.

Cutler (1996) points out that the market for long-term care insurance is limited by the intertemporal risk that comes into play when insurers establish premiums. Recall from the earlier discussion on insurance in Chapter 11 that the insurer is responsible for managing the financial risk associated with establishing premiums. Relying on the law of large numbers, the insurer estimates the expected medical costs for a given population over a specified period of time. With that information in hand, the insurer sets the insurance premium to equal the expected benefits to be paid out plus any marketing and administration costs, taxes, and profits. Overall risk, which is reflected in profits in terms of the classic risk-return trade-off, is minimized through diversification across a given population of potential policyholders.

With long-term care insurance, insurers are forced to assess risk over an extended period of time when the average cost of an insured event is likely to increase over time.[6] With this increase in cost over time comes increasing price risk because the insurer finds it progressively more difficult to predict medical payments well into the future. The problem is that in this situation the insurer cannot diversify risk across policyholders because everyone faces the same potential increase in costs due to higher input prices. Faced with the inability to lower risk through cross-sectional diversification, the insurer has no alternative but to increase premiums in excess of the

6. Take the case of an individual who purchases a long-term health care policy at age 55. It may be 25 years or more before benefits are paid out for the first time.

expected payout or offer an indemnity-type insurance policy. In the first case, the insurer increases the premium to compensate for the added risk of predicting health care costs well into the future by requiring a higher rate of profit. In the second case, the insurer forces policyholders to bear some of the risk of higher long-term care costs. For example, the policy may call for the insurer to pay up to $200 a day if the policyholder enters a nursing home. If the cost of nursing home care is in excess of that amount, then the policyholder must pay the added expense out-of-pocket. To illustrate his point, Cutler notes that for a sample of 73 long-term health care policies in 1991, 72 had indemnity payments. In either case, the demand for long-term care insurance is likely to decrease because of intertemporal risk.

The theoretical and empirical research in this area clearly indicates that the decision to purchase long-term insurance is complex and involves a host of factors. Other variables found to impact the probability of purchasing a long-term health insurance policy include assets, income, age, and education. The positive and significant results for the assets and income variables make sense and suggest that those with greater wealth and income are more likely to purchase insurance because they have a greater incentive to protect against the possibility of spending down to qualify for Medicaid coverage. The positive and significant results for the age variable indicates that as people get older and the possibility of needing long-term care increases, so does the likelihood of purchasing insurance coverage. Finally, more highly educated people are found to be more likely to purchase insurance coverage (Mellor, 2001).

Prices for Nursing Home Services

Unfortunately, a lack of data prevents a detailed examination of the pricing behavior of nursing home and home health care facilities over time. What little information there is can be obtained from the National Nursing Home Survey that is periodically administered by the National Center for Health Statistics. These data appear in Table 15–4. According to the survey results, the

TABLE 15–4
Average Monthly Charge for Nursing Home Care, Selected Years 1963–1999

	1963	1973/1974	1977	1985	1995	1997	1999
All Facilities	$186	$479	$ 689	$1,456	$3,135	$3,609	$3,891
Annual Rate of Increase*		9.9%	9.5%	9.8%	8.0%	7.3%	3.8%
Funding Source							
Own Income			$ 690	$1,450	$3,081	$3,643	$3,947
Medicare			$1,167	$2,141	$5,546	$6,037	$5,764
Medicaid			$ 720	$1,504	$2,769	$3,081	$3,505

*This is the average annual rate of increase from the previous period. For 1973/1974 the based year is assumed to be 1973.

SOURCE: Various Issues of *Health, United States*, published by the National Center for Health Statistics Health Care Financing Administration. http://www.cms.gov.

average monthly charge for all nursing home facilities was $186 in 1963. By 1985 the monthly charge increased almost eightfold to $1,456, and by the middle of the 1990s it topped $3,000. The most recent figures indicate that the average monthly charge for nursing home care equaled $3,891 in 1999, or $46,692 per year.

The annualized rates of increase, also provided in the table, indicate that price increases for nursing home services were sustained throughout the entire period, hovering at between 9 and 10 percent much of the time. It was not until many of the cost constraints implemented in the mid-1990s began to take hold that the rate of increase began to cool down. By 1999, the average rate of increase fell to a modest 3.8 percent that year.

The information on monthly charges by funding sources in Table 15–4 is interesting and merits a brief discussion. During the 1970s and into the 1980s the average rate of reimbursement for Medicaid patients was higher than that of private-pay patients. It was not until somewhere around 1990 that the situation reversed itself and the average monthly charge for private-pay patients exceeded the average charge for Medicaid patients. While these are only average figures and do not consider a number of factors such as the level and quality of care provided, they do appear to confirm the basic premise of the dual market model that private-pay patients pay a higher price than Medicaid patients for the same nursing home services. The high rate of reimbursement for Medicare patients in all likelihood can be attributed to the level of care received by those patients. For Medicare to cover skilled nursing home care, the patient needs to have a qualifying hospital inpatient stay of three consecutive days or more within 30 days of leaving the hospital. The general intent is to cover the cost of rehabilitation for a short period after hospitalization and such care is likely to be more expensive than custodial care, which is provided on a more long-term basis.

Other points of interest generated by the National Nursing Home Survey (2002) are that for-profit nursing homes appear to charge less than their not-for-profit and public counterparts and that the monthly charge for all facilities appears to be positively correlated with the size of the larger nursing home. For example, in 1999 for-profit nursing homes charged an average of $3,698 per month while not-for-profit and public nursing home charged an average of $4,225. At the same time, facilities with less than 50 beds charged $3,808 per month while nursing homes with 200 or more beds charged an average of $4,281. Unfortunately, these figures are difficult to interpret without additional information about the intensity of care provided.

The Utilization of Long-Term Care Facilities

Nursing Homes. Tables 15–5 and 15–6 supply information about the users of nursing home care based on a national survey of nursing homes conducted in 1997 and again in 1999 by the National Center for Health Statistics. Included in Table 15–5 is an age profile of nursing home residents in 1999. In general, the data confirm our earlier point that the need for long-term care is heavily concentrated among the elderly population. According to the table more than 9 out of 10 nursing home residents were 65 years old or older, and almost 430 out of every 10,000 elderly people resided in a nursing home in 1999. To no one's surprise, data in the table also indicate that the need for nursing home care increases rapidly with age among the elderly population. Almost half of all nursing home residents were 85 years old or older and more than one of six elderly above age 84 resided in a nursing home in 1999.

Table 15–6 provides additional information about the representative nursing home resident in 1999. Approximately three-quarters of all nursing home residents were female. This finding is not surprising given that females tend to outlive their male counterparts and are more likely to require assistance in older age either in nursing homes or in private residences. In addition, about

TABLE 15–5
Distribution of Nursing Home Residents According to Age, 1999

Age Group	Percent of Nursing Home Population
Under 65 Years	9.8%
65 Years and Older	90.3%
65–74 Years	12.0%
75–84 Years	31.8%
85 Years and Older	46.5%
Age Group	**Nursing Home Residents per 10,000 Population**
All residents	59.1
Under 65 Years	6.6
65 Years and Older	429.2
65–74 Years	108.0
75–84 Years	429.7
85 Years and Older	1,825.0

SOURCE: *National Nursing Home Survey: 1999 Summary* (June 2002).

TABLE 15–6
Percentage Distribution of Nursing Home Residents According to Gender, Functional Status, and Length of Stay, 1999

	Percent of Nursing Home Population
Gender	
Male	28.1%
Female	71.9%
Functional Status	
Received no help	5.0%
Received help with 1 ADL	6.7%
Received help with 2 or 3 ADLs	45.2%
Received help with more than 3 ADLs	43.1%
Length of Stay Since Admission	
Less than 3 months	17.8%
Between 3 and 12 months	25.0%
1 year to less than 3 years	30.1%
3 years or more	27.1%

SOURCE: *National Nursing Home Survey: 1999 Summary* (June 2002).

90 percent of all residents needed assistance with at least two ADLs. The information on the length of stay since admission is telling because it provides us with an understanding of the extent to which medical care is needed on a long-term basis. At the time when the survey was taken, only 17.8 percent of nursing home residents were at the facility for less than three months. More than half of the residents were in a facility in excess of one year, while more than one in four resided in a nursing home for more than three years. Overall, the average length of stay since admission was 892 days, or slightly more than two years and five months. This is in sharp contrast to a 7.3-day average length of stay for inpatient hospital care in 1997.

While these utilization figures paint an interesting profile of the current users of nursing home services, they do not tell the whole story. Some interesting trends beginning to emerge are likely to have a profound impact on the market for long-term services (Bishop, 1999). First, the extent to which the elderly rely on nursing homes for long-term care is diminishing. According to the most recent figures, while the number of elderly nursing home residents increased from slightly more than 1.32 million in 1985 to 1.47 million in 1999, the proportion of elderly in nursing homes has diminished from 46.2 to 42.9 per 10,000 population over the same time period.[7] Second, the intensity of care provided to nursing home residents has increased because of an increase in disabilities among elderly residents. In 1985, 74.8 percent of elderly residents had dependent mobility while 40.5 percent had dependent eating. Those percentages grew to 80.4 and 47.4, respectively, in 1999. Bishop (1999) contends that these changes are the result of a decrease in disabilities among the elderly and an increased desire among the elderly to seek care in alternative settings such as home health care, adult day care facilities, or assisted living facilities. According to Cutler (2001), the steady decline in disability among the elderly can be attributed to enhanced medical technology and lifestyle changes. Other contributing factors may be improved socioeconomic status, diminished exposure to diseases, and the development and use of medical aids that allow the elderly to live independently for a longer period of time.

Thus, it appears that the nursing home industry has been simultaneously experiencing a significant decline in its patient population and an increase in the disability rate among those patients who require nursing home care. These trends may help explain some of the changes that have taken place in the nursing home industry over the past decades. For example, the increase in the level of care provided may in part explain the significant increase in the price of nursing home services that took place from the mid-1980s to the present. As noted earlier, the average monthly charge for nursing home care increased from $1,456 in 1985 to $3,891 in 1999. The decrease in the proportion of elderly in need of nursing home facilities may also help explain the recent decrease in the occupancy rate for nursing homes. From 1987 to 1999 the occupancy rate for nursing homes fell from 92.3 percent to 86.6 percent. Faced with a shrinking patient base coupled with increased competition from alternative long-term care providers, nursing homes have been forced to operate with some excess capacity.

Home Health Care and Hospice Care. A variety of demographic characteristics for home health care and hospice patients appear in Table 15–7. More than 1.3 million patients used some form of home health care in 2000, which is in sharp contrast to the 2.4 million who received home health care in 1996. This decrease reflects the cost containment and utilization controls mandated by the Balanced Budget Act of 1997 for home health care. Only a tiny fraction of that total, 105,496, utilized hospice care in 2000.

---

7. Bishop (1999) points out that some evidence suggests that the average length of stay has also decreased.

TABLE 15–7
Home Health Care and Hospice Patient Characteristics, 2000

	Home Health Care Providers	Hospice Patients
Number of Patients	1,355,290	105,496
	Percentage Distribution	
Gender		
Male	35.2%	42.6%
Female	64.8%	57.4%
Age Group		
Under 65	29.5%	18.6%
65 and older	70.5%	81.4%
65–74	17.3%	17.2%
75–84	31.3%	37.0%
85 and older	21.9%	27.3%

SOURCE: NCHS, *Health, United States, 2004*. Hyattsville, Md.: 2004, Tables 90 and 91.

In total this means that almost 3 million people used some type of formal long-term care from either a nursing home, a home health agency, or a hospice facility in the late 1990s. The data also indicate that females use formal long-term care more frequently than males, with the degree of gender imbalance being greatest for nursing home care. Finally, it appears that the elderly use formal care most intensively, with the heaviest users being between ages 75 and 84 for home and hospice care, and over age 84 for nursing home care.

What Do the Demographics Tell Us about the Future of Long-Term Care?

Predicting what the future holds in store for the long-term care market is, as you can imagine, a speculative task. However, longer life expectancies coupled with an aging baby boom generation should translate into a substantial increase in the demand for long-term care services.[8] At the turn of the new millennium, between 12 and 13 percent of the total population was age 65 or older and less than 2 percent was age 85 or older. By 2050 the number of elderly is projected to make up 20 percent of the total population, with 1 out of 20 citizens being over age 85. Keeping in mind that more than 90 percent of nursing home residents were over 65 years old in 1999, these projections indicate that the demand for long-term care is likely to dramatically increase over the next few decades.

These demographic changes notwithstanding, a number of factors may cause the demand for long-term care to increase at a rate lower than otherwise would be the case. For one thing, increased longevity does not appear to have a major impact on health expenditures. Lubitz et al.

8. For example, recent population projections estimate that the average life expectancies for males and females are expected to increase from 74.1 and 79.8 in 1999 to 81.2 and 86.7 in 2050, respectively (Hollmann et al., 2000).

(1995) estimate the lifetime Medicare expenses for a sample of beneficiaries and find total health expenditures to be only modestly impacted by longevity. Long-term expenditures are also likely to be impacted by overall health, everything else constant. It stands to reason that long-term care expenses will fall as the proportion of life spent in a relatively healthy state increases. Cutler explains earlier that disability among the elderly has decreased by approximately 1 percent per year since the 1950s. If this trend were to continue into the future, it would have a significant impact on the individual demand for long-term care (Cutler, 2001).

Picking up on this point, Lakdawalla and Philipson (2002) argue that improved health coupled with increased life expectancy will impact the mix of formal and informal care provided along with the total amount spent on formal long-term care. The reason is relatively straightforward: a healthy elderly individual may become an informal supplier of long-term care. What is most interesting, however, is that the authors argue that impact on the supply of informal care depends on the degree to which increases in longevity and health impact men relative to women. If the increase in health and longevity impacts men more than women, then the individual demand for long-term care may diminish, on average. If the opposite occurs, the individual demand for long-term care may increase.

Since women live longer than men on average, they generally spend more years alone and, therefore, have a greater need for formal care. Recall from Table 15–6 that women made up 72 percent of all nursing home residents in 1999. When the relative supply of healthy men increases, elderly couples stay married longer and husbands become informal suppliers of care. As a result, the demand for formal care among women should diminish. If, on the other, hand, the increase in health and longevity is concentrated among women, the demand for formal long-term care should increase because women will spend even more time alone and without a spouse to provide informal care. Lakdawalla and Philipson test their hypothesis using panel data for 1971 through 1991. Their results generally support the contention that healthy aging is inversely related to the per capita demand for formal long-term care. Healthy aging decreases the amount of formal care provided directly by "shrinking the base of people who need care, and indirectly, by raising the supply of healthy elderly who can provide care at home" (p. 305).

While improved health and longevity may dampen the individual demand for long-term care,[9] the sheer number of baby boomers reaching retirement age over the next few decades will ensure that the market demand for long-term care increases. One estimate has 76 million baby boomers born between 1946 and 1964 reaching retirement age by 2035 (GAO, 2002). With this anticipated increase in market demand comes a great many challenges concerning the availability of public and private funding and the relative mix of informal and formal care provided.

SUMMARY

Monopolistic competition best describes the market structure of the long-term care industry. A large availability of substitute providers exists in the industry and entry barriers are very low. The typical nursing home most likely faces a downward-sloping demand because people prefer

9. Of course, increased income, enhanced quality, and changes in tastes and preferences may have the opposite effect on the individual demand for long-term care. The increased prevalence of long-term care insurance will also increase demand because it decreases the out-of-pocket price of formal long-term care.

convenient locations near former neighbors, relatives, and friends. The buyer side of the market is relatively concentrated, with the federal and state governments representing highly influential buyers of both home health care and nursing home care.

Pricing and quality are two important conduct issues pertaining to long-term care. Empirical studies continue to sort the impact of reimbursement policies on the behavior of nursing homes. Recent studies indicate that there may no longer be an excess demand for nursing home services because of the elimination of CON laws and increased availability of alternative ways to acquire long-term care. Research also points out that reimbursement methods faced by nursing homes influence firm behavior because of financial incentives. It appears that more restrictive reimbursement schemes not only lower costs but also adversely impact the quality of care provided. Finally, the empirical evidence also corroborates the property rights theory as for-profit nursing homes appear to produce care at a lower cost than their not-for-profit counterparts but by providing lower quality of care when asymmetrical information exists.

Market competition also appears to impact both the price and quality of nursing home care. While more research needs to be done on the relationship between market competition and price in the nursing home industry before definitive conclusions can be drawn, economic theory suggests that ability of the firm to exercise control over price is dictated by market concentration. The empirical evidence does suggest, however, that greater market concentration is linked to improved quality of nursing home care.

The market for long-term care services has experienced profound changes over the last few decades and these changes are likely to continue into the near future. In the coming years, we are likely to see a significant increase in the demand for long-term care as baby boomers reach retirement age. While improved health and longevity may moderate the overall increase in the demand, the steep increase in the absolute number of retirees will place a significant strain on funding sources for long-term care.

On the supply side of the market, the delivery system for long-term care has become increasingly more diversified and has an almost endless list of community-based and institutional providers. For example, in recent years a host of community-based long-term care programs have been aimed at augmenting the level of informal care provided by assisting patients who have difficulty maintaining an independent lifestyle. Meals on wheels, home health care, and adult day care are but three examples of such programs. These community-based programs represent a low-cost alternative to skilled nursing home care because they either delay or avert altogether the decision to institutionalize an individual in need of long-term care. Institutional care is now provided in a number of alternative settings aside from skilled nursing homes. For example, assisted living residences and continuing care retirement communities have become very popular in recent years.

While this can be considered only a cursory look at the supply side of the long-term care market, it does indicate that individual providers of long-term care are likely to face increasing competition in the coming years. This increase in competition will likely have an impact on the mix of informal and formal care as well as the total expenditures on long-term care.

Case Studies

15-1 Long-Term Care Insurance in the United States[10]

Insurers have been increasing their efforts to sell long-term care policies, offering new products and working with employers to make the policies available in the workplace. One reason for the

10. Source: Jeff Opdyke, "Insurers Push Policies for Long-Term Care," *The Wall Street Journal*, December 27, 2005.

renewed interest in marketing long-term care policies is Congress's recent passage of new rules tightening Medicaid eligibility. Many seniors rely on Medicaid to pay for long-term care once they have spent down their assets. But the new rules have tightened the financial eligibility requirement, which means that more Americans will have to fund a greater share on their own. The result, insurers are hoping, is that more middle-class Americans will be cognizant of the need for long-term care coverage, and may also be willing to pay more for that coverage if they suspect that they will not meet the new eligibility criteria when they are in need. Some carriers, such as Genworth Financial, market long-term care policies to groups of workers through employers, much as group life insurance has typically been sold. The costs of long-term care are increasing nearly twice as fast as the consumer price index. The average cost for one year in a nursing home is nearly $70,000, while the average hourly rate for a home health aide tops $18 an hour, equivalent to more than $37,000 a year. Private health insurance and Medicare generally do not cover these expenses.

Questions for Discussion

1. *Describe some demographic changes in the United States that might make lawmakers tighten Medicaid eligibility and make Americans more likely to consider long-term care insurance.*
2. *Is long-term care insurance a good idea? What are the alternatives?*

15-2 Long-Term Care in Germany

The United States is not the only country wrestling with long-term care issues. In fact, U.S. citizens appear relatively young when compared to individuals residing in other OECD countries. Reinhardt et al. (2002) report that the percentage of people age 65 and older averaged 14.7 among OECD countries in 1999; the comparable statistic for the United States was only 12.3. Canada (12.4), Germany (16.7), and the United Kingdom (15.7), countries whose health care systems are typically compared to the U.S. system, all face a higher elderly population rate. While industrialized countries around the world face similar problems relating to long-term care, they have taken different paths toward meeting the needs of the elderly. Germany adopted universal social insurance for long-term care in 1994. The program provides extensive coverage for nursing home and home care for people of all ages without regard to their financial status. The social insurance is administered by the sickness funds and is financed by a uniform long-term care insurance premium fixed by law at 1.7 percent of salary. Employers and employees are responsible for paying an equal share. Retirees pay half of the premium and pension funds pay the other half. To control program expenditures, both revenues and benefits are capped to some degree, with revenues fixed by the predetermined contribution rate. Benefits are legislatively determined and therefore do not automatically adjust with inflation. Benefits are fixed by the disability level of individuals and the setting in which the long-term care takes place, as discussed shortly. People are eligible for long-term care benefits if they have a mental or physical condition requiring a need for assistance that is expected to last at least six months. Eligible people, at any level of disability, can choose institutional or home care. In 1998, 2.3 percent of the total population participated in the program, including 29.6 percent of the population age 80 and older. Long-term care in noninstitutional settings accounted for about half of all program expenditures. Roughly three-quarters of all beneficiaries received care in noninstitutional settings. Nursing home coverage includes basic care, medical care, and social activities, but not room and board or capital costs. Residents must pay any difference between actual costs and program benefits and are responsible for at least 25 percent of nursing home care costs. Individuals with the highest levels of disability may have the greatest disincentive to live in institutions because they pay a greater proportion of costs given that program costs do not rise as sharply as nursing home costs with respect to disability level. Social assistance, based on means-tested eligibility, is available for individuals unable to afford out-of-pocket costs for either home or institutional care.

Supply appeared adequate to meet need, at least within the first two years of the program. Both the number of home health care providers and nursing homes increased during the first two years. Waiting lists virtually disappeared. The new program, however, has not been very successful at fostering competition. Although communities may not prevent new providers from entering markets, sickness funds must contract with all providers, both not-for-profit and for-profit, that meet minimal standards rather than on the basis of price. Consumers can freely choose among the listed long-term care providers. While the plan is not flawless, experts agree that the long-term care program in Germany has made substantial progress toward achieving its goals.

Questions for Discussion

1. *Compare and contrast the strengths and weaknesses of the U.S. and German approaches to providing long-term care to seniors. Consider how each approach might address costs and access.*
2. *Should the U.S. government consider adopting the German approach to providing long-term care? Why or why not?*

Review Questions and Problems

1. Explain the various differences between the demand for long-term care and medical services.
2. List the different providers of long-term care.
3. Explain the profile of the typical informal long-term caregiver.
4. Identify the structural characteristics of the typical nursing home. Think in terms of ownership status, size, chain membership, entry barriers, and so on.
5. Who is the main purchaser of nursing home services?
6. Discuss the role that entry barriers play in the nursing home industry.
7. Explain why the number of home health care agencies increased so dramatically in recent years.
8. Who is the largest payer for home health care services?
9. What role do Medicare and Medicaid serve in the home health care industry?
10. What does the empirical evidence suggest about scale economies in the home health care industry?
11. Use the Scanlon model to identify the impact of an increase of the Medicaid reimbursement rate on the private price for nursing home care and the number of private-pay and Medicaid patients.
12. Use the Scanlon model to identify the impact of an increase of the Medicaid reimbursement rate on the private price for nursing home care and the number of private-pay and Medicaid patients given a completely vertical marginal cost curve.
13. Explain theoretically how the method of reimbursement influences costs, quality, and patient case-mix. Note the trade-offs typically involved.
14. Explain why returns to scale are so important when it comes to quality improvements.
15. Discuss theoretically how a nondistribution constraint may influence costs and quality differences among nursing homes with different ownership structures. What are the general

findings of studies examining the relation between ownership status and the costs and quality of nursing home care?

16. Explain why the relation between market concentration and the quality of care is theoretically unclear.
17. Identify and explain the intuition behind the Lerner index of monopoly power.
18. Suppose the price elasticity of market demand for nursing home care equals −3 and the individual nursing home's price elasticity of demand equals −6. The Medicaid reimbursement rate facing the nursing home equals $100 per day. Also suppose that because of a few nursing homes in the market and high barriers, the nursing home expects that other nursing homes will match its behavior with perfect certainty. Calculate the price charged to private payers by the individual nursing home. How would the results change if the individual nursing home expected offsetting behavior with perfect certainty? How about with a 50 percent probability of offsetting behavior?
19. Discuss the factors that researchers must consider when estimating the cost of informal care.
20. Approximately what fraction of long-term care expenditures is informal care?
21. Identify and explain the reasons why so few people purchase long-term care insurance.
22. Provide a profile of the typical nursing home resident. How is this profile likely to change in the future and why?
23. Discuss the demographic changes taking place that are likely to impact the future of long-term care.
24. Consult the Nursing Home Compare web site developed by Medicare at http://www.medicare.gov/NHCompare. Choose two different nursing home markets in the same state as defined by two distinct zip code areas that have both for-profit and not-for-profit nursing homes and compute the four-firm concentration ratio, CR_4, and Herfindahl-Hirschman Index, HHI, for each market based on the number of licensed beds for a market area of 10 miles. What percentage of the nursing homes is for-profit? What do the figures tell you about the degree of market concentration in each market? What do the figures tell you about any potential price differences that may exist across the two markets? Now recalculate the CR_4 and HHI for a market area of 25 miles. Have the figures changed? Why?

Online Resources

To access Internet links related to the topics in this chapter, please visit our web site at **www.thomsonedu.com/economics/santerre**.

References

AARP. *AARP Caregiver Identification Study*. Washington D.C.: AARP, February 2001.

Arno, Peter S., "Economic Value of Informal Caregiving: 2000." Presented at the American Association for Geriatric Psychiatry, Orlando, Florida, February 24, 2002.

Arno, Peter S., Carol Levine, and Margaret M. Memmott. "The Economic Value of Informal Caregiving." *Health Affairs* 18 (March/April 1999), pp. 182–88.

Bishop, Christine. "Where Are the Missing Elders? The Decline in Nursing Home Use, 1985 and 1995." *Health Affairs* 18 (July/August 1999), pp. 146–55.

Chattopadhyay, Sajal, and Dennis Heffley. "Are For-Profit Nursing Homes More Efficient? Data Envelope Analysis with a Case-Mix Constraint." *Eastern Economic Journal* 20 (Spring 1994), pp. 171–86.

Chen, Li-Wu, and Dennis G. Shea. "Does Prospective Payment Really Contain Nursing Home

Costs?" *Health Services Research* 37 (April 2002), pp. 251–71.

______. "The Economies of Scale for Nursing Home Care." *Medical Care Research and Review* 61 (March 2004), pp. 38–63.

Chou, Shin-Yi. "Asymmetric Information, Ownership and Quality of Care: An Empirical Analysis of Nursing Homes." *Journal of Health Economics* 21 (2002), pp. 293–311.

Christensen, Eric W. "Scale and Scope Economies in Nursing Homes: A Quantile Regression Approach." *Health Economics* 13 (April 2004), pp. 363–77.

Coburn, Andrew F., Richard Fortinsky, Catherine McGuire, and Thomas P. McDonald. "Effect of Prospective Reimbursement on Nursing Home Costs." *Health Services Research* 28 (April 1993), pp. 45–68.

Cohen, Joel W., and L. C. Dubay. "The Effect of Medicaid Reimbursement Method and Ownership on Nursing Home Costs, Case Mix, and Staffing." *Inquiry* 27 (1990), pp. 183–200.

Cohen, Joel W., and William D. Spector. "The Effect of Medicaid Reimbursement on Quality of Care in Nursing Homes." *Journal of Health Economics* 15 (1996), pp. 23–48.

Cutler, David M. "Declining Disability among the Elderly." *Health Affairs* 20 (November/December 2001), pp. 11–27.

______. "Why Don't Markets Insure Long-Term Risk?" Working paper, *National Bureau of Economic Research* 1996.

Fizel, J., and T. Nunnikhoven. "Technical Efficiency of For-Profit and Non-Profit Nursing Homes." *Managerial and Decision Economics* (September/October 1992), pp. 429–39.

Frech, H. E., and Paul B. Ginsburg. "The Cost of Nursing Home Care in the United States: Government, Financing, Ownership, and Efficiency." In *Health, Economics, and Health Economics*, eds. J. van der Gang and M. Perlman. Amsterdam: North-Holland, 1981.

General Accounting Office. *Long-Term Care, Current Issues and Future Directions*. GAO/HEHS-95-109. Washington, D.C.: GAO, April 1995.

______. *Long-Term Care—Baby Boom Generation Presents Financing Challenges*. (Testimony 3/9/98.) Washington, D.C.: GAO, April 1998.

______. *Long-Term Care Aging Baby Boom Generation Will Increase Demand and Burden on Federal and State Budgets*. Washington, D.C.: GAO, March 2002.

Gertler, Paul J. "Subsidies, Quality, and Regulation in Nursing Homes." *Journal of Public Economics* 39 (1989), pp. 33–53.

Gertler, Paul J., and Donald M. Waldman. "Quality-Adjusted Cost Functions and Policy Evaluation in the Nursing Home Industry." *Journal of Political Economy* 100 (1992), pp. 1232–56.

Gonzales, Theresa I. "An Empirical Study of Economies of Scope in Home Healthcare." *Health Services Review* 32 (August 1997), pp. 313–24.

Grabowski, David C. "Medicaid Reimbursement and the Quality of Nursing Home Care." *Journal of Health Economics* 20 (2001), pp. 549–69.

Grabowski, David C., and Richard A. Hirth. "Competitive Spillovers across Nonprofit and For-Profit Nursing Homes." *Journal of Health Economics* 22 (January 2003), pp. 1–22.

Grabowski, David C., Robert L. Ohsfeldt, and Michael A. Morrisey. "The Effects of CON Repeal on Medicaid Nursing Home and Long-Term Care Expenditures." *Inquiry* 40 (summer 2003), pp. 146–57.

Gulley, O. David, and Rexford E. Santerre. "The Effect of Public Policies on the Availability of Nursing Home Care in the United States." *Eastern Economics Journal* 29 (winter 2003), pp. 93–104.

Hansmann, Henry. *The Ownership of Enterprise.* Cambridge, Mass.: Harvard University Press, 1996.

Harrington, Charlene, James H. Swan., John A. Nyman, and Helen Carrillo. "The Effect of Certificate of Need and Moratoria Policy on Change in Nursing Home Beds in the United States." *Medical Care* 35 (1997), pp. 574–88.

Harrington, Charlene, Steffie Woolhandler, Joseph Mullan, Helen Carrillo, and David U. Himmelstein. "Does Investor Ownership of Nursing Homes Compromise the Quality of Care?" *American Journal of Public Health* 91 (September 2001), pp. 1452–55.

Haupt, Barbara J. "An Overview of Home Health and Hospice Care Patients: 1996 National Home and Hospice Care Survey." U.S. Department of Health and Human Services, National Center for Health Statistics, Advance Data No. 297, April 16, 1998.

Hillmer, Michael P., Walter P. Wodchis, Sudeep S. Gill, Geoffrey M. Anderson, and Paula A. Rochon. "Nursing Home Profit Status and Quality of Care: Is There Any Evidence of an Association?" *Medical Care Research and Review* 62 (April 2005), pp. 139–66.

Ho, Alice, Sara R. Collins, Karen Davis, and Michelle M. Doty. "A Look at Working-Age Caregivers' Roles, Health Concerns, and Need for Support." Issue Brief. *The Commonwealth Fund*, publication no. 854 (August 2005), http://www.cmwf.org.

Holahan, John F., and Joel W. Cohen. "Nursing Home Reimbursement: Implications for Cost Containment, Access, and Quality." *Millbank Quarterly* 65 (1987), pp. 112–47.

Hollmann, Frederick, Tammany J. Mulder, and Jeffrey E. Kallan. *Methodology and Assumptions for the Population Projections of the United States: 1999 to 2000*. Washington, D.C.: U.S. Census Bureau, January 13, 2000.

Kass, D. J. "Economies of Scale and Scope in the Provision of Home Health Services." *Journal of Health Economics* 6 (June 1987), pp. 129–46.

Lakdawalla, Darius, and Tomas Philipson. "The Rise of Old-Age Longevity and the Market for Long-Term Care." *American Economic Review* 92 (March 2002), pp. 295–306.

Lerner, Abba P. "The Concept of Monopoly and the Measurement of Monopoly Power." *Review of Economic Studies* 1 (1934), pp. 157–75.

Levit, Katherine, et al. "Inflation Spurs Health Spending in 2000." *Health Affairs* 21 (January/February 2002), pp. 172–81.

Lubitz, James, James Beebe, and Colin Baker. "Longevity and Medicare Expenditures." *The New England Journal of Medicine* 332 (April 13, 1995), pp. 999–1003.

Medicare Payment Advisory Commision, (MedPAC). *Report to the Congress; Selected Medicare Issues*. Washington, D.C., June 1999.

———. *Report to the Congress; Medicare. Payment Policy*, Washington, D.C., March 2000.

———. *Medicare Payment Policy Report to Congress*. Washington D.C., March 2005.

Mellor, Jennifer C. "Long-Term Care and Nursing Home Coverage: Are Adult Children Substitutes for Insurance Policies?" *Journal of Health Economics* 20 (2001), pp. 527–47.

Metropolitan Life Insurance Company. *The MetLife Study of Employer Costs for Working Caregivers*. June 1997.

Mukamel, Dana B., and William D. Spector. "The Competitive Nature of the Nursing Home Industry: Price Mark Ups and Demand Elasticities." *Applied Economics* 34 (2002), pp. 413–20.

National Alliance for Caregiving and AARP. "Family Caregiving in the U.S. Findings from a National Survey," Bethesda, Md., June 1997.

———. *Caregiving in the U.S.* Bethesda, Md., April 2004.

National Center for Health Statistics. *Health, United States, 2004*. Hyattsville, Md.: NCHS, 2004.

National Home and Hospice Survey: 1996 Summary. Series 13, Number 141. U.S. Department of Health and Human Services. Washington D.C., October 1999.

National Nursing Home Survey, 1999 Summary. Series 13, Number 152. U.S. Department of Health and Human Services. Washington D.C., June 2002.

Norton, Edward C. "Long-Term Care." In *Handbook of Health Economics*, Volume 1, eds. A. J. Culyer and J. P. Newhouse. Amsterdam: Elsevier Science, 2000.

Nyman, John A. "Medicaid Reimbursement, Excess Medicaid Demand, and the Quality of Nursing Home Care." *Journal of Health Economics* 4 (1985), pp. 237–59.

———. "Testing for Excess Demand in Nursing Home Care Markets." *Medical Care* 31 (1993), pp. 680–93.

———. "The Effects of Market Concentration and Excess Demand on the Price of Nursing Home Care." *Journal of Industrial Economics* 17 (June 1994), pp. 193–204.

Nyman, John A., and Dennis L. Bricker. "Profit Incentives and Technical Efficiency in the Production of Nursing Home Care." *Review of Economics and Statistics* 71 (November 1989), pp. 586–94.

Nyman, John A., Dennis L. Bricker, and D. Link. "Technical Efficiency in Nursing Homes." *Medical Care* 28 (June 1990), pp. 541–51.

Nyman, John A., and Robert A. Connor. "Do Case-Mix Adjusted Nursing Home Reimbursements Actually

Reflect Costs? Minnesota's Experience." *Journal of Health Economics* 13 (1994), pp. 145–62.

Pauly, Mark. "The Rational Nonpurchase of Long-Term-Care Insurance." *Journal of Political Economy* 98 (1990), pp. 153–68.

Pauly, Mark, and M. Satterthwaite. "The Pricing of Primary Care Physician Services: A Test of the Role of Consumer Information." *Bell Journal of Economics* 12 (1981), pp. 488–506.

Reschovsky, James D. "The Roles of Medicaid and Economic Factors in the Demand for Nursing Home Care." *Health Services Research* 33 (October 1998), pp. 787–813.

Rosko, Michael D., and Robert W. Broyles. *The Economics of Health Care: A Reference Handbook*. New York: Greenwood Press, 1988.

Scanlon, William J. "A Theory of the Nursing Home Market." *Inquiry* 17 (spring 1980), pp. 25–41.

Sloan, Frank A., and Edward C. Norton. "Adverse Selection, Bequests, Crowding Out, and Private Demand for Insurance, Evidence from the Long-Term Care Insurance Market." *Journal of Risk and Uncertainty* 15 (1997), pp. 201–9.

Temkin-Greener, Helena, Dana B. Mukamel, and Mark R. Meimers. "Long-Term Care Insurance Underwriting: Understanding Eventual Claims Experience." *Inquiry* 37 (winter 2000/2001), pp. 348–58.

Wagner, Donna A. *Comparative Analysis of Caregiver Data for Caregivers to the Elderly 1987 and 1997*. Bethesda, Md.: National Alliance for Caregiving, June 1997.

White-Means, Shelly, and Deborah Chollet. "Opportunity Wages and Workforce Adjustments: Understanding the Cost of In-Home Elder Care." *Journal of Gerontology Social Sciences* 51B (1996), pp. S82–S90.

Zinn, Jacqueline S. "Market Competition and the Quality of Nursing Home Care." *Journal of Health Care Politics, Policy and Law* 19 (fall 1994), pp. 555–82.

PART 4

HEALTH CARE REFORM

CHAPTER 16

HEALTH CARE REFORM

Hospital Fees Hit the Middle Class Hard: Present System Favors the Rich and the Poor—Medical Men Suggest Ways to Lower the Cost of Illness
—*The New York Times*

Many people today are dissatisfied with the performance of the U.S. health care system. The cost of health care in the United States is alleged to be higher and rising faster than in any other country. Many worry that the health care monster will continue to devour an increasingly large slice of the economic pie. Moreover, at any one point in time, critics note that one out of every six non-elderly citizens lacks insurance coverage for acute care. Many others in the United States are seriously underinsured or lack proper long-term care insurance coverage.

The title of the newspaper article above captures the U.S. health care system's failure to provide universal coverage and contain health care costs. One indeed might argue (perhaps wrongly) that poor people either receive free care at public institutions or are provided with medical and long-term care coverage through the Medicaid program, while rich individuals can afford to self-insure. Middle-income individuals, then, are hit hardest by hospital fees because they face the prospects of rising copayments, reduced wage income, benefit denial, job lock, or other problems pertaining to private health insurance coverage.

The fascinating thing about the newspaper article cited above is that it originally appeared in The New York Times *more than 80 years ago, proving that the more things change, the more they remain the same.*[1] *Private health insurance was just barely in its embryonic stage in 1924 when the article was first published. Without health insurance, a large fraction of a middle-class family's income was subject to the vagaries of health status. In fact, at a well-known hospital, the cost of maintaining one patient for one day rose from \$2.65 in 1919 to \$4.71 in 1929, an average annual increase of nearly 9 percent.*[2] *The quest for financial security in the 1920s most likely resulted in the eventual birth and growth of private health insurance in the United States. Interestingly enough, William Chenery, the journalist who wrote the* New York Times *article, suggested that the United States copy the private health insurance system with which Cuba was experimenting with at the time rather than the British or German social health insurance systems. The U.S. private health insurance industry, in fact, began to emerge about five years later, in 1929, as discussed at the beginning of Chapter 11.*

1. See Chenery (1924). Incidentally, the next article on the same page was titled "When Russian Empire Tottered—An Inside Picture." Go figure!

2. Caldwell (1930), as cited by Stevens (1987). According to Stevens, the 1920s represented the flowering of consumerism in the hospital services industry. Stevens notes that "there was a running joke in the late 1920s that there were two classes of people in hospitals, those who entered poor and those who left poor" (p. 134). Apparently, the joke is still running!

Today the health care crisis has taken on a different shape. Only a small percentage of the population is currently uninsured compared to the 1920s. However, everyone is affected by the rising cost of health care services, not just the middle-income class. A rising share of compensation going toward health insurance premiums affects employers and employees alike. The poor and elderly populations, as well as the state and federal governments, are affected by Medicaid and Medicare budgets that are being squeezed due to escalating medical costs. Health care analysts and policy makers are searching for ways to improve the American health care system.

Not surprisingly, various groups have advanced a large number of health care reform plans. The plans differ in a number of respects, especially concerning the role the individual, employer, and government play in the financing of medical insurance and the functions the government and marketplace serve in the allocation of health care resources. To help us better understand what health care reform is all about, this chapter

- summarizes the performance of the U.S. health care system and conducts an international comparison
- examines why there is so much disagreement concerning the design of health care reform
- examines the various proposals for health care reform at the national level
- analyzes the experiences of selected states at implementing health care reform
- briefly reviews President Clinton's National Health Security Act of 1993

The Performance of the U.S. Health Care System: A Summary and an International Comparison

Thus far, the structure, conduct, and performance of the U.S. health care system has been examined in piecemeal fashion. Chapter 11 analyzed the private health insurance industry, and Chapters 12 through 15 discussed the individual markets for physician services, hospital services, pharmaceutical products, and long-term care. In this section, we summarize what is known about the structure, conduct, and performance of each individual medical care market. After the summary of the individual markets, the aggregate performance of the entire health care economy is assessed and compared to the performance of a select group of health care systems around the world.

Summarizing the Structure, Conduct, and Performance of the Various Medical Care Markets

Private Health Insurance Industry. The structure of the private health insurance industry appears to be reasonably competitive. Although highly concentrated in most geographical markets, a large competitive fringe exists in the industry and large employers have the alternative of self-insurance. These two structural features of the industry help to constrain the conduct of the dominant insurers. Nevertheless, antitrust officials might want to keep a watchful eye on future organizational developments in this market. Barriers to entry appear low so potential competition must be considered by the existing firms, and products appear to be reasonably homogeneous. Consumer information in the group buyer market is relatively complete; however, some information imperfections exist in the market for individual insurance.

As economic theory suggests, the conduct of the insurance industry reflects its competitive structure. That is, firms in the industry have followed undesirable practices because of the intense competition. Benefit denial, cherry picking, and high premiums charged to the medically indigent are among some of the undesirable practices observed. On the performance side, a large percentage of people remain uninsured in the United States, even after allowing for Medicaid and Medicare coverage. A family without health insurance coverage faces substantial financial insecurity.

Physician Services Industry. Because convenience is valued by consumers (and thus the individual demand curves are downward sloping) and given the vast number of sellers in the market, the physician services industry can be considered monopolistically competitive with relatively low barriers to entry. Medical licensure represents the primary barrier to entry into the physician market. The question, from a societal point of view, is whether the benefits of quality improvements resulting from medical licensing outweigh the higher prices from entry restrictions. With the development of large, institutional suppliers of physician services, the necessity of medical licensing may diminish in the future as enterprise liability plays a greater role. The limited nature of the entry barrier has meant that the number of physicians per capita has grown substantially over time. One important structural issue is whether there are too many specialists and not enough primary care givers in the United States. It should not be forgotten that any ability of physicians to raise prices has been seriously compromised, both by MCOs and by the government, which have increasingly used their bargaining powers to extract price concessions from physicians.

The prevalence of an asymmetry of information between patients and physicians has influenced conduct in the physician services market. Health economists continue to analyze whether physicians play on the asymmetry of information, especially in competitive markets, by unnecessarily increasing the quantity supplied of their services. This type of behavior was developed and analyzed within the context of the supplier-induced-demand model and the McGuire quantity-setting model.

Practice variations have also been observed across geographic regions of the United States (and in other countries as well). Policy analysts continue to sort out the reasons behind practice variations. Medical malpractice reform continues to be a concern for many individuals. At issue is whether the rise in liability premiums is the result of fundamental flaws in the overall system, structural changes, or the insurance profitability cycle. Tort reform in the form of damage caps appeal to have the desired effect on liability premiums. In terms of performance, the growth in physician prices and expenditures continues to outpace the growth in the general price level and the overall economy, although the differential has moderated in recent years. However, in real terms, physician income growth has stalled in recent years, and the rate of return of physician education is reasonably close to the rates of return observed on comparable types of educational investments.

Hospital Services Industry. Because economies of scale are exhausted at about the two hundred-bed level, most areas in the United States cannot support more than two or three hospitals. Moreover, people are reluctant to travel far for hospital services, so most markets tend to be local. Certificate-of-need laws, the huge sunk costs of building a hospital, and learning curve effects cause substantial barriers to entry into the hospital services industry. While most hospitals tend to offer standardized products, some large teaching hospitals are often perceived as offering better quality. Given that the out-of-pocket price for hospital services is around 3 cents on the dollar, most patients/consumers tend to be relatively uninformed about price and have little incentive to comparison shop for hospital services. Countervailing these monopoly-like characteristics is the fact that institutional buyers, such as MCOs and the government, have taken on a greater buyer role in the hospital services industry. All these considerations suggest that the hospital services industry can best be described structurally as a mild or loose (standardized) oligopoly.

Conduct issues pertaining to the hospital services industry include the effects of ownership and competition on pricing and the charitable function of hospitals. Earlier studies, prior to the 1980s, found that increased competition caused hospitals, especially nonprofit hospitals, to increase quality by adopting new cost-enhancing technologies and thus raising prices. This type of behavior was referred to as the *medical arms race*. Newer studies based on more recent data have tended to find that greater competition has not led to higher hospital prices and, in some cases, has led to lower prices. Given the many complex factors affecting hospital pricing, more careful studies on the effects of competition in this industry are needed before we can comfortably conclude that competition leads to lower hospital prices and improved quality of care, however.

The effect of MCOs on the cost of hospital services and the growth of integrated delivery systems (IDSs) are two other important conduct issues concerning the hospital services industry. Studies conclude that MCOs tend to lower hospital costs by about 15 to 20 percent compared to otherwise identical fee-for-service insurance plans. Quality of care in MCOs and in fee-for-service insurance plans is very similar, although some evidence indicates that MCOs may provide poor individuals with inferior care. This is another important area in which additional research is required. IDSs, in which physicians, hospitals, and other medical organizations integrate their organizations either legally or by contract, have been evolving over time. These integrated systems have been developing in large part to counteract the powerful institutional buyer side (such as MCOs and the government) in the hospital services market. IDSs may offer cost savings and quality-of-care improvements, but studies have not consistently provided evidence for these benefits.

As far as performance is concerned, hospital expenditures make up a large percentage of GDP. While hospital care expenditures exploded from 1.8 percent of GDP in 1960 to 4.9 percent in 1992, the good news is that the rate has stabilized in recent years and was 4.7 percent in 2003. The hospital price inflation rate continues to outstrip the general price inflation rate, although recent years have witnessed a narrowing of the gap. Staffing ratios at hospitals continue to burgeon, most likely reflecting the more severe case-mix associated with inpatient services, as more people are directed toward outpatient services. Any dramatic attempts at further cost reductions for inpatient hospital services may be futile as a smaller percentage of critically ill patients account for an increasingly greater fraction of costs. Most likely, only rationing of care to the severely ill will further reduce the cost of hospital inpatient services in the future.

Pharmaceutical Industry. Substantial barriers to entry brought on by patents and promotion expenditures, differentiated products resulting from promotion expenditures, and a few dominant firms in the therapeutic markets are the key structural characteristics associated with the pharmaceutical industry. The demand side of the pharmaceutical market has become more concentrated over time due to institutional buyers, but their ability to affect the operation and performance of the industry is still somewhat limited. Recall that consumers' out-of-pocket expenditures currently stand at about 30 percent for drugs compared to 3 percent for hospital services. All these characteristics lead to the conclusion that the pharmaceutical industry can be roughly labeled as a tight, differentiated oligopoly.

Despite its oligopolistic nature, the pharmaceutical industry shows ample signs of price competition. During the patent period, branded drugs often compete against other branded drugs treating the same illness but based on different chemical compositions. After the legal patent period, branded drugs face considerable competition from generic drugs, and generic drugs compete among themselves, as well. Although the price competition is not perfect, it has tended to be much more rigorous since the passing of the Hatch-Waxman Act in 1984. The high promotion expenditures of pharmaceutical companies simultaneously play both an informative and a persuasive role. For example, studies suggest that the promotion expenditures of leading firms tend to preserve their market shares while the promotion expenditures of follower firms reduce the leaders' market shares. Research and development expenditures, the source of product competition among pharmaceutical companies, have been found to depend on cash flows. It appears from the literature that an assortment of firm sizes, some relatively large and some relatively small, are desirable for innovation purposes.

At first blush, the U.S. pharmaceutical industry appears to allocate resources inefficiently. Since the late 1970s, real drug prices have risen, although once again the gap between the drug price inflation rate and the general price inflation rate has narrowed in recent years. In addition, pharmaceutical profit rates are much greater than the manufacturing industry average even after allowing for the amortization of promotion and R&D expenditures. It is interesting to note that these high profits may be financing new drug discoveries because the innovation and commercial introduction of new drugs tend to be risky endeavors. Most pharmaceutical companies have a series of costly misses before a commercial hit. Rather than signal a misallocation of society's resources, the high profits may reflect the high risks and provide the source of financing for R&D ventures. New drug discoveries have increased tremendously in the United States since the late 1970s as a result.

Long-Term Care Industry. The long-term care industry is somewhat unusual because of the nature of the care provided and the wide range of organizational settings that offer long-term care. In terms of care, the emphasis is on enhancing the quality of life rather than curing a particular medical problem. Given that long-term medical needs vary widely, a whole range of services are provided in a multitude of organizational settings. For example, long-term care can be provided by a loved one on an informal basis, or on a more formal basis by a home health care agency, at an assisted living facility, or at a skilled nursing home. Overall, the market for long-term care can best be treated as a monopolistically competitive industry with rather modest barriers to entry. On the demand side, estimates indicate that between 12 and 14 million people are currently in need of some type of long-term care. The supply side of the market is composed of an amalgam of health care providers with the three most important being informal providers, nursing homes, and home health care agencies.

Pricing and quantity are two important issues in the market for long-term care. With regard to price, the empirical evidence indicates that the demand for nursing home care appears to be highly elastic with respect to price and that reimbursement policies impact the behavior of nursing homes. Lower reimbursement appears to result in decreased costs and diminished quality. In addition, the market for nursing home care may no longer be characterized by excess demand due to the removal of CON laws and the increased availability of alternative providers. Research also indicates that for-profit nursing homes are more technically efficient and produce at a lower cost than their not-for-profit counterparts, supporting the property rights theory. However, quality of care tends to be higher in not-for-profit settings.

Expenditures on long-term care are substantial and account for approximately one-quarter of all health care outlays when the economic cost of informal care is factored into the equation. Public funding sources play an important role in the market for long-term care, accounting for approximately 60 percent of all formal expenditures. The implication is that the government has considerable power to control prices and affect resource allocation in this industry. Private insurance, however, accounts for less than 8 percent of total formal long-term care expenditures and researchers are somewhat at a loss to explain why so few individuals purchase long-term care insurance. Moral hazard, adverse selection, and Medicaid crowding out are all factors that are likely to come into play.

Overall, the market for long-term care is changing rapidly with a number of demographic and institutional factors coming into play. Market competition is likely to intensify in the future as providers became more numerous and varied. As a result, the average skilled nursing home is likely to face a highly elastic demand curve for its services and, therefore, have only limited ability to raise price without losing a substantial number of patients. At the same time, the aggregate demand for long-term care is likely to increase as baby boomers reach retirement age in the coming years. However, improved health coupled with longevity may dampen the overall increase.

Overall Health Care Economy. The preceding discussion suggests that the prices and expenditures on various medical services continue to rise, albeit at a slower rate than in the past. The transition to a managed care health care system has helped promote some cost savings in various medical care markets but has also resulted in some rationing of care. Choice of physician, physician autonomy and income, hospital inpatient admissions, and selection among pharmaceutical products have all been greatly limited by the movement to a managed care health care system in the United States. The limitations pertain not only to private managed care insurance plans but also to managed care plans under the auspices of the Medicare and Medicaid programs. Whether MCOs have properly curbed the excesses brought on by the unlimited fee-for-service plans of the past or have unnecessarily and unfairly denied care remains a heated issue and an important area for future research.

From the preceding discussion, it also seems that competition in the health care sector may have sown the seeds of its own destruction. For example, benefit denial and cherry-picking behavior take place in the private health insurance industry because of competition. Quantity-setting behavior in the physician services industry and the medical arms race in the hospital industry are argued to occur because of competition. Indeed, one who thinks medical care is unique would certainly subscribe to that opinion. Others might argue, however, that competition cannot function properly until more medical firms are organized on a for-profit basis and consumers pay a greater proportion of the price of medical services, two properties of perfect competition that were described at the beginning of Chapter 8.

About the only thing that is clear from this discussion is that the debate over the relative merits of competition in the health care industry is likely to continue in the future. A portion of that debate is taken up in the remainder of the chapter. Before we tackle that issue, however, let us examine how the U.S. health care system stacks up against other health care systems around the world. For example, we saw in Chapter 4 that the health care systems in Canada, Germany, and the United Kingdom involve a single-payer system rather than a multiple-payer system like that of the United States. Also, their health care systems provide nearly universal access to medical care services and involve a greater financing and regulatory role for the federal government and less reliance on competition in health care matters. Thus it would be interesting and informative to examine how the United States compares to these and other countries in terms of health care expenditures, the utilization of medical care, and health care outcomes. To that we now turn our attention.

The U.S. Health Care Economy: An International Comparison

Table 16–1 compares health care spending, medical utilization, and demographic data for seven of the G-8 countries: Canada, France, Germany, Italy, Japan, the United Kingdom, and

TABLE 16–1
Comparative Health Care System States for the G-8 Countries Excluding the Russian Federation

	Per Capita Health Care Expenditures	Per Capita GDP	MRIs per Million Persons	Percent of Obese Adults	Alcohol Consumption Liters per Adult Pop.	Per Capita Nitrogen Oxides	Hospital Beds per 1,000 Pop.	Practicing Physicians per 1,000 Pop.
	(2004)	(2004)	(2003)	(2003)	(2003)	(2002)	(2003)	(2003)
Canada	$3,003	$30,600	4.5	14.3	7.8*	78	3.2*	2.1
France	2,903	32,900	2.8	9.4	14.8*	23	3.8	3.4
Germany	2,996	33,300	6.0	12.9	10.2	17	6.6*	3.4
Italy	2,258	28,900	11.6	8.5	8.0	22	3.9*	4.1
Japan	2,139	36,500	35.3	3.2*	7.6	16	8.5	2.0*
United Kingdom	2,231	35,600	5.2	23.0*	11.2	26	3.7	2.2
United States	5,635	39,700	8.6	30.6	8.3*	65	2.8*	2.3*

* Data are for 2002.

SOURCE: Organization for Economic Cooperation and Development, http://www.oecd.org.

the United States. The Federation of Russia is excluded for lack of current data. These countries possess highly developed market economies and share many similar circumstances. (Like the other countries, with the exception of the United States, France and Italy provide nearly universal access to medical services and have a single-payer system.) Data for health care spending on a per capita basis are shown in column 1 of the table. The next five columns contain comparative data on per capita income, the availability of technology, lifestyle and the environment. Data for hospital beds and practicing physicians are reported in the last two columns and are intended as measures of medical utilization. All these data are collected and based on definitions established by the Organization for Economic Cooperation and Development.

Before discussing the figures in the tables, we should point out that data from different countries may not be directly comparable for several reasons and, therefore, should be accepted with some skepticism. For example, no standard taxonomy exists across countries. Medical authorities in, say, France might distinguish among inpatient and outpatient services differently than do their counterparts in the United States. Also, in practice it is often difficult to draw a line separating medical services, such as acute care and long-term care services. In addition, monetary values for health care expenditures and gross domestic product must be converted to a common denominator, such as U.S. dollars, before meaningful comparisons can be made. Any conversion factor, such as purchasing power parities or currency exchange rates, is not without measurement error. Nevertheless, many comparative system analysts believe these data paint a reasonable picture of the health care situation in various countries.

The figures in column 1 suggest that the United States spends more on medical care in absolute and relative terms than do the other countries. Per capita health care spending in the United States ($5,635) was more than double the average of the other six countries in 2003 ($2,588). Three countries—Italy, Japan, and the United Kingdom—had per capita health care expenditures below $2,500. The United States also appears to spend more in relative terms than the other countries on medical care. As a fraction of GDP, medical care expenditures topped 15 percent of GDP in the United States in 2003; this is almost four percentage points higher than Germany, the next largest spender. The remaining five countries held medical expenditures at or below 10 percent of GDP in 2003, with the United Kingdom spending the smallest fraction of total domestic income on medical care at 7.7 percent of GDP (not shown in the table).

Data in the next seven columns provide some explanation for the higher health care spending in the United States. According to the data, per capita income was higher in the United States ($39,700) in 2004 than in every other country. Japan had the next-highest per capita GDP in 2004 at $36,500. As discussed in Chapter 5, the income elasticity of demand in the aggregate is greater than one, indicating that health care spending is highly responsive to income at the aggregate level. Income (GDP) per capita in the United States is about 20 percent higher than the average of the other countries and, therefore, supports a greater proportion of health care spending.

In addition, we saw in Chapters 7 and 8 that a greater availability of cost-enhancing medical technologies raises the demand and also reduces the supply of medical services. The shifts in demand and supply both lead to a greater amount of spending on health care services, provided both curves are inelastic with respect to price. According to the data in the table, the United States has more MRIs per million people than all the countries under consideration, with the exceptions of Japan and Italy. Data not shown in the table also indicate that the United States has the third-highest number of CT scanners per million population, behind both Japan and Italy. If availability of technology offers a complete explanation, Japan and Italy should also experience high health care costs, as both countries have more MRIs and scanners than the United States. That is not the case, however.

We learned in Chapter 2 that lifestyle and environmental factors play an important role in determining health status and demand for medical care. People may try to compensate for risky lifestyle behaviors, such as poor diet or excessive drinking, by consuming more health care services. That would cause the demand for medical care to increase and result in an increase in overall expenditures on health care. The percentage of obese adults shown in column 4 is taken as a crude measure of dietary behavior. It is generally agreed in the medical community that excessive weight could result in a number of medical problems such as high blood pressure, diabetes, and heart failure. According to the figures, 30 percent of all adults in the United States are considered obese, which is more than twice the average of the remaining six countries. Column 5 indicates that the United States is at the median when it comes to yearly alcohol consumption per adult population. Excessive consumption of alcohol can also lead to a number of health complications such as cirrhosis of the liver, stroke, and high blood pressure. While these two measures together may be considered crude measures of lifestyle, they do suggest that lifestyle may play a role in explaining the high medical care costs in the United States.

Environmental factors as measured by per capita nitrogen oxide emissions may also play a role in explaining high medical care costs in the United States. Nitrogen oxides result when fuel is burned to power motor vehicles, electric utilities, and industrial and commercial plants. According to column 6, nitrogen oxide emissions in the United States are far higher than in the other six countries, with the exception of Canada. Emission levels in the United States are more than twice the levels in France, Italy, and the United Kingdom and three times the levels in Germany and Japan. High levels of nitrogen oxides contribute to respiratory ailments, formation of acid rain, deterioration of water quality, and global warming. To counter the negative impact of these environmental factors, Americans may consume more medical care than otherwise would be the case, thereby causing an increase in medical care expenditures.

Columns 7 and 8 provide information on medical resources to see what health dollars may buy besides medical technology. Perhaps the high health care spending in the United States shows up in a relatively large number of acute hospital beds and physicians. An examination of the medical resources data in the table suggests just the opposite, however. In particular, the United States had only 2.8 hospital beds per 1,000 population in 2003, compared to 6.6 in Germany and 8.5 in Japan. The data for the supply of physicians also allows us to draw a similar conclusion: the availability of medical resources does not explain the high health care cost in the United States.

Comparatively high health care expenditures coupled with low medical utilization rates have led some analysts to believe that medical prices must be significantly higher in the United States than in other countries. Others argue, however, that this may not be a legitimate conclusion to draw from these data due to quality differences in medical services across countries. Specifically, the quality of medical care may be higher in the United States and account for higher medical prices. Unfortunately, good indicators of the quality of care are unavailable because of measurement issues. Anecdotal evidence does suggest that waiting times are shorter for most medical services in the United States.

Figure 16–1 indicates the level of health in the United States relative to the other countries. The infant mortality rate (deaths per thousand live births) is thought to be highly correlated with other measures of health status, making it a reasonable benchmark for the general state of health of all population segments. The data in the figure imply that all other G-8 countries (excluding Russia) have an infant mortality rate much lower than that of the United States. The discrepancy is not a trivial one. In the United States, about 2.6 more infants out of every 1,000 children born alive never get a chance to blow out the candles on their first birthday cake. Think about that!

FIGURE 16–1
Infant Mortality 2003 (Deaths per 1,000 Live Births)

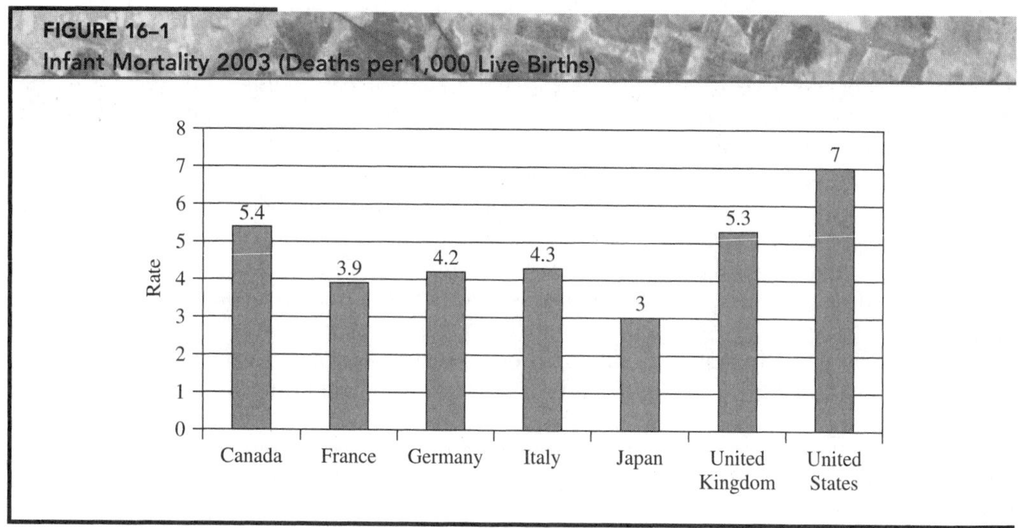

SOURCE: Organization for Economic Cooperation and Development, http://www.oecd.org.

In summary, around 15 to 16 percent of the U.S. population is without health insurance coverage throughout the year. In contrast, nearly universal health insurance coverage exists in the other countries studied. Government in the United States is responsible for financing about 60 percent of all health care spending. The comparable figure for the other six countries was well over 75 percent in 2003, according to OECD figures. Health care spending as a fraction of GDP is higher, medical utilizations rates are lower, and the infant mortality rate is higher in the United States than in the typical G-8 country (excluding Russia). Many analysts have concluded from such data that health care costs and infant mortality are lower in other countries because the government plays a more dominant role in the health care sector and because there is universal access to health insurance. In fact, many health care policy analysts believe that a similar approach can produce better results in the United States.

Why Is There So Much Disagreement Concerning How Health Care Reform Should Be Designed?

In the following sections of this chapter, we examine various plans for reforming the U.S. health care system at the national level and review health reform taking place in a select group of states. One may wonder why so much disagreement exists concerning health care reform. Some advocates for reform argue vehemently for more government controls on health care providers and a greater role for government in the financing of health care. Others shout, "Let the market work!" Musgrave (1993) argues that the disagreement over health care reform can best be explained by theories X and Y of health economics. Table 16–2 summarizes his arguments, presenting theories X and Y as they pertain to five dimensions of health economics. Notice the essential differences.

On the one hand, theory X views illnesses as occurring randomly. That is, some people get sick or become involved in accidents, and others do not; some live long and healthy lives, whereas others live abnormally short lives plagued with illness. On the other hand, theory Y

TABLE 16–2
The X and Y Theories of Health Economics

View of	Theory X	Theory Y
Health	Health and disease occur randomly	Health is determined by people's lifestyle choices
Medical care	Special	No different from any other good or service
The practice of medicine	A science	An art
Economics	Financial rewards reduce the quality of caring	Financial rewards are responsible for generating high-quality medicine
Policy	Regulations are needed to mitigate economic forces	Reduce regulations and encourage market forces
	Tax the healthy; subsidize the sick	Tax the sick, not the healthy
	Discourage new medical technologies	Encourage new medical technologies

SOURCE: Based on Gerald L. Musgrave, "Health Economics Outlook: Two Theories of Health Economics," *Business Economics* (April 1995), pp. 7–13.

treats illnesses and accidents as being determined largely by lifestyle choices. Choices concerning cigarette smoking, excessive drinking, safe sex, wearing safety belts, occupation, and the like can affect the probability of entering a state of sickness or suffering a harmful accident. Individuals who choose healthy lifestyles enjoy long lives free of sickness, according to theory Y.

Theory X treats medical care as being special. Necessity, consumer ignorance, the dominance of not-for-profit hospitals and other medical institutions, highly inelastic demand, and the preponderance of government intervention all make medical care unique. Theory X says that because of uniqueness, medical care "is not and cannot be treated in the same fashion as other economic commodities whose allocation is left to relatively unregulated markets" (Aaron, 1991, p. 6). In fact, greedy, profit-oriented doctors, insurance companies, and pharmaceutical companies as well as the unfettered forces of the marketplace are the root cause of rising health care costs, according to theory X.

Theory Y, in contrast, perceives medical care to be no different from any other good or service. Health care is not more important than food, clothing, or shelter. Consumers probably know more about health care than they do about the engines in their cars, Musgrave asserts, because the benefit of possessing information is greater. Just as no one blames carpenters for homelessness, according to theory Y, health care providers should not be held responsible for the failure of the U.S. health care system. High profits in the health care sector reflect success, not failure. Theory Y'ers believe that markets have not been allowed to work because of excessive government regulations.

Theory X also views medicine as a science. Someday experts will arrive at the best way to treat each and every illness. Conversely, theory Y treats medicine as an art. Health care providers will never find the best cure for a given illness, especially because many illnesses are patient specific and newer, less painful, and lower-cost treatments will always be in demand.

Regarding economics, theory X proposes that financial rewards diminish the quality of care. Economics and medicine, like oil and water, do not mix. Profit seeking gets in the way of proper patient care. For example, theory X'ers claim that personal investments in MRI facilities create an incentive for physicians to overprescribe their diagnostic services to patients. Theory Y, in contrast, views financial rewards as the reason for high-quality medicine in the United States. Health care providers are in the best position to determine the true needs for health care capital. Ownership provides health care providers with an incentive to ensure that needed capital is supplied.

Given the difference between the two views regarding health, medical care, the practice of medicine, and the role of economics, it should not be surprising that theories X and Y take a different stance on policy as well. Table 16–2 lists three policy stances. According to theory X, because financial rewards are the source of system failure, further regulations are needed to curb the profit appetites of health care providers. Government planning is necessary to control the number of hospitals, physicians, and other health care providers and establishments. Government requires more information on health care markets for planning purposes.

Theory Y asserts that health care markets are already overregulated as mentioned earlier. Excessive regulations are partly accountable for some of the observed health care problems. Competitive economic forces should be allowed to function such that health care providers have incentives to produce with least-cost methods and satisfy consumer wants. Consumers need information to make more informed decisions.

Theory X further proposes that taxes should be levied on healthy individuals to pay for the health care costs of unhealthy ones. Because bad health or illness occurs randomly, it is fair to tax the lucky and not the unlucky. In contrast, theory Y argues that subsidizing sickness rewards it. Taxing health reduces the number of people who will remain healthy. It is not efficient to tax the healthy to subsidize the unhealthy.

Finally, theories X and Y differ on their positions concerning medical technology. New technology and health care spending are undesirable, according to theory X. Global budgets and other spending controls are necessary to curb technologies offering high-cost, low-benefit medicine. Theory Y asserts just the opposite. New technologies advance medical care. More health care services, just like more clothing or food, are good. When expenditures rise in the computer or automobile industry, for example, people point to success, not failure.

Given these two extreme views, it should not be surprising that many issues pertaining to health economics are hotly debated. Of course, it is constructive to remember that most issues, especially as they pertain to a social science field like health economics, are never truly black or white, but, as Billy Joel reminds us, are only different "shades of grey."[3] Hence, many people adopt an intermediate view of health economics somewhere in the XY theory plane.

An Overview of Health Care Reform in the United States

The debate over health care reform in the United States has been heated, and the volume of the discussion in the popular press attests to the liveliness of the issue. While the list of concerns with the U.S. health care system is almost endless, most would agree that the two most glaring problems have to do with access problems faced by the uninsured and escalating health care costs. We learned in Chapter 11 that approximately one out of six Americans is without health insurance

3. "Shades of Grey" written by Billy Joel © 1992 Impulsive Music (ASCAP).

and millions more are underinsured.[4] And the future does not look very bright either, as Gilmer and Kronick (2005) estimate that the number of uninsured Americans will increase by another 11 million by 2013 if the current trend continues. At the same time, currently 15 cents out of every dollar spend in the United States is devoted to health care and that figure is anticipated to grow to more than 18 cents out of every dollar by 2014 (Heffler et al., 2005).

Given these rather bleak figures, it is not too difficult to figure out why there is so much dissatisfaction with the U.S. health care system. Facing a bewildering number of proposals and counterproposals from every interest group imaginable, health care professionals and consumers alike have a difficult time keeping abreast of the issues. The debate is further complicated by a vast array of new terminology. Terms with which many of us are unfamiliar, such as *global budgeting*, *health alliances*, and *play-or-pay*, are bandied about regularly. This section attempts to help you sort through this maze by reviewing the efficiency and equity implications of four generic health care reform proposals: managed competition, national health insurance, medical savings accounts, and individual mandates. These four proposals were chosen primarily because they include the basic elements of the majority of the proposals typically considered.

Following this discussion, we examine health care reform at the state level. State governments are a frequently overlooked player in the health care debate. We review the health care reform packages of four states to get a flavor of the various strategies at the state level. Finally, we examine the basic features of the Clinton health care plan, or the National Health Security Act of 1993.

Health Care Reform at the Federal Level

To bring some consistency to the discussion, each plan is evaluated using four economic criteria:

1. ***Universal coverage:*** Does the plan achieve universal coverage, and, if so, how?
2. ***Financing and budgetary implications:*** How is the plan financed, and to what extent does it affect the federal deficit?
3. ***Cost containment:*** How does the plan contain the growth of medical care expenditures over time?
4. ***Employment:*** To what extent does the plan influence overall employment opportunities?

Note that the first criterion deals with the issue of vertical equity, while the last two concern efficiency. A summary of how each plan measures up to the four criteria appears in Table 16–3, on the following two pages, which the reader is urged to consult throughout the discussion. In addition, the discussion refers to the generalized model of a health care system discussed in Chapter 4.

Managed Competition[5]

The managed-competition plan has received tremendous publicity primarily because it was used as the basis for the Clinton health care plan. The attractive feature of the plan is that it builds on the existing system of employer-provided medical insurance coverage. Employers are mandated

4. To put these figures in perspective, Hadley and Holahan (2003) estimate that health care costs in 2001 would have increased by between $34 and $69 billion if the uninsured were fully insured. Some would consider this a rather modest sum.

5. This discussion is based on Enthoven and Kronick (1989) and Enthoven (1993).

TABLE 16–3
A Summary of the Four Health Care Plans

	Managed Competition	National Health Insurance
Universal coverage	Employers are required to provide medical coverage to all full-time workers. Subsidies are provided to make it possible for low-income families to purchase medical insurance. Medicaid and Medicare are maintained. Near-universal coverage is possible.	Universal coverage is achieved through a national health insurance plan that covers all citizens.
Financing	Medical coverage is financed primarily through employer mandates so employees most likely pay through forgone wages. Government expenditures are paid through a payroll tax. The impact on the deficit should not be too significant.	Medical coverage is financed out of an income tax. Also, funds for Medicare and Medicaid are diverted to partially offset the cost of the plan. An employer tax equal to the cost of employer-financed medical insurance is also levied.
Cost containment	Cost containment results from the maintenance of a highly competitive private insurance market. A uniform benefit package is offered, and employers are required to pay for 80 percent of the representative plan. The remaining 20 percent provides an incentive for consumers to shop wisely.	Costs are contained through the utilization of a single-payer system that decreases the administration and billing costs that are the by-product of a multipayer system. Also, global budgeting is used to establish a constant relation between gross domestic product and health care expenditures.
Employment	Likely to have a significant effect because employer mandates may create substantial distortions in labor markets, especially among low-wage workers.	Employment effects will be concentrated in the private insurance market and health care administration.

to provide medical coverage for basic medical services and pay, for example, an 8 percent payroll tax on the first $22,500 of wages for employees not covered.[6] Self-employed individuals and early retirees must pay for health care coverage with an 8 percent tax on adjusted income up to a preset maximum. The tax is collected through the income tax system.

6. Other health care proposals give employers the option to pay a tax in lieu of providing medical coverage to full-time employees. In the popular literature, this is referred to as the "pay-or-play" option.

TABLE 16–3 *(continued)*

	Medical Savings Accounts	Individual Mandates
Universal coverage	This program is not designed to achieve universal coverage. However, health insurance premiums should become more affordable when they become tax deductible and apply mainly to catastrophic plans. Tax credits and subsidies are used to make health insurance more affordable for poor individuals.	The plan is implemented through mandated insurance coverage and a guarantee by the government that basic medical coverage is available across the country. Tax credits and subsidies are available to make coverage affordable to all. Near-universal coverage is attainable.
Financing	The plan is financed primarily out of individual contributions to medical savings accounts. Because government expenditures on Medicare and Medicaid end, the deficit should diminish.	The plan is financed largely by premium payments by consumers either directly or through employers. A tax increase is necessary. Medicare and Medicaid programs are ended.
Cost containment	Because consumers pay for most health care expenditures out of their own Medisave accounts, they have the incentive to minimize waste and shop around for competitive prices. A reduction in administrative expenses also translates into cost savings.	Costs are contained through the maintenance of a highly competitive medical insurance market. Private insurance vendors are disciplined by the marketplace to provide competitive prices to consumers.
Employment	Minimal impact because labor market distortions are kept to a minimum.	Minor impact because labor market distortions are kept to a minimum.

The most novel portion of this plan is the creation across the country of government insurance buyer organizations called **health alliances.** These public or not-for-profit agencies use their purchasing power to negotiate competitive prices for health insurance from private insurance companies. Individuals without employer-provided insurance and small employers may purchase competitively priced health insurance through one of these alliances. The alliances also serve as brokers that collect premiums, manage enrollment, and carry out other administrative duties. The intent is to have each alliance offer a number of competing plans to its enrollees.

Universal coverage is ensured through employer mandates and subsidies provided to low-income families to pay for medical coverage. Medicaid and Medicare are maintained and eventually take advantage of the alliances to provide medical insurance coverage. The plan is financed primarily with employer-mandated health insurance premiums and consumer payments. Government expenditures are financed primarily by the payroll tax and other revenues resulting from the plan. The impact on the deficit is not likely to be significant.

Cost containment results from competition among private insurers as they vie for customers through the alliances. This is why the term **managed competition** was coined. The health alliances "manage" the various health care plans to ensure sufficient "competition" at the insurance end of the medical care market. To simplify matters for consumers and intensify competition, all plans must offer a uniform benefit package. This puts consumers in a better position to make informed choices. As further encouragement for cost-conscious behavior, employers are required to make a fixed contribution toward medical coverage for each employee equal to 80 percent of the average plan's cost in the area. The remaining 20 percent is the employee's responsibility. A limit is also placed on the tax deduction employees can take for premium payments. This encourages consumers to pick less expensive health plans that provide less generous benefits, since they must pay for more costly plans with after-tax dollars.

One criticism of managed competition is that rural areas may lack enough private insurance companies. The scarcity of suppliers may make it difficult to promote price competition (Kronick et al., 1993). Another complaint is that the government-sponsored health alliances may result in "one-size-fits-all" health insurance plans, and, as a result, consumers will lose the benefits of variety. Finally, one of the more controversial elements of employer mandates is the fact that they create labor market distortions and lead to unemployment of unskilled workers.

Who Pays for Employer-Mandated Health Insurance? Most proposals for employer-mandated health insurance in the United States call for employers to finance at least 80 percent of the premiums. The remaining 20 percent of the premiums would be paid by employees, presumably in the form of payroll deductions.

Economic principles suggest, however, that the actual economic incidence of a mandate (or tax) may differ from its statutory or legal incidence. For example, in the case of employer-mandated health insurance, it might be the case that the employer may simply pass on their legal share of the mandate to the employee in the form of lower wages. If so, the employee could actually pay the entire cost of the mandate.

Summers (1989) provides a conceptual model that can be used to examine who pays for an employer-mandated health insurance program. The model is presented graphically in Figure 16–2. The figure depicts a competitive labor market in equilibrium where W stands for the annual money wage and L represents the number of full-time workers. Assuming no health insurance benefits are initially provided, equilibrium is at point W_0, L_0, where the supply and demand curves intersect. We will now compare this initial equilibrium to one with a mandated health insurance program.

According to Summers's analysis, the mandate potentially shifts both the supply and demand curves. The demand curve shifts downward by the amount of the per-employee cost of the insurance program, M. The shift of the demand curve from D_0 to D_1 reflects that any insurance costs must be potentially offset by wage reductions given that each worker generates a particular amount of revenues for a company as discussed at the beginning of chapter 6. The interesting question then becomes: What happens to the supply of labor?

Just as the shift in demand reflects the per-employee cost of the health insurance, the shift in the supply curve captures the benefit of the mandated insurance to the typical employee. If the supply curve shifts downward by the dollar amount of the mandated benefit, it means that the typical employee values the health insurance by exactly the same amount that it costs. That is, the employee is willing to give up wage income equal to the cost of the mandated health

FIGURE 16–2
The Impact of an Employer Mandate on a Labor Market

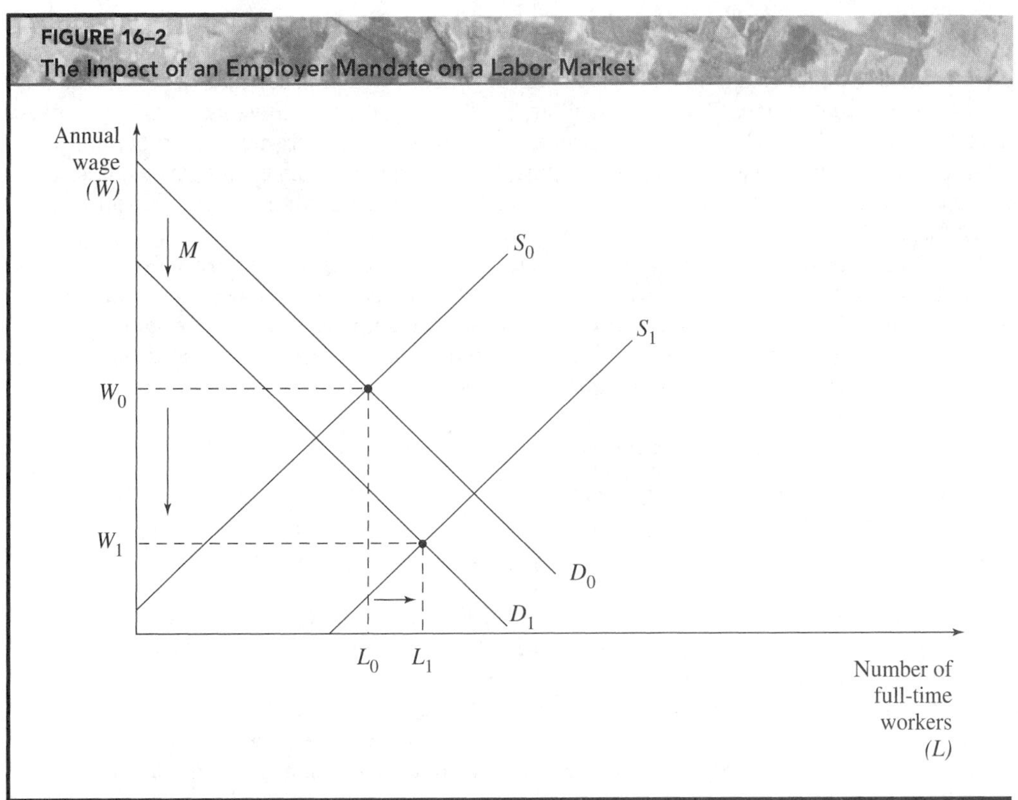

Assuming no health insurance benefits, equilibrium in the labor market initially occurs at point W_0L_0 where the supply and demand curves intersect. Now, assume that government mandates that employers provide health insurance to their employees. In this case, the demand curve shifts to the left from D_0 to D_1 because the cost of health insurance must be offset by a lower wage offer. But the supply curve of labor also potentially shifts rightward to reflect the wage income that workers are willing to give up because of the value they attach to health insurance benefits. Supposing that supply shifts from S_0 to S_1 the next equilibrium point is at W_1L_1. Notice that in this case, the wage rate falls by more than the cost of the health insurance because workers perceive that the benefits of health insurance outweigh its cost.

insurance. A supply curve that shifts downward by less than the mandated cost suggests that the value of the health insurance is less than its cost.

For discussion purposes, let us suppose that the supply curve shifts downward by more than demand from S_0 to S_1. That would mean that the new equilibrium wage becomes W_1 and that the employee pays more than the full cost of the mandated benefit. The implication is that the mandated health insurance is efficient since its benefit exceeds its cost. That is, the mandate makes employees better off, and it shows in the form of a much lower wage.

If, on the other hand, the supply curve shifts downward by less than the mandated insurance costs, wages decline but by less than the mandated cost, reflecting that wage income is more important than health insurance at the margin. (You may want to work through this exercise.) Workers would be made worse off by the mandated benefit in this case. In fact, if the supply of labor increases less than demand declines, the analysis suggests that the level of employment decreases in the market. Moreover, economic theory indicates that the costs of the resulting unemployment are likely to fall disproportionately upon unskilled workers for three reasons. First, unskilled workers possess low productivity levels. Hence, assuming all other factors remain constant, low skilled workers are the first to be laid off if employers are required to incur higher labor costs (i.e., wages and health insurance costs). Second, unskilled workers, because of their low income, may place less value on the health insurance benefits and assign greater costs to the forgone wages associated with the mandate. The lower net benefits serve as a disincentive for unskilled workers to remain at their jobs. Third, unskilled workers may be paid a government set minimum wage. As a result, their wages cannot legally be adjusted downward to compensate for the added cost of the insurance mandate. In this case, employers have no other recourse than to lay-off workers when faced with the added expense of providing health insurance.

In sum, the degree to which employees gain from health insurance coverage determines the economic incidence of a mandate. When they benefit more, employees pay a greater amount for mandated benefits in the form of lower wages. However, if employees place little value on health insurance coverage or are subject to a minimum wage constraint, economic theory suggests that mandated benefits may inhibit employment, particularly among low skilled workers.

National Health Insurance[7]

The national health insurance plan calls for the implementation of a national health insurance system similar to the one presently existing in Canada. As such, the current multipayer system in the United States is replaced by a single-payer public medical insurance program. In terms of the generalized model of a health care system, this means the role of third-party payer is completely taken over by the government sector, and the private market for medical insurance is almost completely eliminated (some specific services, such as dental and optical care, may continue to be covered by private insurance).

Universal coverage is guaranteed with this plan because everyone is covered for all necessary medical services, with no coinsurance, copayments, or deductibles. The plan achieves vertical equity because it is financed out of general taxes, with a heavy reliance on the income tax system. A tax increase is necessary to provide the additional funding needed to broaden coverage to uninsured individuals. Since currently funded medical programs, such as Medicare and Medicaid, are no longer needed, funds earmarked for these programs would be used to finance a national health insurance program. Employer taxes increase by the amount currently spent on health care benefits. The implication is that employer-provided funds are diverted from the private insurance market to a publicly run health insurance program.

Cost containment is based primarily on the efficiencies associated with using a single-payer system. Billing and administration costs are reduced because health care providers no longer need to contend with the complex set of insurance forms and billing procedures that result from a multipayer system. In addition, overall expenditures are controlled by establishing a link between gross domestic product and health care costs. Once the proportion between the two is established, overall health care costs are allowed to grow only as fast as the overall economy. Global budgets and simplified fee schedules are utilized to compensate health care providers, such as hospitals and physicians, for services provided. The role of managed care with a national insurance plan is difficult to determine, because most of the impetus for managed care comes from the private health insurance market, which the plan eliminates.

Finally, the employment effects are likely to be most noticeable in the private health insurance market and health care administration. With the elimination of the private health insurance market and the decrease in administrative services, some job displacement is likely to occur, particularly in the short run.

---

7. This discussion is based on Himmelstein and Woolhandler (1989).

While the national health insurance plan comes closest to providing universal health insurance, a general criticism has been levied against the plan. The extensive involvement of government and the elimination of private insurers alarm those who believe that government enterprise is monopoly enterprise. Critics claim that the creation of financial innovations to control medical costs would be weakened in a government-run health insurance program. Critics also argue that because a competitive incentive is missing, a public monopoly insurer may offer little variety and be unresponsive to consumer wants.

Medical Savings Accounts

This plan takes a distinctly market-oriented approach to reforming health care by calling for the development of individual tax-free medical savings accounts (MSAs) to pay for routine medical care. Proponents claim that routine care accounts for a significant fraction of medical expenditures.[8] The program is purely voluntary in that individuals have the option to make yearly contributions to their MSAs up to a specified amount, and any funds left in the account at the end of the year can be carried over to the next year and earn interest. Catastrophic health insurance plans to finance major medical expenses can also be purchased with pretax income. Premiums for the catastrophic plans are generally cheap due to the high deductibles involved.

An example may help clarify the structure of the MSA proposal. Suppose your employer presently pays $7,000 for your family's major medical and routine care insurance coverage. Under the MSA plan, your employer would purchase catastrophic health insurance coverage worth, say, $3,500 for your family. The catastrophic plan covers expensive major illnesses and has a sizeable deductible. In addition, the employer deposits the remaining $3,500 into a tax-free MSA. Your family can use the funds in the MSA to pay for routine care or to finance the deductible on major medical illnesses during the year. The routine care services could be purchased as needed or on a prepaid basis through a health care provider like an HMO. Your family makes the choice by considering relative prices, income, health status, degree of risk aversion, and other demand-side factors. Any unused funds in the MSA are rolled over and used for similar purposes in future years.

The MSA plan does not call for universal health care coverage, but it does give the public freedom of choice. A person can elect to create an MSA and contribute as much as desired up to a preset limit. Because contributions to the MSAs are tax deductible, the price of medical care is reduced, making it affordable for more people. Tax credits also further reduce the price for low-income families, and government subsidies are available for truly needy individuals. Horizontal equity is achieved because all premiums or contributions to the MSAs are tax deductible whether paid by the employee or the employer.[9] Elderly individuals finance health care expenditures with the introduction of medical IRAs. Like traditional IRAs, these accounts grow tax-free and can be used to cover medical expenses during retirement. Eventually they will take the place of Medicare.

Under this plan, consumers individually finance a major proportion of medical expenditures by drawing from the MSAs. The impact on the federal deficit is minimal because the current Medicare and Medicaid programs are eventually ended. The increase in the deficit results primarily from forgone tax revenues because of the tax-exempt nature of the MSAs and because of the tax credits and subsidies to needy individuals.

Cost containment is achieved through enhanced price competition. Since consumers are directly responsible for purchasing medical care out of their MSAs, they have the incentive to reduce waste and comparison shop. Realizing this, health care providers, such as physicians and

8. This discussion is based on Goodman and Musgrave (1992) and Tripoli (1993). See Heffley and Miceli (1998) for an advanced treatment of the impact of incentive plans on medical care utilization.

9. If only medical premiums paid by employers are tax deductible, horizontal inequities exist because the price of medical coverage depends on employment status rather than income.

hospitals, are forced to provide high-quality, competitively priced medical care. This point is made clear if we look at MSAs in terms of the generalized model of a health care system presented in Chapter 4. It is apparent that MSAs minimize the impact of third-party payers because most transactions take place directly between consumers and health care providers. As a result, fewer market distortions occur because third-party payers play a less influential role in the MSA plan. In addition, costs are reduced due to administrative savings. With high deductibles on catastrophic health care plans, insurance companies are no longer bogged down with thousands of small claims that are relatively expensive to process. Managed care is likely to thrive under the MSA plan as health care providers and insurance companies strive to control costs and remain competitive. The employment effect of this plan is minimal because labor market incentives are not distorted (see the previous discussion on employer mandates).

Several criticisms of MSAs have been raised (Tanner, 1995). First, critics claim that consumers are not sufficiently informed to make cost-conscious decisions regarding medical treatments. Opponents argue that due to the lack of information, physicians will continue to induce the demand for their services and health care costs will continue to rise. Second, critics argue that consumers will forgo necessary or preventive care to save money in the MSAs for other purposes. Less medical care, in turn, will lead to poorer health and higher health care costs in the long run. Third, opponents allege that the plan will lead to adverse selection as healthy people select MSAs while sick individuals choose conventional insurance. Eventually, the price of insurance will increase and create financial access problems as more and sicker members enroll in conventional insurance plans. Fourth, critics point out that the deductible on catastrophic insurance will be insufficient to control expenditures on high-cost, low-benefit medicine. That is, once a person is hospitalized for a major illness, the size of the deductible will not matter. Since critically sick patients account for most of the spending on health care, the MSA plan will be ineffective in containing health care costs. Finally, critics argue that an MSA plan is regressive since the benefits accrue primarily to wealthy individuals.

The advocates of medical saving accounts have responded to each of these criticisms. Basically, proponents point to demand studies showing that consumers are conscious of health care prices, even very small out-of-pocket prices. MSAs will make consumers more responsive and cost conscious, since they will consider the full price of medical services. Further, proponents point to the success of MSA plans currently in use in producing medical cost savings and preventing adverse selection. Finally, advocates claim that the current tax break for employer-provided insurance is far more regressive than an MSA plan available for all. The MSA plan has recently become a hot item as the Medicare Modernization Act of 2003 encourages health insurance plans of that kind.

Individual Mandates[10]

Like the MSA plan, the individual mandate plan places the responsibility for medical coverage squarely on the shoulders of consumers. Individuals are required by law to purchase a basic medical insurance plan as defined by the government. They still have the option to purchase more comprehensive coverage, and nothing precludes employers from providing medical insurance to their employees.

Universal coverage is achieved through a combination of mandated medical coverage and the government's guarantee that basic medical coverage is available at a competitive price for those unable to pay for a private plan. Tax credits are offered to ensure affordability, and for those who still cannot afford insurance, government vouchers are available. The Medicaid and Medicare programs are eventually phased out.

10. This overview is based on Pauly et al. (1991).

To make sure competitively priced medical coverage for the basic plan is available to all, the government solicits bids from private insurance vendors throughout the country. At least one basic plan is offered in every geographic region of the country to serve as "fallback" coverage for any consumer who did not purchase a plan in the private market. The plan also moves toward achieving horizontal equity because tax credits depend on income status rather than employment status.

The plan is financed primarily by individual contributions; however, tax credits and subsidies are available for eligible individuals. Although Pauly et al. (1991) do not provide figures, they believe a modest tax increase is necessary to extend medical coverage to the uninsured. The extent of the increase depends on the magnitude of the tax credits and subsidies provided.

Cost containment is ensured through the maintenance of a highly competitive medical insurance market. Private insurance companies find it in their self-interest to provide high-quality, low-cost insurance to consumers who must purchase and pay for their own medical coverage. Competition is also enhanced because the government plays no role as a third-party insurer since the market for medical insurance is completely private. Employment ramifications are likely to be kept to a minimum because labor market incentives are minimally disturbed. In this type of market environment, managed care is likely to be relied on extensively to control costs.

As with the MSA plan, critics of the individual mandate argue that consumers lack the necessary information to shop wisely. Medical insurance plans contain numerous complex terms and conditions, and therefore are difficult for the average person to comprehend. In addition, some argue that the individual mandate provides less incentive than the MSA plan for consumers to consider the full price of the medical services they buy because third-party payers continue to play an influential role under the individual mandate plan. Finally, critics claim that the individual mandate imposes a serious restraint on an individual's freedom of choice (although it should be kept in mind that Social Security and car insurance in many states are presently mandatory).

Attempts at State Health Care: Successes and Failures

Unlike most countries, the United States follows a more decentralized approach to health care policy that allows individual states a certain degree of latitude in developing their own health care policies. The reason is largely historic and has its roots in our federalist form of government, which provides states with limited discretion to govern. Coupled with this tradition has been the general belief in the United States that issues relating to health, education, and poverty are best addressed at the local or community level. A case in point is the Medicaid program, which is jointly financed by the federal and state governments. Since states foot a portion of the bill, they have been given some say as to how those tax dollars are spent. As a result, vastly different Medicaid programs have developed across states over time.

Advocates for a decentralized approach to health care reform point out that this approach is more democratic. This is because states are in a better position than the federal government to address the unique needs of the local population. Another advantage is that states can be seen as "laboratories" or "guinea pigs" where alternative policies can be tried out to see whether they should be adopted at the national level or in other states. Finally, advocates of the decentralized approach are fond of pointing out that the issue of whether health care reform should take place at the state or federal level is largely moot because our system of government allows states to block any major reforms if they desire. All this suggests that states are likely to continue playing a critical role in the formation of U.S. health care policy for years to come.

Confronted with the burden of rising health care costs, a growing number of individuals who lack health care coverage, and a citizenry in no mood for further tax increases, most states have been forced to reexamine their health care insurance programs. Many states are aggressively investigating various policy options aimed at reforming the financing and delivery of medical care. Naturally, space limitations prohibit a discussion of the health care reform taking place in each state. With this constraint in mind, we now provide a brief overview of the health care reform packages that were adopted in Hawaii, Maryland, Minnesota, and Oregon over the last several years. These states were chosen because they represent the broad spectrum of policies currently under consideration in other states.

Hawaii: The Case of Employer Mandates

Hawaii's health care system achieved a certain level of recognition a few years ago, primarily because the state succeeded in achieving near-universal health insurance coverage. When the percentage of uninsured in the nation averaged 14.9 percent during the three-year period from 1991–1993, it barely topped 8 percent in Hawaii (Bureau of the Census). Much of this success can be attributable to the Prepaid Health Act of 1974, which requires employers to provide health insurance to all full-time employees. At the moment, all employers, with few exceptions, are required to provide health insurance coverage to all employees who work a minimum of 20 hours a week. Each medical plan must provide a minimum number of benefits, and the employee's annual premium contribution is limited to 1.5 percent of his maximum salary.

Low-income residents who do not receive employer-provided health insurance may qualify for government-subsidized health insurance. The Fee-for-Service Medicaid Program primarily serves qualifying individuals who are over age 65, or who are blind or disabled. The Hawaii QUEST program offers subsidized health insurance through a variety of managed care plans for those who qualify. The premium payment depends on employment status and asset limits. (Pollitz et al., 2005).

Despite the mandate that employers provide insurance to certain employees, the uninsured rate in Hawaii has increased significantly in recent years, jumping to a 10 percent average for the period 2002 to 2004 while the national average rose to 15.5 percent. A number of factors have been offered to explain this increase in the uninsured. First, the high cost of the QUEST program has forced the state in recent years to tighten eligibility requirements. Currently, the state has a cap of 125,000 enrollees in the program. Second, a growing number of employers provide health insurance only to employees and not their families. Third and probably the most controversial, a growing number of workers do not qualify for employer-provided health insurance because they work fewer than 20 hours a week (Health Trends in Hawaii). Economic incentives may account for the growing share of employees working less than 20 hours a week as employers attempt to avoid the requirement of the state mandate.

Maryland: The Case of Regulation

Over the years, the state of Maryland has taken a decidedly regulatory approach to health care policy. Beginning in the 1970s the Health Services Cost Review Commission (HSCRC) was established and given the responsibility of reviewing and approving the rates hospitals can charge for their services. After receiving a permanent waiver in 1980 from the federal government exempting Maryland from Medicare and Medicaid reimbursement policies, the state was free to implement an "all-payor system" whereby the HSCRC sets the hospital reimbursement rate for all private insurance companies, HMOs, Medicare, and Medicaid (Maryland Hospital Association, 2002). In 2000 Maryland's hospital payment system went through a significant overhaul and a DRG-based system was implemented. The five major goals of the overhaul were to develop a payment system that was more formulaic and predictable, prospective, able to accommodate input inflation, streamlined, and reflective of the national experience (Maryland Hospital Association, 2002).

The HSCRC also plays a major role in Maryland's health insurance system. Of particular importance is the maintenance of the Comprehensive Standard Health Benefit Plan, which was established in 1994 to provide small to medium-sized firms with access to health insurance. Any health insurance company doing business in Maryland must offer a standard health insurance package to all businesses employing 50 or fewer workers. Coverage cannot be denied for any medical precondition or because of frequency of claims submitted. To control costs, the average community-rated premium cannot be greater than 10 percent of the average wage in the states. However, this legislation does not mandate that employers finance health insurance. The hope was that once employers with few workers have improved access to reasonably priced plans and can comparison shop, they will voluntarily provide insurance for their employees. Unfortunately for Maryland, however, the uninsured rate rose from an average of 12.7 percent during the 1991 to 1993 period to 14 percent during the 2002 to 2004 period.

Disappointed because only 58 percent of the eligible firms in the state were taking advantage of the health plan, the HSCRC recently made available a Limited Benefit Plan. The actuarial value of the limited plan cannot exceed 70 percent of the Comprehensive Standard Health Benefit Plan and is available only to small employers with an average wage that does not exceed 75 percent of the state average (Maryland Health Care Commission, 2005). The hope is that creating a "bare-bones" insurance plan with a lower premium will induce more small firms to offer health insurance to their employees.

Minnesota: The Case of Regulated Competition

In contrast to Maryland, Minnesota had taken a more free market approach to health care through the years, except for a relatively brief period in the early 1990s. In 1992 Minnesota approved MinnesotaCare (originally called HealthRight), which addressed the issues of cost containment and access. The cost containment plan placed great emphasis on competition along with some degree of regulation (Blewett, 1994). The competitive aspect focused on integrated service networks (ISNs), which were prepaid health plans that competed on the basis of price and quality. Competition was made possible by the mandatory disclosure of price and quality information and standardization of health benefits coverage.

The regulatory component called for the state commissioner of health to set a cap on the growth of ISN premiums and controlled fees of out-of-network providers through an all-payer rate-setting system. Other cost containment mechanisms included targets for health care expenditure growth, statewide and regional limits on health care spending, health care planning, retrospective review of capital expenditures for new technologies that cost more than $500,000, restrictions on physician referrals, and a ban on balance-billing for Medicare charges (Leichter, 1993).

The act addressed the problem of uninsured people primarily by offering state-subsidized coverage based on a sliding-fee scale to children, their parents, and eventually others not covered by Medicaid. The subsidized insurance was financed through a variety of taxes on health care providers and a 5-cent-per-pack increase in the state cigarette tax. The legislation also called for significant changes in the small-group insurance market similar to those adopted in Maryland. Any insurance company offering health insurance policies in Minnesota must guarantee coverage regardless of health conditions, and policies cannot be canceled due to excessive claims or health reasons. In addition, a modified community rating system was put in place, and small businesses were offered low-cost insurance plans that do not include selected high-cost medical services (Intergovernment Health Policy Project, 1993).

In 1995, the Minnesota legislature began to repeal or modify many of the reforms enacted earlier. For example, the legislature repealed the all-payer rate-setting regulations. In addition, the state repealed revenue limits placed on health care providers and changed the growth limits on health care expenditures to cost containment goals that are now voluntary (Minnesota Department of Health, 1998).

One of the few major reforms still in place is the retrospective review of capital expenditures that was recently raised from a threshold of $500,000 to $1 million. The law requires health care providers to submit a justification of all capital expenditures over the $1 million level to the Minnesota Department of Health for a retrospective review. If the review fails, the provider may be required to submit any major capital expenditures for prospective approval for the next five years. The law is not without its critics. For one thing, the Department of Health never fully articulated the review criteria and providers are expected to justify any capital expenditure in terms of its impact on health care costs, quality and access (the so-called three-legged stool of health care policy). Given the vagueness of the criteria, many health care providers have not taken the review process very seriously when filing applications. In addition, the Department of Health has done a poor job monitoring capital expenditure projects throughout the state. As a result, it is difficult if not impossible to determine whether the capital expenditure reporting law has had any impact on overall health care costs or the quality of care provided. It is open for debate as to whether the state should repeal or strengthen the capital expenditure reporting law (Joint Task Force on Health Care Costs and Quality, 2003).

Despite the recent movement to repeal much of the reform legislation of the early 1990s, Minnesota has remained committed to expanding health insurance to low-income individuals. "The state supports a comprehensive Medicaid program, characterized by liberal eligibility policies and a rich set of benefits as well as a subsidized health insurance program for low-income population" (Long and Kendall, 2002). The Minnesota Care program provides subsidized health insurance for low-income state residents, and premiums are on a sliding scale based on income and family size (Pollitz et al., 2004). The commitment to health insurance reform in Minnesota shows up in the reduction of the uninsured rate from 9.2 percent during the 1991 to 1993 period to 8.5 percent during the 2002 to 2004 period.

Oregon: The Case of Rationing Medicaid Services

Confronted with the conflicting problems of rising Medicaid expenditures and a growing number of people without medical insurance, Oregon developed one of the more controversial health care reform packages. At issue was a plan that rationed medical care to those on Medicaid. The Oregon Health Plan was troubling to many because it represented the first time a government authority had taken such an active role in the explicit rationing of medical services in the United States.

The focal point of the program was a prioritized list of approximately 740 medical procedures. The list was developed after an exhaustive process that measured the relative value of each medical procedure. Each medical procedure was ranked based on its ability to improve health, its cost, and perceived community value. Based on the list, treatment for appendicitis was ranked 12 and medical therapy for a stroke was ranked 287, for example.

Once the legislature has determined the level of funding for the program, the health services commission determines the number of medical procedures the state can finance. According to recent estimates (January 2006), the state covers 530 out of 710 illnesses or disorders. A lack of funds precludes coverage for the remaining 180. For example, any Medicaid recipient in need of repair of an uncomplicated hernia (ranked 606) would be denied coverage under the Oregon plan.[11]

11. This information is available on the Oregon Health Services Commission's web site at http://egov.oregon.gov.

Proponents of the Oregon plan argue that the state is trading off comprehensive coverage for a few to make greater access available to many. Prior to the plan, the Oregon Medicaid program covered only individuals with incomes at or below 58 percent of the poverty level as established by the federal government. When the plan was implemented, individuals with incomes at or below 100 percent of the poverty level became eligible for Medicaid coverage. In addition, pregnant women and children below age 6 can also qualify if family income does not exceed 133 percent of the poverty level. For a fixed budget, greater coverage can be achieved only by denying services to a relatively few individuals who need very costly medical care relative to the benefits received. The Oregon Plan also attempted to control cost through the use of managed care (Bodenheimer, 1997).

As you can imagine, criticism of the program emanated from all corners of the health care field. From an economic perspective, the program was criticized on both equity and efficiency grounds. Equity questions revolved around the fact that the burden of rationing falls exclusively on the poor while more affluent individuals are left untouched. Regarding efficiency there is concern about whether the state can objectively determine the relative values of alternative medical procedures. Tanner (1993) argues that such determinations are better off left to the marketplace.

This criticism is not without merit. When the list was originally put together, cost effectiveness values were determined for each medical treatment; treatments with lower cost per medical benefit were ranked the highest. Unfortunately, because of a number of methodological problems in determining the benefit scale and political stumbling blocks, the first list was met with considerable resistance. As a result, the list was revamped to consider a number of subjective criteria. For example, higher priority was given to preventive medical services and those that cured potentially acute and/or fatal conditions. Lower priority was given to medical treatments that had little impact on quality or quantity of life, such as end-stage cancer treatments (Dranove, 2003). The revised list was approved by the Department of Health and Human Services in 1993. In 2003 legislation was passed that directed the Health Services Commission to consider the cost effectiveness of health services in terms of evidence-based studies when determining relative rankings (Oregon Health Services Commission, 2005).

The desire to control costs and extend health care coverage has resulted in additional changes to the Oregon Plan. Effective in February 2003, two different plans or benefits packages were made available: the Oregon Health Plan Plus and the Oregon Health Plan Standard. The Oregon Health Plan Plus, or OHP Plus, provides health care coverage to those eligible for Medicaid and other select populations with incomes up to 185 percent of the federal poverty level. The Oregon Health Plan Standard provides fewer benefits than the OHP Plus package and covers some adults who are not eligible for traditional Medicaid programs. Most individuals who quality for the OHP standard plan are required to pay a premium based on income and size of family. Another program available is the Family Health Insurance Assistance Program, which helps uninsured residents pay part of their health insurance premiums (Oregon Health Services Commission, 2005). Although some of these programs may be too recent to matter, it should be noted that the average uninsured rate in Oregon increased from an average of 14.3 percent in the early 1990s to an average of 16.1 percent in the early 2000s.

What Can Be Gained from State Attempts at Health Care Reform?

After reviewing the tremendous diversity in the strategies adopted by states to reform health care, one is left to question what knowledge can be gained from all of this. Barrand and Schroeder (1994) suggest that four basic lessons can be gleaned from health care reform at the state level. First, the tremendous diversity in health care reform reflects the diversity in our health care system across states and the differing views concerning the appropriate role of government. Reform at the national level must be broad enough to consider diversity. Second, attempts at state health care reform reveal that the political process is as complicated at the state level as it is at the federal level. It appears that the political gridlock impeding health care reform at the federal level is also present at the state level. Third, "implementing" health care reform may be more difficult than "designing" reform. With the implementation of such items as new billing procedures, price controls, and quality reviews, states face an enormous set of practical problems in getting the reform up and running. These problems should be kept in mind when changes are made at the federal level. Finally, the need for public education is paramount. Confusion on the part of the public concerning various policies under review only clouds the issue and makes the task of reforming health care even more difficult.

An Overview of the Clinton Health Care Plan

The National Health Security Act proposed by former president Bill Clinton drew extensively on the managed-competition model of health care reform. Each region of the country would be represented by one not-for-profit health alliance that would utilize its purchasing power to negotiate premiums for health insurance with private insurance companies. Employers and individuals would be able to purchase health insurance through these alliances at rates that would be lower than those under the present decentralized, fragmented system. Large firms with more than 5,000 employees would be able to form their own corporate alliances.[12]

Universal coverage was to be accomplished primarily through employer-mandated health insurance. Each employer would be required to provide health insurance to its full-time employees and finance at least 80 percent of the premium of the average plan in the health alliance. The remaining portion would be the responsibility of the employee. To make the cost affordable for employers, total premium contributions would be capped at 3.5 to 7.9 percent of total payroll. Additional reductions in premiums would be made available to small firms. Also, adjustments in premiums would be made for unemployed people, part-time workers, and self-employed individuals.

The plan would be financed from a combination of savings from existing public health insurance programs and additional taxes. Savings from Medicaid would result as that program was merged into the Clinton plan. Presumably, the rate of growth of expenditures for the Medicaid program would diminish over time as the cost containment policies of the Clinton plan took hold. Savings in the Medicare program would emanate from a variety of sources, including more extensive use of managed care and a reduction in payments to providers. There would also be savings from other federal medical programs as they were integrated into the system. Additional taxes would include an increase in the cigarette tax of 75 cents per pack and a 1 percent payroll tax on all corporate alliances.

Cost containment would be achieved primarily through the creation of a national health board. Among other duties, that agency would be responsible for determining the maximum rate of growth of health insurance premiums from year to year. Indirectly, that would give the national health board control over the growth of health care expenditures by allowing it to establish global budgets for each health alliance.

12. The notion of one alliance per region differs slightly from the managed-competition plan developed by Enthoven and Kronick (1989). Under that plan, multiple alliances would be set up in different regions. The argument against multiple alliances is that such an arrangement would add unwanted complexity to the structure. Enthoven and Singer (1995) counter with the argument that health alliances would become too strong under the Clinton plan. Health alliances are meant "to be market makers, not regulating agencies" (p. 117). With only one alliance per region, power may become too concentrated on the demand side and result in numerous mergers on the supply side of the market. The result would be less competition, not more. In addition, with only one health alliance, it may become too easy for interest groups to exert political pressure on the system.

The Collapse of the Clinton Health Care Plan

When former president Bill Clinton unveiled his plan to reform the U.S. health care system on September 22, 1993, public support was initially strong.[13] Early public opinion polls reported twice as many people supporting as opposing the Clinton plan (Rockman, 1995). By the summer of 1994, support for the Clinton plan had dipped to about 40 percent, and it was highly unlikely that any comprehensive health care package would be enacted. The final blow was the election of November 1994, which gave the Republican party control of the House of Representatives. The question now becomes: Why did support for the Clinton health care reform plan erode so rapidly?

The most obvious explanation is that the Clinton health care plan lacked the necessary political support in Congress. Brady and Buckley (1995) utilize the median voter hypothesis to address that possibility. The median position is the middle position at which an equal number is above or below it. As a result, the median position represents the decisive or swing position under a simple majority voting rule (that is, 51 percent agreement). By observing the characteristics of the median voter, we can identify whether a policy under consideration is likely to pass or fail.

Brady and Buckley rank each member of the 103rd Congress from most to least liberal (or most to least conservative) and argue that the Clinton plan would pass only if it mustered the support of the median voter in each house of Congress. Without the support of those members of Congress, the Clinton health care plan had little or no chance of becoming law. After reviewing the voting records of those legislators at or near the 50th position in the Senate and the 218th position in the House (there are 435 representatives), Brady and Buckley conclude that the Clinton plan was politically to the left of the median voter in both houses of Congress and therefore would not be enacted.

Other analysts attribute the demise of the plan to its complexity and the failure of the Clinton administration to articulate the plan to the public in clear and precise terms. Many people found it difficult to understand, and, as debate over reform progressed, they began to worry more about its ill effects than the problem of health care reform. As a result, public support dwindled out of a fear of the unknown.

Steinman and Watts (1995) point to the political institutions in the United States that are biased against reform. Our political system is based on the federalist model, in which political power is fragmented and shared among many groups. This situation "yields enormous power to intransigent interest groups and thus makes efforts" at reform extremely difficult (p. 329). With our system of government, political interest groups have the ability to put pressure on the political process to effectively block any meaningful reform. Also, because the period of debate was so protracted, opponents of reform had time to muster a public relations campaign to turn public opinion against the plan.

Navarro (1995) looks at the entire episode from the perspective of class relations. The corporate or capitalist class in the United States rejected the Clinton reform package because it would weaken their hold over the working class. Any program that guarantees universal medical coverage infringes on the ability of the corporate class to dictate the terms of employment to the working class. To maintain a strong hold, it is preferable that the working class depend on the corporate class for medical coverage rather than on a government entity.

These are just a few of the many reasons being offered to explain why the Clinton health care plan collapsed. It is safe to say that a multitude of social, political, and economic factors

13. For a more comprehensive look at why the Clinton plan failed, consult the spring 1995 issues of either *Health Affairs* or the *Journal of Health Politics, Policy and Law.*

contributed to the failure of the plan. Yankelovich (1995) summarizes the entire process best: "Technical experts designed it, special interests argued it, political leaders sold it, journalists more interested in the political ramifications than its contents kibitzed it, and advertising attacked it. There was no way for the average American to understand what it meant for them" (p. 9).

Summary

The advanced state of technology is the greatest strength of the U.S. health care system. Premature babies, sometimes weighing much less than 2 pounds, face a relatively good chance of surviving if they are born in the United States because of the state of technology. A relatively high life expectancy after age 80 is another reflection of the advanced state of health care technology in the United States. That is, people age 80 and older in the United States tend to live longer than their counterparts in most other countries because of the abundance of advanced medical technologies. Also, the United States continues to be the world leader in pharmaceutical innovation. As mentioned in the text, pharmaceutical products save, extend, and improve the quality of lives.

Unfortunately, the U.S. health care system is not without weaknesses. Its most glaring weakness is exemplified by the fact that nearly 16 percent of the population is without health insurance. The lack of health insurance creates medical access problems and subjects a family's income to the vagaries of health status. The inability to successfully control costs is another major weakness of the U.S. health care system. The growth of health care costs continues unabated, although the pace has slowed in recent years mostly due to the influence of managed care organizations. Whether managed care can continue to slow the growth of health care costs remains questionable.

Eliminating the weaknesses while maintaining the strengths is a challenge faced by any plan for changing the U.S. health care system. Indeed, much of the debate on health care reform reflects that dilemma. This chapter presented four generic health care reform plans to provide insight into the health care reform debate in the United States.

The managed-competition plan calls for government intervention. The key to this plan is the formation of health alliances, government-sponsored organizations that negotiate with private insurance companies for competitively priced medical insurance. Also, employers are mandated to provide health insurance to employees.

The national health insurance plan calls for the most extensive level of government involvement in medical markets. With this plan, the government replaces the private insurance market by offering a national health insurance plan that covers all citizens for medical expenses. Furthermore, global budgets and price controls are utilized to contain the growth of medical costs over time.

The MSA plan is the most market oriented of the four plans. With this plan, consumers are allowed to contribute to medical savings accounts with pretax income to pay for routine medical expenses. Low-cost catastrophic medical insurance with high deductibles is also available to pay for major medical expenses.

The individual mandate plan also relies heavily on the market mechanism to allocate medical resources. Consumers are required to purchase a private medical insurance plan that covers basic medical care. To make this possible, the government guarantees that basic insurance coverage is available throughout the country at a competitive price through a government-sponsored fallback plan. In addition, tax credits and subsidies are available to further lower the price for those who cannot afford health insurance.

These four plans capture the essence of most of the health care reform plans currently being considered. The vast differences among the plans indicate the many opinions concerning what ails the U.S. health care system and what needs to be done to correct those ailments.

We also saw that the states have taken a very active role in health care reform. Almost every state has wrestled with health care reform. Despite the fact that the policies vary immensely across states, the goal is always the same: to simultaneously contain the growth of health care costs while improving access to quality care.

The chapter closed with a basic blueprint of the Clinton health care plan. The Clinton health care plan represents the sixth time during the 20th century that the United States has debated a greatly expanded role for government in health care. Previous debates took place in the late 1910s, the 1930s, the late 1940s, the 1960s, the 1970s, and the 1990s. Only once—during the 1960s, when the Medicaid and Medicare programs were instituted—were proponents of government involvement in medical care successful (Skocpol, 1995).

Case Studies

16-1 Medicare Prescription Drug Benefits[14]

A new Medicare prescription drug benefit took effect in January 2006. The plan is designed to allow seniors to buy private policies, subsidized and regulated by Medicare, to help cover the costs of prescription drugs. There is considerable variation in the costs and benefits of the private policies. Insurers view their participation as a way to sell insurance to a new group of customers. To aid seniors in choosing a plan, the government developed a web site that allows seniors to enter their medications and preferred pharmacies in order to find a plan that best suits their needs. Health experts encourage seniors to sign up on time because for each month a person is late signing up, she will automatically pay 1 percent more in monthly premiums. Seniors are also advised to weigh costs carefully, as they will be responsible for a substantial amount of the costs in the form of monthly premiums, deductibles, and copayments. In most locations, seniors can find plans for less than $20 a month, but these plans do not always offer the most coverage. Seniors are also confronted with the "doughnut hole" problem: after beneficiaries meet their deductible, they must pay 25 percent of the medical costs until their bill reaches $2,250 in one year. After that threshold is met, beneficiaries pay all the costs until the bill reaches $3,600, when the benefits kick in again and cover 95 percent of the costs for the rest of the year. Plans that eliminate the "doughnut hole" have higher monthly premiums. Seniors are also directed to contact their former employers because many will continue to get drug coverage through their existing retirement benefits. Finally, seniors are encouraged to consider all alternatives and find out whether they have Medigap, or Medicare supplement policies that cover deductibles and other out-of-pocket costs Medicare does not cover. Seniors who had Medigap plans when the new benefit was implemented may choose to keep them, but the government does not subsidize those policies.

14. Source: Sarah Lueck, "Medicare's Drug Plan: What to Do Now," *The Wall Street Journal,* September 14, 2005.

Questions for Discussion

1. *Describe the selection issues with a voluntary program like this. Who is most likely to enroll or not enroll?*
2. *Why are large pharmaceutical companies opposed to this program, even if a large proportion of the program expenditures will ultimately flow to those companies?*
3. *Speculate as to why this program was not structured like the other Medicare benefit programs, which essentially offer first-dollar reimbursement for most inpatient and outpatient services.*

16-2 Can Quebec Ban Private Health Plans?[15]

In June 2005, Canada's Supreme Court ruled that Quebec's prohibition on private insurance for services that the public system covers violated Quebec's bill of rights. The public system in Canada has long provided health care to all citizens for no charge beyond their already existing taxes. Some health care professionals saw the ruling as recognition that Canadians should have the right to pay for privately insured medical services as a way to alleviate backlogs in the public system, which included waiting hours in an emergency room or waiting months for cancer treatment and other scheduled procedures. Experts anticipated that the ruling would lead to business opportunities for U.S. health care providers. The demand for private services was expected to center on non-urgent care, with the most urgent and life-threatening cases continuing to be routed through the public system. The Quebec government indicated it would ask the Supreme Court to stay the ruling so it could make adjustments in the system that may include changing the existing law or attempting to reduce the waiting times for many services. Policy experts believed the ruling would spawn legal challenges in other provinces, but it was not clear whether such challenges would have the same success.

Questions for Discussion

1. *Why is there a market for private insurance in a country with a national health care system offering coverage to all individuals?*
2. *Assume that the ruling results in the entry of private health insurers into health insurance markets. Discuss the potential role, if any, of adverse selection.*
3. *Discuss how the Canadian health system is likely to evolve in Quebec and other provinces if the entry of private health insurers is permitted. In addition to considering your answer to the previous question, also consider issues pertaining to financing, such as a voucher system for those "opting out" of the national system.*

16-3 A Single-Payer System in California?

In 2005, the California legislature debated a bill, Senate Bill 840, which would have created a statewide single-payer system similar to that of Canada's. Unlike previous attempts at similar legislation, the bill was not immediately dismissed, and was modified and carried over to be voted on in the 2006 legislative session. One reason that the bill survived the first cut was likely a favorable report by the Lewin Group, which found that the net effects of the legislation were positive; new costs incurred by the program would be more than offset by savings from reduced administrative expenses and bulk purchasing from providers and pharmaceutical companies. At the beginning of the 2006 legislative session, the Health Economics Consulting Group released its

15. Source: Christopher J. Chipello, "Shock Treatment for Canadian Health Care," *The Wall Street Journal*, June 13, 2005.

own evaluation of the legislation, and found that, contrary to the Lewin report, the new program would incur net losses in the first five years, and possibly longer, mainly because SB 840 would essentially eliminate the $64 billion health insurance industry in California and would face many, if not all, of the same forces applying upward pressure on health care costs nationwide.

Questions for Discussion

1. *During debates over the bill, and in single-payer debates in general, the success of the Canadian system is touted by single-payer supporters. Assuming that a single-payer plan like SB 840 was politically viable enough to become law, discuss some of the likely challenges that the plan would face in the United States. In other words, one key question is, "It works in Canada, but will it work here?" Consider differences between the United States and Canada in medical care prices and organization, per capita income, and demographics.*
2. *The two delivery models—a government single-payer or a private "system"—each have strengths and weaknesses. Using a table format, compare the two systems in how they might address access, quality, costs, and adaptation. Does a clear winner emerge?*

Review Questions and Problems

1. Discuss the four generic plans for health care reform in terms of the general model of a health care system presented in Chapter 4. Pay particular attention to the role third-party payers play in each plan.
2. Discuss each of the four generic plans for health care reform in terms of theories X and Y.
3. Which of the four generic plans of health care reform appeals to you the most? Substantiate your opinion using economic theory.
4. Which generic health care plan would best correct moral hazard? Why? Which generic plan would best achieve scale economies in health insurance administration? Why? Which plan would provide the most variety? Why?
5. Choose a state other than one of the four discussed in the chapter, and research any basic changes in health care policy that have been made or are currently being considered.
6. Discuss the main features of the Clinton health care reform plan, and provide some reasons why it was not enacted.
7. Use economic theory to explain how employees may end up paying for at least a portion of mandated health insurance in terms of forgone wages.

Online Resources

To access Internet links related to the topics in this chapter, please visit our web site at **www.thomsonedu.com/economics/santerre**.

References

Aaron, Henry J. *Serious and Unstable Condition: Financing America's Health Care.* Washington, D.C.: The Brookings Institution, 1991.

Barrand, Nancy L., and Steven Schroeder. "Lessons from the States." *Inquiry* 31 (spring 1994), pp. 10–13.

Blewett, Lynn A. "Reforms in Minnesota: Forging the Path." *Health Affairs* 13 (fall 1994), pp. 200–9.

Bodenheimer, Thomas. "The Oregon Health Plan—Lessons for the Nation." *New England Journal of Medicine* 337 (August 28, 1997), pp. 651–55.

Brady, David W., and Kara M. Buckley. "Health Care Reform in the 103d Congress: A Predictable Failure." *Journal of Health Politics, Policy and Law* 20 (spring 1995), pp. 447–84.

Bureau of the Census, Statistical Abstract of the United States (various years), http://www.census.gov/statab/www/(accessed March 8, 2006).

Caldwell, Bert W. "The Cost of Medical Care from the Viewpoint of the Hospital." In *Hospitals and the Cost of Medical Care*. Papers of the American Conference of Hospital Services. Chicago: American Hospital Association, February 18, 1930.

Chenery, William L. "Hospital Fees Hit the Middle Class Hard." *The New York Times*, November 9, 1924, p. 7.

Dranove, David. *What's Your Life Worth?* Upper Saddle River, N.J.: Prentice Hall, 2003.

Enthoven, Alain C. "The History and Principles of Managed Competition." *Health Affairs* (supplement 1993), pp. 24–48.

Enthoven, Alain C., and Richard Kronick. "A Consumer-Choice Health Plan for the 1990s." Parts 1 and 2. *New England Journal of Medicine* 320 (January 5, 1989), pp. 29–37, and (January 12, 1989), pp. 94–101.

Enthoven, Alain C., and Sara J. Singer. "Market-Based Reform: What to Regulate and by Whom?" *Health Affairs* 14 (spring 1995), pp. 105–19.

Gilmer, Todd, and Richard Kronick. "It's the Premiums, Stupid: Projections of the Uninsured through 2013." *Health Affairs*, Web Exclusive, http://www.healthaffairs.org, April 5, 2005.

Goodman, John C., and Gerald L. Musgrave. *Patient Power: Solving America's Health Care Crisis*. Washington, D.C.: Cato Institute, 1992.

Hadley, Jack, and John Holahan. "Covering the Uninsured: How Much Would It Cost?" *Health Affairs*, Web Exclusive, June 4, 2003.

Health Trends in Hawaii, http://www.healthtrends.org.

Heffley, Dennis R., and Thomas J. Miceli. "The Economics of Incentive-Based Health Plans." *Journal of Risk and Insurance* 65 (September 1998), pp. 445–65.

Heffler, Stephen, Sheila Smith, Sean Keehan, Christine Borger, M. Kent Clemens, and Christopher Truffer. "Trends: U.S. Health Spending Projections for 2004–2014." *Health Affairs*, Web Exclusive, http://www.healthaffairs.org, February 23, 2005.

Himmelstein, David, and Steffie Woolhandler. "A National Health Program for the United States." *New England Journal of Medicine* 320 (January 12, 1989), pp. 102–8.

Intergovernment Health Policy Project. *Profiles of the States and Health Care Reform*. Washington, D.C.: George Washington University, July 1993.

Joint Task Force on Health Care Costs and Quality. "The Health Care Capital Expenditure Reporting Law: Report to the Minnesota Legislature." St. Paul: Minnesota Department of Health, February 2003.

Kronick, Richard, David C. Goodman, John Wennberg, and Edward Wagner. "The Marketplace in Health Care Reform: The Demographic Limitations of Managed Competition." *New England Journal of Medicine* 328 (January 14, 1993), pp. 148–52.

Leichter, Howard M. "Minnesota: The Trip from Acrimony to Accommodation." *Health Affairs* 12 (summer 1993), pp. 48–57.

Long, Sharon K., and Stephanie J. Kendall. "Recent Changes in Health Policy for Low-Income People in Minnesota." Washington, D.C.: Urban Institute, March 2002.

Maryland Health Care Commission. "Ensuring the Viability of the CSHBP and the Small Group Market: Options for Reform." Baltimore: MHCC, November 22, 2005.

Maryland Hospital Association. "Achievement, Access and Accountability: A Guide to Hospital Rate Regulation in Maryland." Elkridge: MHA, January 2002.

Minnesota Department of Health. *MinnesotaCare Interim Growth Limits Changed to Cost Containment*. February 1998.

Musgrave, Gerald L. "Health Economics Outlook: Two Theories of Health Economics." *Business Economics* (April 1993), pp. 7–13.

Navarro, Vincente. "Why Congress Did Not Enact Health Care Reform." *Journal of Health Politics, Policy and Law* 20 (spring 1995), pp. 455–62.

Oregon Health Services Commission. "Prioritization of Health Services: A Report to the Governor and the 73rd Oregon Legislative Assembly." Salem: OHSC, March 2005.

Organization for Economic Cooperation and Development, http://www.oecd.org.

Pauly, Mark, Patricia Danzon, Paul Feldstein, and John Hoff. "A Plan for Responsible National Health Insurance." *Health Affairs* 10 (spring 1991), pp. 5–25.

Pollitz, Karen, Eliza Bangit, Kevin Lucia, Jennifer Libster, Nadja Ruzica, and Mila Kofman. "A Consumer's Guide to Getting and Keeping Health Insurance in Minnesota." Washington, D.C.: Georgetown University Health Policy Institute, December 2004.

Pollitz, Karen, Kevin Lucie, Eliza Bangit, and Mila Kofman. "A Consumer's Guide to Getting and Keeping Health Insurance in Hawaii." Washington, D.C.: Georgetown University Health Policy Institute, October 2005.

Rockman, Bert A. "The Clinton Presidency and Health Care Reform." *Journal of Health Politics, Policy and Law* 20 (spring 1995), pp. 399–402.

Skocpol, Theda. "The Rise and Resounding Demise of the Clinton Plan." *Journal of Health Politics, Policy and Law* 19 (spring 1995), pp. 86–98.

Steinman, Sven, and Jon Watts. "It's the Institutions, Stupid! Why Comprehensive National Health Insurance Always Fails in America." *Journal of Health Politics, Policy and Law* 19 (spring 1995), pp. 329–72.

Stevens, Rosemary. *In Sickness and in Wealth*. New York: Basic Books, 1987.

Summers, Lawrence H. "Some Simple Economics of Mandated Benefits." *American Review* 79 (May 1989), pp. 177–83.

Tanner, Michael. "Medical Savings Accounts: Answering the Critics." *Policy Analysis*, no. 228 (May 25, 1995).

_____. "Laboratory Failures: States Are No Model for Health Care Reform." *Policy Analysis*, no. 207 (September 23, 1993).

Tripoli, Leigh. "Agoraphobia: What Ails Most of the Conservative Proposals to Reform Health Care." *Business Economics* (April 1993), pp. 30–35.

Yankelovich, Daniel. "The Debate That Wasn't: The Public and the Clinton Plan." *Health Affairs* 14 (spring 1995), pp. 7–23.

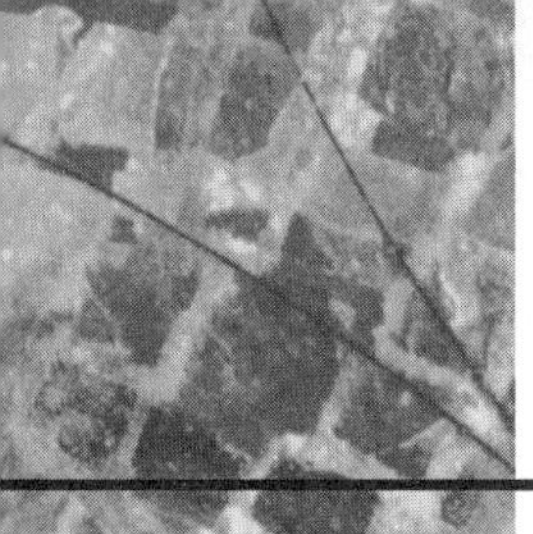

GLOSSARY

activities of daily living (ADL) A predetermined list of everyday activities used to assess whether an individual needs long-term health care.

actual competition The level of competition or rivalry as determined by the number of firms currently operating in the market.

adverse selection Occurs when an individual with poor health acquires low-risk medical insurance meant for healthy consumers. Results when an asymmetry of information develops between the insurer and the subscriber concerning the subscriber's true health status.

advertising Promotional activities undertaken by a firm to either manipulate the demand for its product or provide more information to consumers. (See *informational advertising, persuasive advertising*, and *reminder advertising*.)

advertising intensity Advertising expenditures divided by sales.

Agency for Health Policy Research A government agency established to develop outcomes research and medical care guidelines for physician services.

agency theory Models a situation in which a principal (say external stockholders) hires a manager (an agent) to run the affairs of the business. Because the principal may be rationally ignorant of the current policies of the company, the agent may pursue goals that conflict with the objectives of the principal. To better align the interests of the agent with those of the principal, the proper design of the compensation package is an important consideration. For medical care, an important agency relationship holds between the patient and physician.

allocative efficiency The condition in which the optimal amount of output is produced given the underlying structure of social benefits and costs. (See *production possibilities curve*.)

American Medical Association (AMA) A national organization founded in 1897 that represents the collective interests of physicians.

antitrust laws A body of legislation aimed at promoting competition in the U.S. economy.

applied research See *technology*.

assignment A policy under Medicare in which physicians agree to accept a guaranteed payment for their services and in return forgo the right to balance-bill Medicare patients.

asymmetry of information The situation in which two economic agents in a market transaction have different amounts of relevant information. Asymmetry may allow the agent with more information to practice opportunistic behavior.

average fixed costs Total fixed costs divided by the quantity of output.

average product Total output divided by the level of a factor input, such as labor.

average total costs Total costs divided by the quantity of output.

average variable costs Total variable costs divided by the quantity of output.

balance-billing A situation in which medical care providers bill patients in excess of the price established by a third-party payer.

Balanced Budget Act of 1997 (BBA) An act passed by Congress in 1997 that significantly expands the role of managed care in the Medicare Program. (See also *Medicare + Choice*.)

Balanced Budget Refinement Act of 1999 (BBRA) An act passed by Congress in 1999 that allowed health care providers more time to accommodate many of the changes called for in the Balanced Budget Act of 1997.

barrier to entry An obstacle that prevents firms from costlessly entering a particular market. In the health care field, barriers can exist because of cost structure or legal restrictions.

basic research See *technology*.

Blue Cross/Blue Shield A traditionally not-for-profit insurance company that provides medical insurance for hospital (Blue Cross) and physician (Blue Shield) services.

bounded rationality The notion that people, in general, have a limited ability to formulate and solve problems at a point in time.

boycott An agreement among competitors in a given input or output market not to do business with a particular supplier or customer. Boycotting is prohibited by the Sherman Antitrust Act.

brand loyalty advantage See *first mover*.

capitation payment A method of payment for medical services in which medical care providers receive a fixed payment per person in return for providing medical care services regardless of the quantity of medical care delivered.

Centers for Medicare & Medicaid Services Formerly known as the Health Care Financing Administration; a federal agency responsible for administering the Medicare, Medicaid, and SCHIP programs.

certificate of need (CON) laws State laws requiring health care providers to receive permission from a state agency before making a capital purchase above a stipulated amount.

ceteris paribus A Latin phrase meaning "all other factors remaining constant."

cherry picking A practice by private insurance companies of offering medical insurance to individuals they believe to be healthy while denying coverage to those they believe to be unhealthy.

clinical investigation See *technology*.

clinical need The quantity of medical care that a clinical expert prescribes as though medical care were a free good.

coinsurance A component of a medical insurance plan in which consumers pay a fixed percentage of the cost of medical care.

collusive oligopoly An oligopolistic-type market structure in which all the firms in the industry jointly maximize profits as if they all acted collectively as a monopolist.

community rating A method used by third-party payers to establish insurance premiums based on the average benefits paid out for the total population served. In this case, premiums reflect the average health risk factors for the entire population served.

comparative static analysis A comparison of the initial and new equilibrium points after an external change alters the model.

compensating wage differential The increase in wages needed to attract the marginal worker to a given occupation because there is an added cost to entering the occupation, such as a professional license.

competitive oligopoly A product market characterized by a few dominant sellers that act competitively and do not coordinate their activities. (See *oligopoly.*)

complements Two goods that are used together in consumption. Two goods are complements in consumption if an increase in the price of one good causes a decrease in the demand for the other.

compulsory licensing The situation in which one firm is required by law to grant to another firm the opportunity to import or manufacture a patented drug for a royalty.

concentration ratio Measures the percentage of industry output produced by the largest firms in an industry. For example, the four firm concentration ratio identifies the percentage of industry output produced by the four largest firms.

concurrent utilization review A program to contain medical costs that evaluates the necessity of continual care. (See *utilization review programs.*)

conjectural variations The beliefs a firm has regarding how its rivals will react to its own price and output decisions.

constant returns to scale Exist when a percentage increase in all factor inputs leads to a proportionately equal increase in output. The long-run average cost curve is horizontal if constant returns to scale exist.

consumer price index (CPI) A price index that measures the cost of purchasing a fixed market basket of consumer goods and services over time. The CPI is used to measure the consumer price inflation rate from one period to the next.

consumer surplus The difference between what consumers are willing to pay for a product and the market clearing price. As such, consumer surplus is represented by the area under the demand curve but above market price.

copayment A fixed amount paid by consumers for medical care that is independent of the market price.

cost-benefit analysis A method of analysis used for decision making that estimates the total costs and benefits of an activity.

cost effectiveness analysis A method of analysis used for decision making that estimates the total costs of achieving a defined health care objective, such as a life-year saved, from a medical treatment or health behavior.

cost identification study A study that measures the total costs of a particular medical condition. Cost identification considers direct medical costs, direct nonmedical costs, and indirect costs.

cost shifting The practice of charging a higher price for a medical service in one market to compensate for a lower administered price.

cost-utility analysis A method of analysis used to make policy decisions that considers the quantity as well as the quality of life-years saved from a medical intervention. (See *cost effectiveness analysis.*)

credence attributes The characteristics of a good or service that can be assessed only after repeated purchases. Most medical care products possess credence characteristics.

cross-price elasticity An elasticity measure of the extent to which the quantity demanded of one product changes with respect to a change in the price of an alternative product. In precise terms, it equals the percentage change in the quantity demanded of one product divided by the percentage change in the price of another product. If the value of the ratio is negative, the two products are complements; if the ratio is positive, the two products are substitutes.

customary, prevailing, and reasonable rate See *usual, customary, and reasonable rate.*

cyclical uninsurance The condition of individuals who are uninsured because of variations in the business cycle.

data envelopment analysis (DEA) A statistical technique used by researchers to estimate the technical efficiency of organizations.

deadweight loss The social surplus not realized because resources are misallocated.

decreasing returns to scale Exist when a percentage increase in all factor inputs leads to a less than proportional increase in output.

deductible An annual out-of-pocket, lump-sum payment for medical services that a consumer must pay before medical insurance provides reimbursement.

defensive medicine The overutilization of medical services by a health care provider in order to prevent a potential medical malpractice suit.

demand The quantities of a good or service that a consumer is willing and able to purchase at various prices at a specific point in time. The market demand for a product equals the total demand for an entire population.

demand curve A graphical depiction of the relationship between quantity demanded and the price of a good or service. The market demand curve equals the horizontal summation of consumers' individual demand curves.

demand function A mathematical expression containing the various factors that influence the quantity demanded of a given product.

demand-side subsidy A payment of funds generally directed at consumers to purchase goods and services.

dependent variable A variable whose value is influenced by the value of one or more independent variables.

deselection The termination of a health care provider in a medical network based on an established set of criteria.

diagnosis-related group (DRG) A prospective reimbursement system developed under Medicare used to compensate hospitals based primarily on the patient's primary diagnosis. (See *prospective payment system.*)

diffusion See *technology.*

direct medical care costs All costs incurred by medical care providers resulting from a particular medical intervention.

direct nonmedical costs All nonmedical costs resulting from a particular medical intervention.

discount rate The rate of interest used to discount a future stream of payments. (See *present value.*)

discovery by design The use of scientific knowledge to discover and develop new drugs.

disease management program A program in which health care interventions are coordinated and patients take an active role in their own care.

diseconomies of scale Exist when the average cost of production increases with the level of output.

disproportionate share hospital payments Additional reimbursement payments received by states from the federal government for the Medicaid program to defer the high cost of providing medical care to a large number of low-income individuals.

distributive justice Achieving fairness in the way that goods and services are distributed to members of society. (See *horizontal equity* and *vertical equity.*)

Dorfman-Steiner model A model of the determinants of advertising expenditures. For a monopolist, the Dorfman-Steiner condition states that optimal advertising intensity is equal to the ratio of the advertising elasticity of demand to the own-price elasticity of demand. It also equals the price-cost margin as a percentage of price times the advertising elasticity of demand.

doughnut hole The portion of the Part D benefit structure in which the enrollee pays 100 percent of the cost of prescription drugs. For 2006, the doughnut hole begins when total annual spending for drugs reaches $2,250 and concludes when total annual spending for drugs surpasses $5,100.

drug utilization review Programs that control costs by reviewing the prescribing behavior of physicians to ensure that formularies are followed and inappropriate medicines are not prescribed.

dual-market model An economic model that illustrates how a producer decides to participate or operate in two different market segments.

economic model A simplified depiction of a complex economic phenomenon used by economists to examine economic behavior.

economic profit Total revenues minus total costs, including both explicit and implicit costs.

economies of scale Exist when the average cost of production decreases with the quantity of output.

economies of scope Exist when the total cost of jointly producing two or more products is cheaper than the total cost of producing each product individually.

elastic Describes a situation in which the absolute value of the elasticity is greater than 1, or the percentage change in the dependent variable is greater than the percentage change in the independent variable, in absolute value terms.

elasticity A measure economists use to gauge the extent to which one variable changes in response to a change in another variable. It equals the percentage change in a dependent variable divided by the percentage change in an independent variable.

elasticity of input substitution An elasticity measure of the extent to which two inputs can be substituted for each other in the production process. In precise terms, it equals the percentage change in the input rate divided by the percentage change in the marginal products of the two inputs.

employer mandate A health care reform plan that requires employers to provide medical care insurance to employees.

endogenous Describes factors that are determined in the economic model, such as price and quantity in the supply-and-demand model.

enthusiasm hypothesis The hypothesis that geographic variations in the utilization of certain types of medical procedures reflect differences in medical preferences among physicians.

equilibrium Exists when there is no tendency for further change. Market equilibrium occurs in the supply-and-demand model when quantity demanded equals quantity supplied at the market clearing price.

excess burden The burden created by a tax when a wedge is driven between marginal benefits and costs and thereby distorts productive incentives.

exclusive dealing contract A situation in which a distributor agrees to sell only the manufacturer's products and not the products of a manufacturer's competitors.

exclusive provider organization (EPO) A type of preferred provider organization that provides zero reimbursement to enrollees who acquire medical care from health care providers not included in the network.

exogenous Describes factors that are determined outside the economic model, such as buyer income or tastes and preferences in the supply-and-demand model.

expected utility model A model that assumes that people maximize their expected utility rather than actual utility. Maximizing expected utility serves as the objective because people often make decisions with imperfect information such that individual events occurring involve some uncertainty. For instance, a person may derive utility from medical care but only when a state of sickness triggers the necessity for medical care. Expected utility represents the weighted average of the actual utility levels, with the probabilities of the actual utility levels occurring serving as the weights.

experience attributes The characteristics of a good or service that can be assessed only after the product has been purchased.

experience rating A method used by third-party payers to establish insurance premiums based on the expected benefits paid out as a result of individual health risk factors.

explicit costs Payments made to nonowners of the firm.

extensive margin The market change in the quantity demanded for a product brought about by a price change because more (fewer) consumers buy the product when its price decreases (increases).

externality Exists when the actions of a market participant affect another participant in either an adverse or a beneficial fashion and no financial compensation takes place. An externality can emanate from either the demand or the supply side of the market.

extra billing The situation in which a health care provider bills a patient in excess of a preset fee established by a third party for health care provided.

fee-for-service payment A method of payment for medical care services in which a medical care provider receives an individual payment for each medical service provided.

firm An organization that is responsible for coordinating the transformation of inputs, such as land, labor, capital, and entrepreneurship, into some final output or outputs.

first-dollar coverage A health insurance plan that reimburses an individual for all medical care expenses, beginning with the first dollar spent on medical care.

first mover A firm that poses a barrier to entry by being the first to introduce a product to a given market. Potential competitors must overcome the problem of name recognition if they wish to enter the market.

fixed costs Costs of production that remain constant regardless of the level of production.

fixed payment A payment that is independent of the actual costs or quantity of medical services delivered.

Flexner Report A report published in 1910 that was highly critical of the medical training physicians received in the United States and Canada. As a result, numerous changes were made in the education and training of physicians.

Food and Drug Administration (FDA) A government agency that regulates the introduction of new drugs in the United States.

formulary A list of low-cost, effective pharmaceutical products that physicians are required to prescribe whenever possible. Hospitals and other health care providers use formularies to control costs.

for-profit organization An organization owned by private individuals. Ownership gives the individuals a claim on any residual profits.

frictional uninsurance The condition of individuals who are uninsured because they are temporarily between jobs or searching for a suitable insurance policy.

function A mathematical expression that establishes a relationship between the value of a dependent variable and a set of values for the independent variables.

fuzzy demand curve A demand curve for medical care reflecting the possibility that the relationship between the price and quantity demanded of medical care may not be exact or precisely known.

gag rules Rules that prohibit a physician in a managed care plan from discussing alternative treatment options not covered by the health insurance plan, providing information on the limitations of the plan, and commenting negatively about the plan to patients.

generic drug A drug that is bioequivalent to a brand-name drug.

global budgeting A method used by third-party payers to control medical care costs by establishing total expenditure limits for medical services over a specified period of time.

group-model health maintenance organization A health maintenance organization (HMO) that contracts with group physician practices. (See *health maintenance organization*.)

guaranteed renewability Contractual feature of an insurance policy that requires the insurer to renew the policy on its anniversary date and not charge a premium for that policy based on an individual's personal loss experience.

Hatch-Waxman Act of 1984 The Drug Price Competition and Patent Term Restoration Act, which extended the effective life of a new drug product and shortened the approval process for generic drugs.

health The condition of being of sound body and mind and free of any disease or physical pain.

health alliance A public agency that uses its bargaining power to negotiate competitive prices for health insurance from the private insurance market. (See *managed competition*.)

Health Care Financing Administration (HCFA) An agency of the U.S. Department of Health and Human Services that was created to oversee the financing and quality-control programs for Medicare and the federal portion of Medicaid. The agency has since been renamed the Centers for Medicaid & Medicare Services.

health care system The organizational and institutional structures through which an economy makes choices regarding the production, consumption, and distribution of health care services.

health economics A field of economics that uses economic theory to study how an economy utilizes scarce health care resources to provide and distribute medical care.

health insurance mandate A requirement that an insurance company or a health plan cover specific benefits, health care providers, or patient populations.

Health Insurance Portability and Accountability Act of 1996 An act of Congress that addresses the nonportability of health insurance by making it more difficult for insurers to segment markets and deny individuals or groups health insurance based on health status.

health maintenance organization (HMO) A health care delivery system that combines the insurer and producer functions. HMOs are prepaid and in return provide comprehensive services to enrollees.

health production function A mathematical expression that shows the relationship between an individual's health and a number of variables, including the amount of health care consumed. (See *production function.*)

health-utility index A scale used to measure the quality of life remaining. (See *rating scale, standard gamble model,* and *time trade-off.*)

Herfindahl-Hirschman index An index used to measure the degree of industry concentration in a given market. It is measured by squaring and then summing the market shares of all of the firms in the same industry.

home health care Health care delivered at the home of the patient by a health care provider.

horizontal equity Equity that is achieved when, for example, individuals with similar incomes pay equal amounts of taxes and receive the same amounts of subsidies; in other words, equals are treated equally.

horizontal merger A merger between two firms in the same market.

hospice care Palliative care provided to a patient who is terminally ill.

Hospital Insurance program See *Part A.*

human capital approach Equates the value of a human life to the discounted market value of the output produced by an individual over an expected lifetime.

image differentiation The use by a firm of promotional activities to differentiate consumers' perceptions of its product relative to other products in the market.

imperfect consumer information The assumption that consumers lack all the information necessary to make informed decisions concerning the appropriate quantity and type of medical care to consume.

implicit costs Costs that measure the opportunity cost of utilizing resources owned by the firm.

income effect The increase (decrease) in quantity demanded brought about by an increase (decrease) in real income when the price of a product decreases (increases). The concept is used to derive a downward-sloping demand curve.

income elasticity of demand An elasticity measure of the extent to which the quantity demanded changes with a change in income. In precise terms, it equals the percentage change in the quantity demanded divided by the percentage change in income.

inconsistency See *service.*

increasing returns to scale Exist when a percentage increase in all factor inputs leads to a greater percentage increase in output.

incremental cost effectiveness ratio (ICER) A measure that gauges the relative value of one medical intervention over another. The numerator of the ratio equals the cost of a new medical intervention minus the cost of an established medical intervention, and the denominator of the ratio equals the difference in effectiveness between the new and established medical intervention. (See *cost effectiveness analysis.*)

indemnity insurance Medical insurance that reimburses the insured a fixed amount for each type of medical service consumed.

independent provider association (IPA) A type of health maintenance organization that contracts with a number of independent medical care providers to deliver medical services at a discounted price or on a capitation basis.

independent variable A variable whose values are predetermined and influence the value of a dependent variable.

indirect costs All nonmonetary costs, such as time costs, incurred from a given medical intervention.

individual mandates A health care reform plan that requires individuals to purchase their own medical insurance. Tax credits and subsidies would be available to those who cannot afford to purchase medical insurance.

inelastic Describes a situation in which the absolute value of the elasticity is less than 1, or the percentage change in the dependent variable is less than the percentage change in the independent variable, in absolute value terms.

inferior good A good for which demand decreases when consumers experience an increase in income.

informational advertising Advertising that provides information to consumers.

in-kind subsidy Specific goods or vouchers provided to a defined population, such as the needy.

inseparability See *service*.

instrumental activities of daily living (IADL) A predetermined list of daily activities used to assess whether an individual needs long-term health care.

insurance premium The cost of medical insurance to the consumer. In the private insurance market, it equals the sum of expected benefits paid out, administrative costs, taxes, and profits. (See also *community rating* and *experience rating*.)

intangibility See *service*.

integrated delivery system (IDS) A legal or contractual combination of buyers and suppliers, such as medical organizations, producing different medical services—for example, physician groups, hospitals, and nursing homes.

intensive margin The market change in the quantity demanded for a product brought about by a price change because consumers buy more (less) of the product when its price decreases (increases).

inventory See *service*.

job lock The situation in which an individual cannot change jobs without potentially losing medical care insurance for a given period of time.

joint probability The probability that two events occur simultaneously. It is calculated by multiplying the individual probabilities of the events occurring.

law of demand An economic principle stating that the quantity demanded of a good or service is inversely related to its price.

law of diminishing marginal product An economic principle stating that as units of an input are used in production, a point is eventually reached at which output increases by a continually smaller amount. In other words, the marginal product of the factor input begins to fall in value.

law of diminishing marginal utility An economic principle stating that as units of a product are consumed, a point is eventually reached at which total utility increases at a continually smaller rate. In other words, the marginal utility of the product begins to fall.

law of increasing opportunity cost An economic principle stating that the opportunity cost of an activity increases as more of that activity is undertaken.

law of supply An economic principle stating that the quantity supplied of a good or service increases with its price.

learning by doing The economies that result from knowledge or experience gained through the cumulative production of a product.

learning by watching Productivity of quality improvements that occur over time because of knowledge or technological change that can be easily transferred across organizations.

Lerner index Measure of market power measured by the difference between price and marginal cost (that is, the price-cost margin) expressed as a percentage of price. For a monopoly this ratio is equal to the reciprocal of the price elasticity of market demand.

lifestyle The adopted health behaviors of an individual or population like diet, exercise, and risky activities. According to economic theory, how a person or group lives impacts overall health.

limit pricing The practice of pricing a product just below the break-even point of a potential entrant as a way to discourage entry.

loading fee The portion of medical insurance premiums in excess of expected benefits paid out. Its value depends on such items as administrative costs, taxes, and the intensity of competition in the insurance market.

long run A time horizon over which all inputs in the production process are variable.

long-run average cost curve An envelope curve comprising the cost-minimizing points from a series of short-run average cost curves. It represents the lowest cost of producing each unit of output in the long run.

long-run economies of scale See *economies of scale*.

long-term care Health care provided to an individual with some disabilities over an extended period of time for the purpose of enhancing the quality of life rather than curing a particular medical problem.

loss distribution The relationship between the magnitude of the loss and its frequency of occurring. Typically, individual loss distributions are heavily skewed to the left, meaning that small (large) losses are much more (less) likely to occur.

managed care organization (MCO) An organization that controls the utilization and cost of medical care by reviewing and monitoring the appropriateness, extensiveness, and costs of medical services.

managed competition A health care reform plan that calls for the establishment of health alliances that would use their bargaining power to negotiate competitively priced medical coverage from a number of alternative private insurance companies.

managerial expense preference model A model of firm behavior positing that managers use a portion of the firm's profits to maximize their own utility.

marginal cost The change in total costs brought about by a one-unit change in the production of a product.

marginal product The change in total output brought about by a one-unit change in a factor input.

marginal rate of technical substitution The rate at which one input can be substituted for another in the production process. In precise terms, it equals the ratio of the marginal products of two inputs.

marginal revenue The addition to total revenue brought about by the sale of one more unit of output.

marginal revenue product The marginal value or worth of an additional input, such as an employee, to a company. In a competitive marketplace, it is calculated by multiplying the price of the good or service by the marginal productivity of the input.

marginal social benefit The change in total social benefit brought about by a one-unit change in the consumption of a good or service.

marginal social cost The change in total social costs resulting from a one-unit change in the production of a good or service.

marginal utility The change in total utility or satisfaction brought about by a one-unit change in the consumption of a good or service.

market allocation A collusive agreement among rival firms not to compete with one another in a given geographical market. This activity is prohibited by the Sherman Antitrust Act.

market concentration Reflects the number and size distribution of firms in an industry.

market conduct The second element in the industrial organization triad, which considers firms in terms of pricing, promotion, and research and development activities.

market failure The situation in which a market outcome fails to produce the socially optimal quantity of output or distribute income fairly.

market performance The third element in the industrial organization triad, which considers firms in terms of production and allocative efficiencies, equity, and technological progress.

market power The ability of a firm to raise the price above the competitive level.

market structure The first element in the industrial organization triad, which considers the overall environment within which each firm operates.

McGuire's quantity-setting model An economic model of physician behavior based on monopolistic competition. The model predicts the quantity-setting behavior of a physician when physicians are considered imperfect substitutes by consumers.

Medicaid A jointly financed public program between federal and state governments that provides medical insurance to certain segments of the poor population without private health insurance.

medical care Goods and services that maintain, improve, or restore an individual's physical, social, or mental well-being.

medical savings accounts A health care reform plan that allows individuals to establish tax-free savings accounts to finance primary medical care.

Medicare A federally financed program that provides medical insurance primarily to elderly individuals.

Medicare + Choice Part of the Balanced Budget Act of 1997 that significantly increased the number of managed care insurance plans available to Medicare recipients, along with altering the method in which Medicare pays for those plans. The program was replaced with Medicare Advantage in 2003.

Medicare Advantage Replaced the Medicare + Choice program with the passage of the Medicare Prescription Drug Improvement and Modernization Act of 2003. This program calls for the creation of regional PPOs and gives Medicare enrollees the option of enrolling in private insurance plans, including managed care plans.

Medicare Payment Advisory Commission (MedPAC) An independent federal agency formed by the Balanced Budget Act of 1997 to advise Congress on issues regarding the Medicare Program.

Medicare Prescription Drug Improvement and Modernization Act of 2003 The piece of legislation that established the prescription drug coverage option, Part D, under Medicare and replaced Medicare + Choice with Medicare Advantage.

Medicare volume performance standards A target rate of growth for physician expenditures under

Medicare used to establish expenditure limits and contain costs. The targets were enacted under the Omnibus Budget Act of 1989 and later repealed under the Balanced Budget Act of 1997.

medigap insurance policies Private insurance policies purchased by elderly individuals to cover some or all of their medical expenses not paid for by Medicare.

merger The combining of two or more firms.

merit good A good provided by the government because it is considered socially desirable.

microeconomics A field of economics that uses economic theory to study how individual consumers and firms make economic decisions.

molecule manipulation A method of drug discovery in which pharmaceutical companies use trial and error to determine the therapeutic value of a large number of chemical entities.

monopolistic competition A product market characterized by numerous sellers, moderate product differentiation, no barriers to entry, and some imperfections in consumer information.

monopoly A product market characterized by one seller and perfect barriers to entry.

monopoly power The ability of a monopolist in a given market to raise the price of its product. The degree of monopoly power is inversely related to the price elasticity of market demand.

monopoly rents Excess of revenues over costs that exceed the competitive rate of return.

monopsony A market characterized by a single buyer that has the ability to influence market price. According to economic theory, a monopsonist lowers price below the competitive level.

moral hazard The situation in which individuals alter their behavior after they have purchased medical insurance because they are no longer liable for the full cost of their actions.

morbidity rate The rate at which a given disease is present in a population.

mortality rate The death rate for a given population measured by the ratio of the number of deaths divided by the average size of the population during a given period.

multihospital system An organization that is made up of two or more hospitals and is managed by a single corporation.

multipayer system A system in which health care providers are reimbursed by numerous third-party payers.

multiple regression A statistical technique used by economists to estimate the relation between a dependent variable and one or more independent variables.

multisource drug A drug that is no longer under patent protection and is available from alternative suppliers.

mutual interdependence The situation in which the behavior of one firm in a given market impacts the pricing and output decisions of other firms in the market.

national health insurance (NHI) A government-sponsored health insurance system covering the entire population and financed by tax revenues. Such a system exists in Canada.

national health system (NHS) A health care system directly operated by the government and financed by general taxes. Such a system exists in Sweden and Finland.

natural monopoly A firm that faces long-run economies of scale over the entire market demand curve.

negative demand-side externality Exists when the actions of a consumer adversely affect other market participants and no financial compensation takes place.

negative supply-side externality Exists when the actions of a producer adversely affect other market participants and no financial compensation takes place.

net benefit calculus The optimizing rule used by economic agents that looks at the expected net benefits of a given activity, defined as the expected benefits minus the expected costs. When net benefits are greater than zero, the economic agent's well-being is enhanced by choosing the activity in question.

net marginal social benefit The difference between marginal social benefit and marginal social cost.

network health maintenance organization An HMO that provides physician services by contracting with more than one physician group practice.

new chemical entities (NCEs) Pharmaceutical products that contain active ingredients not previously marketed in the United States.

nominal Describes an economic measure that is expressed in terms of current market prices.

non-distribution constraint Law stating that non-profit organizations cannot distribute surplus earnings to individuals without regard to the charitable purpose for which the organization was formed.

normal good A good for which demand increases when consumers experience an increase in income.

normal profit Occurs when revenues are just enough to cover the opportunity cost of each and every resource used in production of a medical good or service. According to economic theory, the typical firm earns a normal profit in the long run when the market is perfectly competitive.

normative analysis The use of economic theory and empirical analysis to justify whether an economic outcome is desirable.

not-for-profit An organization that is prohibited from distributing profits.

oligopoly A product market that is characterized by a few dominant sellers and substantial barriers to entry.

Omnibus Budget Reconciliation Act of 1989 An act passed by Congress significantly reforming the method by which physicians are compensated under the Medicare program.

operating margin Earning power on ongoing operations determined by dividing operating revenues by operating expenses expressed as a percentage of operating revenues. The operating margin does not include any interest payments incurred on debt (as an expense) or interest revenues received on investments (as revenues). The operating margin also does not consider any income taxes.

opportunistic behavior The situation in which an individual pursues his or her own self-interests with guile or deceit.

opportunity cost The value of what is given up by not pursuing the next best alternative.

Orphan Drug Act An act providing incentives to pharmaceutical companies to develop drugs to treat rare diseases that are otherwise unprofitable to develop because the potential demand is low.

outcome quality The quality of medical care as measured by its end result, such as patient satisfaction or postcare morbidity or mortality.

out-of-pocket price The price consumers pay for medical care after all third-party payments have been considered.

output maximization See *quantity maximization*.

over-the-counter drug A drug that consumers can purchase without a prescription from a physician.

own-price elasticity of demand An elasticity measure of the responsiveness of quantity demanded to changes in a product's own price. In precise terms, it equals the percentage change in quantity demanded divided by the percentage change in price.

own-price elasticity of supply An elasticity measure of the responsiveness of quantity supplied to changes in price. In precise terms, it equals the percentage change in quantity supplied divided by the percentage change in price.

Part A The Hospital Insurance program under the Medicare program that primarily covers inpatient hospital services.

Part B The Supplementary Medical Insurance program under the Medicare program that primarily covers physician and outpatient medical services.

Part C A program under Medicare that gives Medicare recipients the option of enrolling in private insurance plans, including managed care plans. This program was formerly known as Medicare + Choice and is now known as Medicare Advantage.

Part D The prescription drug coverage option under Medicare established by the Medicare Prescription Drug Improvement and Modernization Act of 2003.

patent A government document that grants the legal right to an innovating firm to be the sole producer of a product for up to 20 years (in the United States).

patient dumping The situation in which a private hospital fails to admit a very sick patient because it fears that the medical bills will exceed a preset limit established by a third-party payer. As a result, the patient is forced to acquire medical care services from a public hospital.

per capita Per unit of the population.

perfect competition A product market characterized by numerous buyers and sellers, a homogeneous product, no barriers to entry, and perfect consumer information.

perfectly elastic The special case in which there is an infinite change in the value of the dependent variable when the independent variable changes in value.

perfectly inelastic The special case in which the value of the dependent variable is unresponsive to changes in the value of the independent variable.

personal health care expenditures Total expenditures by individuals on medical care goods and services.

persuasive advertising Advertising that aims to persuade consumers to purchase one product rather than others.

pharmacy benefit management (PMB) companies Intermediaries that secure favorable prices from drug manufacturers and/or pharmacies at a reduced price and offer that service to health plans for a fee.

Physician Payment Review Commission (PPRC) A commission established in 1985 to advise and make recommendations to Congress regarding physician payment reform. PPRC was replaced by MedPAC.

physician practice hypothesis A hypothesis stating that per capita variations in the use of medical care are explained by systematic differences in clinical opinions concerning the proper type and amount of medical care to prescribe.

physician profiling The process by which a managed care organization selects and monitors the performance of physicians.

point-of-service (POS) plan A type of managed care insurance plan that requires subscribers who go outside the network for medical care to pay higher out-of-pocket expenses. The purpose is to contain costs by encouraging subscribers to acquire medical care from a network of providers.

pooling arrangement An agreement in which people agree to share in each other's losses if and when they occur. Each contributes a fixed amount to a fund based on a prior agreement and draws from that fund when a loss occurs.

positive analysis The analysis of economic behavior that uses economic theory along with empirical analysis to explain what is or what happened.

positive demand-side externality Exists when the actions of a consumer beneficially affect another market participant and no financial compensation takes place.

positive supply-side externality Exists when the actions of a supplier beneficially affect another market participant and no financial compensation takes place.

potential competition The level of competition as determined by the number of firms that may enter a particular market. Potential competition is determined by the height of any barriers to entry.

practice guideline A statement concerning the known costs, benefits, and risks of using a particular medical intervention to bring about a given medical outcome.

preferred provider organization (PPO) A third-party payer that offers financial incentives, such as low out-of-pocket prices, to enrollees who acquire medical care from a preset list of physicians and hospitals.

prescription drug A drug that can be purchased only with a physician's prescription.

present value A technique used to determine today's value of a future stream of cash payments.

price ceiling A government-imposed limit on the price of a product.

price discrimination The practice of charging a different price for the same product in two or more market segments.

price fixing The practice by rival firms in the same market of acting in a collusive manner and setting prices for the purpose of increasing profits. This practice is prohibited by the Sherman Antitrust Act.

price leadership model An oligopolistic-type market structure in which the firms in a given industry agree that one firm will serve as the price leader and the others will follow its pricing and output actions.

price-payoff contract An insurance contract that compensates the consumer through a price reduction rather than a lump sum payment. A price-payoff contract potentially triggers both a substitution and income effect but helps prevent the consumer from engaging in opportunistic behavior.

price taker A firm that has no influence over the market price of its product and treats the price as a given.

primary care Medical care services that deal with the prevention, early detection, and treatment of disease.

primary care physician A physician specializing in family practice, general practice, internal medicine, obstetrics/gynecology, or pediatrics.

process quality The quality of medical care as measured by the quality of treatment.

producer surplus The net benefit producers receive equal to the difference between the price received by the producer and the marginal cost of production.

product differentiation A situation in which firms within a given market sell slightly different products.

production efficiency Achieved when one activity (production or consumption) cannot be increased without a reduction in another activity because the maximum level of output is being produced from a finite amount of inputs. (See *production possibilities curve.*)

production function A mathematical expression that shows the maximum level of output that a firm can produce using various quantities of factor inputs.

production possibilities curve (PPC) An economic model that shows the various combinations of goods an economy can produce when production efficiency is achieved. Allocative efficiency is obtained when society chooses the point on the curve that maximizes overall satisfaction. The model illustrates the economic concepts of scarcity, choice, and opportunity costs.

professional licensure The requirement that a health care professional, such as a doctor or a nurse, obtain a license from the government before being allowed to practice medicine.

profitability cycle See *underwriting cycle.*

profit margin Net income divided by total revenues or sales.

profit maximization A situation in which sellers strive to attain the greatest amount of economic profits.

progressive redistribution scheme The situation in which net taxes as a fraction of income increase with income.

property rights model A model hypothesizing that for-profit organizations are more efficient than their not-for-profit counterparts because the owners of for-profit organizations force managers to act in a cost-efficient manner and strive to maximize profits. Managers of not-for-profit organizations do not face that same pressure and may be free to pursue other objectives, such as quality maximization.

proportional redistribution scheme The situation in which net taxes as a fraction of income remain constant with income.

prospective payment system (PPS) A method of payment used by third-party payers in which payments are made on a case-by-case basis. Congress adopted a prospective payment system in 1983 when it introduced the DRG system for classifying Medicare patients.

prospective utilization review A program to control medical costs that evaluates medical decisions prior to the application of any medical treatments. (See *utilization review programs.*)

public choice model A model postulating that public organizations are less efficient than private organizations because bureaucrats and special interest groups cause public organizations to behave inefficiently and overproduce.

public contracting A health insurance model in which the government contracts with various health care providers for medical services on behalf of the general population.

public enterprise A medical care organization operated by a government authority.

public good A product has the properties of a public good if it can be consumed simultaneously by more than one consumer and it is costly to exclude nonpayers from consuming the good. Public goods are generally provided by a government entity and funded out of tax revenues.

public interest theory A theory of government behavior that hypothesizes that government intervenes in a market-based economy to advance the general interest of its citizens.

pure egalitarian system A system that distributes goods and services equally to all members of a society regardless of their willingness or ability to earn income.

pure market system A system that allocates resources and distributes goods and services based on buying and selling decisions made at an individual or decentralized level within a market economy.

pure monopoly A product market characterized by one seller and perfect barriers to entry.

quality-adjusted life-year (QALY) A measure that reflects the quantity and quality of life-years saved. It equals the product of life expectancy times a measure of the quality of life-years remaining. (See *cost-utility analysis.*)

quality and quantity maximization The assumption that a medical care provider jointly determines quality and quantity of output in the process of maximizing the utility of the decision maker(s).

quality differentiation The situation in which firms attempt to differentiate their products based on quality.

quality maximization Occurs when medical care providers maximize the quality of output produced at the expense of economic profits.

quantity maximization Occurs when medical care providers maximize the amount of output produced at the expense of economic profits.

quaternary-level care State-of-the-art medical care.

rationality The notion that consumers will never purposely make themselves worse off and have the ability to rank preferences and allocate income in a fashion that derives the maximum level of utility.

rationally ignorant The situation in which consumers have less than perfect information concerning a good or service due to the high cost of acquiring additional information.

rating scale A technique used to generate a health-utility index that asks individuals to rate various health outcomes.

regressive redistribution scheme The situation in which net taxes as a fraction of income decrease with income.

relevant geographical market (RGM) Captures the spatial dimension of the relevant market by considering the location of firms that consumers might switch to given a nontrivial and nontemporary change in the price of a product at any one location.

relevant product market (RPM) Captures the product dimension of the relevant market by considering all of the products that consumers might switch to given a nontrivial and nontemporary change in the price of any one product.

reminder advertising Advertising that reinforces consumers' knowledge about the product.

required generic substitution Cost control policies that require physicians and pharmacists to use lower-priced generic drugs whenever medically possible.

resource-based relative value system A method to compensate physicians that bases the payment on the time and effort of physician services necessary to produce the medical service. This system is currently used by the Medicare program.

retrospective utilization review A program to contain medical costs that reviews the medical care provided after the fact to determine whether any of the care provided should be denied reimbursement. (See *utilization review programs.*)

return on assets (ROA) Net income plus interest payments divided by the book value of assets.

return on stockholder equity (ROE) Net income divided by the current market value of stockholder equity.

risk adjustment The process of setting the capitation rate for an insurance policy based on the health status and expected medical costs of an individual or group purchasing the plan.

risk assessment The process of modeling and estimating the expected medical costs of a person or group of people.

risk aversion The quality of preferring less risk to more, all other things held equal.

risk selection Occurs when health plans choose subscribers based on their risk status during the underwriting process.

rule of reason States that courts should weigh the social desirability of a business practice, such as a merger, when determining whether that practice should be allowed to take place. Thus, both the procompetitive and anticompetitive aspects of the business practice are considered.

search attributes The characteristics of a good or service that are easily evaluated prior to its purchase, such as size, color, or design.

secondary care Medical care that consists of more sophisticated treatments than primary care services.

second opinions A utilization review program in which each decision made by a physician concerning the need for surgery is routinely reviewed by another physician.

selective contracting Occurs when a third party contracts exclusively with a preselected set of medical care providers.

service A product that exhibits the four characteristics of intangibility, inseparability, inventory, and inconsistency. Intangibility means that a medical service cannot be evaluated by the five senses. Inseparability means that production takes place at the time of consumption. Inventory refers to the fact that it is impossible for health care providers to maintain an inventory of medical services. Inconsistency reflects the fact that the composition and quality of medical services vary greatly across points of consumption.

Sherman Antitrust Act A law passed in 1890 prohibiting certain forms of anticompetitive behavior. This act is considered the centerpiece of antitrust legislation in the United States.

short run A time horizon over which the quantity of at least one factor input is fixed in the production process. In this case, output can be altered only by changing the quantity of one or more of the variable inputs used in the production process.

short-run economies of scale Exist when average variable costs decline with the level of output.

Sickness Funds Private, not-for-profit insurance companies in Germany that collect premiums from employees and employers. (See *socialized health insurance.*)

single payer The situation in which only one third-party payer is responsible for paying health care providers for medical services.

single-source drug A drug covered by patent protection.

socialized health insurance (SI) A health care system in which the government mandates that employers and employees jointly finance the cost of medical care insurance.

socioeconomic status The overall position of an individual in a given society based on social and economic factors, such as education and income.

spatial differentiation The situation in which firms attempt to differentiate themselves based on location.

special interest group theory A theory of government behavior that hypothesizes that governments intervene in a market-based economy for the purpose of advancing the economic self-interests of a particular interest group.

staff-model health maintenance organization An HMO that directly employs physicians on a salary basis.

standard gamble A technique used to generate a health-utility index that asks individuals with a given medical condition to choose the probability of dying at which they are indifferent between living a healthy life after having a medical procedure and dying because of the medical procedure.

standard gamble model A model of insurance that assumes that people purchase insurance to avoid or transfer risk. That is, people purchase health insurance to avoid the likelihood of irregular and unpredictable medical care expenses.

Standard Industrial Classification (SIC) system A system designed by the U.S. Census Bureau to categorize and code the output of firms into various classes. The code can contain up to seven digits. The four-digit SIC code is considered to represent the industry level. The first digit in the coding system identifies the sector of the economy (0 for agriculture, 2 for manufacturing, 5 for trade). The second digit defines the commodity group in that sector. For example, the two-digit code 28 represents the "chemicals and allied products" group of the manufacturing sector. The third digit represents an industry group. For example, 283 represents the "drugs" industry group and 282 stands for the "plastic materials and synthetics" industry group. The fourth digit identifies a specific segment of an industry group. For example, the four-digit code 2834 represents the "pharmaceutical preparations" industry, and 2833 stands for the "medicinal chemicals and botanical products" industry.

State Children's Health Insurance Program (SCHIP) An act passed by Congress in 1997 that significantly expanded medical insurance coverage to children.

statistical life-year A measure based on the observation that a 1 in 100,000 risk of death to an individual is equivalent in statistical terms to 1 death in a society or community of 100,000 people.

structural quality The quality of medical services as measured by the quality of the inputs used in production, such as credentials of physicians, education of nurses, and vintage and variety of equipment.

structurally uninsured The condition of individuals who are uninsured on a long-run basis because of, for example, chronic illnesses, preexisting conditions, or insufficient income.

structure-conduct-performance paradigm A model used by economists when conducting an industry analysis. It predicts that market structure influences firm conduct, which determines market performance.

substitutes Two goods that are replacements in consumption and fulfill a similar purpose. Two goods are substitutes in consumption if an increase in the price of one good causes an increase in demand for the other.

substitution effect The increase (decrease) in quantity demanded brought about by a relative decrease (increase) in the price of a product. The concept is used to derive a downward-sloping demand curve.

Supplementary Medical Insurance program See *Part B*.

supplier-induced demand (SID) theory A model of firm behavior that hypothesizes that physicians, to further pursue their own economic self-interests, take advantage of the asymmetry of information about medical care to persuade their patients to consume more medical care than is necessary.

supply The quantity of output a firm is willing and able to produce at various prices during a specific time period. The market supply equals the total amount supplied in a given market.

supply curve The short-run supply curve for an individual firm facing a perfectly competitive market equals the part of the short-run marginal cost curve that lies above the average variable cost curve. The market supply curve equals the horizontal summation of the individual firms' supply curves, with adjustments made for factor price changes.

supply-side subsidy A monetary sum received from a third party directed at reducing the cost of producing a good or service.

survivor theory A theory that categorizes firms based on size and hypothesizes that any category that includes a growing number of firms over time represents the most efficient producers in comparison to categories in which the number of firms is decreasing.

technically efficient The condition that exists when the maximum level of output is produced from a given mix of inputs at a point in time.

technology The development and diffusion of medical technology takes place in four stages. During the basic research stage, the investigation of new knowledge is without commercial purpose. In the applied research stage, new scientific knowledge is applied to the solution of a medical problem. The clinical investigation stage occurs with testing of new medical technologies on human subjects. The diffusion stage marks the commercial introduction and adoption of a new medical technology.

tertiary care Highly complex medical care that involves more sophisticated medical treatments than primary or secondary medical care.

theory X of health economics An economic theory stating that health and disease occur randomly and that economic incentives cannot be called on to provide quality medical care at low cost. Government intervention is needed to ensure that individuals have access to quality medical care.

theory Y of health economics An economic theory stating that individuals have significant control over health through lifestyle choices and that the market mechanism will discipline health care providers to provide high-quality medical care at low cost. There is little need for government intervention in health care markets.

third-party payer An organization that provides medical care insurance to individuals in return for taxes or premium payments and then reimburses health care providers on behalf of those individuals.

time cost The monetary cost of travel and waiting resulting from the consumption of a good or service.

time trade-off A technique used to generate a health-utility index that asks individuals to choose the number of years of healthy living at which they are indifferent between living in perfect health followed by death and living a fixed number of years with a given chronic health condition.

total costs The sum of fixed and variable costs associated with the production of a given quantity of output.

total net social benefit The difference between the total social benefit in consuming and total social cost of producing a good or service.

total product curve A curve showing the quantity of output produced by different levels of a specific input, such as labor, given that all other inputs are held constant.

total social benefit The total of the benefits a society receives from the consumption of a particular product. (See *total social surplus*.)

total social cost The total of the costs resulting from the production of a particular product. (See *total social surplus*.)

total social surplus The total social benefit minus the total social cost of producing a given quantity of a good or service.

transaction costs The costs of searching out the best price and the cost associated with negotiating, writing, and enforcing contracts. Transaction cost economics holds the view that contracts may be incomplete and therefore costly to engage in.

tying contract The situation in which a buyer is required to purchase product B (the tied product) to purchase product A (the tying product).

type I error Occurs when an outcome is rejected as false when it is true; for example, when the FDA rejects an application of a drug even though the drug is truly safe and effective.

type II error Occurs when an outcome is accepted as true when it is false; for example, when the FDA accepts an application of a drug even though the drug is unsafe or ineffective.

underwriting cycle (profitability cycle) A profit cycle experienced by firms operating in the group health insurance market that includes three consecutive years of underwriting gains followed by three years of underwriting losses.

unit elastic An elasticity with a value of 1 such that the percentage change in the dependent variable equals the percentage change in the independent variable, in absolute value terms.

universal coverage Achieved when an entire population has medical insurance coverage.

usual, customary, and reasonable rate (UCR) A cost control method used by third-party payers to control the fees paid to medical care providers for medical goods and services. The UCR fee is limited to the lowest of the actual charge of the physician, the customary charge, and the prevailing charge in the local area.

utility The level of satisfaction or pleasure an individual or group receives from consuming a good or service.

utility function A mathematical expression that shows the extent to which various factors affect total utility.

utility maximization model An economic model that assumes that people try to attain the highest possible level of satisfaction through their consumption decisions.

utility-maximizing rule A rule stating that a consumer's utility is maximized when the marginal utility received from the last dollar spent on each commodity is equal across all goods and services purchased.

utilization review Programs implemented to control medical costs by evaluating the medical decisions of hospitals and physicians. These programs can be carried out on a prospective, concurrent, or retrospective basis.

value of life The monetary worth of a human life.

variable costs Costs of production that vary directly with the quantity of output produced.

variable payment Reimbursement that increases with higher costs incurred or a greater quantity of services supplied.

vertical equity Achieved when unequal individuals are treated unequally. For example, people with higher incomes pay higher taxes.

vertical merger A merger between two firms in a supplier–purchaser relationship.

virtual integration A contractual combination of buyers and suppliers.

voluntary performance standard A target rate of growth for physician expenditures financed by the Medicare program. This rate is established by Congress to control the cost of Medicare over time. This cost control method ended in 1997.

willingness-to-pay approach Determines the value of a human life based on a person's willingness to pay for relatively small reductions in the chance of dying.

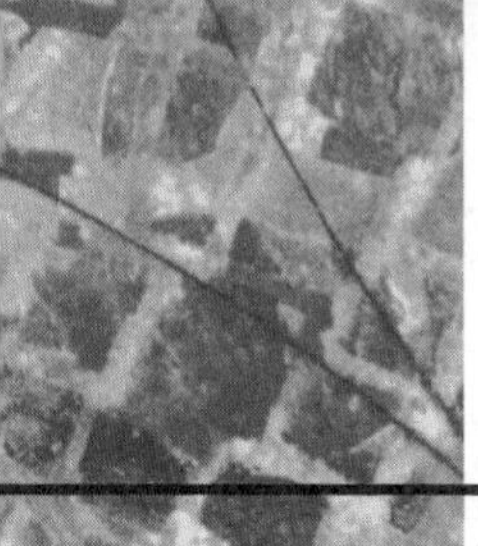

NAME INDEX

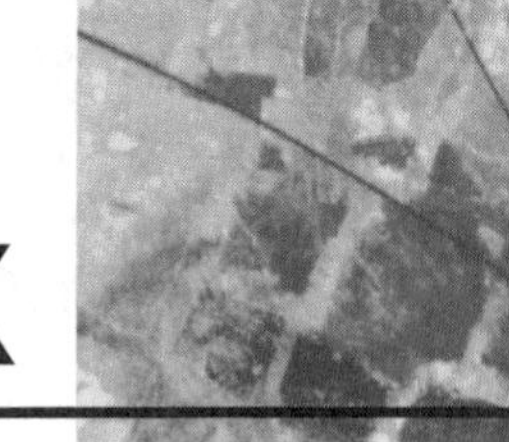

SUBJECT INDEX

Note: Definitions and the appropriate page numbers appear in boldface type. Page numbers followed by "f" and "t," respectively, indicate figures or tables.